The Ruminant Nutrition System

Volume II — Tables of Equations and Coding

Luis Orlindo Tedeschi
Professor and Fellow
Department of Animal Science
Texas A&M University

Danny Gene Fox
Professor Emeritus
Department of Animal Science
Cornell University

XanEdu

Cover illustration and design by Luis Orlindo Tedeschi.

Published in the United States of America

ISBN 978-1-97507-621-4 (perfect bound)
ISBN 978-1-97507-702-0 (case bound)

http://www.nutritionmodels.com
http://nutritionmodels.tamu.edu

XanEdu
4750 Venture Drive
Ann Arbor, MI 48108
800-562-2147
www.xanedu.com

Preface

This book accompanies *The Ruminant Nutrition System: Volume I – An Applied Model for Predicting Nutrient Requirements and Feed Utilization in Ruminants* (**RNS**). It shows the equations and code used to implement the RNS model for use by advanced teaching courses and research by faculty and graduate students at the master or doctoral levels in life sciences, animal science, wildlife and fisheries sciences, veterinary medicine, and biology and zoology, as well as any others who wish to understand the execution of the RNS model.

Since we started writing the first edition of the *Ruminant Nutrition System*, we planned to include the computer model's equations and the calculation logic. The book, however, quickly became a comprehensive document of the published research used to identify essential equations and variables for the underlying calculation logic of the RNS model. It was a rich, dense source of information about the biology and nutrition of ruminants and the mathematical modeling concepts behind the computer model. As a result, we scattered the RNS model equations throughout the book, within the appropriate chapters containing the pertinent scientific discussions, making it difficult for the reader to reconstruct the computer model. Soon after the publication of the first edition of the book, readers wishing to see the RNS model equations, their linkages, the calculation logic, and how they were implemented into the computer software started requesting more details. To meet this need, we needed to produce a companion book focused on describing the RNS model's equations and code. Before releasing it to the public, however, we had to make sure that the equations accurately reflected the concepts (i.e., the validation step in mathematical modeling) delineated in the RNS's *Volume I*.

The RNS's *Volume II – Tables of Equations and Code* arose because of our commitment to document and disseminate the mathematics composing the RNS model clearly and in detail. Each part of *Volume II* presents the RNS model's equations and the calculation logic in two ways. The first, more traditional approach lists the equations in a tabular form, including an equation number, the independent variable with its description, and a mathematical formulation (in the form of the equation) that follows a logical sequence for calculation and execution. The second approach embeds the equations into a modern, highly aggregated method of an actual computer programming language structure, the R script. This second approach presents the sequence and the calculation logic for the equations more systematically and coherently than the first approach for those wishing to understand how the RNS calculations were programmed.

Rumen dynamics, the multitude of variables describing fermentation dynamics, and the steps for each diet ingredient are complex. This complexity, as discussed in the *Mathematical and programming notations* section below, required us to develop a more robust and descriptive way to name variables, specifically for the supply calculations, rather than only using acronyms. Consequently, the variable names presented in this volume are not necessarily the same between these two equation presentation approaches (tabular and scripted), but they follow the same calculation logic and are presented in order of calculation. **Part I** contains the equations and the code of the dietary supply of energy and protein, using common calculations for solution levels 0, 1, and 2 (Chapter 1) and specific calculations for solution level 0 (Chapter 2), solution level 1 (Chapter 3), and solution level 2 (Chapter 4). **Part II** contains the equations and the code of the requirements of energy and other nutrients (Chapter 5) and supplementary calculations (Chapter 6).

We also developed the RNS for R. The RNS calculations are currently executed in R, an interpreted computer program, via scripts that yields slower computational performance than compiled versions, though high-processing capacity computers will not be intimidated. Basic programming skills with R are necessary to execute the RData file created by the RNS for R. We also provided a rudimentary introduction to running the RNS for R without the RNS computer program interface. Chapter 7, in **Part III**, contains additional information to use the RData file created by the RNS for R. Users can modify the source code, add new source code (see Appendix 1 to Appendix 4), and execute the RNS for R. Once the R object is created containing all necessary diet ingredients and the animal groups, seasoned R users can perform simulations with the RNS for R object without having to use the RNS computer program interface. We adopted the R for its convertibility to other computer languages and programming environments. It also has rich programming support: statistics, graphics, computation for operational research capabilities including linear and nonlinear optimization programming, import and export options, easy and intuitive R language scripting, broad usability and accessibility, and programming and scripting environment. The *Software programming* section below provides additional information.

We also received requests for the RNS computer model to interpret the results. While we believe that the interpretation of the results, along with the required inputs to execute the computer model, rely on the user's expertise and knowledge, **Part IV** (Chapter 8) provides some guidance for interpreting some biological indices, including predicting ideal levels of fiber in the diets, adequate balance of degradable protein in the rumen, and nitrogen balance, to help users make decisions about balancing and formulating diets. These biological indices represent the range and the average of ideal values, but users do not necessarily have to strive for the average because the average, as discussed in Chapter 18 of RNS's *Volume I*, does not necessarily represent the real value. For instance, consider the composition of a feedstuff from the feed library. Averages, in general, represent unrelated and independent physicochemical characteristics or properties of the feedstuff that in real life are interrelated. The averaging process breaks their dependencies, often resulting in an unrepresented feed. Averages are unbiased predictors of an independent variable, but when multiple dependent variables need to be taken into account, their average may become impractical as it does not account for intrinsic co-variances among the physicochemical characteristics or properties of the feedstuffs.

Mathematical and programming notations

The great number of variables originally published in the Cornell Net Carbohydrate and Protein System (**CNCPS**) model, and additional variables that were subsequently incorporated into the original CNCPS model, created challenges in describing and organizing variables in a logical way, a task that became even more difficult as the CNCPS-based models expanded. For the RNS, we developed a mechanistic notation scheme to be intuitive, meaningful, and comprehensive yet simple enough to accommodate future additions. This book uses the following notation for the supply submodels: `compartment.source.substrate.form`. The *compartment* indicates the scope and location in which the calculation is being performed, such as `anim` (animal), `git` (gastro-intestinal tract), `rum` (rumen), `si` (small intestine), `li` (large intestine), and `fc` (feces). The *source* describes the origin of the substrate, such as `bact` (bacteria), `diet` (complete ration), and `fd` (ration ingredients). Examples of *substrate* are CHOB3 (carbohydrate fraction B3) and FAC16_0 (fatty acid C16:0: palmitic acid). The *form* characterizes the format and unit of the variable, such as `amt` (amount: kg, lb, L, mL), `rate` (kg/d, lb/d, g/h, L/s), `conc` (concentration, expressed as %) or `perc` (percentage, expressed as %), `ppm` (parts per million), `frac` (fraction, decimal form), `fracrate` (fractional rate, expressed as 1/h), `fracprate` (fractional rate as percent basis, %/h), `time` (time units, expressed as h, s, or min), and `factor` (dimensionless adjustment, usually a multiplier or divider). Variables can represent either a single value or a list of values. For instance, `rum.fd.CHOB3.amt = 5` indicates 5 kg (or lb, depending on the weight unit) of feed carbohydrate B3 in the rumen. Similarly, `rum.fd.CHOB3.rate = (5, 3.4, 2.1)` represents the rates for the first (5 kg/d), second (3.4 kg/d), and third (2.1 kg/d) ration ingredients. Not all variables have the *form* suffix. When the format or unit is too complex to be shown, the *form* suffix might not be specified. A substrate followed by an underscore emphasizes a specific unit (_kg, _lb, or _L) or indicates in which base the substrate is being reported (the default is kg on a dry-matter basis). For instance, `si.fd.Leu_RUP.conc` is the concentration of the amino acid (**AA**) leucine of the ruminally undegraded protein of the ration ingredients in the small intestine; `rum.fd.CHOB3.fracprate = 5.1` indicates 5.1%/h of dietary carbohydrate B3 in the rumen, and `si.diet.CHOB3_CHO.rate = 1` indicates 1 kg/d of dietary carbohydrate B3 in the small intestine on a CHO basis. The suffix *_vector* indicates that the variable is represented in a vector form, meaning there were multiple simulation runs.

Software programming

The graphical user interface and basic calculations of the RNS were created with Visual Basic .NET using Microsoft Visual Studio 2017 Professional[(1)]. Concurrently, we used the R[(2)] version 3.6.2 language and environment for statistical computing and graphics (Crawley, 2007; Everitt and Hothorn, 2010; Horton and Kleinman, 2011; Teetor, 2011; Wickham, 2009) to provide powerful and advanced computing capabilities to the RNS. We developed the R scripts by using the RStudio (Verzani, 2011), and we produced the tables of codes using the TINN-R (Faria et al., 2015). We intended the RNS for R to allow researchers to programmatically modify the standard RNS calculations and add customized calculations (see Appendix 1 to Appendix 4). The RNS invokes RNS for R to perform stochastic modeling. The R software is used under the GNU Project License and is freely distributed. The LP Solve[(3)] version 5.5.2 and GLPK[(4)] version 4.44 packages perform the linear programming optimization. LP Solve is used under the GNU Lesser General Public License (LGPL), and GLPK is used under the GNU General Public License.

---

(1) http://www.microsoft.com/visualstudio

(2) http://cran.r-project.org

(3) http://lpsolve.sourceforge.net/5.5/

(4) http://www.gnu.org/software/glpk

About the Authors

Luis Tedeschi is a professor in the Department of Animal Science at the Texas A&M University. He received his Bachelor of Science degree in Agronomy Engineering from the University of São Paulo (Piracicaba, Brazil) in **1991**, his Master of Science degree in Animal and Forage Sciences from the same university in **1996**, and his Doctor of Philosophy degree in Animal Science from Cornell University (Ithaca, NY) in **2001**. In **2004**, he obtained his Professional Animal Scientist in Beef Cattle certification by the American Registry of Professional Animal Scientists (ARPAS). Prior to joining Texas A&M University in **2005**, he held a research associate position at Cornell University. He teaches several courses related to ruminant animals for undergraduate and graduate students, including Ruminant Nutrition, Precision Diet Formulation, Introduction to System Dynamics for Agriculture and Life Sciences, and Comparative Ruminant Production as a summer study-abroad course. He has served on more than 60 graduate students' committees and mentored more than 35 post-doctorates and international exchange students under the auspices of the U.S. Department of Education. His research focuses on the integration of accumulated scientific knowledge of ruminant nutrition to solve contemporary problems. This integration is achieved through mathematical modeling, more specifically by adopting the System Dynamics methodology. This modeling methodology is used to build nutrition models and reveal how complex systems' underlying structure affects the systems' behavior under different management policies. These nutrition models are being used as valuable tools for solving current and future needs related to environmental pollution and scarcity of resources through the development of efficient production systems. Tedeschi's areas of interest are energy and nutrient requirements of grazing and feedlot animals, growth biology and bioenergetics, chemical composition and kinetics of fermentation of feeds, modeling and simulation of decision support systems, and evaluation of models. He started his research career as an active developer of submodels for the Cornell Net Carbohydrate and Protein System (CNCPS) and the Cattle Value Discovery System (CVDS). He has published more than 250 articles in peer-reviewed journals and book chapters, and presented at more than 80 modeling nutrition conferences and workshops worldwide. He has served as a member of the Modeling Committee of the National Animal Nutrition Program (NANP) and on a committee at the National Research Council (NRC) of the National Academies of Sciences, Engineering, and Medicine (NASEM) to revise the nutrient requirements for beef cattle. He has been an active member of the American Society of Animal Science (ASAS), the American Dairy Science Association (ADSA), the Brazilian Society of Animal Science (SBZ), the American Registry of Professional Animal Scientists (ARPAS), and the System Dynamics Society (SDS). In **2011**, he received the prestigious Sir Frederick McMaster Fellowship to conduct modeling research at the Commonwealth Scientific and Industrial Research Organization Livestock Industries (Australia). In **2012**, Tedeschi received the Texas A&M AgriLife Vice Chancellor's Award in Excellence for International Involvement. In **2013**, he was awarded the distinguished J. William Fulbright Scholarship to collaborate with the Brazilian Research Company (Brazil). In **2016**, Tedeschi was named Texas A&M AgriLife Research Faculty Fellow to acknowledge and reward his exceptional research contributions to the resilience and sustainability in animal agriculture. In **2017**, Tedeschi became a board-certified Diplomate in Animal Nutrition by the American College of Animals Science (ACAS) and he received the respected American Feed Industry Association (AFIA) in Ruminant Nutrition Research award by the American Society of Animal Science (ASAS) for stimulating research excellence in the nutrition of ruminant animals. In **2018**, Tedeschi was recognized for this international involvement by receiving the College of Agriculture and Life Sciences Dean's Outstanding Achievement Award. In **2019**, Tedeschi received the Chancellor EDGES Fellowships for demonstrating significant accomplishment in ruminant nutrition and modeling with recognized national and international impacts. Several industry companies worldwide, including the Performance Cattle Company and Micro Beef Technologies, use Tedeschi's modeling research. His mathematical nutrition model website (http://www.nutritionmodels.com or http://nutritionmodels.tamu.edu) contains 12 computer models that have been visited more than 150,000 times so far.

Danny Fox is a professor emeritus of the Department of Animal Science at Cornell University. He received his Bachelor of Science, Master of Science, and Doctor of Philosophy degrees from The Ohio State University. After coming to Cornell University in **1977**, Fox conducted research in cattle nutrition and taught courses in cattle nutrition and nutrient management. Before joining the faculty at Cornell, he held positions as a beef cattle extension feedlot specialist at South Dakota State University and Michigan State University. His 35 years of research at these three land grant universities focused on the development of data, methods, models, and computer programs to predict cattle nutrient requirements, as well as nutrients derived from feeds to meet cattle requirements in unique production situations. His team at Cornell developed the Cornell Net Carbohydrate and Protein System cattle nutrition model and software, which has users in more than 42 countries, for formulating rations for beef and dairy cattle. His team also developed the Cornell Value Discovery Program for determining the feed requirements of individual cattle fed in groups. This program is being used to identify differences in feed conversion among individual steers, heifers, and bulls fed in feedlot pens. Following the 1990 USDA Farm Bill, which made Sustainable Agriculture a priority, Fox served as team leader for several multidisciplinary programs in the College of Agriculture and Life Sciences at Cornell to address nutrient management on dairy farms, including the Dairy Farm Sustainability project, the New York City Watershed Computer Software Development project, and the Integrated Nutrient Management Work Group. These projects resulted in the development of the Cornell University Nutrient Management Planning System. Fox's research resulted in more than 330 publications, 15 computer programs, presentations at more than 150 conferences, and training of 59 graduate students. He has been a member of numerous national committees, including National Research Council committees on Animal Nutrition, Feed Intake, and the 1996 Nutrient Requirements of Beef Cattle. He provided input on nutrient requirements for growth and body reserves and computer software design to the 2001 National Research Council Nutrient Requirements of Dairy Cattle Committee. His growth and energy reserves models were adapted by both the 1996 Beef Cattle National Research Council committee and the 2001 Dairy Cattle National Research Council committee, and the 2016 National Academies of Sciences, Engineering, and Medicine Beef Cattle Nutrient Requirements Committee. He conducted many workshops on the use of these models in the United States, Canada, South America, and Europe, and he has served as a consultant to Agribrands International, Micro Beef Technologies, and Future Beef Organization on the application of these models in their cattle management systems. For his extensive contributions to research in cattle nutrition, management and computer modeling related to cattle production, Dr. Fox received numerous awards during his 35-year career. In **2019**, he was inducted into The Ohio State University Animal Sciences Hall of Fame and received the Plains Nutrition Council Legends of Feedlot Nutrition Award.

"You don't have to be a mathematician to have a feel for numbers."
John Nash Jr. (2006)

Table of Contents

List of Figures

List of Tables

Part I. Calculations of Energy and Nutrient Supply

"Knowledge is obtained rather by the use of the ear
than of the tongue."
Benjamin Franklin

(This page intentionally left blank)

1 Basic Dietary Chemical Composition and Calculations (L0, L1, L2)

1.1 Equations

1.1.1 Dietary cation-anion balance: calcDCAB()

#	Variable	Description	Equation
1:		mEq/100 g DM	$\left(\frac{Na}{0.023}+\frac{K}{0.039}+\frac{Ca}{0.02}+\frac{Mg}{0.012}\right)-\left(\frac{Cl}{0.0355}+\frac{S}{0.016}+\frac{P}{0.0155}\right)$
2:		mEq/100 g DM	$\left(\frac{Na}{0.023}+\frac{K}{0.039}\right)-\left(\frac{Cl}{0.0355}\right)$
3:		mEq/100 g DM	$\left(\frac{Na}{0.023}+\frac{K}{0.039}\right)-\left(\frac{Cl}{0.0355}+\frac{S}{0.016}\right)$
4:	*DCAB*	mEq/100 g DM	$\left(\frac{Na}{0.023}+\frac{K}{0.039}+0.38*\frac{Ca}{0.02}+0.3*\frac{Mg}{0.012}\right)-\left(\frac{Cl}{0.0355}+0.6*\frac{S}{0.016}+0.5*\frac{P}{0.0155}\right)$
5:		mEq/100 g DM	$\left(\frac{Na}{0.023}+\frac{K}{0.039}+0.15*\frac{Ca}{0.02}+0.15*\frac{Mg}{0.012}\right)-\left(\frac{Cl}{0.0355}+0.2*\frac{S}{0.016}+0.3*\frac{P}{0.0155}\right)$
6:		mEq/100 g DM	$\left(\frac{Na}{0.023}+\frac{K}{0.039}+0.15*\frac{Ca}{0.02}+0.15*\frac{Mg}{0.012}\right)-\left(\frac{Cl}{0.0355}+0.6*\frac{S}{0.016}+0.5*\frac{P}{0.0155}\right)$

1.1.2 Empirical methane production: calcMethane()

#	Variable[(1)]	Description	Equation[(2)]
1:		forage>20%	$GE*0.065*MJ_{PER_{Mcal}}*kg_{PER_{MJ}}*1000$
2:		forage>40%	$45.98*\left(1-\exp\left(-0.003*\left(ME*MJ_{PER_{Mcal}}\right)\right)\right)*L_{PER_{MJ}}*g_{PER_{L}}$
3:		forage>40% & SL=2	$(-1.01+2.76*NDF+0.722*CHOB1)*L_{PER_{MJ}}*g_{PER_{L}}$
4:		forage>40% & SL=2	$\left(2.68-1.14*\left(\frac{CHOB1}{NDF}\right)+0.786*DMI\right)*L_{PER_{MJ}}*g_{PER_{L}}$
5:		forage>40%	$71.5+0.12*FBW+0.1*DMI\text{^}3-244.8*EE\text{^}3)$
6:	*CH4*	forage>40% & female	$\left(-1.487+0.046*GE*MJ_{PER_{Mcal}}+0.032*\left(NDF*\frac{100}{DMI}\right)+0.006*SBW\right)*L_{PER_{MJ}}*g_{PER_{L}}$
7:		forage>40% & female	$\left(-0.163+0.051*GE*MJ_{PER_{Mcal}}+0.038*\left(NDF*\frac{100}{DMI}\right)\right)*L_{PER_{MJ}}*g_{PER_{L}}$
8:		forage>40% & male	$\left(-0.221+0.048*GE*MJ_{PER_{Mcal}}+0.005*SBW\right)*L_{PER_{MJ}}*g_{PER_{L}}$
9:		forage>40% & male	$\left(0.743+0.054*GE*MJ_{PER_{Mcal}}\right)*L_{PER_{MJ}}*g_{PER_{L}}$
10:		20%<forage<40%	$(2.70+1.16*DMI-15.8*EE)*L_{PER_{MJ}}*g_{PER_{L}}$

11:		20%<forage<40% & SL=2	$30.7 + 0.165 * FBW + 0.18 * DMI^2 + 0.05 * DMI^3 - 157 * EE^3 + 6.5 * \frac{CP}{NDF} - 2.45 * \frac{CHOB1}{NDF}$
12:		forage<20%	$GE * 0.03 * MJ_{PER_{Mcal}} * kg_{PER_{MJ}} * 1000$
13:		forage<20%	$\left(0.357 + 0.0591 * \left(ME * MJ_{PER_{Mcal}}\right) + 0.0500 * (Forage)\right) * L_{PER_{MJ}} * g_{PER_L}$
14:		forage<20%	$(-1.02 + 0.681 * DMI + 0.0481 * Forage) * L_{PER_{MJ}} * g_{PER_L}$
15:		forage<20% & SL=2	$(-1.01 + 2.76 * NDF + 0.722 * CHOB1) * L_{PER_{MJ}} * g_{PER_L}$
16:		forage<20% & SL=2	$-10.1 + 0.21 * FBW + 0.36 * DMI^2 - 69.2 * EE^3 + 13 * \frac{CP}{NDF} - 4.9 * \frac{CHOB1}{NDF}$

(1) ***CHOB1*** is starch, kg/d; ***CH4*** is methane, g/d; ***CP*** is crude protein, kg/d; ***DMI*** is dry matter intake, kg/d; ***EE*** is ether extract, kg/d; ***FBW*** is full body weight, kg; ***Forage*** is percent of dietary forage (DM basis); ***GE*** is gross energy, Mcal/d; ***ME*** is metabolizable energy, Mcal/d; ***NDF*** is neutral detergent fiber, kg/d; ***SBW*** is shrunk body weight, kg; and ***SL*** is solution level. All variables are at the diet level.

(2) $MJ_{PER_{Mcal}} = 4.1868$; $kg_{PER_{MJ}} = \frac{1}{55.65}$; $kg_{PER_{Mcal}} = kg_{PER_{MJ}} * MJ_{PER_{Mcal}}$; $L_{PER_{MJ}} = 1000 * \frac{kg_{PER_{MJ}}}{0.6556}$; $L_{PER_{Mcal}} = 1000 * \frac{kg_{PER_{Mcal}}}{0.6565}$; $kg_{PER_L} = \frac{0.6556}{1000}$; $g_{PER_L} = 0.6556$

1.1.3 Empirical dry matter intake: calcDMI()

#	Variable[1]	Description[2]	Equation
1:		dry	$12.5 - 0.0299 * FBW + 2e-05 * FBW^2 - 0.05531 * aOMD + 0.00032 * FBW * aOMD$
2:	*OMI (cattle)*	growing or finishing or replacement heifers	$4.56 + 0.0053 * FBW - 2e-05 * FBW^2 - 0.05531 * aOMD + 0.00032 * FBW * aOMD$
3:		lactating	$27.9 - 0.0902 * FBW + 9e-05 * FBW^2 - 0.05531 * aOMD + 0.00032 * FBW * aOMD$
4:		CETI≥29 & LNT≥20	$a = 0.9;\ b = 0.1;\ c = 24.7;\ d = -0.00145;\ e = 0.96$
5:		CETI≥29 & LNT<20	$a = 0.65;\ b = 0.25;\ c = 35.5;\ d = 0.33;\ e = -1.21$
6:		10>CETI≥20	$a = 0.9;\ b = 0.1;\ c = 24.7;\ d = -0.00145;\ e = -0.96$
7:		0>CETI≥10	$a = 1;\ b = 0.03;\ c = 14.5;\ d = -0.0019;\ e = -0.9$
8:		-10>CETI≥0	$a = 1.03;\ b = 0.02;\ c = 4.5;\ d = -0.0019;\ e = -0.9$
9:	*DMIft*	CETI≥-10	$a = 1.05;\ b = 0.02;\ c = -5.5;\ d = -9.7 * 10^{-5};\ e = -0.85$
10:		CETI<-10	$a = 1.07;\ b = 0.09;\ c = -14.4;\ d = 0.0046;\ e = -1.04$
11:			$a + b * \frac{2 * e * \left(\log\left(\exp\left(\frac{CETI + \frac{d}{2}}{e}\right) + \exp\left(\frac{c}{e}\right)\right) - \log\left(\exp\left(\frac{c + \frac{d}{2}}{e}\right) + \exp\left(\frac{CETI}{e}\right)\right)\right) + d}{2 * d}$
12:	*DMImf*		$1 - 0.01 * MudDepth$
13:		growing or finishing & straightbred & Holstein	1.08
14:	*DMIbif*	growing or finishing & 2-way & (dam or sire) is Holstein	1.04
15:		otherwise	1
16:	*DMIbf*	growing or finishing and EqSBW>350	$0.7714 + 0.00196 * EqSBW - 3.71e-06 * EqSBW^2$
17:		otherwise	1
18:	*DMIfaf*	ionophore & forage>10%	1
19:		otherwise	0.97
20:	*FCM*		$0.4 * MY + 0.15 * MkFat * MY$
21:	*DMI (cattle)*	lactating dairy & WOL>16	$(0.0185 * FBW + 0.305 * FCM) * DMItf * DMImf * DMIfaf$

#	Variable[1]	Description[2]	Equation
22:		lactating dairy & WOL≤16	$(0.0185 * FBW + 0.305 * FCM) * DMItf * DMImf * DMIfaf * (1 - \exp(-(0.564 - 0.124 * 2) * (WOL + 3.67)))$
23:		lactating dairy	$(0.372 * FCM + 0.0968 * FBW^{0.75}) * (1 - \exp(-0.192 * (WOL + 3.67)))$
24:		lactating dairy	$(0.4762 * FCM + 0.07219 * FBW^{0.75}) * (1 - \exp(-0.03202 * (WOL * 7 + 24.9576)))$
25:		dry dairy & DG≥260	$0.016 * FBW * DMItf * DMImf * DMIfat$
26:		dry dairy & DG<260	$0.02 * FBW * DMItf * DMImf * DMIfat$
27:		dry dairy	$\left(\frac{FBW}{100}\right) * (1.97 - 0.75 * \exp(0.16 * (DG - 280)))$
28:		replacement dairy & DG>210	$-29.864 + 0.1575 * FBW^{0.75} - 1.5425e - 05 * FBW^2 + aTDN * (0.7296 - 0.0048178 * aTDN) + SWG * (2.0895 - 0.1177 * SWG - 0.001363 * FBW - 0.01908 * aTDN)$
29:		replacement dairy & DG>210 & age≤12	$FBW^{0.75} * (0.2435 * NEma - 0.0466 * NEma^2 - 0.1128) * DMItf * DMImf * \frac{1 + (210 - DG) * 0.0025}{if(NEma \geq 1, NEma, 0.95)}$
30:		replacement dairy & DG>210 & age>12	$FBW^{0.75} * (0.2435 * NEma - 0.0466 * NEma^2 - 0.0869) * DMItf * DMImf * \frac{1 + (210 - DG) * 0.0025}{if(NEma \geq 1, NEma, 0.95)}$
31:		replacement dairy & straightbred & Holstein	$15.79 * \left(1 - \exp\left(-2.1 * \frac{FBW}{1000}\right)\right) - \left(\frac{8.2}{100}\right) * \left(NDF - 22.07 - 87.14 * \frac{FBW}{1000} + 7.383 * \frac{FBW^2}{1e} + 05\right)$
32:		replacement dairy	$13.48 * \left(1 - \exp\left(-2.71 * \frac{FBW}{1000}\right)\right) - \left(\frac{8.24}{100}\right) * \left(NDF - 23.11 - 79.68 * \frac{FBW}{1000} + 6.252 * \frac{FBW^2}{1e} + 05\right)$
33:		replacement dairy	$0.1175 * FBW^{0.75} - 3.4984 * \exp(-2.469 * SWG)$
34:		growing or finishing & age≤12	$FBW^{0.75} * (0.2435 * NEma - 0.0466 * NEma^2 - 0.1128) * DMItf * DMImf * DMIbif * DMIbff * \frac{DMIfaf}{if(NEma \geq 1, NEma, 0.95)}$
35:		growing or finishing & age>12	$FBW^{0.75} * (0.2435 * NEma - 0.0466 * NEma^2 - 0.0869) * DMItf * DMImf * DMIbif * DMIbff * \frac{DMIfaf}{if(NEma \geq 1, NEma, 0.95)}$
36:		growing or finishing	$\left(\frac{FBW}{100}\right) * (1.2425 + 1.9218 * NEma - 0.7259 * NEma^2) * DMItf * DMImf * DMIbif * DMIbff * DMIfaf$
37:		growing or finishing & Nellore	$-2.6098 + 0.08844 * FBW^{0.75} + 4.4672 * SWG - 1.3579 * SWG^2$
38:		growing or finishing & not Nellore	$-2.7878 + 0.08789 * FBW^{0.75} + 5.0487 * SWG - 1.6835 * SWG^2$
39:		lactating dual-purpose & DG≤93	$SBW^{0.75} * (0.04997 * NEma^2 + 0.0384) * DMItf * \frac{DMImf}{if(NEma \geq 1, NEma, 0.95)} + 0.2 * MY$
40:		lactating dual-purpose & DG>93	$SBW^{0.75} * (0.04997 * NEma^2 + 0.04631) * DMItf * \frac{DMImf}{if(NEma \geq 1, NEma, 0.95)} + 0.2 * MY$
41:		lactating dual-purpose	$FBW^{0.75} * (0.1462 * NEma - 0.0517 * NEma^2 - 0.0074) + 0.305 * FCM + if(MY \geq 15, 1.7, 0)$
42:		lactating dual-purpose	$FBW * 0.024$
43:		dry dual-purpose	$SBW^{0.75} * (0.04997 * NEma^2 + 0.04631) * DMItf * \frac{DMImf}{if(NEma \geq 1, NEma, 0.95)}$
44:		dry dual-purpose	$FBW * 0.019$
45:		dry dual-purpose	$FBW * \frac{0.012}{\frac{NDF}{DMI}}$
46:		replacement dual-purpose & age≤12	$FBW^{0.75} * (0.2435 * NEma - 0.0466 * NEma^2 - 0.1128) * DMItf * DMImf * \frac{DMIfaf}{if(NEma \geq 1, NEma, 0.95)}$

#	Variable[(1)]	Description[(2)]	Equation
47:		replacement dual-purpose & age>12	$FBW^{0.75} * (0.2435 * NEma - 0.0466 * NEma^2 - 0.0869) * DMItf * DMImf * \frac{DMIfaf}{if(NEma \geq 1, NEma, 0.95)}$
48:	*k (sheep[(3)])*	DG>0 & lamb weight≤4	$ca = 0.66;\ t = DG - 150$ $if\left(t \leq -35, (a = 0.97; b = 1 - a; c = -42; d = 0.04; e = -1.3), if\left(t \leq -21, (a = 0.93; b = 0.97 - a; c = -28; d = 0.04; e = -1.3), if\left(\leq -7, (a = 0.88; b = 0.93 - a; c = -14; d = 0.04; e = -1.3), \left(a = \frac{1}{1 + ca}; b = 0.88 - a; c = 0; d = 0.04; e = -1.3\right)\right)\right)\right)$
49:		DG>0 & lamb weight>4	$ca = 0.88;\ t = DG - 150$ $if\left(t \leq -35, (a = 0.96; b = 1 - a; c = -42; d = 0.04; e = -1.3), if\left(t \leq -21, (a = 0.9; b = 0.96 - a; c = -28; d = 0.04; e = -1.3), if\left(\leq -7, (a = 0.82; b = 0.9 - a; c = -14; d = 0.04; e = -1.3), \left(a = \frac{1}{1 + ca}; b = 0.82 - a; c = 0; d = 0.04; e = -1.3\right)\right)\right)\right)$
50:		DG>0	$a + b * \frac{2 * e * \left(\log\left(\exp\left(\frac{t + \frac{d}{2}}{e}\right) + \exp\left(\frac{c}{e}\right)\right) - \log\left(\exp\left(\frac{c + \frac{d}{2}}{e}\right) + \exp\left(\frac{t}{e}\right)\right)\right) + d}{2 * d}$
51:		lactating & lamb weight≤4	$ca = 0.66; cc = 28$ $if\left(DIM \leq cc, if\left(DIM = 0, \frac{1}{1 + ca}, \frac{1 + ca * \left(\left(\frac{DIM}{cc}\right)^{1.4}\right) * \exp\left(1.4 * \left(1 - \frac{DIM}{cc}\right)\right)}{1 + ca}\right), 1\right)$
52:		lactating & lamb weight>4	$ca = 0.88; cc = 28$ $if\left(DIM \leq cc, if\left(DIM = 0, \frac{1}{1 + ca}, \frac{1 + ca * \left(\left(\frac{DIM}{cc}\right)^{1.4}\right) * \exp\left(1.4 * \left(1 - \frac{DIM}{cc}\right)\right)}{1 + ca}\right), 1\right)$
53:	*FCM*	MY>0	$0.3688 * MY + 0.0971 * MkFat * MY$
54:	*DMI (sheep)*	lactating	$(-0.545 + 0.095 * FBW^{0.75} + 0.65 * FCM + 0.0025 * SWG) * k$
55:		dry	$(-0.545 + 0.095 * FBW^{0.75} + 0.005 * SWG) * k$
56:		ram or sheep wether & age>12	$0.065 * FBW^{0.75}$
57:		lamb & age<12	$-0.124 + 0.0711 * FBW^{0.75} + 0.0015 * SWG$
58:	*DMI (goats)*	lactating	$0.42 * MY + 0.024 * FBW^{0.75} + 0.4 * SWG + 0.7 * \left(\frac{Forage}{100}\right)$
59:		dry	$\left(130.9 * \frac{ME}{GE} + 0.384 * FBW - 18.75\right) * \frac{FBW^{0.75}}{1000}$

#	Variable[(1)]	Description[(2)]	Equation
60:		billy or goat wether	$0.522 + 0.0135 * FBW$
61:		Kid	$\left(104.7 * \frac{ME}{GE} + 0.307 * FBW - 15\right) * \frac{FBW^{0.75}}{1000}$

[(1)] ***aOMD*** is apparent organic matter digestibility, %; ***aTDN*** is apparent total digestible nutrient, %; ***CETI*** is current effective temperature index, °C; ***DG*** is days pregnant; ***DIM*** is days in milk; ***DMIbf*** is dry matter intake factor due to body fat; ***DMIbif*** is dry matter intake factor due to breed type; ***DMIfaf*** is dry matter intake factor due to feed additives; ***DMIft*** is dry matter intake factor due to temperature; ***DMImf*** is dry matter intake factor due to mud; ***EqSBW*** is equivalent shrunk body weight, kg; ***FBW*** is full body weight, kg; ***FCM*** is fat corrected milk, kg/d; ***GE*** is gross energy, Mcal/kg; ***LNT*** is least night temperature, °C; ***ME*** is metabolizable energy, Mcal/kg; ***MkFat*** is milk fat content, %; ***MudDepth*** is mud depth, cm; ***MY*** is milk yield, kg/d; ***NEma*** is dietary net energy for maintenance, Mcal/kg; ***OMI*** is organic matter intake, kg/d; ***SWG*** is shrunk weight gain, kg/d; and ***WOL*** is week of lactation.

[(2)] Equations 1 to 47 are for cattle, Equations 48 to 57 are for sheep, and Equations 58 to 61 are for goats.

[(3)] Showing the continuous adjustment for DMI, assuming gestation length is 150 days, based on Gallo and Tedeschi (2021).

1.1.4 Empirical water intake: calcWI()

#	Variable[(1)]	Description	Equation
1:		lactating dairy	$15.9 + 1.58 * DMI + 0.9 * MY + 0.05 * NaI + 1.2 * LCT$
2:		nonlactating dairy	$-10.34 + 0.2296 * DM + 2.212 * DMI + 0.03944 * CP$
3:	*WI (cattle)*	nonfinishing beef	$7.3 + 0.0805 * SBW - 0.00008 * SBW^2 - 1.225 * CETI + 0.0411 * CETI^2 + 0.0023268 * SBW * CETI$
4:		finishing beef	$6.336 + 0.1057 * SBW - 0.0000963 * SBW^2 - 1.6 * CETI + 0.056 * CETI^2 + 0.00226 * SBW * CETI$
5:	*WI (sheep)*		$0.429 + 0.073 * CETI - 0.014 * rain$
6:	*WI (goats)*		$\left(\frac{0.159}{1000}\right) * \left(\frac{FBW}{1000}\right)^{0.946}$

[(1)] ***CETI*** is current effective temperature index, °C; ***CP*** is crude protein, % DM; ***DM*** is dry matter, %; ***DMI*** is dry matter intake, kg/d; ***FBW*** is full body weight, kg/d; ***LNT*** is least night temperature, °C; ***MY*** is milk yield, kg/d; ***NaI*** is sodium intake, g/d; ***Rain*** is rain rate, mm/d; ***SBW*** is shrunk body weight, kg; and ***WI*** is water intake, kg/d.

1.2 Code

1.2.1 Carbohydrate, protein, ether extract, minerals, and organic matter [5]

```
getBasicChemistry1 <- function(fds = feeds3, genRPT = TRUE)
{
  rum.N_balance.rate <<- 0
  rum.Recycled_N.rate <<- 0
  anim.diet.Forage.frac <<- sum(anim.fd.Forage.conc * anim.fd.DMI.rate/100)/anim.diet.DMI.rate
  anim.diet.Concentrate.frac <<- 1 - anim.diet.Forage.frac

  # CHO (DM)
  anim.fd.NDF.conc <<- as.numeric(fds[, "AdjNDF_DM"])
  anim.fd.UnAdjNDF.conc <<- as.numeric(fds[, "NDF_DM"])
  anim.fd.ADF.conc <<- as.numeric(fds[, "ADF_DM"])
  anim.fd.lignin.conc <<- as.numeric(fds[, "Lignin_DM"])
  anim.fd.peNDF.conc <<- as.numeric(fds[, "peNDF_DM"])
  anim.fd.CHO.conc <<- as.numeric(fds[, "CHO_DM"])
  anim.fd.NFC.conc <<- as.numeric(fds[, "NFC_DM"])
  anim.fd.NDF.rate <<- anim.fd.NDF.conc * anim.fd.DMI.rate/100
  anim.fd.UnAdjNDF.rate <<- anim.fd.UnAdjNDF.conc * anim.fd.DMI.rate/100
  anim.fd.ADF.rate <<- anim.fd.ADF.conc * anim.fd.DMI.rate/100
  anim.fd.lignin.rate <<- anim.fd.lignin.conc * anim.fd.DMI.rate/100
  anim.fd.peNDF.rate <<- anim.fd.peNDF.conc * anim.fd.DMI.rate/100
  anim.fd.CHO.rate <<- anim.fd.CHO.conc * anim.fd.DMI.rate/100
  anim.fd.NFC.rate <<- anim.fd.NFC.conc * anim.fd.DMI.rate/100
  anim.fd.FC.rate <<- anim.fd.CHO.rate - anim.fd.NFC.rate
  anim.diet.NDF.rate <<- sum(anim.fd.NDF.rate)
  anim.diet.NDF.conc <<- isz(anim.diet.NDF.rate*100, anim.diet.DMI.rate)
  anim.diet.UnAdjNDF.rate <<- sum(anim.fd.UnAdjNDF.rate)
  anim.diet.UnAdjNDF.conc <<- isz(anim.diet.UnAdjNDF.rate*100, anim.diet.DMI.rate)
  anim.diet.ADF.rate <<- sum(anim.fd.ADF.rate)
  anim.diet.ADF.conc <<- isz(anim.diet.ADF.rate*100, anim.diet.DMI.rate)
  anim.diet.lignin.rate <<- sum(anim.fd.lignin.rate)
  anim.diet.lignin.conc <<- isz(anim.diet.lignin.rate*100, anim.diet.DMI.rate)
  anim.diet.peNDF.rate <<- sum(anim.fd.peNDF.rate)
  anim.diet.peNDF.conc <<- isz(anim.diet.peNDF.rate*100, anim.diet.DMI.rate)
  anim.diet.CHO.rate <<- sum(anim.fd.CHO.rate)
  anim.diet.CHO.conc <<- isz(anim.diet.CHO.rate*100, anim.diet.DMI.rate)
  anim.diet.NFC.rate <<- sum(anim.fd.NFC.rate)
  anim.diet.NFC.conc <<- isz(anim.diet.NFC.rate*100, anim.diet.DMI.rate)
  anim.diet.FC.rate <<- anim.diet.CHO.rate - anim.diet.NFC.rate
  anim.diet.FC.conc <<- isz(anim.diet.FC.rate*100, anim.diet.DMI.rate)
  # Protein
  anim.fd.CP.conc <<- as.numeric(fds[, "CP_DM"])
```

[5] Applies to L0 and L1 only.

```
    anim.fd.NDIP.conc <<- as.numeric(fds[, "NDIP_DM"])
    anim.fd.ADIP.conc <<- as.numeric(fds[, "ADIP_DM"])
    anim.fd.CP.rate <<- anim.fd.CP.conc * anim.fd.DMI.rate/100
    anim.fd.NDIP.rate <<- anim.fd.NDIP.conc * anim.fd.DMI.rate/100
    anim.fd.ADIP.rate <<- anim.fd.ADIP.conc * anim.fd.DMI.rate/100
    anim.diet.CP.rate <<- sum(anim.fd.CP.rate)
    anim.diet.CP.conc <<- isz(anim.diet.CP.rate*100, anim.diet.DMI.rate)
    anim.diet.NDIP.rate <<- sum(anim.fd.NDIP.rate)
    anim.diet.NDIP.conc <<- isz(anim.diet.NDIP.rate*100, anim.diet.DMI.rate)
    anim.diet.ADIP.rate <<- sum(anim.fd.ADIP.rate)
    anim.diet.ADIP.conc <<- isz(anim.diet.ADIP.rate*100, anim.diet.DMI.rate)
    # Ether Extract
    anim.fd.EE.conc <<- as.numeric(fds[, "EE_DM"])
    anim.fd.EE.rate <<- anim.fd.EE.conc * anim.fd.DMI.rate/100
    anim.diet.EE.rate <<- sum(anim.fd.EE.rate)
    anim.diet.EE.conc <<- isz(anim.diet.EE.rate*100, anim.diet.DMI.rate)
    # Ash
    anim.fd.ash.conc <<- as.numeric(fds[, "Ash_DM"])
    anim.fd.ash.rate <<- anim.fd.ash.conc * anim.fd.DMI.rate/100
    anim.diet.ash.rate <<- sum(anim.fd.ash.rate)
    anim.diet.ash.conc <<- isz(anim.diet.ash.rate*100, anim.diet.DMI.rate)
    if (genRPT)
    {
      # %DM
      rptNutrientComposition_DM <- fds["FeedName.x"]
      names(rptNutrientComposition_DM) <- "FeedName"
      rptNutrientComposition_DM["CP"] <- anim.fd.CP.conc
      rptNutrientComposition_DM["NDIP"] <- anim.fd.NDIP.conc
      rptNutrientComposition_DM["ADIP"] <- anim.fd.ADIP.conc
      rptNutrientComposition_DM["NFC"] <- anim.fd.NFC.conc
      rptNutrientComposition_DM["NDF"] <- anim.fd.NDF.conc
      rptNutrientComposition_DM["ADF"] <- anim.fd.ADF.conc
      rptNutrientComposition_DM["Lignin"] <- anim.fd.lignin.conc
      rptNutrientComposition_DM["peNDF"] <- anim.fd.peNDF.conc
      rptNutrientComposition_DM["EE"] <- anim.fd.EE.conc
      rptNutrientComposition_DM["Ash"] <- anim.fd.ash.conc
      rptNutrientComposition_DM2 <- data.frame(FeedName = "Ration")
      rptNutrientComposition_DM2["CP"] <- isz(anim.diet.CP.rate * 100, anim.diet.DMI.rate)
      rptNutrientComposition_DM2["NDIP"] <- isz(anim.diet.NDIP.rate * 100, anim.diet.DMI.rate)
      rptNutrientComposition_DM2["ADIP"] <- isz(anim.diet.ADIP.rate * 100, anim.diet.DMI.rate)
      rptNutrientComposition_DM2["NFC"] <- isz(anim.diet.NFC.rate * 100, anim.diet.DMI.rate)
      rptNutrientComposition_DM2["NDF"] <- isz(anim.diet.NDF.rate * 100, anim.diet.DMI.rate)
      rptNutrientComposition_DM2["ADF"] <- isz(anim.diet.ADF.rate * 100, anim.diet.DMI.rate)
      rptNutrientComposition_DM2["Lignin"] <- isz(anim.diet.lignin.rate * 100, anim.diet.DMI.rate)
      rptNutrientComposition_DM2["peNDF"] <- isz(anim.diet.peNDF.rate * 100, anim.diet.DMI.rate)
      rptNutrientComposition_DM2["EE"] <- isz(anim.diet.EE.rate * 100, anim.diet.DMI.rate)
      rptNutrientComposition_DM2["Ash"] <- isz(anim.diet.ash.rate * 100, anim.diet.DMI.rate)
      rptNutrientComposition_DM <- rbind(rptNutrientComposition_DM, rptNutrientComposition_DM2)
      report(rptNutrientComposition_DM, "Nutrient Composition, %DM", "", "", 3, 3, 1, 10, FALSE, FALSE, FALSE, FALSE, FALSE,
FALSE, TRUE)
      # %Nutrient
```

```
    rptNutrientComposition_ <- fds["FeedName.x"]
    names(rptNutrientComposition_) <- "FeedName"
    rptNutrientComposition_["NDIP, %CP"] <- isz(anim.fd.NDIP.rate * 100, anim.fd.CP.rate)
    rptNutrientComposition_["ADIP, %CP"] <- isz(anim.fd.ADIP.rate * 100, anim.fd.CP.rate)
    rptNutrientComposition_["NFC, %CHO"] <- isz(anim.fd.NFC.conc * 100, anim.fd.CHO.conc)
    rptNutrientComposition_["NDF, %CHO"] <- isz(anim.fd.NDF.conc * 100, anim.fd.CHO.conc)
    rptNutrientComposition_["ADF, %CHO"] <- isz(anim.fd.ADF.conc * 100, anim.fd.CHO.conc)
    rptNutrientComposition_["Lignin, %CHO"] <- isz(anim.fd.lignin.rate * 100, anim.fd.CHO.rate)
    rptNutrientComposition_["peNDF, %CHO"] <- isz(anim.fd.peNDF.rate * 100, anim.fd.CHO.rate)
    rptNutrientComposition_["Lignin(1), %NDF"] <- isz(anim.fd.lignin.rate * 100, anim.fd.UnAdjNDF.rate)
    rptNutrientComposition_["Lignin(2), %NDF"] <- isz(anim.fd.lignin.rate * 100, anim.fd.NDF.rate)
    rptNutrientComposition_["peNDF, %NDF"] <- isz(anim.fd.peNDF.rate * 100, anim.fd.NDF.rate)
    rptNutrientComposition_2 <- data.frame(FeedName = "Ration")
    rptNutrientComposition_2["NDIP, %CP"] <- isz(anim.diet.NDIP.rate * 100, anim.diet.CP.rate)
    rptNutrientComposition_2["ADIP, %CP"] <- isz(anim.diet.ADIP.rate * 100, anim.diet.CP.rate)
    rptNutrientComposition_2["NFC, %CHO"] <- isz(anim.diet.NFC.rate * 100, anim.diet.CHO.rate)
    rptNutrientComposition_2["NDF, %CHO"] <- isz(anim.diet.NDF.rate * 100, anim.diet.CHO.rate)
    rptNutrientComposition_2["ADF, %CHO"] <- isz(anim.diet.ADF.rate * 100, anim.diet.CHO.rate)
    rptNutrientComposition_2["Lignin, %CHO"] <- isz(anim.diet.lignin.rate * 100, anim.diet.CHO.rate)
    rptNutrientComposition_2["peNDF, %CHO"] <- isz(anim.diet.peNDF.rate * 100, anim.diet.CHO.rate)
    rptNutrientComposition_2["Lignin(1), %NDF"] <- isz(anim.diet.lignin.rate * 100, anim.diet.UnAdjNDF.rate)
    rptNutrientComposition_2["Lignin(2), %NDF"] <- isz(anim.diet.lignin.rate * 100, anim.diet.NDF.rate)
    rptNutrientComposition_2["peNDF, %NDF"] <- isz(anim.diet.peNDF.rate * 100, anim.diet.NDF.rate)
    rptNutrientComposition_ <- rbind(rptNutrientComposition_, rptNutrientComposition_2)
    if (any(as.logical(fds[, "AdjCHOforNPN"])) == TRUE)
    {
      footnote1 <- paste(which(as.logical(fds[, "AdjCHOforNPN"]) == T), collapse = ",")
      footnote <- paste("(1) User-entered NDF\n", "(2) RNS-adjusted NDF (RNS uses this value)\nWhen sodium sulfite is used, NDF and adjusted NDF values are identical\n", "(3) The following feedstuffs had total CHO adjusted for non-protein N: ", footnote1, sep = "")
      rm(footnote1)
    } else
    {
      footnote <- paste("(1) User-entered NDF\n", "(2) RNS-adjusted NDF (RNS uses this value)\nWhen sodium sulfite is used, NDF and adjusted NDF values are identical", sep = "")
    }
    report(rptNutrientComposition_, "Nutrient Composition, %Nutrient", "", footnote, 3, 3, 1, 7, FALSE, FALSE, FALSE, FALSE, FALSE, FALSE, TRUE)
    # g/d
    rptNutrientComposition_DMI <- fds["FeedName.x"]
    names(rptNutrientComposition_DMI) <- "FeedName"
    rptNutrientComposition_DMI["CP"] <- anim.fd.CP.rate
    rptNutrientComposition_DMI["NDIP"] <- anim.fd.NDIP.rate
    rptNutrientComposition_DMI["ADIP"] <- anim.fd.ADIP.rate
    rptNutrientComposition_DMI["NFC"] <- anim.fd.NFC.rate
    rptNutrientComposition_DMI["NDF"] <- anim.fd.NDF.rate
    rptNutrientComposition_DMI["ADF"] <- anim.fd.ADF.rate
    rptNutrientComposition_DMI["Lignin"] <- anim.fd.lignin.rate
    rptNutrientComposition_DMI["peNDF"] <- anim.fd.peNDF.rate
    rptNutrientComposition_DMI["EE"] <- anim.fd.EE.rate
    rptNutrientComposition_DMI["Ash"] <- anim.fd.ash.rate
```

```
        rptNutrientComposition_DMI2 <- data.frame(FeedName = "Ration")
        rptNutrientComposition_DMI2["CP"] <- anim.diet.CP.rate
        rptNutrientComposition_DMI2["NDIP"] <- anim.diet.NDIP.rate
        rptNutrientComposition_DMI2["ADIP"] <- anim.diet.ADIP.rate
        rptNutrientComposition_DMI2["NFC"] <- anim.diet.NFC.rate
        rptNutrientComposition_DMI2["NDF"] <- anim.diet.NDF.rate
        rptNutrientComposition_DMI2["ADF"] <- anim.diet.ADF.rate
        rptNutrientComposition_DMI2["Lignin"] <- anim.diet.lignin.rate
        rptNutrientComposition_DMI2["peNDF"] <- anim.diet.peNDF.rate
        rptNutrientComposition_DMI2["EE"] <- anim.diet.EE.rate
        rptNutrientComposition_DMI2["Ash"] <- anim.diet.ash.rate
        rptNutrientComposition_DMI <- rbind(rptNutrientComposition_DMI, rptNutrientComposition_DMI2)
        report(rptNutrientComposition_DMI, "Nutrient Intake, kg/d", "", "", 3, 3, 1, 10, FALSE, FALSE, FALSE, FALSE, FALSE,
FALSE, TRUE)
    }
    # Minerals and vitamins
    anim.fd.Ca.conc <<- as.numeric(fds[, "Ca_DM"])
    anim.fd.P.conc <<- as.numeric(fds[, "P_DM"])
    anim.fd.Mg.conc <<- as.numeric(fds[, "Mg_DM"])
    anim.fd.K.conc <<- as.numeric(fds[, "K_DM"])
    anim.fd.S.conc <<- as.numeric(fds[, "S_DM"])
    anim.fd.Cl.conc <<- as.numeric(fds[, "Cl_DM"])
    anim.fd.Na.conc <<- as.numeric(fds[, "Na_DM"])
    anim.fd.Fe_ppm.conc <<- as.numeric(fds[, "Fe_ppmDM"])
    anim.fd.Zn_ppm.conc <<- as.numeric(fds[, "Zn_ppmDM"])
    anim.fd.Cu_ppm.conc <<- as.numeric(fds[, "Cu_ppmDM"])
    anim.fd.Mn_ppm.conc <<- as.numeric(fds[, "Mn_ppmDM"])
    anim.fd.Se_ppm.conc <<- as.numeric(fds[, "Se_ppmDM"])
    anim.fd.Co_ppm.conc <<- as.numeric(fds[, "Co_ppmDM"])
    anim.fd.I_ppm.conc <<- as.numeric(fds[, "I_ppmDM"])
    anim.fd.Cr_ppm.conc <<- as.numeric(fds[, "Cr_ppmDM"])
    anim.fd.VitA.conc <<- as.numeric(fds[, "VitA_kIU"])
    anim.fd.VitD.conc <<- as.numeric(fds[, "VitD_kIU"])
    anim.fd.VitE.conc <<- as.numeric(fds[, "VitE_IU"])
    anim.fd.Ca.rate <<- anim.fd.Ca.conc * anim.fd.DMI.rate/100
    anim.fd.P.rate <<- anim.fd.P.conc * anim.fd.DMI.rate/100
    anim.fd.Mg.rate <<- anim.fd.Mg.conc * anim.fd.DMI.rate/100
    anim.fd.K.rate <<- anim.fd.K.conc * anim.fd.DMI.rate/100
    anim.fd.S.rate <<- anim.fd.S.conc * anim.fd.DMI.rate/100
    anim.fd.Cl.rate <<- anim.fd.Cl.conc * anim.fd.DMI.rate/100
    anim.fd.Na.rate <<- anim.fd.Na.conc * anim.fd.DMI.rate/100
    anim.fd.Fe.rate <<- anim.fd.Fe_ppm.conc * anim.fd.DMI.rate/1e+06
    anim.fd.Zn.rate <<- anim.fd.Zn_ppm.conc * anim.fd.DMI.rate/1e+06
    anim.fd.Cu.rate <<- anim.fd.Cu_ppm.conc * anim.fd.DMI.rate/1e+06
    anim.fd.Mn.rate <<- anim.fd.Mn_ppm.conc * anim.fd.DMI.rate/1e+06
    anim.fd.Se.rate <<- anim.fd.Se_ppm.conc * anim.fd.DMI.rate/1e+06
    anim.fd.Co.rate <<- anim.fd.Co_ppm.conc * anim.fd.DMI.rate/1e+06
    anim.fd.I.rate <<- anim.fd.I_ppm.conc * anim.fd.DMI.rate/1e+06
    anim.fd.Cr.rate <<- anim.fd.Cr_ppm.conc * anim.fd.DMI.rate/1e+06
    anim.fd.VitA.rate <<- anim.fd.VitA.conc * anim.fd.DMI.rate
    anim.fd.VitD.rate <<- anim.fd.VitD.conc * anim.fd.DMI.rate
```

```
    anim.fd.VitE.rate <<- anim.fd.VitE.conc * anim.fd.DMI.rate
    anim.diet.Ca.rate <<- sum(anim.fd.Ca.rate)
    anim.diet.P.rate <<- sum(anim.fd.P.rate)
    anim.diet.Mg.rate <<- sum(anim.fd.Mg.rate)
    anim.diet.K.rate <<- sum(anim.fd.K.rate)
    anim.diet.S.rate <<- sum(anim.fd.S.rate)
    anim.diet.Cl.rate <<- sum(anim.fd.Cl.rate)
    anim.diet.Na.rate <<- sum(anim.fd.Na.rate)
    anim.diet.Fe.rate <<- sum(anim.fd.Fe.rate)
    anim.diet.Zn.rate <<- sum(anim.fd.Zn.rate)
    anim.diet.Cu.rate <<- sum(anim.fd.Cu.rate)
    anim.diet.Mn.rate <<- sum(anim.fd.Mn.rate)
    anim.diet.Se.rate <<- sum(anim.fd.Se.rate)
    anim.diet.Co.rate <<- sum(anim.fd.Co.rate)
    anim.diet.I.rate <<- sum(anim.fd.I.rate)
    anim.diet.Mo.rate <<- 0
    anim.diet.Cr.rate <<- sum(anim.fd.Cr.rate)
    anim.diet.VitA.rate <<- sum(anim.fd.VitA.rate)
    anim.diet.VitD.rate <<- sum(anim.fd.VitD.rate)
    anim.diet.VitE.rate <<- sum(anim.fd.VitE.rate)
    if (genRPT)
    {
      rptMinerals_DM <- fds["FeedName.x"]
      names(rptMinerals_DM) <- "FeedName"
      rptMinerals_DM["Ash, %DM"] <- fds[, "Ash_DM"]
      rptMinerals_DM["Ca, %DM"] <- fds[, "Ca_DM"]
      rptMinerals_DM["P, %DM"] <- fds[, "P_DM"]
      rptMinerals_DM["Mg, %DM"] <- fds[, "Mg_DM"]
      rptMinerals_DM["K, %DM"] <- fds[, "K_DM"]
      rptMinerals_DM["S, %DM"] <- fds[, "S_DM"]
      rptMinerals_DM["Cl, %DM"] <- fds[, "Cl_DM"]
      rptMinerals_DM["Na, %DM"] <- fds[, "Na_DM"]
      rptMinerals_DM["Fe, ppm"] <- fds[, "Fe_ppmDM"]
      rptMinerals_DM["Zn, ppm"] <- fds[, "Zn_ppmDM"]
      rptMinerals_DM["Cu, ppm"] <- fds[, "Cu_ppmDM"]
      rptMinerals_DM["Mn, ppm"] <- fds[, "Mn_ppmDM"]
      rptMinerals_DM["Se, ppm"] <- fds[, "Se_ppmDM"]
      rptMinerals_DM["Co, ppm"] <- fds[, "Co_ppmDM"]
      rptMinerals_DM["I, ppm"] <- fds[, "I_ppmDM"]
      rptMinerals_DM["Cr, ppm"] <- fds[, "Cr_ppmDM"]
      rptMinerals_DM2 <- data.frame(FeedName = "Ration")
      rptMinerals_DM2["Ash, %DM"] <- isz(anim.diet.ash.rate * 100, anim.diet.DMI.rate)
      rptMinerals_DM2["Ca, %DM"] <- isz(anim.diet.Ca.rate * 100, anim.diet.DMI.rate)
      rptMinerals_DM2["P, %DM"] <- isz(anim.diet.P.rate * 100, anim.diet.DMI.rate)
      rptMinerals_DM2["Mg, %DM"] <- isz(anim.diet.Mg.rate * 100, anim.diet.DMI.rate)
      rptMinerals_DM2["K, %DM"] <- isz(anim.diet.K.rate * 100, anim.diet.DMI.rate)
      rptMinerals_DM2["S, %DM"] <- isz(anim.diet.S.rate * 100, anim.diet.DMI.rate)
      rptMinerals_DM2["Cl, %DM"] <- isz(anim.diet.Cl.rate * 100, anim.diet.DMI.rate)
      rptMinerals_DM2["Na, %DM"] <- isz(anim.diet.Na.rate * 100, anim.diet.DMI.rate)
      rptMinerals_DM2["Fe, ppm"] <- isz(anim.diet.Fe.rate * 1e+06, anim.diet.DMI.rate)
      rptMinerals_DM2["Zn, ppm"] <- isz(anim.diet.Zn.rate * 1e+06, anim.diet.DMI.rate)
```

```
    rptMinerals_DM2["Cu, ppm"] <- isz(anim.diet.Cu.rate * 1e+06, anim.diet.DMI.rate)
    rptMinerals_DM2["Mn, ppm"] <- isz(anim.diet.Mn.rate * 1e+06, anim.diet.DMI.rate)
    rptMinerals_DM2["Se, ppm"] <- isz(anim.diet.Se.rate * 1e+06, anim.diet.DMI.rate)
    rptMinerals_DM2["Co, ppm"] <- isz(anim.diet.Co.rate * 1e+06, anim.diet.DMI.rate)
    rptMinerals_DM2["I, ppm"] <- isz(anim.diet.I.rate * 1e+06, anim.diet.DMI.rate)
    rptMinerals_DM2["Cr, ppm"] <- isz(anim.diet.Cr.rate * 1e+06, anim.diet.DMI.rate)
    rptMinerals_DM <- rbind(rptMinerals_DM, rptMinerals_DM2)
    report(rptMinerals_DM, "Macromineral and Micromineral Composition, %DM or ppm", "", "", 3, 3, 1, 8, FALSE, FALSE, FALSE,
FALSE, FALSE, FALSE, TRUE)
    rptMinerals_Ash <- fds["FeedName.x"]
    names(rptMinerals_Ash) <- "FeedName"
    rptMinerals_Ash["Ca"] <- fds[, "Ca_Ash"]
    rptMinerals_Ash["P"] <- fds[, "P_Ash"]
    rptMinerals_Ash["Mg"] <- fds[, "Mg_Ash"]
    rptMinerals_Ash["K"] <- fds[, "K_Ash"]
    rptMinerals_Ash["S"] <- fds[, "S_Ash"]
    rptMinerals_Ash["Cl"] <- fds[, "Cl_Ash"]
    rptMinerals_Ash["Na"] <- fds[, "Na_Ash"]
    rptMinerals_Ash["Fe"] <- fds[, "Fe_Ash"]
    rptMinerals_Ash["Zn"] <- fds[, "Zn_Ash"]
    rptMinerals_Ash["Cu"] <- fds[, "Cu_Ash"]
    rptMinerals_Ash["Mn"] <- fds[, "Mn_Ash"]
    rptMinerals_Ash["Se"] <- fds[, "Se_Ash"]
    rptMinerals_Ash["Co"] <- fds[, "Co_Ash"]
    rptMinerals_Ash["I"] <- fds[, "I_Ash"]
    rptMinerals_Ash["Cr"] <- fds[, "Cr_Ash"]
    rptMinerals_Ash2 <- data.frame(FeedName = "Ration")
    rptMinerals_Ash2["Ca"] <- isz(anim.diet.Ca.rate * 100, anim.diet.ash.rate)
    rptMinerals_Ash2["P"] <- isz(anim.diet.P.rate * 100, anim.diet.ash.rate)
    rptMinerals_Ash2["Mg"] <- isz(anim.diet.Mg.rate * 100, anim.diet.ash.rate)
    rptMinerals_Ash2["K"] <- isz(anim.diet.K.rate * 100, anim.diet.ash.rate)
    rptMinerals_Ash2["S"] <- isz(anim.diet.S.rate * 100, anim.diet.ash.rate)
    rptMinerals_Ash2["Cl"] <- isz(anim.diet.Cl.rate * 100, anim.diet.ash.rate)
    rptMinerals_Ash2["Na"] <- isz(anim.diet.Na.rate * 100, anim.diet.ash.rate)
    rptMinerals_Ash2["Fe"] <- isz(anim.diet.Fe.rate * 100, anim.diet.ash.rate)
    rptMinerals_Ash2["Zn"] <- isz(anim.diet.Zn.rate * 100, anim.diet.ash.rate)
    rptMinerals_Ash2["Cu"] <- isz(anim.diet.Cu.rate * 100, anim.diet.ash.rate)
    rptMinerals_Ash2["Mn"] <- isz(anim.diet.Mn.rate * 100, anim.diet.ash.rate)
    rptMinerals_Ash2["Se"] <- isz(anim.diet.Se.rate * 100, anim.diet.ash.rate)
    rptMinerals_Ash2["Co"] <- isz(anim.diet.Co.rate * 100, anim.diet.ash.rate)
    rptMinerals_Ash2["I"] <- isz(anim.diet.I.rate * 100, anim.diet.ash.rate)
    rptMinerals_Ash2["Cr"] <- isz(anim.diet.Cr.rate * 100, anim.diet.ash.rate)
    rptMinerals_Ash <- rbind(rptMinerals_Ash, rptMinerals_Ash2)
    description <- paste("Least % of ash accounted for by the sum of macromineral and microminerals of feeds    : ",
formatC(min(rowSums(rptMinerals_Ash[2:length(rptMinerals_Ash)])), format = "f", digits = 3, width = 7), "% \n",
                        "Greatest % of ash accounted for by the sum of macromineral and microminerals of feeds: ",
formatC(max(rowSums(rptMinerals_Ash[2:length(rptMinerals_Ash)])), format = "f", digits = 3, width = 7), "% \n",
                        "% of ash accounted for by the sum of macromineral and microminerals of the ration    : ",
formatC(rowSums(rptMinerals_Ash[nrow(rptMinerals_Ash), 2:length(rptMinerals_Ash)]), format = "f", digits = 3, width = 7), "%
\n\n", sep = "")
    report(rptMinerals_Ash, "Macromineral and Micromineral Composition, %Ash", description, "", 3, 3, 1, 7, FALSE, FALSE,
```

```
    TRUE, FALSE, FALSE, FALSE, TRUE)
        rptMinerals_DMI <- fds["FeedName.x"]
        names(rptMinerals_DMI) <- "FeedName"
        rptMinerals_DMI["Ash"] <- anim.fd.ash.rate
        rptMinerals_DMI["Ca"] <- anim.fd.Ca.rate
        rptMinerals_DMI["P"] <- anim.fd.P.rate
        rptMinerals_DMI["Mg"] <- anim.fd.Mg.rate
        rptMinerals_DMI["K"] <- anim.fd.K.rate
        rptMinerals_DMI["S"] <- anim.fd.S.rate
        rptMinerals_DMI["Cl"] <- anim.fd.Cl.rate
        rptMinerals_DMI["Na"] <- anim.fd.Na.rate
        rptMinerals_DMI["Fe"] <- anim.fd.Fe.rate
        rptMinerals_DMI["Zn"] <- anim.fd.Zn.rate
        rptMinerals_DMI["Cu"] <- anim.fd.Cu.rate
        rptMinerals_DMI["Mn"] <- anim.fd.Mn.rate
        rptMinerals_DMI["Se"] <- anim.fd.Se.rate
        rptMinerals_DMI["Co"] <- anim.fd.Co.rate
        rptMinerals_DMI["I"] <- anim.fd.I.rate
        rptMinerals_DMI["Cr"] <- anim.fd.Cr.rate
        rptMinerals_DMI["VitA, kIU"] <- anim.fd.VitA.rate
        rptMinerals_DMI["VitD, kIU"] <- anim.fd.VitD.rate
        rptMinerals_DMI["VitE, IU"] <- anim.fd.VitE.rate
        rptMinerals_DMI2 <- data.frame(FeedName = "Ration")
        rptMinerals_DMI2["Ash"] <- anim.diet.ash.rate
        rptMinerals_DMI2["Ca"] <- anim.diet.Ca.rate
        rptMinerals_DMI2["P"] <- anim.diet.P.rate
        rptMinerals_DMI2["Mg"] <- anim.diet.Mg.rate
        rptMinerals_DMI2["K"] <- anim.diet.K.rate
        rptMinerals_DMI2["S"] <- anim.diet.S.rate
        rptMinerals_DMI2["Cl"] <- anim.diet.Cl.rate
        rptMinerals_DMI2["Na"] <- anim.diet.Na.rate
        rptMinerals_DMI2["Fe"] <- anim.diet.Fe.rate
        rptMinerals_DMI2["Zn"] <- anim.diet.Zn.rate
        rptMinerals_DMI2["Cu"] <- anim.diet.Cu.rate
        rptMinerals_DMI2["Mn"] <- anim.diet.Mn.rate
        rptMinerals_DMI2["Se"] <- anim.diet.Se.rate
        rptMinerals_DMI2["Co"] <- anim.diet.Co.rate
        rptMinerals_DMI2["I"] <- anim.diet.I.rate
        rptMinerals_DMI2["Cr"] <- anim.diet.Cr.rate
        rptMinerals_DMI2["VitA, kIU"] <- anim.diet.VitA.rate
        rptMinerals_DMI2["VitD, kIU"] <- anim.diet.VitD.rate
        rptMinerals_DMI2["VitE, IU"] <- anim.diet.VitE.rate
        rptMinerals_DMI <- rbind(rptMinerals_DMI, rptMinerals_DMI2)
        report(rptMinerals_DMI, "Macromineral and Micromineral (g/d) and Vitamin (IU/d) Intake", "", "", 3, 3, 1000, 8, FALSE,
    FALSE, FALSE, FALSE, FALSE, FALSE, TRUE)
      }
      # Organic matter
      anim.fd.OMI.rate <<- anim.fd.CP.rate + anim.fd.CHO.rate + anim.fd.EE.rate
      anim.diet.OMI.rate <<- sum(anim.fd.OMI.rate)
    }
```

1.2.2 Absorbable minerals

```
calcAbsorbableMinerals <- function(fds = feeds3, genRPT = TRUE)
{
  # +++++++++++++++++++++++++
  # Mineral bioavailability
  # +++++++++++++++++++++++++
  if (anim.species == "Cattle")
  {
    if (anim.type == "Milk")
    {
      # Dairy cattle
      anim.fd.CaBio.conc <<- as.numeric(fds[, "Ca_BioAvail"])
      anim.fd.PBio.conc <<- as.numeric(fds[, "P_BioAvail"])
      anim.fd.MgBio.conc <<- as.numeric(fds[, "Mg_BioAvail"])
      anim.fd.KBio.conc <<- as.numeric(fds[, "K_BioAvail"])
      anim.fd.SBio.conc <<- as.numeric(fds[, "S_BioAvail"])
      anim.fd.ClBio.conc <<- as.numeric(fds[, "Cl_BioAvail"])
      anim.fd.NaBio.conc <<- as.numeric(fds[, "Na_BioAvail"])
      anim.fd.FeBio.conc <<- as.numeric(fds[, "Fe_BioAvail"])
      anim.fd.ZnBio.conc <<- as.numeric(fds[, "Zn_BioAvail"])
      anim.fd.CuBio.conc <<- as.numeric(fds[, "Cu_BioAvail"])
      anim.fd.MnBio.conc <<- as.numeric(fds[, "Mn_BioAvail"])
      anim.fd.SeBio.conc <<- as.numeric(fds[, "Se_BioAvail"])
      anim.fd.CoBio.conc <<- as.numeric(fds[, "Co_BioAvail"])
      anim.fd.IBio.conc <<- as.numeric(fds[, "I_BioAvail"])
      anim.fd.CrBio.conc <<- as.numeric(fds[, "Cr_BioAvail"])
    } else
    {
      # Beef cattle
      anim.fd.CaBio.conc <<- rep(50, nrow(fds))
      anim.fd.PBio.conc <<- rep(68, nrow(fds))
      anim.fd.MgBio.conc <<- rep(100, nrow(fds))
      anim.fd.KBio.conc <<- rep(100, nrow(fds))
      anim.fd.SBio.conc <<- rep(100, nrow(fds))
      anim.fd.ClBio.conc <<- rep(100, nrow(fds))
      anim.fd.NaBio.conc <<- rep(100, nrow(fds))
      anim.fd.FeBio.conc <<- rep(100, nrow(fds))
      anim.fd.ZnBio.conc <<- rep(100, nrow(fds))
      anim.fd.CuBio.conc <<- rep(100, nrow(fds))
      anim.fd.MnBio.conc <<- rep(100, nrow(fds))
      anim.fd.SeBio.conc <<- rep(100, nrow(fds))
      anim.fd.CoBio.conc <<- rep(100, nrow(fds))
      anim.fd.IBio.conc <<- rep(100, nrow(fds))
      anim.fd.CrBio.conc <<- rep(100, nrow(fds))
    }
  } else
  {
    # Sheep and goats
    anim.fd.CaBio.conc <<- rep(100, nrow(fds))
```

```
        anim.fd.PBio.conc <<- rep(100, nrow(fds))
        anim.fd.MgBio.conc <<- rep(100, nrow(fds))
        anim.fd.KBio.conc <<- rep(100, nrow(fds))
        anim.fd.SBio.conc <<- rep(100, nrow(fds))
        anim.fd.ClBio.conc <<- rep(100, nrow(fds))
        anim.fd.NaBio.conc <<- rep(100, nrow(fds))
        anim.fd.FeBio.conc <<- rep(100, nrow(fds))
        anim.fd.ZnBio.conc <<- rep(100, nrow(fds))
        anim.fd.CuBio.conc <<- rep(100, nrow(fds))
        anim.fd.MnBio.conc <<- rep(100, nrow(fds))
        anim.fd.SeBio.conc <<- rep(100, nrow(fds))
        anim.fd.CoBio.conc <<- rep(100, nrow(fds))
        anim.fd.IBio.conc <<- rep(100, nrow(fds))
        anim.fd.CrBio.conc <<- rep(100, nrow(fds))
    }
    # kg/d
    si.fd.GCa.rate <<- anim.fd.Ca.rate * (anim.fd.CaBio.conc/100)
    si.fd.GP.rate <<- anim.fd.P.rate * (anim.fd.PBio.conc/100)
    si.fd.GMg.rate <<- anim.fd.Mg.rate * (anim.fd.MgBio.conc/100)
    si.fd.GK.rate <<- anim.fd.K.rate * (anim.fd.KBio.conc/100)
    si.fd.GS.rate <<- anim.fd.S.rate * (anim.fd.SBio.conc/100)
    si.fd.GCl.rate <<- anim.fd.Cl.rate * (anim.fd.ClBio.conc/100)
    si.fd.GNa.rate <<- anim.fd.Na.rate * (anim.fd.NaBio.conc/100)
    si.fd.GFe.rate <<- anim.fd.Fe.rate * (anim.fd.FeBio.conc/100)
    si.fd.GZn.rate <<- anim.fd.Zn.rate * (anim.fd.ZnBio.conc/100)
    si.fd.GCu.rate <<- anim.fd.Cu.rate * (anim.fd.CuBio.conc/100)
    si.fd.GMn.rate <<- anim.fd.Mn.rate * (anim.fd.MnBio.conc/100)
    si.fd.GSe.rate <<- anim.fd.Se.rate * (anim.fd.SeBio.conc/100)
    si.fd.GCo.rate <<- anim.fd.Co.rate * (anim.fd.CoBio.conc/100)
    si.fd.GI.rate <<- anim.fd.I.rate * (anim.fd.IBio.conc/100)
    si.fd.GCr.rate <<- anim.fd.Cr.rate * (anim.fd.CrBio.conc/100)
    si.diet.GCa.rate <<- sum(si.fd.GCa.rate)
    si.diet.GP.rate <<- sum(si.fd.GP.rate)
    si.diet.GMg.rate <<- sum(si.fd.GMg.rate)
    si.diet.GK.rate <<- sum(si.fd.GK.rate)
    si.diet.GS.rate <<- sum(si.fd.GS.rate)
    si.diet.GCl.rate <<- sum(si.fd.GCl.rate)
    si.diet.GNa.rate <<- sum(si.fd.GNa.rate)
    si.diet.GFe.rate <<- sum(si.fd.GFe.rate)
    si.diet.GZn.rate <<- sum(si.fd.GZn.rate)
    si.diet.GCu.rate <<- sum(si.fd.GCu.rate)
    si.diet.GMn.rate <<- sum(si.fd.GMn.rate)
    si.diet.GSe.rate <<- sum(si.fd.GSe.rate)
    si.diet.GCo.rate <<- sum(si.fd.GCo.rate)
    si.diet.GI.rate <<- sum(si.fd.GI.rate)
    si.diet.GMo.rate <<- 0
    si.diet.GCr.rate <<- sum(si.fd.GCr.rate)

    anim.diet.CaBio.conc <<- ifelse(anim.diet.DMI.rate > 0, sum(anim.fd.CaBio.conc * anim.fd.DMI.rate)/anim.diet.DMI.rate, 100)
    anim.diet.PBio.conc <<- ifelse(anim.diet.DMI.rate > 0, sum(anim.fd.PBio.conc * anim.fd.DMI.rate)/anim.diet.DMI.rate, 100)
    anim.diet.MgBio.conc <<- ifelse(anim.diet.DMI.rate > 0, sum(anim.fd.MgBio.conc * anim.fd.DMI.rate)/anim.diet.DMI.rate, 100)
```

```
  anim.diet.KBio.conc <<- ifelse(anim.diet.DMI.rate > 0, sum(anim.fd.KBio.conc * anim.fd.DMI.rate)/anim.diet.DMI.rate, 100)
  anim.diet.SBio.conc <<- ifelse(anim.diet.DMI.rate > 0, sum(anim.fd.SBio.conc * anim.fd.DMI.rate)/anim.diet.DMI.rate, 100)
  anim.diet.ClBio.conc <<- ifelse(anim.diet.DMI.rate > 0, sum(anim.fd.ClBio.conc * anim.fd.DMI.rate)/anim.diet.DMI.rate, 100)
  anim.diet.NaBio.conc <<- ifelse(anim.diet.DMI.rate > 0, sum(anim.fd.NaBio.conc * anim.fd.DMI.rate)/anim.diet.DMI.rate, 100)
  anim.diet.FeBio.conc <<- ifelse(anim.diet.DMI.rate > 0, sum(anim.fd.FeBio.conc * anim.fd.DMI.rate)/anim.diet.DMI.rate, 100)
  anim.diet.ZnBio.conc <<- ifelse(anim.diet.DMI.rate > 0, sum(anim.fd.ZnBio.conc * anim.fd.DMI.rate)/anim.diet.DMI.rate, 100)
  anim.diet.CuBio.conc <<- ifelse(anim.diet.DMI.rate > 0, sum(anim.fd.CuBio.conc * anim.fd.DMI.rate)/anim.diet.DMI.rate, 100)
  anim.diet.MnBio.conc <<- ifelse(anim.diet.DMI.rate > 0, sum(anim.fd.MnBio.conc * anim.fd.DMI.rate)/anim.diet.DMI.rate, 100)
  anim.diet.SeBio.conc <<- ifelse(anim.diet.DMI.rate > 0, sum(anim.fd.SeBio.conc * anim.fd.DMI.rate)/anim.diet.DMI.rate, 100)
  anim.diet.CoBio.conc <<- ifelse(anim.diet.DMI.rate > 0, sum(anim.fd.CoBio.conc * anim.fd.DMI.rate)/anim.diet.DMI.rate, 100)
  anim.diet.IBio.conc <<- ifelse(anim.diet.DMI.rate > 0, sum(anim.fd.IBio.conc * anim.fd.DMI.rate)/anim.diet.DMI.rate, 100)
  anim.diet.MoBio.conc <<- 100
  anim.diet.CrBio.conc <<- ifelse(anim.diet.DMI.rate > 0, sum(anim.fd.CrBio.conc * anim.fd.DMI.rate)/anim.diet.DMI.rate, 100)

  if (genRPT)
  {
    # Bioavailability
    rptMinerals_Absorbable <- fds["FeedName.x"]
    names(rptMinerals_Absorbable) <- "FeedName"
    rptMinerals_Absorbable["Ca Bio"] <- anim.fd.CaBio.conc
    rptMinerals_Absorbable["P Bio"] <- anim.fd.PBio.conc
    rptMinerals_Absorbable["Mg Bio"] <- anim.fd.MgBio.conc
    rptMinerals_Absorbable["K Bio"] <- anim.fd.KBio.conc
    rptMinerals_Absorbable["S Bio"] <- anim.fd.SBio.conc
    rptMinerals_Absorbable["Cl Bio"] <- anim.fd.ClBio.conc
    rptMinerals_Absorbable["Na Bio"] <- anim.fd.NaBio.conc
    rptMinerals_Absorbable["Fe Bio"] <- anim.fd.FeBio.conc
    rptMinerals_Absorbable["Zn Bio"] <- anim.fd.ZnBio.conc
    rptMinerals_Absorbable["Cu Bio"] <- anim.fd.CuBio.conc
    rptMinerals_Absorbable["Mn Bio"] <- anim.fd.MnBio.conc
    rptMinerals_Absorbable["Se Bio"] <- anim.fd.SeBio.conc
    rptMinerals_Absorbable["Co Bio"] <- anim.fd.CoBio.conc
    rptMinerals_Absorbable["I Bio"] <- anim.fd.IBio.conc
    rptMinerals_Absorbable["Cr Bio"] <- anim.fd.CrBio.conc
    rptMinerals_Absorbable2 <- data.frame(FeedName = "Ration")
    rptMinerals_Absorbable2["Ca Bio"] <- anim.diet.CaBio.conc
    rptMinerals_Absorbable2["P Bio"] <- anim.diet.PBio.conc
    rptMinerals_Absorbable2["Mg Bio"] <- anim.diet.MgBio.conc
    rptMinerals_Absorbable2["K Bio"] <- anim.diet.KBio.conc
    rptMinerals_Absorbable2["S Bio"] <- anim.diet.SBio.conc
    rptMinerals_Absorbable2["Cl Bio"] <- anim.diet.ClBio.conc
    rptMinerals_Absorbable2["Na Bio"] <- anim.diet.NaBio.conc
    rptMinerals_Absorbable2["Fe Bio"] <- anim.diet.FeBio.conc
    rptMinerals_Absorbable2["Zn Bio"] <- anim.diet.ZnBio.conc
    rptMinerals_Absorbable2["Cu Bio"] <- anim.diet.CuBio.conc
    rptMinerals_Absorbable2["Mn Bio"] <- anim.diet.MnBio.conc
    rptMinerals_Absorbable2["Se Bio"] <- anim.diet.SeBio.conc
    rptMinerals_Absorbable2["Co Bio"] <- anim.diet.CoBio.conc
    rptMinerals_Absorbable2["I Bio"] <- anim.diet.IBio.conc
    rptMinerals_Absorbable2["Cr Bio"] <- anim.diet.CrBio.conc
    rptMinerals_Absorbable <- rbind(rptMinerals_Absorbable, rptMinerals_Absorbable2)
```

```
    description <- paste("Bio = bioavailability or absorption coefficient\n",
                         "Abs = absorbable nutrient (intake x bioavailability or intake x absorption coefficient)\n",
                         "Absorbable macrominerals are in g/d and microminerals are in mg/d\n\n", sep = "")
    report(rptMinerals_Absorbable, "Macromineral and Micromineral Bioavailability (%) and Absorbable Amounts", description,
"", 3, 2, 1, 10,
           FALSE, FALSE, FALSE, FALSE, FALSE, FALSE, FALSE, , , , TRUE,"-", TRUE)
    # Absorbed minerals
    rptMinerals_Absorbable <- fds["FeedName.x"]
    names(rptMinerals_Absorbable) <- "FeedName"
    rptMinerals_Absorbable["Abs Ca"] <- si.fd.GCa.rate * 1000
    rptMinerals_Absorbable["Abs P"] <- si.fd.GP.rate * 1000
    rptMinerals_Absorbable["Abs Mg"] <- si.fd.GMg.rate * 1000
    rptMinerals_Absorbable["Abs K"] <- si.fd.GK.rate * 1000
    rptMinerals_Absorbable["Abs S"] <- si.fd.GS.rate * 1000
    rptMinerals_Absorbable["Abs Cl"] <- si.fd.GCl.rate * 1000
    rptMinerals_Absorbable["Abs Na"] <- si.fd.GNa.rate * 1000
    rptMinerals_Absorbable["Abs Fe"] <- si.fd.GFe.rate * 1000000
    rptMinerals_Absorbable["Abs Zn"] <- si.fd.GZn.rate * 1000000
    rptMinerals_Absorbable["Abs Cu"] <- si.fd.GCu.rate * 1000000
    rptMinerals_Absorbable["Abs Mn"] <- si.fd.GMn.rate * 1000000
    rptMinerals_Absorbable["Abs Se"] <- si.fd.GSe.rate * 1000000
    rptMinerals_Absorbable["Abs Co"] <- si.fd.GCo.rate * 1000000
    rptMinerals_Absorbable["Abs I"] <- si.fd.GI.rate * 1000000
    rptMinerals_Absorbable["Abs Cr"] <- si.fd.GCr.rate * 1000000
    rptMinerals_Absorbable2 <- data.frame(FeedName = "Ration")
    rptMinerals_Absorbable2["Abs Ca"] <- si.diet.GCa.rate * 1000
    rptMinerals_Absorbable2["Abs P"] <- si.diet.GP.rate * 1000
    rptMinerals_Absorbable2["Abs Mg"] <- si.diet.GMg.rate * 1000
    rptMinerals_Absorbable2["Abs K"] <- si.diet.GK.rate * 1000
    rptMinerals_Absorbable2["Abs S"] <- si.diet.GS.rate * 1000
    rptMinerals_Absorbable2["Abs Cl"] <- si.diet.GCl.rate * 1000
    rptMinerals_Absorbable2["Abs Na"] <- si.diet.GNa.rate * 1000
    rptMinerals_Absorbable2["Abs Fe"] <- si.diet.GFe.rate * 1000000
    rptMinerals_Absorbable2["Abs Zn"] <- si.diet.GZn.rate * 1000000
    rptMinerals_Absorbable2["Abs Cu"] <- si.diet.GCu.rate * 1000000
    rptMinerals_Absorbable2["Abs Mn"] <- si.diet.GMn.rate * 1000000
    rptMinerals_Absorbable2["Abs Se"] <- si.diet.GSe.rate * 1000000
    rptMinerals_Absorbable2["Abs Co"] <- si.diet.GCo.rate * 1000000
    rptMinerals_Absorbable2["Abs I"] <- si.diet.GI.rate * 1000000
    rptMinerals_Absorbable2["Abs Cr"] <- si.diet.GCr.rate * 1000000
    rptMinerals_Absorbable <- rbind(rptMinerals_Absorbable, rptMinerals_Absorbable2)
    report(rptMinerals_Absorbable, "\n", "", "", 3, 2, 1, 10,
           FALSE, FALSE, FALSE, FALSE, FALSE, FALSE, TRUE, , FALSE, , TRUE, , FALSE)
  }
}
```

1.2.3 Dietary cation-anion balance

```
calcDCAB <- function()
{
  # Dietary Cation-Anion Balance (DCAB), or
  # Dietary Cation-Anion Difference (DCAD)
  # Equivalent (eq) is atomic gram-atomic weight divided by valence = (g/mol)/(eq/mol)
  # Milliequivalent (meq) = eq/1000
  DMI <- anim.diet.DMI.rate
  if (DMI == 0) return(invisible(NULL))
  # Intake basis
  Ca <- anim.diet.Ca.rate * 100/DMI  # 40 g/mol, 2 eq/mol, 20 g/eq
  Mg <- anim.diet.Mg.rate * 100/DMI  # 24 g/mol, 2 eq/mol, 12 g/eq
  Na <- anim.diet.Na.rate * 100/DMI  # 23 g/mol, 1 eq/mol, 23 g/eq
  K <- anim.diet.K.rate * 100/DMI  # 39 g/mol, 1 eq/mol, 39 g/eq
  Cl <- anim.diet.Cl.rate * 100/DMI  # 35.5 g/mol, 1 eq/mol, 35.5 g/eq
  S <- anim.diet.S.rate * 100/DMI  # 32 g/mol, 2 eq/mol, 16 g/eq
  P <- anim.diet.P.rate * 100/DMI  # 31 g/mol, 2 eq/mol, 15.5 g/eq
  # Absorbed basis
  GCa <- si.diet.GCa.rate * 100/DMI
  GMg <- si.diet.GMg.rate * 100/DMI
  GNa <- si.diet.GNa.rate * 100/DMI
  GK <- si.diet.GK.rate * 100/DMI
  GCl <- si.diet.GCl.rate * 100/DMI
  GS <- si.diet.GS.rate * 100/DMI
  GP <- si.diet.GP.rate * 100/DMI
  # meq/100 g DM
  # Intake basis
  anim.DCAB1.rate <<- (Na/0.023 + K/0.039 + Ca/0.02 + Mg/0.012) - (Cl/0.0355 + S/0.016 + P/0.0155)
  anim.DCAB2.rate <<- (Na/0.023 + K/0.039) - (Cl/0.0355)
  anim.DCAB3.rate <<- (Na/0.023 + K/0.039) - (Cl/0.0355 + S/0.016)
  anim.DCAB4.rate <<- (Na/0.023 + K/0.039 + 0.38 * Ca/0.02 + 0.3 * Mg/0.012) - (Cl/0.0355 + 0.6 * S/0.016 + 0.5 * P/0.0155)
  anim.DCAB5.rate <<- (Na/0.023 + K/0.039 + 0.15 * Ca/0.02 + 0.15 * Mg/0.012) - (Cl/0.0355 + 0.2 * S/0.016 + 0.3 * P/0.0155)
  anim.DCAB6.rate <<- (Na/0.023 + K/0.039 + 0.15 * Ca/0.02 + 0.15 * Mg/0.012) - (Cl/0.0355 + 0.6 * S/0.016 + 0.5 * P/0.0155)
  # Absorbed basis
  anim.DCAB7.rate <<- (GNa/0.023 + GK/0.039 + GCa/0.02 + GMg/0.012) - (GCl/0.0355 + GS/0.016 + GP/0.0155)
  anim.DCAB8.rate <<- (GNa/0.023 + GK/0.039) - (GCl/0.0355)
  anim.DCAB9.rate <<- (GNa/0.023 + GK/0.039) - (GCl/0.0355 + GS/0.016)
  return(invisible(TRUE))
}
```

1.2.4 Empirical methane production

```
calcMethane <- function()
{
  CH4 <- vector()
  # Empirical predictions of methane production
  # 55.65 MJ/kg
  # 13.3 Mcal/kg
  # 890 kJ/mol
  # 16 g/mol
  # 0.6556 g/L (kg/m^3) at 25 oC and 1 atm
  # 0.716 g/L (kg/m^3) at 0 oC and 1 atm
  MJ_PER_Mcal<-4.1868
  kg_PER_MJ<-1/55.65
  kg_PER_Mcal<-kg_PER_MJ*MJ_PER_Mcal
  L_PER_MJ<-1000*kg_PER_MJ/0.6556 # 25 oC and 1 atm
  L_PER_Mcal<-1000*kg_PER_Mcal/0.6565
  kg_PER_L<-0.6556/1000
  g_PER_L<-0.6556
  if (anim.diet.Forage.frac > 0.2)
  {
    # IPCC (2006)
    CH4 <- c(CH4, anim.diet.GE.rate*0.065*MJ_PER_Mcal*kg_PER_MJ*1000)
    if (anim.diet.Forage.frac > 0.4)
    {
      # Mills et al. (2003)
      CH4 <- c(CH4, 45.98*(1-exp(-0.003*(anim.diet.ME.rate*MJ_PER_Mcal)))*L_PER_MJ*g_PER_L)
      if (SolutionLevel == 2)
      {
        # Ellis et al. (2009), Eq. G
        CH4 <- c(CH4, (-1.01+2.76*anim.diet.NDF.rate+0.722*anim.diet.CHOB1.rate)*L_PER_MJ*g_PER_L)
        # Ellis et al. (2009), Eq. N
        CH4 <- c(CH4, (2.68-1.14*(anim.diet.CHOB1.rate/anim.diet.NDF.rate)+0.786*anim.diet.DMI.rate)*L_PER_MJ*g_PER_L)
      }
      # Escobar-Bahamondes and Beauchemin (2017)
      CH4 <- c(CH4, 71.5+0.12*anim.FBW+0.1*anim.diet.DMI.rate^3-244.8*anim.diet.EE.rate^3)
      # Moraes et al. (2014)
      if (anim.sex=="Female")
      {
        CH4 <- c(CH4, (-1.487+0.046*anim.diet.GE.rate*MJ_PER_Mcal+0.032*(anim.diet.NDF.rate*100/anim.diet.DMI.rate)+0.006*anim.SBW)*L_PER_MJ*g_PER_L)
        CH4 <- c(CH4, (-0.163+0.051*anim.diet.GE.rate*MJ_PER_Mcal+0.038*(anim.diet.NDF.rate*100/anim.diet.DMI.rate))*L_PER_MJ*g_PER_L)
      } else
      {
        CH4 <- c(CH4, (-0.221+0.048*anim.diet.GE.rate*MJ_PER_Mcal+0.005*anim.SBW)*L_PER_MJ*g_PER_L)
        CH4 <- c(CH4, (0.743+0.054*anim.diet.GE.rate*MJ_PER_Mcal)*L_PER_MJ*g_PER_L)
      }
    } else
    {
```

```
        # Ellis et al. (2007), Eq. 12b
        CH4 <- c(CH4, (2.70+1.16*anim.diet.DMI.rate-15.8*anim.diet.EE.rate)*L_PER_MJ*g_PER_L)
        if (SolutionLevel == 2)
        {
          # Escobar-Bahamondes and Beauchemin (unpublished)
          CH4 <- c(CH4, 30.7+0.165*anim.FBW+0.18*anim.diet.DMI.rate^2+0.05*anim.diet.DMI.rate^3-
157*anim.diet.EE.rate^3+6.5*anim.diet.CP.rate/anim.diet.NDF.rate-2.45*anim.diet.CHOB1.rate/anim.diet.NDF.rate)
        }
      }
    } else
    {
      # IPCC (2006)
      CH4 <- c(CH4, anim.diet.GE.rate*0.03*MJ_PER_Mcal*kg_PER_MJ*1000)
      # Ellis et al. (2007), Eq. 9b
      CH4 <- c(CH4, (0.357+0.0591*(anim.diet.ME.rate*MJ_PER_Mcal)+0.0500*(anim.diet.Forage.frac*100))*L_PER_MJ*g_PER_L)
      # Ellis et al. (2007), Eq. 10b
      CH4 <- c(CH4, (-1.02+0.681*anim.diet.DMI.rate+0.0481*(anim.diet.Forage.frac*100))*L_PER_MJ*g_PER_L)
      if (SolutionLevel ==2 )
      {
        # Ellis et al. (2009), Eq. G
        CH4 <- c(CH4, (-1.01+2.76*anim.diet.NDF.rate+0.722*anim.diet.CHOB1.rate)*L_PER_MJ*g_PER_L)
        # Escobar-Bahamondes and Beauchemin (unpublished)
        CH4 <- c(CH4, -10.1+0.21*anim.FBW+0.36*anim.diet.DMI.rate^2-
69.2*anim.diet.EE.rate^3+13*anim.diet.CP.rate/anim.diet.NDF.rate-4.9*anim.diet.CHOB1.rate/anim.diet.NDF.rate)
      }
    }
    # g -> kg
    CH4<-CH4/1000
    rum.diet.methane.rate <<- rum.diet.methane.rate_mean <<- mean(CH4)
    rum.diet.methane.rate_median <<- median(CH4)
    rum.diet.methane.rate_SD <<- sd(CH4)
    return(invisible(TRUE))
  }
```

1.2.5 Empirical dry matter intake

```
calcDMI <- function()
{
  # Dry matter intake
  NEma <- anim.diet.NEm.frac
  if (anim.species == "Cattle")
  {
    # Coleman et al. (2014), grazing animals Dry cows
    anim.OMI.rate_Coleman <<- 12.5 - 0.0299 * anim.FBW + 2e-05 * anim.FBW^2 - 0.05531 * anim.diet.aOMD.conc + 0.00032 * anim.FBW * anim.diet.aOMD.conc
    if (anim.stage_type == "Growing/Finishing" | anim.stage_type == "Replacement")
      anim.OMI.rate_Coleman <<- 4.56 + 0.0053 * anim.FBW - 2e-05 * anim.FBW^2 - 0.05531 * anim.diet.aOMD.conc + 0.00032 * anim.FBW * anim.diet.aOMD.conc
    if (anim.stage_type == "Lactating")
      anim.OMI.rate_Coleman <<- 27.9 - 0.0902 * anim.FBW + 9e-05 * anim.FBW^2 - 0.05531 * anim.diet.aOMD.conc + 0.00032 * anim.FBW * anim.diet.aOMD.conc
    if (anim.diet.OMI.rate != 0 & anim.diet.DMI.rate != 0)
      anim.DMI.rate_Coleman <<- anim.OMI.rate_Coleman/(anim.diet.OMI.rate/anim.diet.DMI.rate)
    # Temperature effect on DMI
    anim.DMI.temperature.factor <<- calcDMItf(env.CETI, env.temp_night)
    # Mud effect on DMI
    anim.DMI.mud.factor <<- 1 - 0.01 * env.mud.depth
    # Breed effect on DMI
    anim.DMI.breed.factor <<- 1
    if (anim.stage_type == "Growing/Finishing")
    {
      if (anim.breeding == "Straightbred" & anim.breed == "Holstein")
        anim.DMI.breed.factor <<- 1.08
      if (anim.breeding == "2-way" & (anim.breed.dam == "Holstein" | anim.breed.sire == "Holstein"))
        anim.DMI.breed.factor <<- 1.04
    }
    # Body fat effect on DMI
    anim.DMI.bf.factor <<- 1
    if (anim.stage_type == "Growing/Finishing" & anim.EqSBW >= 350)
      anim.DMI.bf.factor <<- 0.7714 + 0.00196 * anim.EqSBW - 3.71e-06 * anim.EqSBW^2
    # Feed additives effect on DMI
    anim.DMI.additives.factor <<- 1
    if (anim.diet.ionophore == TRUE & anim.diet.Forage.frac > 0.1)
      anim.DMI.additives.factor <<- 0.97
    # Pregnancy factor for replacement heifers
    anim.DMI.pregnancy.factor <<- 1
    # Dairy cattle, lactating cows
    if (anim.type == "Milk" & anim.stage_type == "Lactating")
    {
      MY <- anim.lactation.milk.rate  # Milk yield
      MkFat <- anim.lactation.milk.fat.conc  # Milk fat %
      FCM <- anim.lactation.FCM.rate <<- 0.4 * MY + 0.15 * MkFat * MY
      WOL <- anim.lactation.days/7
      PKMK <- 2
```

```
        P <- 3.67
        anim.DMI.rate_Roseler1997 <<- (0.0185 * anim.FBW + 0.305 * FCM) * anim.DMI.temperature.factor * anim.DMI.mud.factor * anim.DMI.additives.factor * ifelse(WOL > 16, 1, 1 - exp(-(0.564 - 0.124 * PKMK) * (WOL + P)))
        anim.DMI.rate_NRC2001 <<- (0.372 * FCM + 0.0968 * anim.FBW^0.75) * (1 - exp(-0.192 * (WOL + 3.67)))
        anim.DMI.rate_Souza2014 <<- (0.4762 * FCM + 0.07219 * anim.FBW^0.75) * (1 - exp(-0.03202 * (WOL * 7 + 24.9576)))
        anim.DMI.rate_min <<- min(c(anim.DMI.rate_Roseler1997, anim.DMI.rate_NRC2001, anim.DMI.rate_Souza2014),na.rm=TRUE)
        anim.DMI.rate_max <<- max(c(anim.DMI.rate_Roseler1997, anim.DMI.rate_NRC2001, anim.DMI.rate_Souza2014),na.rm=TRUE)
        anim.DMI.rate_avg <<- mean(c(anim.DMI.rate_Roseler1997, anim.DMI.rate_NRC2001, anim.DMI.rate_Souza2014),na.rm=TRUE)
      }
      # Dairy cattle, dry cows
      if (anim.type == "Milk" & anim.stage_type == "Dry")
      {
        anim.DMI.rate_Milligan1981 <<- ifelse(anim.pregnancy.days >= 260, 0.016, 0.02) * anim.FBW * anim.DMI.temperature.factor * anim.DMI.mud.factor * anim.DMI.additives.factor
        anim.DMI.rate_NRC2001 <<- (anim.FBW/100) * (1.97 - 0.75 * exp(0.16 * (anim.pregnancy.days - 280)))
        anim.DMI.rate_min <<- min(c(anim.DMI.rate_Milligan1981, anim.DMI.rate_NRC2001),na.rm=TRUE)
        anim.DMI.rate_max <<- max(c(anim.DMI.rate_Milligan1981, anim.DMI.rate_NRC2001),na.rm=TRUE)
        anim.DMI.rate_avg <<- mean(c(anim.DMI.rate_Milligan1981, anim.DMI.rate_NRC2001),na.rm=TRUE)
      }
      # Dairy cattle, replacement heifers
      if (anim.type == "Milk" & anim.stage_type == "Replacement")
      {
        if (anim.pregnancy.days > 210)
          anim.DMI.pregnancy.factor <<- 1 + (210 - anim.pregnancy.days) * 0.0025
        anim.DMI.rate_Quigley1986 <<- -29.864 + 0.1575 * anim.FBW^0.75 - 1.5425e-05 * anim.FBW^2 + anim.diet.aTDN.conc * (0.7296 - 0.0048178 * anim.diet.aTDN.conc) + anim.SWG * (2.0895 - 0.1177 * anim.SWG - 0.001363 * anim.FBW - 0.01908 * anim.diet.aTDN.conc)
        if (anim.age <= 12)
        {
          anim.DMI.rate_NRC2001 <<- anim.FBW^0.75 * (0.2435 * NEma - 0.0466 * NEma^2 - 0.1128) * anim.DMI.temperature.factor * anim.DMI.mud.factor * anim.DMI.pregnancy.factor/ifelse(NEma >= 1, NEma, 0.95)
        } else
        {
          anim.DMI.rate_NRC2001 <<- anim.FBW^0.75 * (0.2435 * NEma - 0.0466 * NEma^2 - 0.0869) * anim.DMI.temperature.factor * anim.DMI.mud.factor * anim.DMI.pregnancy.factor/ifelse(NEma >= 1, NEma, 0.95)
        }
        NDF <- isz(anim.diet.NDF.rate * 100, anim.diet.DMI.rate)
        if (anim.breeding == "Straightbred" & anim.breed == "Holstein")
        {
          anim.DMI.rate_Hoffman2008 <<- 15.79 * (1 - exp(-2.1 * anim.FBW/1000)) - (8.2/100) * (NDF - 22.07 - 87.14 * anim.FBW/1000 + 7.383 * anim.FBW^2/1e+05)
        } else
        {
          anim.DMI.rate_Hoffman2008 <<- 13.48 * (1 - exp(-2.71 * anim.FBW/1000)) - (8.24/100) * (NDF - 23.11 - 79.68 * anim.FBW/1000 + 6.252 * anim.FBW^2/1e+05)
        }
        anim.DMI.rate_OliveiraFerreira2016 <<- 0.1175 * anim.FBW^0.75 - 3.4984 * exp(-2.469 * anim.SWG)
        anim.DMI.rate_min <<- min(c(anim.DMI.rate_Quigley1986, anim.DMI.rate_NRC2001, anim.DMI.rate_Hoffman2008, anim.DMI.rate_OliveiraFerreira2016),na.rm=TRUE)
        anim.DMI.rate_max <<- max(c(anim.DMI.rate_Quigley1986, anim.DMI.rate_NRC2001, anim.DMI.rate_Hoffman2008, anim.DMI.rate_OliveiraFerreira2016),na.rm=TRUE)
```

```
    anim.DMI.rate_avg <<- mean(c(anim.DMI.rate_Quigley1986, anim.DMI.rate_NRC2001, anim.DMI.rate_Hoffman2008, anim.DMI.rate_OliveiraFerreira2016),na.rm=TRUE)
  }
  # Beef, dairy, or dual-purpose cattle, feedlot
  if (anim.stage_type == "Growing/Finishing")
  {
    if (anim.age <= 12)
    {
      anim.DMI.rate_NRC2000 <<- anim.FBW^0.75 * (0.2435 * NEma - 0.0466 * NEma^2 - 0.1128) * anim.DMI.temperature.factor * anim.DMI.mud.factor * anim.DMI.breed.factor * anim.DMI.bf.factor * anim.DMI.additives.factor/ifelse(NEma >= 1, NEma, 0.95)
    } else
    {
      anim.DMI.rate_NRC2000 <<- anim.FBW^0.75 * (0.2435 * NEma - 0.0466 * NEma^2 - 0.0869) * anim.DMI.temperature.factor * anim.DMI.mud.factor * anim.DMI.breed.factor * anim.DMI.bf.factor * anim.DMI.additives.factor/ifelse(NEma >= 1, NEma, 0.95)
    }
    anim.DMI.rate_NASEM2016 <<- (anim.FBW/100) * (1.2425 + 1.9218 * NEma - 0.7259 * NEma^2) * anim.DMI.temperature.factor * anim.DMI.mud.factor * anim.DMI.breed.factor * anim.DMI.bf.factor * anim.DMI.additives.factor
    if (anim.breed == "Nellore")
    {
      anim.DMI.rate_Azevedo2010 <<- -2.6098 + 0.08844 * anim.FBW^0.75 + 4.4672 * anim.SWG - 1.3579 * anim.SWG^2
    } else
    {
      anim.DMI.rate_Azevedo2010 <<- -2.7878 + 0.08789 * anim.FBW^0.75 + 5.0487 * anim.SWG - 1.6835 * anim.SWG^2
    }
    anim.DMI.rate_min <<- min(c(anim.DMI.rate_Coleman, anim.DMI.rate_NRC2000, anim.DMI.rate_NASEM2016, anim.DMI.rate_Azevedo2010),na.rm=TRUE)
    anim.DMI.rate_max <<- max(c(anim.DMI.rate_Coleman, anim.DMI.rate_NRC2000, anim.DMI.rate_NASEM2016, anim.DMI.rate_Azevedo2010),na.rm=TRUE)
    anim.DMI.rate_avg <<- mean(c(anim.DMI.rate_Coleman, anim.DMI.rate_NRC2000, anim.DMI.rate_NASEM2016, anim.DMI.rate_Azevedo2010),na.rm=TRUE)
  }
  # Beef or dual-purpose cattle, lactating
  if ((anim.type == "Meat/Beef" | anim.type == "Dual-purpose") & anim.stage_type == "Lactating")
  {
    MY <- anim.lactation.milk.rate
    MkFat <- anim.lactation.milk.peak.fat.conc
    FCM <- 0.4 * MY + 0.15 * MkFat * MY
    if (anim.pregnancy.days <= 93)
    {
      anim.DMI.rate_NRC2000 <<- anim.SBW^0.75 * (0.04997 * NEma^2 + 0.0384) * anim.DMI.temperature.factor * anim.DMI.mud.factor/ifelse(NEma >= 1, NEma, 0.95) + 0.2 * MY
    } else
    {
      anim.DMI.rate_NRC2000 <<- anim.SBW^0.75 * (0.04997 * NEma^2 + 0.04631) * anim.DMI.temperature.factor * anim.DMI.mud.factor/ifelse(NEma >= 1, NEma, 0.95) + 0.2 * MY
    }
    if (anim.type == "Meat/Beef")
      anim.DMI.rate_Traxler1997 <<- anim.FBW^0.75 * (0.1462 * NEma - 0.0517 * NEma^2 - 0.0074) + 0.305 * FCM + ifelse(MY >= 15, 1.7, 0)
    anim.DMI.rate_Lardy2004 <<- anim.FBW * 0.024
    anim.DMI.rate_min <<- min(c(anim.DMI.rate_Coleman, anim.DMI.rate_NRC2000, anim.DMI.rate_Lardy2004),na.rm=TRUE)
```

```
        anim.DMI.rate_max <<- max(c(anim.DMI.rate_Coleman, anim.DMI.rate_NRC2000, anim.DMI.rate_Lardy2004),na.rm=TRUE)
        anim.DMI.rate_avg <<- mean(c(anim.DMI.rate_Coleman, anim.DMI.rate_NRC2000, anim.DMI.rate_Lardy2004),na.rm=TRUE)
      }
      # Beef or dual-purpose cattle, dry
      if ((anim.type == "Meat/Beef" | anim.type == "Dual-purpose") & anim.stage_type == "Dry")
      {
        anim.DMI.rate_NRC2000 <<- anim.SBW^0.75 * (0.04997 * NEma^2 + 0.04631) * anim.DMI.temperature.factor *
anim.DMI.mud.factor/ifelse(NEma >= 1, NEma, 0.95)
        anim.DMI.rate_Lardy2004 <<- anim.FBW * 0.019
        anim.DMI.rate_NASEM2016 <<- ifelse(anim.diet.NDF.rate != 0 & anim.diet.DMI.rate != 0, anim.FBW *
0.012/(anim.diet.NDF.rate/anim.diet.DMI.rate), 0)
        anim.DMI.rate_min <<- min(c(anim.DMI.rate_Coleman, anim.DMI.rate_NRC2000, anim.DMI.rate_Lardy2004),na.rm=TRUE)
        anim.DMI.rate_max <<- max(c(anim.DMI.rate_Coleman, anim.DMI.rate_NRC2000, anim.DMI.rate_Lardy2004),na.rm=TRUE)
        anim.DMI.rate_avg <<- mean(c(anim.DMI.rate_Coleman, anim.DMI.rate_NRC2000, anim.DMI.rate_Lardy2004),na.rm=TRUE)
      }
      # Beef or dual-purpose cattle, replacement heifers
      if ((anim.type == "Meat/Beef" | anim.type == "Dual-purpose") & anim.stage_type == "Replacement")
      {
        if (anim.age <= 12)
        {
          anim.DMI.rate_NRC2000 <<- anim.FBW^0.75 * (0.2435 * NEma - 0.0466 * NEma^2 - 0.1128) * anim.DMI.temperature.factor *
anim.DMI.mud.factor * anim.DMI.additives.factor/ifelse(NEma >= 1, NEma, 0.95)
        } else
        {
          anim.DMI.rate_NRC2000 <<- anim.FBW^0.75 * (0.2435 * NEma - 0.0466 * NEma^2 - 0.0869) * anim.DMI.temperature.factor *
anim.DMI.mud.factor * anim.DMI.additives.factor/ifelse(NEma >= 1, NEma, 0.95)
        }
        anim.DMI.rate_min <<- min(c(anim.DMI.rate_Coleman, anim.DMI.rate_NRC2000),na.rm=TRUE)
        anim.DMI.rate_max <<- max(c(anim.DMI.rate_Coleman, anim.DMI.rate_NRC2000),na.rm=TRUE)
        anim.DMI.rate_avg <<- mean(c(anim.DMI.rate_Coleman, anim.DMI.rate_NRC2000),na.rm=TRUE)
      }
    } else
    {
      if (anim.species == "Sheep")
      {
        # Sheep
        k <- 1
        if (anim.pregnancy.days > 0)
        {
          # Assuming that gestation length is 150 days
          t<-anim.pregnancy.days - 150
          # Pulina et al. (1996) and Cannas et al. (2004)
          if (anim.pregnancy.lamb.body.weight_birth <= 4)
          {
            if (t/7 >= -6)
              k <- 0.96
            if (t/7 >= -4 & t/7 < -2)
              k <- 0.90
            if (t/7 >= -2)
              k <- 0.82
          } else
```

```
      {
        if (t/7 >= -6)
          k <- 0.97
        if (t/7 >= -4 & t/7 < -2)
          k <- 0.93
        if (t/7 >= -2)
          k <- 0.88
      }
      # Continuous adjustment
      k <- calcDMIk(t,anim.pregnancy.lamb.body.weight_birth)
      #x1 <- -50:0
      #y1 <- 1
      #for (i in x1[2]:x1[length(x1)]) y1 <- c(y1,calcDMIk(i,3))
      #plot(x1,y1)
    }
    if (anim.stage_type == "Lactating")
    {
      #Meat-type sheep
      t <- anim.lactation.days
      cc <- 28
      ca <- 0.66
      if (anim.pregnancy.lamb.body.weight_birth>4)
        ca <- 0.88
      if (t <= cc)
      {
        if (t == 0)
        {
          k <- 1/(1+ca)
        } else
        {
          k <- (1 + ca*((t/cc)^1.4)*exp(1.4*(1-t/cc)))/(1 + ca)
        }
      } else k <- 1
      #x2 <- 0:50
      #y2 <- ifelse(x2<cc,(1 + ca*((x2/cc)^1.4)*exp(1.4*(1-x2/cc)))/(1 + ca),1)
      #plot(c(x1,x2),c(y1,y2),type="b")
      MY <- anim.lactation.milk.rate
      MkFat <- anim.lactation.milk.fat.conc
      FCM <- 0.3688 * MY + 0.0971 * MkFat * MY
      SWG <- ifelse(anim.EB.SWG.rate < 0, 0, anim.EB.SWG.rate)
      anim.DMI.rate_Pulina1996 <<- (-0.545 + 0.095 * anim.FBW^0.75 + 0.65 * FCM + 0.0025 * SWG) * k
    } else
    {
      SWG <- anim.SWG
      if (anim.stage_type == "Dry")
      {
        anim.DMI.rate_Pulina1996 <<- (-0.545 + 0.095 * anim.FBW^0.75 + 0.005 * SWG) * k
      } else
      {
        if (anim.sex == "Male" | (anim.sex == "Castrated male" & anim.age > 12))
        {
```

```
            # Ram or sheep wether (> 12 mo old)
            anim.DMI.rate_Pulina1996 <<- 0.065 * anim.FBW^0.75
          } else
          {
            # Male lamb or female lamb (< 12 mo old)
            anim.DMI.rate_Pulina1996 <<- -0.124 + 0.0711 * anim.FBW^0.75 + 0.0015 * SWG
          }
        }
      }
    } else
    {
      # Goats
      ME <- anim.diet.ME.rate
      GE <- anim.diet.GE.rate
      if (anim.stage_type == "Lactating")
      {
        MY <- anim.lactation.milk.rate
        FOR <- anim.diet.Forage.frac
        SWG <- ifelse(anim.EB.SWG.rate < 0, 0, anim.EB.SWG.rate)
        anim.DMI.rate_Pulina1996 <<- 0.42 * MY + 0.024 * anim.FBW^0.75 + 0.4 * SWG + 0.7 * FOR
      } else
      {
        if (anim.stage_type == "Dry")
        {
          anim.DMI.rate_Pulina1996 <<- (130.9 * ME/GE + 0.384 * anim.FBW - 18.75) * anim.FBW^0.75/1000
        } else
        {
          if (anim.sex == "Male" | (anim.sex == "Castrated male" & anim.age > 12))
          {
            # Billy or goat wether (> 12 mo old)
            anim.DMI.rate_Pulina1996 <<- 0.522 + 0.0135 * anim.FBW
          } else
          {
            # Male kid or female kid (< 12 mo old)
            anim.DMI.rate_Pulina1996 <<- (104.7 * ME/GE + 0.307 * anim.FBW - 15) * anim.FBW^0.75/1000
          }
        }
      }
    }
    anim.DMI.rate_min <<- min(c(anim.DMI.rate_Pulina1996),na.rm=TRUE)
    anim.DMI.rate_max <<- max(c(anim.DMI.rate_Pulina1996),na.rm=TRUE)
    anim.DMI.rate_avg <<- mean(c(anim.DMI.rate_Pulina1996),na.rm=TRUE)
  }
  return(invisible(TRUE))
}
```

1.2.6 Empirical water intake

```
calcWI <- function()
{
  anim.WI.rate <<- 0
  if (anim.species == "Cattle")
  {
    if (anim.type == "Milk")
    {
      if (anim.stage_type == "Lactating")
      {
        MY <- anim.lactation.milk.rate # kg/d
        DMI <- anim.diet.DMI.rate # kg/d
        LNT <- env.temp_night # oC
        NaI <- anim.diet.Na.rate * 1000 # g/d
        anim.WI.rate <<- 15.99 + 1.58 * DMI + 0.9 * MY + 0.05 * NaI + 1.2 * LNT # L/d
      } else
      {
        # Mainly for dry cows, but used for all other class of animals in the RNS
        DMI <- anim.diet.DMI.rate # kg/d
        DM <- anim.diet.DM.conc # % DM
        CP <- anim.diet.CP.conc # % CP
        anim.WI.rate <<- -10.34 + 0.2296 * DM + 2.212 * DMI + 0.03944 * CP # L/d
      }
    } else
    {
      # Beef cattle
      if (anim.body.weight.gain_shrunk < 0.9)
      {
        # used for all classes of animals in the RNS other than finishing
        anim.WI.rate <<- 7.3 + 0.0805 * anim.SBW - 8e-05 * anim.SBW^2 - 1.225 * env.CETI + 0.0411 * env.CETI^2 + 0.0023268 *
anim.SBW * env.CETI
      } else
      {
        # used for finishing cattle with SWG > 0.9 kg/d
        anim.WI.rate <<- 6.336 + 0.1057 * anim.SBW - 9.63e-05 * anim.SBW^2 - 1.6 * env.CETI + 0.056 * env.CETI^2 + 0.00226 *
anim.SBW * env.CETI
      }
    }
  } else
  {
    if (anim.species == "Sheep")
    {
      # CSIRO (2007) uses maximum temperature, not CETI
      anim.WI.rate <<- 0.429 + 0.073 * env.CETI - 0.013 * env.rain.rate
    } else
    {
      # Goats, confined animals
      anim.WI.rate <<- (0.159/1000) * (anim.FBW * 1000)^0.946
    }
```

```
  }
  return(invisible(TRUE))
}
```

2 Level of Solution 0

2.1 Flowchart of the calculation logic

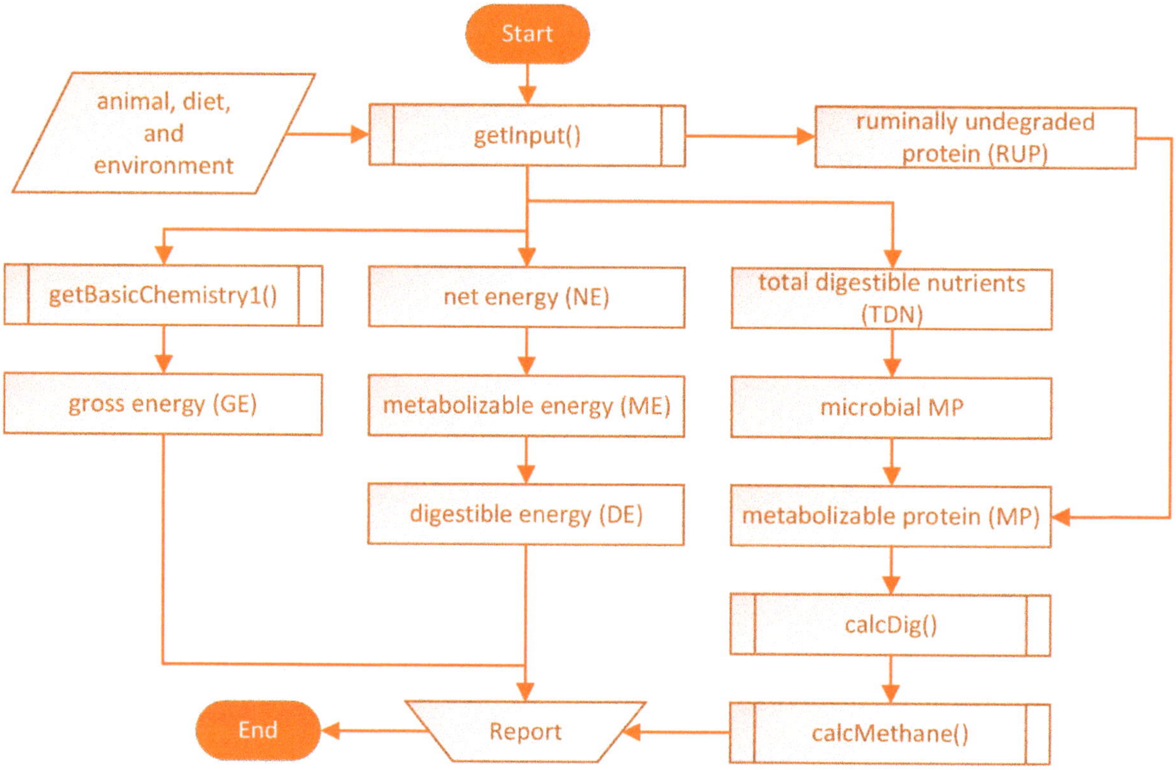

Figure 1.1. Flowchart of the calculation logic for the level of solution 0. The steps in the calcSolutionLevel0() function includes the energy and protein calculations as well as calcDig() and calcMethane() functions.

2.2 Equations

2.2.1 Total digestible nutrients, metabolizable energy and protein, and net energy: calcSolution-Level0()

#	Variable[1]	Description	Equation
1:	GE_f		$9.4 * EE_f + 5.65 * CP_f + 4.1 * (NFC_f + FC_f)$
2:	$tTDN_f$		$aTDN_f + 7.32$
3:	$[MEm]_f$		$findroots(1.37 * [MEm]_f - 0.138 * [MEm]_f^2 + 0.0105 * [MEm]_f^3 - 1.12 - [NEm]_f = 0)$

4:	*[MEg]$_f$*		$findroots(1.42 * [MEg]_f - 0.174 * [MEg]_f^2 + 0.0122 * [MEg]_f^3 - 1.65 - [NEg]_f = 0)$
5:	*[MEl]$_f$*		$findroots(0.644 * [MEl]_f - [NEl]_f = 0)$
6:	*[DEm]$_f$*	lactating or dry dairy	$\frac{[MEm]_f + 0.45}{1.01}$
7:		otherwise	$\frac{[MEm]_f}{0.82}$
8:	*[DEg]$_f$*	lactating or dry dairy	$\frac{[MEg]_f + 0.45}{1.01}$
9:		otherwise	$\frac{[MEg]_f}{0.82}$
10:	*[DEl]$_f$*	lactating or dry dairy	$\frac{[MEl]_f + 0.45}{1.01}$
11:		otherwise	$\frac{[MEl]_f}{0.82}$
12:	*BactCP$_f$*		$0.13 * aTDN_f$
13:	*Bact$_f$*		$\frac{BactCP_f}{0.625}$
14:	*BactMP$_f$*		$0.8 * 0.8 * BactCP_f$
15:	*MP$_f$*		$RUPID_f * RUP_f * DMI_f + BactMP_f$
16:	*k_m*		$\frac{\sum_{f=1}^{nf}(DMI_f * [NEm]_f)}{\sum_{f=1}^{nf}(DMI_f * [MEm]_f)}$
17:	*k_g*		$\frac{\sum_{f=1}^{nf}(DMI_f * [NEg]_f)}{\sum_{f=1}^{nf}(DMI_f * [MEm]_f)}$
18:	*k_l*		$\frac{\sum_{f=1}^{nf}(DMI_f * [NEl]_f)}{\sum_{f=1}^{nf}(DMI_f * [MEm]_f)}$

(1) ***aTDN*** is apparent total digestible nutrients, % DM; ***Bact*** is bacteria mass, kg/d; ***BactCP*** is bacteria crude protein, kg/d; ***BactMP*** is bacteria metabolizable protein, kg/d; ***CP*** is crude protein, kg/d; ***[DEg]*** is dietary content of digestible energy for growth, Mcal/kg; ***DEl*** is digestible energy for lactation, Mcal/kg; ***[DEm]*** is dietary content of digestible energy for maintenance, Mcal/kg; ***DMI*** is dry matter intake, kg/d; ***EE*** is ether extract, kg/d; ***f*** is the jth feed; ***FC*** is fiber carbohydrate, kg/d; ***GE*** is gross energy, Mcal/d; ***k_g*** is the partial efficiency of utilization of metabolizable energy for net energy for growth, dimensionless; ***k_l*** is the partial efficiency of utilization of metabolizable energy for net energy for lactation, dimensionless; ***k_m*** is the partial efficiency of utilization of metabolizable energy for net energy for maintenance, dimensionless; ***[MEg]*** is dietary content of metabolizable energy for growth, Mcal/kg; ***[MEl]*** is metabolizable energy for lactation, Mcal/kg; ***[MEm]*** is dietary content of metabolizable energy for maintenance, Mcal/kg; ***MP*** is metabolizable protein, kg/d; ***[NEg]*** is dietary content of net energy for growth (also called ***NEga***), Mcal/kg; ***[NEl]*** is dietary content of net energy for lactation (also called ***NEla***), Mcal/kg; ***[NEm]*** is dietary content of net energy for maintenance (also called ***NEma***), Mcal/kg; ***nf*** is the number of feeds; ***NFC*** is nonfiber carbohydrate, kg/d; ***RUP*** is ruminally degradable protein, kg/d; ***RUPID*** is ruminally degradable protein intestinal digestibility, %; and ***tTDN*** is true total digestible nutrients, % DM.

2.3 Code

2.3.1 Total digestible nutrients, metabolizable energy and protein, and net energy

```
calcSolutionLevel0 <- function(fds = feeds3, genRPT = TRUE)
{
  # SolutionLevel 0 is computed backwards: NE -> ME -> DE
  # Ration NE are weighted averages rather than from ration ME TDN is computed using the user-inputted values
  # There is a 'disconnection' between TDN and NE, ME, and DE Ionophores effect on NEm is not included
  # ++++++++++++++
  # Gross Energy
  # ++++++++++++++
  # Atwater factors
  anim.fd.GE.rate <<- anim.fd.EE.rate * 9.4 + anim.fd.CP.rate * 5.65 + (anim.fd.NFC.rate + anim.fd.FC.rate) * 4.1
  anim.fd.GE.frac <<- isz(anim.fd.GE.rate, anim.fd.DMI.rate)
  anim.diet.GE.rate <<- sum(anim.fd.GE.rate)
  anim.diet.GE.frac <<- isz(anim.diet.GE.rate, anim.diet.DMI.rate)
  # ++++++++++++++++++++++++++++
  # Total Digestible Nutrients
  # ++++++++++++++++++++++++++++
  # Apparent TDN
  anim.fd.aTDN.conc <<- as.numeric(feeds3[, "TDN_1x"])
  anim.fd.aTDN.rate <<- (anim.fd.aTDN.conc/100) * anim.fd.DMI.rate
  anim.diet.aTDN.rate <<- sum(anim.fd.aTDN.rate)
  anim.diet.aTDN.conc <<- isz(anim.diet.aTDN.rate * 100, anim.diet.DMI.rate)
  # True TDN
  # Assuming a fixed 7.32% as metabolic fecal TDN (Tedeschi and Fox, 2018; p. 62)
  anim.fd.tTDN.conc <<- anim.fd.aTDN.conc + 7.32
  anim.fd.tTDN.rate <<- (anim.fd.tTDN.conc/100) * anim.fd.DMI.rate
  anim.diet.tTDN.rate <<- sum(anim.fd.tTDN.rate)
  anim.diet.tTDN.conc <<- isz(anim.diet.tTDN.rate * 100, anim.diet.DMI.rate)
  # ++++++++++++
  # Net Energy
  # ++++++++++++
  # Feeds
  if (anim.species == "Cattle")
  {
    if (anim.type == "Milk")
    {
      # Dairy cattle
      anim.fd.NEm.frac <<- as.numeric(feeds3[, "NEm_Dairy"])
      anim.fd.NEg.frac <<- as.numeric(feeds3[, "NEg_Dairy"])
      anim.fd.NEl.frac <<- as.numeric(feeds3[, "NEl_Dairy"])
    } else
    {
      # Beef cattle
      anim.fd.NEm.frac <<- as.numeric(feeds3[, "NEm_Beef"])
```

```
        anim.fd.NEg.frac <<- as.numeric(feeds3[, "NEg_Beef"])
        anim.fd.NEl.frac <<- as.numeric(feeds3[, "NEl_Beef"])
      }
    }
    if (anim.species == "Sheep")
    {
      anim.fd.NEm.frac <<- as.numeric(feeds3[, "NEm_Sheep"])
      anim.fd.NEg.frac <<- as.numeric(feeds3[, "NEg_Sheep"])
      anim.fd.NEl.frac <<- as.numeric(feeds3[, "NEl_Sheep"])
    }
    if (anim.species == "Goats")
    {
      anim.fd.NEm.frac <<- as.numeric(feeds3[, "NEm_Goat"])
      anim.fd.NEg.frac <<- as.numeric(feeds3[, "NEg_Goat"])
      anim.fd.NEl.frac <<- as.numeric(feeds3[, "NEl_Goat"])
    }
    anim.fd.NEm.rate <<- anim.fd.NEm.frac * anim.fd.DMI.rate
    anim.fd.NEg.rate <<- anim.fd.NEg.frac * anim.fd.DMI.rate
    anim.fd.NEl.rate <<- anim.fd.NEl.frac * anim.fd.DMI.rate
    # Ration NE values by weighted average
    anim.diet.NEm.rate <<- sum(anim.fd.NEm.rate)
    anim.diet.NEg.rate <<- sum(anim.fd.NEg.rate)
    anim.diet.NEl.rate <<- sum(anim.fd.NEl.rate)
    anim.diet.NEm.frac <<- isz(anim.diet.NEm.rate, anim.diet.DMI.rate)
    anim.diet.NEg.frac <<- isz(anim.diet.NEg.rate, anim.diet.DMI.rate)
    anim.diet.NEl.frac <<- isz(anim.diet.NEl.rate, anim.diet.DMI.rate)
    # ++++++++++++++++++++++
    # Metabolizable Energy
    # ++++++++++++++++++++++
    getMEm <- function(NEm)
    {
      resp <- uniroot(function(MEm, NEm)
      {
        1.37 * MEm - 0.138 * MEm^2 + 0.0105 * MEm^3 - 1.12 - NEm
      }, c(0, 10), tol = 1e-04, NEm = NEm)
      return(resp$root)
    }
    getMEg <- function(NEg)
    {
      resp <- uniroot(function(MEg, NEg)
      {
        1.42 * MEg - 0.174 * MEg^2 + 0.0122 * MEG^3 - 1.65 - NEg
      }, c(0, 10), tol = 1e-04, NEg = NEg)
      return(resp$root)
    }
    getMEl <- function(NEl)
    {
      resp <- uniroot(function(MEl, NEl)
      {
        0.644 * MEl - NEl
      }, c(0, 10), tol = 1e-04, NEl = NEl)
```

```
      return(resp$root)
    }
    # Feeds
    anim.fd.MEm.frac <<- pmax(0, unlist(lapply(anim.fd.NEm.frac, getMEm)))   # Mcal/kg
    anim.fd.MEg.frac <<- pmax(0, unlist(lapply(anim.fd.NEg.frac, getMEg)))   # Mcal/kg
    anim.fd.MEl.frac <<- pmax(0, unlist(lapply(anim.fd.NEl.frac, getMEl)))   # Mcal/kg
    anim.fd.MEm.rate <<- anim.fd.MEm.frac * anim.fd.DMI.rate   # Mcal/d
    anim.fd.MEg.rate <<- anim.fd.MEg.frac * anim.fd.DMI.rate   # Mcal/d
    anim.fd.MEl.rate <<- anim.fd.MEl.frac * anim.fd.DMI.rate   # Mcal/d
    # Ration
    anim.diet.MEm.rate <<- sum(anim.fd.MEm.rate)   # Mcal/d
    anim.diet.MEg.rate <<- sum(anim.fd.MEg.rate)   # Mcal/d
    anim.diet.MEl.rate <<- sum(anim.fd.MEl.rate)   # Mcal/d
    anim.diet.MEm.frac <<- isz(anim.diet.MEm.rate, anim.diet.DMI.rate)   # Mcal/kg
    anim.diet.MEg.frac <<- isz(anim.diet.MEg.rate, anim.diet.DMI.rate)   # Mcal/kg
    anim.diet.MEl.frac <<- isz(anim.diet.MEl.rate, anim.diet.DMI.rate)   # Mcal/kg
    # Assuming that ME = MEm
    anim.fd.ME.frac <<- anim.fd.MEm.frac
    anim.fd.ME.rate <<- anim.fd.MEm.rate
    anim.diet.ME.frac <<- anim.diet.MEm.frac
    anim.diet.ME.rate <<- anim.diet.MEm.rate
    # +++++++++++++++++++
    # Digestible Energy
    # +++++++++++++++++++
    # Feeds
    if (anim.type == "Milk" & (anim.stage_type == "Lactating" | anim.stage_type == "Dry"))
    {
      # Dairy
      anim.fd.DEm.frac <<- (anim.fd.MEm.frac + 0.45)/1.01   # Mcal/kg
      anim.fd.DEg.frac <<- (anim.fd.MEg.frac + 0.45)/1.01   # Mcal/kg
      anim.fd.DEl.frac <<- (anim.fd.MEl.frac + 0.45)/1.01   # Mcal/kg
    } else
    {
      anim.fd.DEm.frac <<- anim.fd.MEm.frac/0.82   # Mcal/kg
      anim.fd.DEg.frac <<- anim.fd.MEg.frac/0.82   # Mcal/kg
      anim.fd.DEl.frac <<- anim.fd.MEl.frac/0.82   # Mcal/kg
    }
    anim.fd.DEm.rate <<- anim.fd.DEm.frac * anim.fd.DMI.rate   # Mcal/d
    anim.fd.DEg.rate <<- anim.fd.DEg.frac * anim.fd.DMI.rate   # Mcal/d
    anim.fd.DEl.rate <<- anim.fd.DEl.frac * anim.fd.DMI.rate   # Mcal/d
    # Ration
    anim.diet.DEm.rate <<- sum(anim.fd.DEm.rate)   # Mcal/d
    anim.diet.DEg.rate <<- sum(anim.fd.DEg.rate)   # Mcal/d
    anim.diet.DEl.rate <<- sum(anim.fd.DEl.rate)   # Mcal/d
    anim.diet.DEm.frac <<- isz(anim.diet.DEm.rate, anim.diet.DMI.rate)   # Mcal/kg
    anim.diet.DEg.frac <<- isz(anim.diet.DEg.rate, anim.diet.DMI.rate)   # Mcal/kg
    anim.diet.DEl.frac <<- isz(anim.diet.DEl.rate, anim.diet.DMI.rate)   # Mcal/kg
    # Assuming that DE = DEm
    anim.fd.DE.frac <<- anim.fd.DEm.frac
    anim.fd.DE.rate <<- anim.fd.DEm.rate
    anim.diet.DE.rate <<- anim.diet.DEm.rate
```

```
  anim.diet.DE.frac <<- anim.diet.DEm.frac
  if (genRPT)
  {
    rptBioValues <- feeds3["FeedName.x"]
    names(rptBioValues) <- "FeedName"
    rptBioValues["aTDN, kg/d"] <- anim.fd.aTDN.rate
    rptBioValues["aTDN, % DM"] <- anim.fd.aTDN.conc
    rptBioValues["NEm, Mcal/kg"] <- anim.fd.NEm.frac
    rptBioValues["NEg, Mcal/kg"] <- anim.fd.NEg.frac
    rptBioValues["NEl, Mcal/kg"] <- anim.fd.NEl.frac
    rptBioValues2 <- data.frame(FeedName = "Ration")
    rptBioValues2["aTDN, kg/d"] <- anim.diet.aTDN.rate
    rptBioValues2["aTDN, % DM"] <- anim.diet.aTDN.conc
    rptBioValues2["NEm, Mcal/kg"] <- anim.diet.NEm.frac
    rptBioValues2["NEg, Mcal/kg"] <- anim.diet.NEg.frac
    rptBioValues2["NEl, Mcal/kg"] <- anim.diet.NEl.frac
    rptBioValues <- rbind(rptBioValues, rptBioValues2)
    description <- paste("# a    = apparent\n", "# m    = maintenance\n", "# g    = growth\n", "# l    = lactation\n", "# TDN = total digestible nutrients\n", "# NE   = net energy\n", sep = "")
    footnote <- "Ration NE values are computed using weighted average"
    report(rptBioValues, "Total Digestible Nutrients and Net Energy (user inputted)", description, footnote, 3, 3, 1, 6, FALSE, FALSE, FALSE, FALSE, FALSE, FALSE, FALSE)
    rptBioValues <- feeds3["FeedName.x"]
    names(rptBioValues) <- "FeedName"
    rptBioValues["aTDN, kg/d"] <- anim.fd.DEm.rate/4.409
    rptBioValues["aTDN, % DM"] <- (anim.fd.DEm.frac/4.409) * 100
    rptBioValues2 <- data.frame(FeedName = "Ration")
    rptBioValues2["aTDN, kg/d"] <- anim.diet.DEm.rate/4.409
    rptBioValues2["aTDN, % DM"] <- (anim.diet.DEm.frac/4.409) * 100
    rptBioValues <- rbind(rptBioValues, rptBioValues2)
    description <- paste("# aTDN = apparent total digestible nutrients\n", sep = "")
    footnote <- ""
    report(rptBioValues, "\nTotal Digestible Nutrients (computed from DE for maintenance)", description, footnote, 3, 3, 1, 6, FALSE, FALSE, FALSE, FALSE, FALSE, FALSE, TRUE)
    rptBioValues <- feeds3["FeedName.x"]
    names(rptBioValues) <- "FeedName"
    rptBioValues["GE, Mcal/kg"] <- anim.fd.GE.frac
    rptBioValues["DEm, Mcal/kg"] <- anim.fd.DEm.frac
    rptBioValues["DEg, Mcal/kg"] <- anim.fd.DEg.frac
    rptBioValues["DEl, Mcal/kg"] <- anim.fd.DEl.frac
    rptBioValues["GE, Mcal/d"] <- anim.fd.GE.rate
    rptBioValues["DEm, Mcal/d"] <- anim.fd.DEm.rate
    rptBioValues["DEg, Mcal/d"] <- anim.fd.DEg.rate
    rptBioValues["DEl, Mcal/d"] <- anim.fd.DEl.rate
    rptBioValues2 <- data.frame(FeedName = "Ration")
    rptBioValues2["GE, Mcal/kg"] <- anim.diet.GE.frac
    rptBioValues2["DEm, Mcal/kg"] <- anim.diet.DEm.frac
    rptBioValues2["DEg, Mcal/kg"] <- anim.diet.DEg.frac
    rptBioValues2["DEl, Mcal/kg"] <- anim.diet.DEl.frac
    rptBioValues2["GE, Mcal/d"] <- anim.diet.GE.rate
    rptBioValues2["DEm, Mcal/d"] <- anim.diet.DEm.rate
```

```
    rptBioValues2["DEg, Mcal/d"] <- anim.diet.DEg.rate
    rptBioValues2["DEl, Mcal/d"] <- anim.diet.DEl.rate
    rptBioValues <- rbind(rptBioValues, rptBioValues2)
    description <- paste("# m   = maintenance\n", "# g   = growth\n", "# l   = lactation\n", "# GE  = gross energy\n", "# DE
  = digestible energy\n", sep = "")
    report(rptBioValues, "Digestible Energy", description, "", 3, 3, 1, 4, FALSE, FALSE, FALSE, FALSE, FALSE, FALSE, TRUE)
    rptBioValues <- feeds3["FeedName.x"]
    names(rptBioValues) <- "FeedName"
    rptBioValues["MEm, Mcal/kg"] <- anim.fd.MEm.frac
    rptBioValues["MEg, Mcal/kg"] <- anim.fd.MEg.frac
    rptBioValues["MEl, Mcal/kg"] <- anim.fd.MEl.frac
    rptBioValues["MEm, Mcal/d"] <- anim.fd.MEm.rate
    rptBioValues["MEg, Mcal/d"] <- anim.fd.MEg.rate
    rptBioValues["MEl, Mcal/d"] <- anim.fd.MEl.frac
    rptBioValues2 <- data.frame(FeedName = "Ration")
    rptBioValues2["MEm, Mcal/kg"] <- anim.diet.MEm.frac
    rptBioValues2["MEg, Mcal/kg"] <- anim.diet.MEg.frac
    rptBioValues2["MEl, Mcal/kg"] <- anim.diet.MEl.frac
    rptBioValues2["MEm, Mcal/d"] <- anim.diet.MEm.rate
    rptBioValues2["MEg, Mcal/d"] <- anim.diet.MEg.rate
    rptBioValues2["MEl, Mcal/d"] <- anim.diet.MEl.rate
    rptBioValues <- rbind(rptBioValues, rptBioValues2)
    description <- paste("# m   = maintenance\n", "# g   = growth\n", "# l   = lactation\n", "# ME  = metabolizable energy\n",
sep = "")
    report(rptBioValues, "Metabolizable Energy", description, "", 3, 3, 1, 6, FALSE, FALSE, FALSE, FALSE, FALSE, FALSE, FALSE)
  }
  # ++++++++++++++++++++++
  # Metabolizable Protein
  # ++++++++++++++++++++++
  # The RUP for solution level 0 is not discounted for level of dry matter intake above maintenance
  # Therefore RUPx = RUP1x (or UIPx = UIP1x) Ruminally undegradable protein (RUP aka UIP)
  rum.fd.RUCP.conc <<- as.numeric(feeds3[, "RUP_1x"])
  rum.fd.RUCP.rate <<- (rum.fd.RUCP.conc/100) * anim.fd.CP.rate
  rum.diet.RUCP.rate <<- sum(rum.fd.RUCP.rate)
  rum.diet.RUCP.conc <<- isz(rum.diet.RUCP.rate * 100, anim.diet.DMI.rate)
  # Ruminal bacteria protein
  rum.fd.bact.CP.rate <<- Parm_rum.bact.CPY_L1 * anim.fd.aTDN.rate
  rum.diet.bact.CP.rate <<- sum(rum.fd.bact.CP.rate)
  # Ruminal bacteria mass
  if (Parm_rum.bact.CP != 0) rum.fd.bact.rate <<- rum.fd.bact.CP.rate/(Parm_rum.bact.CP/100) else rum.fd.bact.rate <<- 0
  rum.diet.bact.rate <<- sum(rum.fd.bact.rate)
  rum.fd.RUPID.conc <<- as.numeric(feeds3[, "RUPID"]) * 100
  rum.fd.RUPID.frac <<- rum.fd.RUPID.conc/100
  anim.fd.bact.MP.rate <<- Parm_rum.bact.TP_CP_L1 * Parm_rum.bact.IDTP_L1 * rum.fd.bact.CP.rate
  anim.fd.fd.MP.rate <<- rum.fd.RUPID.frac * rum.fd.RUCP.rate
  anim.fd.MP.rate <<- anim.fd.bact.MP.rate + anim.fd.fd.MP.rate
  anim.diet.bact.MP.rate <<- sum(anim.fd.bact.MP.rate)
  anim.diet.fd.MP.rate <<- sum(anim.fd.fd.MP.rate)
  anim.diet.MP.rate <<- sum(anim.fd.MP.rate)
  anim.fd.MP.rate <<- rum.fd.RUPID.frac * rum.fd.RUCP.rate + Parm_rum.bact.TP_CP_L1 * Parm_rum.bact.IDTP_L1 *
rum.fd.bact.CP.rate
```

```
  anim.diet.MP.rate <<- sum(anim.fd.MP.rate)
  if (genRPT)
  {
    rptBioValues <- feeds3["FeedName.x"]
    names(rptBioValues) <- "FeedName"
    rptBioValues["RDP, g/d"] <- (anim.fd.CP.rate - rum.fd.RUCP.rate) * 1000
    rptBioValues["RDP, %CP"] <- isz((anim.fd.CP.rate - rum.fd.RUCP.rate) * 100, anim.fd.CP.rate)
    rptBioValues["RUP, g/d"] <- rum.fd.RUCP.rate * 1000
    rptBioValues["RUP, %CP"] <- isz(rum.fd.RUCP.rate * 100, anim.fd.CP.rate)
    rptBioValues["MP Bact, g/d"] <- anim.fd.bact.MP.rate * 1000
    rptBioValues["MP Fd, g/d"] <- anim.fd.fd.MP.rate * 1000
    rptBioValues["MP, g/d"] <- anim.fd.MP.rate * 1000
    rptBioValues2 <- data.frame(FeedName = "Ration")
    rptBioValues2["RDP, g/d"] <- (anim.diet.CP.rate - rum.diet.RUCP.rate) * 1000
    rptBioValues2["RDP, %CP"] <- isz((anim.diet.CP.rate - rum.diet.RUCP.rate) * 100, anim.diet.CP.rate)
    rptBioValues2["RUP, g/d"] <- rum.diet.RUCP.rate * 1000
    rptBioValues2["RUP, %CP"] <- isz(rum.diet.RUCP.rate * 100, anim.diet.CP.rate)
    rptBioValues2["MP Bact, g/d"] <- anim.diet.bact.MP.rate * 1000
    rptBioValues2["MP Fd, g/d"] <- anim.diet.fd.MP.rate * 1000
    rptBioValues2["MP, g/d"] <- anim.diet.MP.rate * 1000
    rptBioValues <- rbind(rptBioValues, rptBioValues2)
    description <- paste("# MP  = metabolizable protein\n", "# RDP = ruminally degraded protein (DIP: digestible intake protein)\n", "# RUP = ruminally undegradable protein (UIP: undegradable intake protein)\n", sep = "")
    report(rptBioValues, "\nMetabolizable Protein, RDP, and RUP", description, "", 3, 3, 1, 7, FALSE, FALSE, FALSE, FALSE, FALSE, FALSE, TRUE)
  }
  # Digested Amino Acids - Feeds
  si.fd.GMet.rate <<- (fds[, "Met_RUP"]/100) * anim.fd.fd.MP.rate
  si.fd.GLys.rate <<- (fds[, "Lys_RUP"]/100) * anim.fd.fd.MP.rate
  si.fd.GArg.rate <<- (fds[, "Arg_RUP"]/100) * anim.fd.fd.MP.rate
  si.fd.GThr.rate <<- (fds[, "Thr_RUP"]/100) * anim.fd.fd.MP.rate
  si.fd.GLeu.rate <<- (fds[, "Leu_RUP"]/100) * anim.fd.fd.MP.rate
  si.fd.GIle.rate <<- (fds[, "Ile_RUP"]/100) * anim.fd.fd.MP.rate
  si.fd.GVal.rate <<- (fds[, "Val_RUP"]/100) * anim.fd.fd.MP.rate
  si.fd.GHis.rate <<- (fds[, "His_RUP"]/100) * anim.fd.fd.MP.rate
  si.fd.GPhe.rate <<- (fds[, "Phe_RUP"]/100) * anim.fd.fd.MP.rate
  si.fd.GTrp.rate <<- (fds[, "Trp_RUP"]/100) * anim.fd.fd.MP.rate
  si.diet.GMet.rate <<- sum(si.fd.GMet.rate)
  si.diet.GLys.rate <<- sum(si.fd.GLys.rate)
  si.diet.GArg.rate <<- sum(si.fd.GArg.rate)
  si.diet.GThr.rate <<- sum(si.fd.GThr.rate)
  si.diet.GLeu.rate <<- sum(si.fd.GLeu.rate)
  si.diet.GIle.rate <<- sum(si.fd.GIle.rate)
  si.diet.GVal.rate <<- sum(si.fd.GVal.rate)
  si.diet.GHis.rate <<- sum(si.fd.GHis.rate)
  si.diet.GPhe.rate <<- sum(si.fd.GPhe.rate)
  si.diet.GTrp.rate <<- sum(si.fd.GTrp.rate)
  if (genRPT)
  {
    rptIDAA_DMI <- fds["FeedName.x"]
    names(rptIDAA_DMI) <- "FeedName"
```

```
      rptIDAA_DMI["Met"] <- si.fd.GMet.rate
      rptIDAA_DMI["Lys"] <- si.fd.GLys.rate
      rptIDAA_DMI["Arg"] <- si.fd.GArg.rate
      rptIDAA_DMI["Thr"] <- si.fd.GThr.rate
      rptIDAA_DMI["Leu"] <- si.fd.GLeu.rate
      rptIDAA_DMI["Ile"] <- si.fd.GIle.rate
      rptIDAA_DMI["Val"] <- si.fd.GVal.rate
      rptIDAA_DMI["His"] <- si.fd.GHis.rate
      rptIDAA_DMI["Phe"] <- si.fd.GPhe.rate
      rptIDAA_DMI["Trp"] <- si.fd.GTrp.rate
      footnote <- "The Digested AA is also the Metabolizable AA."
      report(rptIDAA_DMI, "Metabolizable Feed Amino Acids, g/d", "", footnote, 3, 3, 1000, 7, TRUE, FALSE, TRUE, FALSE, TRUE,
FALSE, TRUE)
    }
    calcDIG(feeds3, genRPT)
    calcMethane()
  }
```

3 Level of Solution 1

3.1 Flowchart of the calculation logic

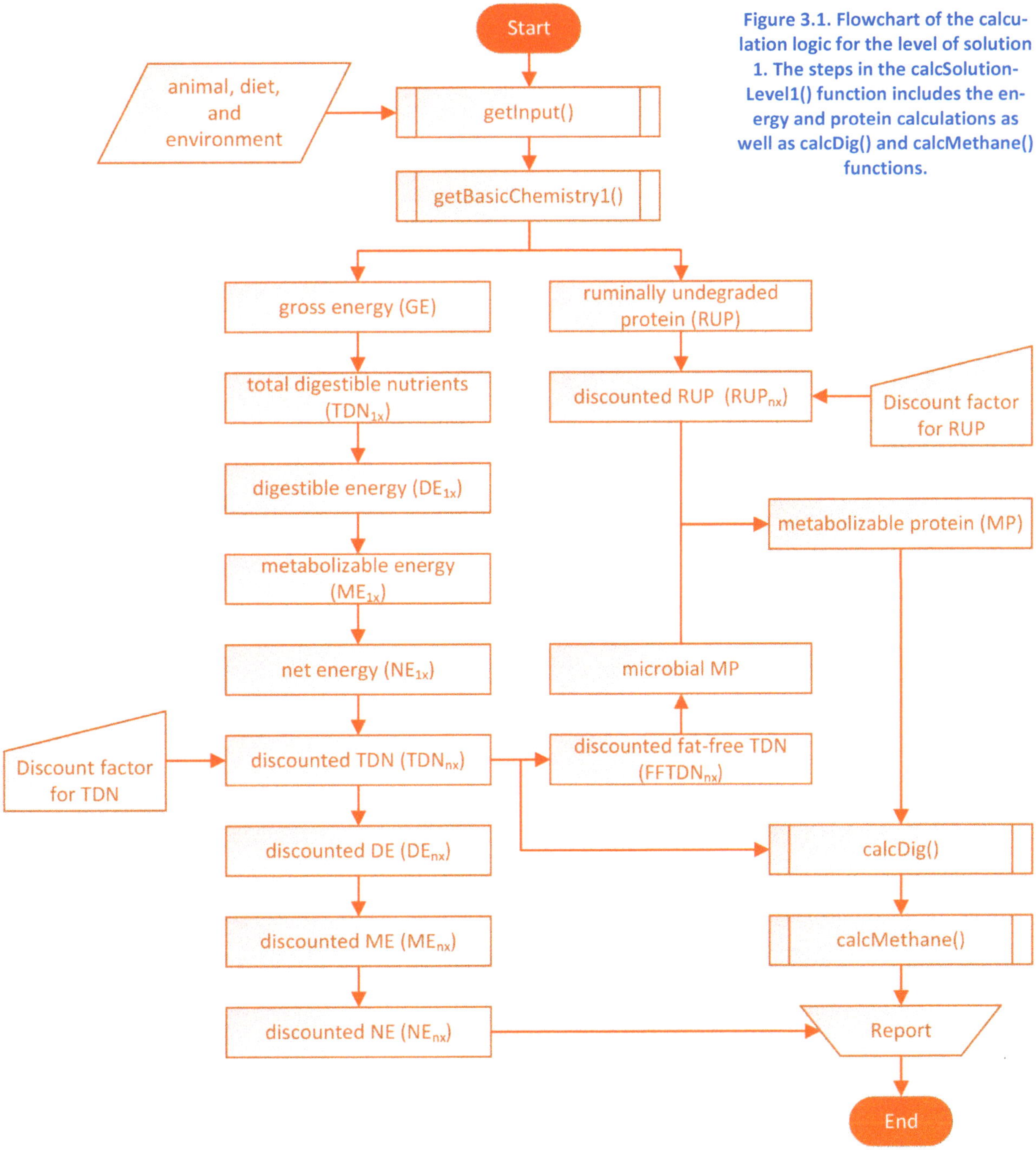

Figure 3.1. Flowchart of the calculation logic for the level of solution 1. The steps in the calcSolutionLevel1() function includes the energy and protein calculations as well as calcDig() and calcMethane() functions.

3.2 Equations

3.2.1 Total digestible nutrients, metabolizable energy and protein, and net energy: calcSolutionLevel1()

#	Variable[1]	Description	Equation
1:	$[GE]_f$		$9.4 * EE_f + 5.65 * CP_f + 4.1 * (NFC_f + FC_f)$
2:	dEE_f	EED>0	$2.25 * EED_f * EE_f$
3:		EED=0 & EE>1	$2.25 * (EE_f - 1) * (1 - 0.0314 * (EE_f - 1))$
4:		otherwise	$2.25 * EE_f$
5:	dCP_f	CPD>0	$CPD_f * CP_f$
6:		CPD=0 & forage>50%	$CP_f * \exp\left(-0.012 * \left(ADIP_f * \frac{100}{CP_f}\right)\right)$
7:		CPD=0 & forage≤ 50%	$CP_f * \left(1 - 0.004 * \left(ADIP_f * \frac{100}{CP_f}\right)\right)$
8:	$IADIP_f$	forage>50%	$0.7 * ADIP_f$
9:		otherwise	$0.4 * ADIP_f$
10:	$NDFn_f$		$NDF_f - NDIP_f + IADIP_f$
11:	$dNDF_f$	NDFn>0	$0.75 * (NDFn_f - Lignin_f) * \left(1 - \varphi_f * \left(\frac{Lignin_f}{NDFn_f}\right)^{\frac{2}{3}}\right)$
12:		otherwise	0
13:	$tTDN_{1x,f}$	EED>0	dEE_f
14:		EED=0 & CPD>0	$0.98 * (100 - CP_f - Ash_f - EE_f) + dCP_f + dEE_f$
15:		EED=0 & CPD=0	$0.98 * (100 - NDFn_f - CP_f - Ash_f - EE_f + IADIP_f) * PAF_f + dCP_f + dEE_f + dNDF_f$
16:	$aTDN_{1x,f}$	EED>0	$tTDN_f - 1.4$
17:		EED=0 & CPD>0	$tTDN_f - 4.13$
18:		EED=0 & CPD=0	$tTDN_f - 7$
19:	$DE_{1x,f}$		$4.409 * aTDN_{1x,f}$
20:	$[ME]_{1x,f}$	lactating or dry dairy	$1.01 * \left(\frac{DE_{1x,f}}{DMI_f}\right) - 0.45$
21:		otherwise	$0.82 * \left(\frac{DE_{1x,f}}{DMI_f}\right)$
22:	$[NEl]_{1x,f}$		$0.644 * ME_{1x,f}$
23:	$[NEm]_{1x,f}$	lactating dairy	$NEl_{1x,f}$
24:		otherwise	$1.37 * [ME]_{1x,f} - 0.138 * [ME]_{1x,f}^2 + 0.105 * [ME]_{1x,f}^3 - 1.12$
25:	$[NEg]_{1x,f}$		$1.42 * [ME]_{1x,f} - 0.174 * [ME]_{1x,f}^2 + 0.122 * [ME]_{1x,f}^3 - 1.65$
26:	L[2]	level of intake	$\frac{\sum_{f=1}^{nf} DMI_f}{FFM} - 1$
27:	D_f	forage<50% & beef & BW ≈ 250	$0.073 - 4.051 * L + 0.05 * TDN_{1x,f} * L + 0.093 * NDF_f * L - 0.0002 * TDN_{1x,f} * NDF_f * L$
28:		forage<50% & beef & BW ≈ 550	$0.086 - 4.653 * L + 0.055 * TDN_{1x,f} * L + 0.101 * NDF_f * L - 0.0001 * TDN_{1x,f} * NDF_f * L$
29:		forage<50% & dairy	$0.1 - 4.853 * L + 0.06 * TDN_{1x,f} * L + 0.122 * NDF_f * L - 0.0005 * TDN_{1x,f} * NDF_f * L$
30:		forage>50% & beef & BW ≈ 250	$0.15 - 17.371 * L + 0.21 * TDN_{1x,f} * L + 0.341 * NDF_f * L - 0.0031 * TDN_{1x,f} * NDF_f * L$
31:		forage>50% & beef & BW ≈ 550	$0.118 - 15.809 * L + 0.195 * TDN_{1x,f} * L + 0.298 * NDF_f * L - 0.0025 * TDN_{1x,f} * NDF_f * L$
32:		forage>50% & dairy	$0.209 - 20.37 * L + 0.249 * TDN_{1x,f} * L + 0.398 * NDF_f * L - 0.0036 * TDN_{1x,f} * NDF_f * L$
33:	$aTDN_{nx,f}$		$aTDN_{1x,f} * \frac{100 - D_f}{100}$

#	Variable[1]	Description	Equation
34:	$DE_{nx,f}$		$4.409 * aTDN_{nx,f}$
35:		lactating or dry dairy & EE>3 & EED=0	$1.01 * \left(\frac{DE_{nx,f}}{DMI_f}\right) - 0.45 + 0.0046 * (EE_f - 3)$
36:	$[ME]_{nx,f}$	lactating or dry dairy	$1.01 * \left(\frac{DE_{nx,f}}{DMI_f}\right) - 0.45$
37:		otherwise	$0.82 * \left(\frac{DE_{nx,f}}{DMI_f}\right)$
38:	$[NEl]_{nx,f}$		$0.644 * [ME]_{nx,f}$
39:	$[NEm]_{nx,f}$	lactating dairy	$[NEl]_{nx,f}$
40:		otherwise	$1.37 * [ME]_{nx,f} - 0.138 * [ME]_{nx,f}^2 + 0.105 * [ME]_{nx,f}^3 - 1.12$
41:	$[NEg]_{nx,f}$		$1.42 * [ME]_{nx,f} - 0.174 * [ME]_{nx,f}^2 + 0.122 * [ME]_{nx,f}^3 - 1.65$
42:	$RUP_{nx,f}$	forage>50%	$0.167 + RUP_{1x,f} + 4.3 * L - 0.032 * RUP_{1x,f} * L$
43:		otherwise	$0.097 + 1.01 * RUP_{1x,f} + 4.47 * L + 0.058 * RUP_{1x,f} * L$
44:	$peNDF_{adj,f}$	peNDF<20	$1 - 0.025 * (20 - peNDF_f)$
45:		otherwise	1
46:	$BactCP_f$		$0.13 * FSFaTDN_f * peNDF_{adj,f}$
47:	$Bact_f$		$\frac{BactCP_f}{0.625}$
48:	$BactMP_f$		$0.8 * 0.8 * BactCP_f$
49:	MP_f		$RUPID_f * RUP_{nx,f} * DMI_f + BactMP_f$
50:	k_m		$\frac{\sum_{f=1}^{nf}(DMI_f * [NEm]_{nx,f})}{\sum_{f=1}^{nf}(DMI_f * [MEm]_{nx,f})}$
51:	k_g		$\frac{\sum_{f=1}^{nf}(DMI_f * [NEg]_{nx,f})}{\sum_{f=1}^{nf}(DMI_f * [MEm]_{nx,f})}$
52:	k_l		$\frac{\sum_{f=1}^{nf}(DMI_f * [NEl]_{nx,f})}{\sum_{f=1}^{nf}(DMI_f * [MEm]_{nx,f})}$

(1) ***1x*** is at maintenance level of intake; ***ADIP*** is acid detergent insoluble protein (also known as acid detergent insoluble nitrogen, ADIN), % DM; ***Ash*** is ash, % DM; ***aTDN*** is apparent total digestible nutrients, % DM; ***Bact*** is bacteria mass, kg/d; ***BactCP*** is bacteria crude protein, kg/d; ***BactMP*** is bacteria metabolizable protein, kg/d; ***CP*** is crude protein, % DM; ***CPD*** is crude protein digestibility, %; ***D*** is the TDN discount for production level of intake (nx); ***dCP*** is digestible crude protein, %; ***dEE*** is digestible ether extract (fat), kg/d; ***DMI*** is dry matter intake, kg/d; ***EE*** is ether extract (fat), % DM; ***EED*** is ether extract (fat) digestibility, %; ***f*** is the jth feed; ***FFM*** is feed required for maintenance, kg/d; ***FSFaTDN*** is the apparent total digestible nutrients of the diet without fat supplements (ingredients with EE > 50% DM); ***[GE]*** is gross energy, Mcal/kg; ***IADIP*** is indigestible ADIP, % DM; $\boldsymbol{k_g}$ is the partial efficiency of utilization of metabolizable energy for net energy for growth, dimensionless; $\boldsymbol{k_l}$ is the partial efficiency of utilization of metabolizable energy for net energy for lactation, dimensionless; $\boldsymbol{k_m}$ is the partial efficiency of utilization of metabolizable energy for net energy for maintenance, dimensionless; ***[ME]*** is dietary content of metabolizable energy, Mcal/kg; ***MP*** is metabolizable protein, kg/d; ***NDF*** is neutral detergent fiber, % DM; ***NDIP*** is neutral detergent insoluble protein (also known as neutral detergent insoluble nitrogen, NDIN), % DM; ***[NEg]*** is dietary content of net energy for growth (also called ***NEga***), Mcal/kg; ***[NEl]*** is dietary content of net energy for lactation (also called ***NEla***), Mcal/kg; ***[NEm]*** is dietary content of net energy for maintenance (also called ***NEma***), Mcal/kg; ***nf*** is the number of feeds; ***nx*** is at production level of intake; ***PAF*** is processing adjustment factor; ***peNDF*** is physically effective neutral detergent fiber, % DM; ***RUP*** is ruminally undegraded protein, % DM; ***RUPID*** is ruminally degradable protein intestinal digestibility, %; and ***tTDN*** is true total digestible nutrients, % DM.

(2) *L* is computed iteratively, see Code 3.3.1.

3.3 Code

3.3.1 Total digestible nutrients, metabolizable energy and protein, and net energy

```
calcSolutionLevel1 <- function(fds = feeds3, genRPT)
{
  # ++++++++++++++
  # Gross Energy
  # ++++++++++++++
  # Atwater factors
  anim.fd.GE.rate <<- anim.fd.EE.rate * 9.4 + anim.fd.CP.rate * 5.65 + (anim.fd.NFC.rate + anim.fd.FC.rate) * 4.1
  anim.fd.GE.frac <<- isz(anim.fd.GE.rate, anim.fd.DMI.rate)
  anim.diet.GE.rate <<- sum(anim.fd.GE.rate)
  anim.diet.GE.frac <<- isz(anim.diet.GE.rate, anim.diet.DMI.rate)
  # ++++++++++++++++++++++++++++++++
  # Total Digestible Nutrients 1x
  # ++++++++++++++++++++++++++++++++
  # Apparent and True TDN 1x based on Weiss et al. 1992, Anim. Feed Sci. Technol. 39:95-110) and NRC (2001)
  anim.fd.TDNAdjFactor.frac <<- as.numeric(fds[, "TDNAdjFactor"])/100
  anim.fd.PAF.frac <<- as.numeric(fds[, "PAF"])
  anim.fd.Phi.frac <<- as.numeric(fds[, "Phi"])
  anim.fd.EED.frac <<- as.numeric(fds[, "EED"])/100
  anim.fd.CPD.frac <<- as.numeric(fds[, "CPD"])/100
  # RNS assumes it is a fat supplement if anim.fd.EED.frac is greater than zero
  anim.fd.dEE.conc <<- ifelse(anim.fd.EED.frac > 0, 2.25 * anim.fd.EED.frac * anim.fd.EE.conc,
                           ifelse(anim.fd.EE.conc > 1, 2.25 * (anim.fd.EE.conc - 1) * (1 - 0.0314 * (anim.fd.EE.conc - 1)),
                               2.25 * anim.fd.EE.conc))
  # RNS assumes it is an animal protein meal if anim.fd.CPD.frac is greater than zero
  anim.fd.dCP.conc <<- ifelse(anim.fd.CPD.frac > 0, anim.fd.CPD.frac * anim.fd.CP.conc,
                           ifelse(anim.fd.Forage.conc > 50, ifelse(anim.fd.CP.conc > 0, anim.fd.CP.conc * exp(-0.012 * (anim.fd.ADIP.conc * 100/anim.fd.CP.conc)), 0),
                               ifelse(anim.fd.CP.conc > 0, anim.fd.CP.conc * (1 - 0.004 * (anim.fd.ADIP.conc * 100/anim.fd.CP.conc)), 0)))
  anim.fd.iADIP.conc <<- ifelse(anim.fd.Forage.conc > 50, 0.7 * anim.fd.ADIP.conc, 0.4 * anim.fd.ADIP.conc)
  anim.fd.NDFn.conc <<- pmax(0, (anim.fd.UnAdjNDF.conc - anim.fd.NDIP.conc + anim.fd.iADIP.conc))
  anim.fd.dNDF.conc <<- ifelse(anim.fd.NDFn.conc > 0, 0.75 * (anim.fd.NDFn.conc - anim.fd.lignin.conc) * (1 - anim.fd.Phi.frac * (anim.fd.lignin.conc/anim.fd.NDFn.conc)^(2/3)), 0)
  anim.fd.tTDNUnAdj.conc <<- ifelse(anim.fd.EED.frac > 0, anim.fd.dEE.conc,
                              ifelse(anim.fd.CPD.frac > 0, 0.98 * (100 - anim.fd.CP.conc - anim.fd.ash.conc - anim.fd.EE.conc) +
                                  anim.fd.dCP.conc + anim.fd.dEE.conc, 0.98 * (100 - anim.fd.NDFn.conc - anim.fd.CP.conc -
                                  anim.fd.ash.conc - anim.fd.EE.conc + anim.fd.iADIP.conc) *
                                  anim.fd.PAF.frac + anim.fd.dCP.conc + anim.fd.dEE.conc + anim.fd.dNDF.conc))
  # RNS discounts true TDN by 1.4 (13*0.15*0.3*2.25) for fat supplements, 4.13 (13*0.15*0.3*2.25+13*0.3*0.7) for animal protein meal, and 7 (13*0.15*0.3*2.25+13*0.3*0.7+13*0.25*0.98) for other feedstuffs
```

```
anim.fd.aTDNUnAdj.conc <<- ifelse(anim.fd.EED.frac > 0, anim.fd.tTDNUnAdj.conc - 1.4,
                                   ifelse(anim.fd.CPD.frac > 0, anim.fd.tTDNUnAdj.conc - 4.13, anim.fd.tTDNUnAdj.conc - 7))
# Remove negative TDN
anim.fd.tTDN1x.conc <<- pmax(0, anim.fd.tTDNUnAdj.conc * anim.fd.TDNAdjFactor.frac)
anim.fd.aTDN1x.conc <<- pmax(0, anim.fd.aTDNUnAdj.conc * anim.fd.TDNAdjFactor.frac)
anim.fd.tTDN1x.rate <<- (anim.fd.tTDN1x.conc/100) * anim.fd.DMI.rate
anim.fd.aTDN1x.rate <<- (anim.fd.aTDN1x.conc/100) * anim.fd.DMI.rate
anim.diet.tTDN1x.rate <<- sum(anim.fd.tTDN1x.rate)
anim.diet.tTDN1x.conc <<- isz(anim.diet.tTDN1x.rate * 100, anim.diet.DMI.rate)
anim.diet.aTDN1x.rate <<- sum(anim.fd.aTDN1x.rate)
anim.diet.aTDN1x.conc <<- isz(anim.diet.aTDN1x.rate * 100, anim.diet.DMI.rate)
# ++++++++++++++++++++++
# Digestible Energy 1x
# ++++++++++++++++++++++
anim.fd.DE1x.rate <<- 4.409 * pmax(0, anim.fd.aTDN1x.rate)  # Mcal/d
anim.diet.DE1x.rate <<- sum(anim.fd.DE1x.rate)  # Mcal/d
anim.fd.DE1x.frac <<- isz(anim.fd.DE1x.rate, anim.fd.DMI.rate)  # Mcal/kg
anim.diet.DE1x.frac <<- isz(anim.diet.DE1x.rate, anim.diet.DMI.rate)  # Mcal/kg
# +++++++++++++++++++++++++
# Metabolizable Energy 1x
# +++++++++++++++++++++++++
if (anim.type == "Milk" & (anim.stage_type == "Lactating" | anim.stage_type == "Dry"))
{
  # Dairy Remove negative values
  anim.fd.ME1x.frac <<- pmax(0, 1.01 * anim.fd.DE1x.frac - 0.45)  # Mcal/kg
} else
{
  # Remove negative values
  anim.fd.ME1x.frac <<- pmax(0, 0.82 * anim.fd.DE1x.frac)  # Mcal/kg
}
if (anim.diet.ionophore == TRUE & flag_Ionophore == 1) anim.fd.ME1x.frac <<- 1.023 * anim.fd.ME1x.frac
anim.fd.ME1x.rate <<- anim.fd.ME1x.frac * anim.fd.DMI.rate  # Mcal/d
anim.diet.ME1x.rate <<- sum(anim.fd.ME1x.rate)  # Mcal/d
anim.diet.ME1x.frac <<- isz(anim.diet.ME1x.rate, anim.diet.DMI.rate)  # Mcal/kg
# +++++++++++++++
# Net Energy 1x
# +++++++++++++++
# Feeds
anim.fd.NEm1x.frac <<- ifelse(anim.fd.ME1x.frac > 0, 1.37 * anim.fd.ME1x.frac - 0.138 *
                              anim.fd.ME1x.frac^2 + 0.0105 * anim.fd.ME1x.frac^3 - 1.12, 0)
anim.fd.NEg1x.frac <<- ifelse(anim.fd.ME1x.frac > 0, 1.42 * anim.fd.ME1x.frac - 0.174 *
                              anim.fd.ME1x.frac^2 + 0.0122 * anim.fd.ME1x.frac^3 - 1.65, 0)
anim.fd.NEl1x.frac <<- ifelse(anim.fd.ME1x.frac > 0, 0.644 * anim.fd.ME1x.frac, 0)
if (anim.type == "Milk" & anim.stage_type == "Lactating") anim.fd.NEm1x.frac <<- anim.fd.NEl1x.frac
# Adjustment for ionophores
if (anim.diet.ionophore == TRUE & flag_Ionophore == 0) anim.fd.NEm1x.frac <<- 1.12 * anim.fd.NEm1x.frac
anim.fd.NEm1x.rate <<- anim.fd.NEm1x.frac * anim.fd.DMI.rate
anim.fd.NEg1x.rate <<- anim.fd.NEg1x.frac * anim.fd.DMI.rate
anim.fd.NEl1x.rate <<- anim.fd.NEl1x.frac * anim.fd.DMI.rate
# Ration
anim.diet.NEm1x.frac <<- ifelse(anim.diet.ME1x.frac > 0, 1.37 * anim.diet.ME1x.frac - 0.138 *
```

```
                                  anim.diet.ME1x.frac^2 + 0.0105 * anim.diet.ME1x.frac^3 - 1.12, 0)
  anim.diet.NEg1x.frac <<- ifelse(anim.diet.ME1x.frac > 0, 1.42 * anim.diet.ME1x.frac - 0.174 *
                                  anim.diet.ME1x.frac^2 + 0.0122 * anim.diet.ME1x.frac^3 - 1.65, 0)
  anim.diet.NEl1x.frac <<- ifelse(anim.diet.ME1x.frac > 0, 0.644 * anim.diet.ME1x.frac, 0)
  if (anim.type == "Milk" & anim.stage_type == "Lactating") anim.diet.NEm1x.frac <<- anim.diet.NEl1x.frac
  # Adjustment for ionophores
  if (anim.diet.ionophore == TRUE & flag_Ionophore == 0) anim.diet.NEm1x.frac <<- 1.12 * anim.diet.NEm1x.frac
  anim.diet.NEm1x.rate <<- anim.diet.NEm1x.frac * anim.diet.DMI.rate
  anim.diet.NEg1x.rate <<- anim.diet.NEg1x.frac * anim.diet.DMI.rate
  anim.diet.NEl1x.rate <<- anim.diet.NEl1x.frac * anim.diet.DMI.rate
  if (genRPT)
  {
    rptBioValues <- fds["FeedName.x"]
    names(rptBioValues) <- "FeedName"
    rptBioValues["GE, Mcal/kg"] <- anim.fd.GE.frac
    rptBioValues["GE, Mcal/d"] <- anim.fd.GE.rate
    rptBioValues["tTDN1x,kg/d"] <- anim.fd.tTDN1x.rate
    rptBioValues["aTDN1x,kg/d"] <- anim.fd.aTDN1x.rate
    rptBioValues["tTDN1x,%DM"] <- anim.fd.tTDN1x.conc
    rptBioValues["aTDN1x,%DM"] <- anim.fd.aTDN1x.conc
    rptBioValues["DE1x,Mcal/d"] <- anim.fd.DE1x.rate
    rptBioValues["DE1x,Mcal/kg"] <- anim.fd.DE1x.frac
    rptBioValues["ME1x,Mcal/d"] <- anim.fd.ME1x.rate
    rptBioValues["ME1x,Mcal/kg"] <- anim.fd.ME1x.frac
    rptBioValues["NEm1x,Mcal/kg"] <- anim.fd.NEm1x.frac
    rptBioValues["NEg1x,Mcal/d"] <- anim.fd.NEg1x.frac
    rptBioValues["NEl1x,Mcal/kg"] <- anim.fd.NEl1x.frac
    rptBioValues2 <- data.frame(FeedName = "Ration")
    rptBioValues2["GE, Mcal/kg"] <- anim.diet.GE.frac
    rptBioValues2["GE, Mcal/d"] <- anim.diet.GE.rate
    rptBioValues2["tTDN1x,kg/d"] <- anim.diet.tTDN1x.rate
    rptBioValues2["aTDN1x,kg/d"] <- anim.diet.aTDN1x.rate
    rptBioValues2["tTDN1x,%DM"] <- anim.diet.tTDN1x.conc
    rptBioValues2["aTDN1x,%DM"] <- anim.diet.aTDN1x.conc
    rptBioValues2["DE1x,Mcal/d"] <- anim.diet.DE1x.rate
    rptBioValues2["DE1x,Mcal/kg"] <- anim.diet.DE1x.frac
    rptBioValues2["ME1x,Mcal/d"] <- anim.diet.ME1x.rate
    rptBioValues2["ME1x,Mcal/kg"] <- anim.diet.ME1x.frac
    rptBioValues2["NEm1x,Mcal/kg"] <- anim.diet.NEm1x.frac
    rptBioValues2["NEg1x,Mcal/d"] <- anim.diet.NEg1x.frac
    rptBioValues2["NEl1x,Mcal/kg"] <- anim.diet.NEl1x.frac
    rptBioValues <- rbind(rptBioValues, rptBioValues2)
    description <- paste("# a    = apparent\n", "# t    = true\n",
                         "# TDN 1x = total digestible nutrients at maintenance level (1x)\n",
                         "# GE     = gross energy\n",
                         "# DE 1x  = digestible energy at maintenance level (1x)\n",
                         "# ME 1x  = metabolizable energy at maintenance level (1x)\n",
                         "# NEm 1x = net energy for maintenance at maintenance level (1x)\n",
                         "# NEg 1x = net energy for growth at maintenance level (1x)\n",
                         "# NEl 1x = net energy for lactation at maintenance level (1x)\n", sep = "")
```

```
    report(rptBioValues, "Gross Energy, Total Digestible Nutrients, Digestible Energy, Metabolizable Energy, Net Energy at 1x",
           description, "", 3, 3, 1, 5, FALSE, FALSE, FALSE, FALSE, FALSE, FALSE, TRUE)
  }
  # ++++++++++++++++++++++++++++++++++++++++++
  # Total Digestible Nutrients - Discounted
  # ++++++++++++++++++++++++++++++++++++++++++
  # DMI multiple of DMI required for maintenance
  temp <- vector(mode = "double", length = 4)
  temp[1] <- 0
  iter_tdn_1x <- 0
  anim.diet.ME.frac <<- anim.diet.ME1x.frac
  anim.diet.NEm.frac <<- anim.diet.NEm1x.frac
  anim.diet.NEg.frac <<- anim.diet.NEg1x.frac
  anim.diet.NEl.frac <<- anim.diet.NEl1x.frac
  while (abs(temp[1] - anim.diet.ME.frac) > temp[1] * diff_iter_tdn_1x & iter_tdn_1x < max_iter_tdn_1x)
  {
    iter_tdn_1x <- iter_tdn_1x + 1
    temp[1] <- anim.diet.ME.frac
    temp[2] <- anim.diet.NEm.frac
    temp[3] <- anim.diet.NEg.frac
    temp[4] <- anim.diet.NEl.frac
    anim.NEmr.rate <<- calcMaintenanceRequirement(T, anim.diet.DMI.rate,
                                                  anim.diet.ME.frac, anim.diet.NEm.frac,
                                                  anim.diet.NEg.frac, anim.diet.NEl.frac)
    # anim.FFM.rate<<-anim.NEmr.rate/anim.diet.NEm.frac
    dmi_factor <- anim.diet.DMI.rate/anim.FFM.rate - 1
    # Discounted TDN (Tedeschi et al., 2005, Prof. Anim. Scient. 21:403-415) discount.coef[1-5] for concentrate dis-
count.coef[6-10] for forage
    discount_coef <- vector(mode = "double", length = 10)
    if (anim.species == "Cattle" & anim.sex == "Female" & anim.type == "Milk" & anim.stage_type == "Lactating")
    {
      # Dairy cow
      discount_coef <- c(0.1, -4.853, 0.06, 0.122, -5e-04, 0.209, -20.37, 0.249, 0.398, -0.0036)
    } else
    {
      if (anim.species == "Cattle")
      {
        # not Dairy cow
        if (anim.FBW <= 250)
        {
          # growing
          discount_coef <- c(0.073, -4.051, 0.05, 0.093, -2e-04, 0.15, -17.371, 0.21, 0.341, -0.0031)
        } else
        {
          # finishing
          discount_coef <- c(0.086, -4.653, 0.055, 0.101, -5e-04, 0.118, -15.809, 0.195, 0.298, -0.0025)
        }
      } else
      {
        discount_coef <- c(0.073, -4.051, 0.05, 0.093, -2e-04, 0.15, -17.371, 0.21, 0.341, -0.0031)
```

```
            }
        }
        # The discount factor is zero for fat supplements. RNS assumes it is a fat supplement if anim.fd.EED.frac is greater than
zero
        discount_factor <- ifelse(anim.fd.EED.frac > 0, 0, ifelse(anim.fd.Forage.conc > 50, discount_coef[1] + discount_coef[2] *
                                  dmi_factor + discount_coef[3] * dmi_factor *
anim.fd.aTDN1x.conc +
                                  discount_coef[4] * dmi_factor * anim.fd.NDF.conc + dis-
count_coef[5] *
                                  dmi_factor * anim.fd.aTDN1x.conc * anim.fd.NDF.conc, dis-
count_coef[6] +
                                  discount_coef[7] * dmi_factor + discount_coef[8] * dmi_factor
*
                                  anim.fd.aTDN1x.conc + discount_coef[9] * dmi_factor *
                                  anim.fd.NDF.conc + discount_coef[10] * dmi_factor *
                                  anim.fd.aTDN1x.conc * anim.fd.NDF.conc))
        # RNS removes the negative discount and aTDN values
        discount_factor <- pmax(discount_factor, 0)
        anim.fd.aTDN.conc <<- pmax(0, anim.fd.aTDN1x.conc * (100 - discount_factor)/100)
        # This is the discount equation for TDN as shown in Table 12 of Fox et al. (2004; Anim. Feed Sci. Technol. 112:29-78)
        # anim.fd.aTDN.conc<<-ifelse(anim.fd.Forage.conc>50,0.53+0.99*anim.fd.aTDN1x.conc-0.009*anim.fd.NDF.conc+
        # 0.00005*anim.fd.aTDN1x.conc*anim.fd.NDF.conc+8.96*dmi_factor-0.1*anim.fd.aTDN1x.conc*dmi_factor-0.13*
        # anim.fd.NDF.conc*dmi_factor+0.0005*anim.fd.aTDN1x.conc*anim.fd.NDF.conc*dmi_factor,1.01*anim.fd.aTDN1x.conc-
1.77*dmi_factor-0.99)
        anim.fd.aTDN.rate <<- (anim.fd.aTDN.conc/100) * anim.fd.DMI.rate
        anim.diet.aTDN.rate <<- sum(anim.fd.aTDN.rate)
        anim.diet.aTDN.conc <<- isz(anim.diet.aTDN.rate * 100, anim.diet.DMI.rate)

        anim.fd.tTDN.conc <<- pmax(0, anim.fd.tTDN1x.conc * (100 - discount_factor)/100)
        anim.fd.tTDN.rate <<- (anim.fd.tTDN.conc/100) * anim.fd.DMI.rate
        anim.diet.tTDN.rate <<- sum(anim.fd.tTDN.rate)
        anim.diet.tTDN.conc <<- isz(anim.diet.tTDN.rate * 100, anim.diet.DMI.rate)
        # +++++++++++++++++++++++++++++++++
        # Digestible Energy - Discounted
        # +++++++++++++++++++++++++++++++++
        anim.fd.DE.rate <<- 4.409 * pmax(0, anim.fd.aTDN.rate)   # Mcal/d
        anim.diet.DE.rate <<- sum(anim.fd.DE.rate)  # Mcal/d
        anim.fd.DE.frac <<- isz(anim.fd.DE.rate, anim.fd.DMI.rate)   # Mcal/kg
        anim.diet.DE.frac <<- isz(anim.diet.DE.rate, anim.diet.DMI.rate)   # Mcal/kg
        # +++++++++++++++++++++++++++++++++++
        # Metabolizable Energy - Discounted
        # +++++++++++++++++++++++++++++++++++
        if (anim.type == "Milk" & (anim.stage_type == "Lactating" | anim.stage_type == "Dry"))
        {
          # Dairy RNS adds 0.0046 Mcal/kg for each EE % unit above 3 for non-fat supplements and feedstuffs with EE greater than
3% RNS also removes negative ME values
          anim.fd.ME.frac <<- pmax(0, ifelse(anim.fd.EE.conc > 3 & anim.fd.EED.frac == 0, 1.01 *
                                     anim.fd.DE.frac - 0.45 + 0.0046 * (anim.fd.EE.conc - 3),
                                   1.01 * anim.fd.DE.frac - 0.45))   # Mcal/kg
        } else
        {
```

```
        # Remove negative values
        anim.fd.ME.frac <<- pmax(0, 0.82 * anim.fd.DE.frac)   # Mcal/kg
      }
      if (anim.diet.ionophore == TRUE & flag_Ionophore == 1) anim.fd.ME.frac <<- 1.023 * anim.fd.ME.frac
      anim.fd.ME.rate <<- anim.fd.ME.frac * anim.fd.DMI.rate   # Mcal/d
      anim.diet.ME.rate <<- sum(anim.fd.ME.rate)   # Mcal/d
      anim.diet.ME.frac <<- isz(anim.diet.ME.rate, anim.diet.DMI.rate)   # Mcal/kg
      # ++++++++++++++++++++++++
      # Net Energy - Discounted
      # ++++++++++++++++++++++++
      # Feeds
      anim.fd.NEm.frac <<- ifelse(anim.fd.ME.frac > 0, 1.37 * anim.fd.ME.frac - 0.138 *
                              anim.fd.ME.frac^2 + 0.0105 * anim.fd.ME.frac^3 - 1.12, 0)
      anim.fd.NEg.frac <<- ifelse(anim.fd.ME.frac > 0, 1.42 * anim.fd.ME.frac - 0.174 *
                              anim.fd.ME.frac^2 + 0.0122 * anim.fd.ME.frac^3 - 1.65, 0)
      anim.fd.NEl.frac <<- ifelse(anim.fd.EE.conc <= 3, 0.644 * anim.fd.ME.frac,
                            ifelse(anim.fd.EE.conc <= 50, ifelse(anim.fd.ME.frac > 0,
                                                             (0.703 * anim.fd.ME.frac - 0.19 +
                                                               (((0.097 * anim.fd.ME.frac + 0.19)/97) *
  (anim.fd.EE.conc - 3))) *
                                                               anim.fd.ME.frac, 0), ifelse(anim.fd.ME.frac > 0, 0.8 *
  anim.fd.ME.frac, 0)))
      if (anim.type == "Milk" & anim.stage_type == "Lactating") anim.fd.NEm.frac <<- anim.fd.NEl.frac
      if (anim.diet.ionophore == TRUE & flag_Ionophore == 0) anim.fd.NEm.frac <<- 1.12 * anim.fd.NEm.frac
      anim.fd.NEm.rate <<- anim.fd.NEm.frac * anim.fd.DMI.rate
      anim.fd.NEg.rate <<- anim.fd.NEg.frac * anim.fd.DMI.rate
      anim.fd.NEl.rate <<- anim.fd.NEl.frac * anim.fd.DMI.rate
      # Ration
      anim.diet.NEm.frac <<- ifelse(anim.diet.ME.frac > 0, 1.37 * anim.diet.ME.frac - 0.138 * anim.diet.ME.frac^2 + 0.0105 *
  anim.diet.ME.frac^3 - 1.12, 0)
      anim.diet.NEg.frac <<- ifelse(anim.diet.ME.frac > 0, 1.42 * anim.diet.ME.frac - 0.174 * anim.diet.ME.frac^2 + 0.0122 *
  anim.diet.ME.frac^3 - 1.65, 0)
      anim.diet.EE.conc <<- anim.diet.EE.rate * 100/anim.diet.DMI.rate
      anim.diet.NEl.frac <<- ifelse(anim.diet.EE.conc <= 3, 0.644 * anim.diet.ME.frac,
                              ifelse(anim.diet.EE.conc <= 50,
                                ifelse(anim.diet.ME.frac > 0, 0.703 * anim.diet.ME.frac - 0.19 +
                                  (((0.097 * anim.diet.ME.frac + 0.19)/97) *
                                    (anim.diet.EE.conc - 3)), 0), 0.8 * anim.diet.ME.frac))
      if (anim.type == "Milk" & anim.stage_type == "Lactating") anim.diet.NEm.frac <<- anim.diet.NEl.frac
      if (anim.diet.ionophore == TRUE & flag_Ionophore == 0) anim.diet.NEm.frac <<- 1.12 * anim.diet.NEm.frac
      anim.diet.NEm.rate <<- anim.diet.NEm.frac * anim.diet.DMI.rate
      anim.diet.NEg.rate <<- anim.diet.NEg.frac * anim.diet.DMI.rate
      anim.diet.NEl.rate <<- anim.diet.NEl.frac * anim.diet.DMI.rate
    }
    if (genRPT)
    {
      rptBioValues <- fds["FeedName.x"]
      names(rptBioValues) <- "FeedName"
      rptBioValues["aTDN, kg/d"] <- anim.fd.aTDN.rate
      rptBioValues["aTDN, % DM"] <- anim.fd.aTDN.conc
      rptBioValues["Disc, %"] <- isz((anim.fd.aTDN1x.conc - anim.fd.aTDN.conc) * 100, anim.fd.aTDN1x.conc)
```

```
    rptBioValues["DE, Mcal/d"] <- anim.fd.DE.rate
    rptBioValues["DE, Mcal/kg"] <- anim.fd.DE.frac
    rptBioValues["ME, Mcal/d"] <- anim.fd.ME.rate
    rptBioValues["ME, Mcal/kg"] <- anim.fd.ME.frac
    rptBioValues["NEm, Mcal/kg"] <- anim.fd.NEm.frac
    rptBioValues["NEg, Mcal/d"] <- anim.fd.NEg.frac
    rptBioValues["NEl, Mcal/kg"] <- anim.fd.NEl.frac
    rptBioValues2 <- data.frame(FeedName = "Ration")
    rptBioValues2["aTDN, kg/d"] <- anim.diet.aTDN.rate
    rptBioValues2["aTDN, % DM"] <- anim.diet.aTDN.conc
    rptBioValues2["Disc, %"] <- isz((anim.diet.aTDN1x.conc - anim.diet.aTDN.conc) * 100, anim.diet.aTDN1x.conc)
    rptBioValues2["DE, Mcal/d"] <- anim.diet.DE.rate
    rptBioValues2["DE, Mcal/kg"] <- anim.diet.DE.frac
    rptBioValues2["ME, Mcal/d"] <- anim.diet.ME.rate
    rptBioValues2["ME, Mcal/kg"] <- anim.diet.ME.frac
    rptBioValues2["NEm, Mcal/kg"] <- anim.diet.NEm.frac
    rptBioValues2["NEg, Mcal/d"] <- anim.diet.NEg.frac
    rptBioValues2["NEl, Mcal/kg"] <- anim.diet.NEl.frac
    rptBioValues <- rbind(rptBioValues, rptBioValues2)
    description <- paste("# a    = apparent\n", "# t    = true\n", "# TDN  = total digestible nutrients at ",
                         formatC(dmi_factor, format = "f", digits = 3, width = 7), "x DMI\n", "# Disc = TDN discount percent-
age (1x - ",
                         formatC(dmi_factor, format = "f", digits = 3, width = 7), "x)/1x\n",
                         "# DE   = digestible energy\n", "# ME   = metabolizable energy\n",
                         "# NEm  = net energy for maintenance\n", "# NEg  = net energy for growth\n",
                         "# NEl  = net energy for lactation\n", sep = "")
    footnote <- paste("Iterations (ME, Mcal/kg): ", iter_tdn_1x, " (Max = ",
                      formatC(max_iter_tdn_1x, format = "f", digits = 0), ")", "\nDifference (ME, Mcal/kg): ",
                      formatC(isz(abs(temp[1] - anim.diet.ME.frac) * 100, temp[1]), format = "f", digits = 3, width = 7), "%
(Max = ", diff_iter_tdn_1x * 100, "%)", sep = "")
    report(rptBioValues, "Total Digestible Nutrients, Digestible Energy, Metabolizable Energy, and Net Energy",
           description, footnote, 3, 3, 1, 6, FALSE, FALSE, FALSE, FALSE, FALSE, FALSE, TRUE)
  }
  # ++++++++++++++++++++++
  # Metabolizable Protein
  # ++++++++++++++++++++++
  # Ruminally undegradable protein (RUP aka UIP) 1x
  rum.fd.RUCP1x.conc <<- as.numeric(fds[, "RUP_1x"])
  rum.fd.RUCP1x.rate <<- (rum.fd.RUCP1x.conc/100) * anim.fd.CP.rate
  rum.diet.RUCP1x.rate <<- sum(rum.fd.RUCP1x.rate)
  rum.diet.RUCP1x.conc <<- isz(rum.diet.RUCP1x.rate * 100, anim.diet.DMI.rate)
  # Ruminally undegradable protein (RUP aka UIP) - Discounted Discounted RUP aka UIP (Tedeschi et al., 2005, Prof. Anim. Sci-
ent. 21:403-415)
  discount_coef <- vector(mode = "double", length = 8)
  discount_coef[1] <- 0
  discount_coef[2] <- 0
  discount_coef[3] <- 0
  discount_coef[4] <- 0
  discount_coef[5] <- -0.07
  discount_coef[6] <- 0.01
  discount_coef[7] <- 0.17
```

```
  discount_coef[8] <- 0.09
  rum.fd.RUCP.conc <<- ifelse(anim.fd.Forage.conc > 50, (0.167 + discount_coef[1]) + (1 + discount_coef[2]) *
                              rum.fd.RUCP1x.conc + (4.3 + discount_coef[3]) * dmi_factor + (-0.032 + discount_coef[4]) *
                              rum.fd.RUCP1x.conc * dmi_factor, (0.167 + discount_coef[5]) + (1 + discount_coef[6]) *
                              rum.fd.RUCP1x.conc + (4.3 + discount_coef[7]) * dmi_factor + (-0.032 + discount_coef[8]) *
                              rum.fd.RUCP1x.conc * dmi_factor)
  rum.fd.RUCP.rate <<- (rum.fd.RUCP.conc/100) * anim.fd.CP.rate
  rum.diet.RUCP.rate <<- sum(rum.fd.RUCP.rate)
  rum.diet.RUCP.conc <<- isz(rum.diet.RUCP.rate * 100, anim.diet.DMI.rate)
  # Ruminal bacteria protein The TDN used to compute the ruminal bacteria protein does not include TDN provided by fat supple-
ments (fat-supplement-free aTDN, FSFaTDN).
  # Hence, RNS uses the discounted apparent TDN for non-fat supplements (EE > 50%) RNS also removes negative FFaTDN
  anim.fd.FSFaTDN.rate <<- pmax(0, ifelse(anim.fd.EED.frac > 0 | anim.fd.EE.conc > 50, 0, (anim.fd.aTDN.conc/100) *
anim.fd.DMI.rate))
  anim.diet.FSFaTDN.rate <<- sum(anim.fd.FSFaTDN.rate)
  anim.diet.FSFaTDN.conc <<- isz(anim.diet.FSFaTDN.rate * 100, sum(ifelse(anim.fd.EED.frac > 0 | anim.fd.EE.conc > 50, 0,
anim.fd.DMI.rate)))
  # A more conservative approach is to remove the fat contribution of the discounted aTDN for feedstuffs with more than 3% EE
  anim.fd.FFaTDN.rate <<- pmax(0, ifelse(anim.fd.EE.conc > 3, anim.fd.aTDN.conc - anim.fd.dEE.conc, anim.fd.aTDN.conc)) *
anim.fd.DMI.rate/100
  anim.fd.FFaTDN.conc <<- ifelse(anim.fd.DMI.rate > 0, anim.fd.FFaTDN.rate * 100/anim.fd.DMI.rate, 0)
  anim.diet.FFaTDN.rate <<- sum(anim.fd.FFaTDN.rate)
  anim.diet.FFaTDN.conc <<- ifelse(anim.diet.DMI.rate > 0, anim.diet.FFaTDN.rate * 100/anim.diet.DMI.rate, 0)
  anim.diet.peNDF.conc <<- anim.diet.peNDF.rate * 100/anim.diet.DMI.rate
  if (anim.diet.peNDF.conc < 20)
  {
    peNDF_factor <<- 1 - 0.025 * (20 - anim.diet.peNDF.conc)
  } else peNDF_factor <- 1
  rum.fd.bact.CP.rate <<- Parm_rum.bact.CPY_L1 * anim.fd.FSFaTDN.rate * peNDF_factor
  rum.diet.bact.CP.rate <<- sum(rum.fd.bact.CP.rate)
  rum.fd.bact.CP.rate_FFaTDN <<- Parm_rum.bact.CPY_L1 * anim.fd.FFaTDN.rate * peNDF_factor
  rum.diet.bact.CP.rate_FFaTDN <<- sum(rum.fd.bact.CP.rate_FFaTDN)
  # Ruminal bacteria mass
  if (Parm_rum.bact.CP != 0)
    rum.fd.bact.rate <<- rum.fd.bact.CP.rate/(Parm_rum.bact.CP/100) else rum.fd.bact.rate <- 0
  rum.diet.bact.rate <<- sum(rum.fd.bact.rate)
  rum.fd.RUPID.conc <<- as.numeric(fds[, "RUPID"]) * 100
  rum.fd.RUPID.frac <<- rum.fd.RUPID.conc/100
  anim.fd.bact.MP.rate <<- Parm_rum.bact.TP_CP_L1 * Parm_rum.bact.IDTP_L1 * rum.fd.bact.CP.rate
  anim.fd.fd.MP.rate <<- rum.fd.RUPID.frac * rum.fd.RUCP.rate
  anim.fd.MP.rate <<- anim.fd.bact.MP.rate + anim.fd.fd.MP.rate
  anim.diet.bact.MP.rate <<- sum(anim.fd.bact.MP.rate)
  anim.diet.fd.MP.rate <<- sum(anim.fd.fd.MP.rate)
  anim.diet.MP.rate <<- sum(anim.fd.MP.rate)
  if (genRPT)
  {
    rptBioValues <- fds["FeedName.x"]
    names(rptBioValues) <- "FeedName"
    rptBioValues["RDP1x, g/d"] <- (anim.fd.CP.rate - rum.fd.RUCP1x.rate) * 1000
    rptBioValues["RDP1x, %CP"] <- isz((anim.fd.CP.rate - rum.fd.RUCP1x.rate) * 100, anim.fd.CP.rate)
    rptBioValues["RUP1x, g/d"] <- rum.fd.RUCP1x.rate * 1000
```

```
      rptBioValues["RUP1x, %CP"] <- isz(rum.fd.RUCP1x.rate * 100, anim.fd.CP.rate)
      rptBioValues["RDP, g/d"] <- (anim.fd.CP.rate - rum.fd.RUCP.rate) * 1000
      rptBioValues["RDP, %CP"] <- isz((anim.fd.CP.rate - rum.fd.RUCP.rate) * 100, anim.fd.CP.rate)
      rptBioValues["RUP, g/d"] <- rum.fd.RUCP.rate * 1000
      rptBioValues["RUP, %CP"] <- isz(rum.fd.RUCP.rate * 100, anim.fd.CP.rate)
      rptBioValues["MP Bact, g/d"] <- anim.fd.bact.MP.rate * 1000
      rptBioValues["MP Fd, g/d"] <- anim.fd.fd.MP.rate * 1000
      rptBioValues["MP, g/d"] <- anim.fd.MP.rate * 1000
      rptBioValues2 <- data.frame(FeedName = "Ration")
      rptBioValues2["RDP1x, g/d"] <- (anim.diet.CP.rate - rum.diet.RUCP1x.rate) * 1000
      rptBioValues2["RDP1x, %CP"] <- isz((anim.diet.CP.rate - rum.diet.RUCP1x.rate) * 100, anim.diet.CP.rate)
      rptBioValues2["RUP1x, g/d"] <- rum.diet.RUCP1x.rate * 1000
      rptBioValues2["RUP1x, %CP"] <- isz(rum.diet.RUCP1x.rate * 100, anim.diet.CP.rate)
      rptBioValues2["RDP, g/d"] <- (anim.diet.CP.rate - rum.diet.RUCP.rate) * 1000
      rptBioValues2["RDP, %CP"] <- isz((anim.diet.CP.rate - rum.diet.RUCP.rate) * 100, anim.diet.CP.rate)
      rptBioValues2["RUP, g/d"] <- rum.diet.RUCP.rate * 1000
      rptBioValues2["RUP, %CP"] <- isz(rum.diet.RUCP.rate * 100, anim.diet.CP.rate)
      rptBioValues2["MP Bact, g/d"] <- anim.diet.bact.MP.rate * 1000
      rptBioValues2["MP Fd, g/d"] <- anim.diet.fd.MP.rate * 1000
      rptBioValues2["MP, g/d"] <- anim.diet.MP.rate * 1000
      rptBioValues <- rbind(rptBioValues, rptBioValues2)
      description <- paste("# MP      = metabolizable protein\n",
                           "# RDP1x   = ruminally degraded protein (DIP: digestible intake protein)\n",
                           "# RUP1x   = ruminally undegradable protein (UIP: undegradable intake protein)\n",
                           "# FFaTDN  = fat-free apparent total digestible nutrients\n",
                           "# FSFaTDN = Fat-supplement-free apparent total digestible nutrients\n",
                           "# RDP    = discounted RDP at ", formatC(dmi_factor, format = "f", digits = 3, width = 7), "x DMI\n",
                           "# RUP    = discounted RUP at ", formatC(dmi_factor, format = "f", digits = 3, width = 7), "x DMI\n",
                           "# peNDF factor for bacteria adjustment of ", formatC(peNDF_factor * 100, format = "f", digits = 3, width = 7), "% \n\n",
                           "# Ration discounted apparent TDN, % DM                    : ", formatC(anim.diet.aTDN.conc, format = "f", digits = 3, width = 7), "\n",
                           "# Ration discounted apparent TDN, kg/d                    : ", formatC(anim.diet.aTDN.rate, format = "f", digits = 3, width = 7), "\n\n",
                           "# Ration discounted apparent fat-supplement-free TDN, % DM : ",
                           formatC(anim.diet.FSFaTDN.conc, format = "f", digits = 3, width = 7), "\n",
                           "# Ration discounted apparent fat-supplement-free TDN, kg/d : ", formatC(anim.diet.FSFaTDN.rate, format = "f", digits = 3, width = 7), "\n",
                           "# Ration bacteria crude protein (BCP) using FSFaTDN, g/d   : ", formatC(rum.diet.bact.CP.rate * 1000, format = "f", digits = 3, width = 7), "\n",
                           "# Ration bacteria MP using fat-supplement-free aTDN, g/d   : ", formatC(Parm_rum.bact.TP_CP_L1 * Parm_rum.bact.IDTP_L1 * rum.diet.bact.CP.rate * 1000, format = "f", digits = 3, width = 7), "\n\n",
                           "# Ration discounted apparent fat-free TDN, % DM           : ", formatC(anim.diet.FFaTDN.conc, format = "f", digits = 3, width = 7), "\n",
                           "# Ration discounted apparent fat-free TDN, kg/d           : ", formatC(anim.diet.FFaTDN.rate, format = "f", digits = 3, width = 7), "\n",
                           "# Ration bacteria crude protein (BCP) using FFaTDN, g/d    : ", formatC(rum.diet.bact.CP.rate_FFaTDN * 1000, format = "f", digits = 3, width = 7), "\n",
                           "# Ration bacteria MP using fat-free aTDN, g/d             : ", formatC(Parm_rum.bact.TP_CP_L1 * Parm_rum.bact.IDTP_L1 * rum.diet.bact.CP.rate_FFaTDN * 1000, format = "f", digits = 3, width = 7), "\n",
```

```
                         "# Bacteria MP difference between FSFaTDN and FFaTDN, g/d   : ", formatC(Parm_rum.bact.TP_CP_L1 *
Parm_rum.bact.IDTP_L1 * (rum.diet.bact.CP.rate - rum.diet.bact.CP.rate_FFaTDN) * 1000, format = "f", digits = 3, width = 7),
"\n\n", sep = "")
      report(rptBioValues, "Metabolizable Protein, RDP, and RUP", description, "", 3, 3, 1, 6, FALSE, FALSE, FALSE, FALSE,
FALSE, FALSE, TRUE)
    }
    # Digested Amino Acids - Feeds
    si.fd.GMet.rate <<- (fds[, "Met_RUP"]/100) * anim.fd.fd.MP.rate
    si.fd.GLys.rate <<- (fds[, "Lys_RUP"]/100) * anim.fd.fd.MP.rate
    si.fd.GArg.rate <<- (fds[, "Arg_RUP"]/100) * anim.fd.fd.MP.rate
    si.fd.GThr.rate <<- (fds[, "Thr_RUP"]/100) * anim.fd.fd.MP.rate
    si.fd.GLeu.rate <<- (fds[, "Leu_RUP"]/100) * anim.fd.fd.MP.rate
    si.fd.GIle.rate <<- (fds[, "Ile_RUP"]/100) * anim.fd.fd.MP.rate
    si.fd.GVal.rate <<- (fds[, "Val_RUP"]/100) * anim.fd.fd.MP.rate
    si.fd.GHis.rate <<- (fds[, "His_RUP"]/100) * anim.fd.fd.MP.rate
    si.fd.GPhe.rate <<- (fds[, "Phe_RUP"]/100) * anim.fd.fd.MP.rate
    si.fd.GTrp.rate <<- (fds[, "Trp_RUP"]/100) * anim.fd.fd.MP.rate
    si.diet.GMet.rate <<- sum(si.fd.GMet.rate)
    si.diet.GLys.rate <<- sum(si.fd.GLys.rate)
    si.diet.GArg.rate <<- sum(si.fd.GArg.rate)
    si.diet.GThr.rate <<- sum(si.fd.GThr.rate)
    si.diet.GLeu.rate <<- sum(si.fd.GLeu.rate)
    si.diet.GIle.rate <<- sum(si.fd.GIle.rate)
    si.diet.GVal.rate <<- sum(si.fd.GVal.rate)
    si.diet.GHis.rate <<- sum(si.fd.GHis.rate)
    si.diet.GPhe.rate <<- sum(si.fd.GPhe.rate)
    si.diet.GTrp.rate <<- sum(si.fd.GTrp.rate)
    if (genRPT)
    {
      rptIDAA_DMI <- fds["FeedName.x"]
      names(rptIDAA_DMI) <- "FeedName"
      rptIDAA_DMI["Met"] <- si.fd.GMet.rate
      rptIDAA_DMI["Lys"] <- si.fd.GLys.rate
      rptIDAA_DMI["Arg"] <- si.fd.GArg.rate
      rptIDAA_DMI["Thr"] <- si.fd.GThr.rate
      rptIDAA_DMI["Leu"] <- si.fd.GLeu.rate
      rptIDAA_DMI["Ile"] <- si.fd.GIle.rate
      rptIDAA_DMI["Val"] <- si.fd.GVal.rate
      rptIDAA_DMI["His"] <- si.fd.GHis.rate
      rptIDAA_DMI["Phe"] <- si.fd.GPhe.rate
      rptIDAA_DMI["Trp"] <- si.fd.GTrp.rate
      footnote <- "The Digested AA is also the Metabolizable AA."
      report(rptIDAA_DMI, "Metabolizable Feed Amino Acids, g/d", "", footnote, 3, 3, 1000, 7, TRUE, FALSE, TRUE, FALSE, TRUE,
FALSE, TRUE)
    }
    calcDIG(feeds3, genRPT)
    calcMethane()
  }
```

4 Level of Solution 2

4.1 Flowchart of the calculation logic

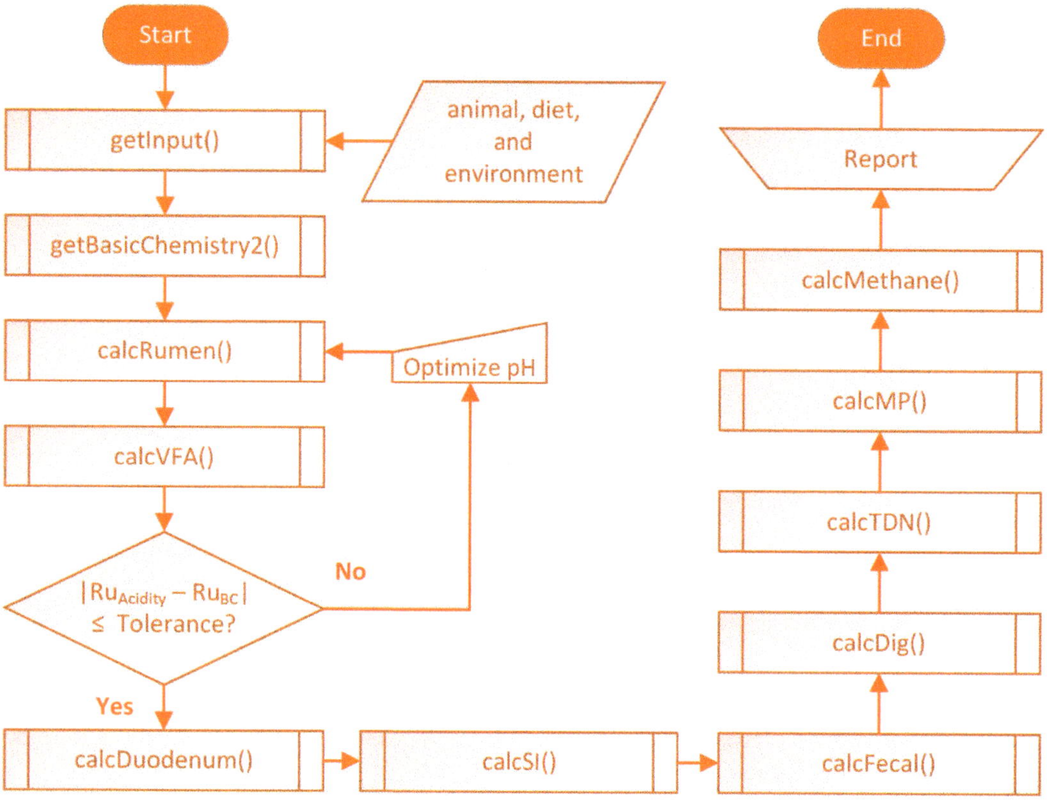

Figure 4.1. Flowchart of the calculation logic for the level of solution 2. The steps in the calcSolutionLevel2() function includes the calcRumen() to calcMethane() functions.

4.2 Equations

4.2.1 Carbohydrate and protein fractionation, fatty acids, minerals, and plant defensive compounds

#	Variable[1]	Description	Equation
1:	CHO_f	adjust for NPN = True	$100 - (Ash_f + EE_f + (CP_f - 0.01 * NPN_f * 0.01 * SP_f * CP_f) + \frac{0.01 * NPN_f * 0.01 * SP_f * CP_f}{6.25}$
2:		adjust for NPN = False	$100 - (Ash_f + EE_f + CP_f)$
3:	TDC_f		$TCT_f + Alkaloids_f + Terpenoids_f + ODC_f$
4:	NFC_f	sodium sulfite = T & adjust for TDC = T	$CHO_f - (NDF_f - 0.01 * CP_f * NDIP_f) - TDC_f$
5:		sodium sulfite = F & adjust for TDC = T	$CHO_f - NDF_f - TDC_f$
6:		adjust for TDC = T &	$CHO_f - (NDF_f - 0.01 * CP_f * NDIP_f)$

#	Variable[(1)]	Description	Equation
		adjust for TDC =F	
7:		adjust for TDC = F & adjust for TDC =F	$CHO_f - NDF_f$
8:	$CHOB2_f$		$NFC_f - (CHOA1_f + CHOA2_f + CHOA3_f + CHOA4_f + CHOB1_f)$
9:	$CHOB3_f$	sodium sulfite = T	$(NDF_f - 0.01 * CP_f * NDIP_f) - CHOC_f$
10:		sodium sulfite = F	$NDF_f - CHOC_f$
11:	$CHOC$	linear adjustment	$2.4 * Lignin_f$
12:		surface adjustment	$NDF_f - (NDF_f - Lignin_f) * \left(1 - \frac{Lignin_f}{NDF_f}\right)^{\frac{2}{3}}$
13:	$ProtB1_f$		$SP_f - ProtA_f$
14:	$ProtB2_f$		$CP_f - (ProtA_f + ProtB1_f + ProtB3_f + ProtC_f)$
15:	$ProtB3_f$		$NDIP_f - ADIP_f$
16:	$ProtC_f$		$ADIP_f$

(1) ***ADIP*** is acid detergent insoluble protein (also known as acid detergent insoluble nitrogen, ADIN), % DM; ***Alkaloids*** is total alkaloids, % DM; ***Ash*** is ash, % DM; ***CHO*** is carbohydrate, % DM; ***CHOA1*** is the sum of acetate, propionate, and butyrate, % DM; ***CHOA2*** is lactate, % DM; ***CHOA3*** is other organic acids, % DM; ***CHOA4*** is sugars, % DM; ***CHOB1*** is starch, % DM; ***CHOB2*** is soluble fiber, % DM; ***CHOB3*** is available neutral detergent fiber, % DM; ***CHOC*** is unavailable carbohydrate, % DM; ***CP*** is crude protein, % DM; ***EE*** is ether extract (fat), % DM; ***f*** is the fth feed in the diet; ***Lignin*** is lignin, % DM; *NDF* is neutral detergent fiber, % DM; ***NDIP*** is neutral detergent insoluble protein (also known as neutral detergent insoluble nitrogen, NDIN), % CP; ***NFC*** is nonfiber carbohydrate, % DM; ***NPN*** is nonprotein nitrogen, % SP; ***ODC*** is other defensive chemicals, % DM; ***ProtA*** is nonprotein nitrogen, % DM; ***ProtB1*** is true protein with fast rate of degradation, % DM; ***ProtB2*** is true protein with medium rate of degradation, % DM; ***ProtB3*** is true protein with slow rate of degradation, % DM; ***ProtC*** is unavailable protein, % DM; ***SP*** is soluble protein, % CP; ***TCT*** is total condensed tannins, % DM; ***TDC*** is total defensive chemicals, % DM; and ***Terpenoids*** is total terpenoids, % DM.

4.2.2 Rumen volume and area: calcRumenVolume() and calcRumenArea()

#	Variable[(1)]	Description	Equation
1:	Vr		$0.0888 * FBW^{1.034}$
2:	Ar	NDF>32	$4.836 * \left(\frac{Vr}{1000}\right)^{\frac{2}{3}}$
3:		NDF≤32	$4.836 * \left(\frac{Vr}{1000}\right)^{\frac{2}{3}} * (3 - 0.062 * NDF)$

(1) ***Ar*** is rumen surface area, m[2]; ***FBW*** is full body weight, kg; ***NDF*** is neutral detergent fiber, % DM; ***Vr*** is rumen volume, liters.

4.2.3 Empirical ruminal pH: calcRumenpH()

#	Variable[(1)]	Description	Equation
1:	pH	broken-line & peNDF≥24.5	6.46
2:		broken-line & peNDF<24.5	$5.425 + 0.04229 * peNDF$
3:		continuous	$\left(1 - \frac{5.418454 + 4.26014 * 0.01 * peNDF}{1 + Exp(-282.77726 * (0.01 * peNDF - 0.2429614))}\right) + \left(\frac{6.459806}{1 + Exp(-282.77726 * (0.01 * peNDF - 0.2429614))}\right)$

(1) ***peNDF*** is physically effective neutral detergent fiber, % DM.

4.2.4 Carbohydrate B3 kd adjustment for ruminal pH: calcCHOB3_kdAdjustment()

#	Variable[(1)]	Description[(2)]	Equation
1:	Y_1'	pH < 5.7	0
2:	Kd_{CB3}'	pH < 5.7	0
3:	Y_1	5.7 < pH < 6.05	$\frac{1}{\frac{km_1}{kd_{CB3} - km_1 * Yg_1} + \frac{1}{Yg_1}}$
4:	Km_1'	5.7 < pH < 6.05	$0.1409 - 0.0135 * pH$
5:	Yg_1'	5.7 < pH < 6.05	$0.0752 * pH - 0.1058$
6:	$RelY$	5.7 < pH < 6.05	$\frac{1 - Exp(-5.624 * (pH - 5.7)^{0.909})}{0.9968}$
7:	Y_1'	5.7 < pH < 6.05	$RelY * Y_1$
8:	Kd_{CB3}'	5.7 < pH < 6.05	$Min\left[kd_{CB3}, \left(\frac{km_1' * Y_1' * Yg_1'}{Yg_1' - Y_1'} + km_1' * Yg_1'\right)\right]$
9:	Y_1'	pH ≥ 6.05	$\frac{1}{\frac{km_1}{kd_{CB3} - km_1 * Yg_1} + \frac{1}{Yg_1}}$
10:	Kd_{CB3}'	pH ≥ 6.05	kd_{CB3}
11:	Kd_{CB3}'	pH < 5.4	0
12:	Kd_{CB3}'	5.4 < pH < 6.6	$Min[kd_{CB3}, kd_{CB3} * (1 - 0.7282 * (6.6 - pH))]$
13:	Kd_{CB3}'	pH > 6.6	kd_{CB3}
14:	Km_1'	all pH values	$0.1409 - 0.0135 * pH$
15:	Yg_1'	all pH values	$0.0752 * pH - 0.1058$
16:	y'	all pH values	$\frac{1 - Exp(-5.624 * (pH - 5.7))}{0.9968}$
17:	g'	all pH values	$\frac{1}{1 + Exp(-8.9094 * (pH - 5.5832))}$
18:	h'	all pH values	$\frac{1}{1 + Exp(-20 * (pH - 5.6988))}$
19:	$RelY$	all pH values	$h' * ((1 - g') + (y' * g'))$
20:	Y_1	all pH values	$\frac{1}{\frac{km_1}{kd_{CB3} - km_1 * Yg_1} + \frac{1}{Yg_1}}$
21:	Y_1'	all pH values	$RelY * Y_1$
22:	Kd_{CHOB3}'	all pH values	$Min\left[kd_{CHOB3}, \frac{1}{1 + Exp(-35 * (pH - 5.6992))} * \left(\frac{km_1' * Y_1' * Yg_1'}{Yg_1' - Y_1'} + km_1' * Yg_1'\right)\right]$

(1) ***kd_{CB3}*** is fractional degradation rate of carbohydrate fraction B3 (available fiber), 1/h; ***kd_{CB3}'*** is the adjusted kd_{CB3}, 1/h; ***Km_1*** is maintenance coefficient for fiber carbohydrate-degrading bacteria, g/(g·h); ***Y_1*** is fiber carbohydrate-degrading bacteria yield, g/d; ***Y_1'*** is the adjusted Y_1, g/d; and ***Yg_1*** is yield of fiber carbohydrate-degrading bacteria for growth, g/g.

(2) Equations 1 to 10 are based on Fox et al. (2004), Equations 11 to 13 are based on Mouriño et al. (2001), and Equations 14 to 22 are based on Boston et al. (2000). Figure 4.2 compares these approaches and Figure 4.4 shows the impact of ruminal pH on the bacteria yield.

4.2.5 Ruminal passage rate: calcPassageRate()

#	Variable[(1)]	Description[(2)]	Equation
1:	Af_{Forage}	adjust for peNDF = T	$\frac{100}{peNDF + 70}$
2:		adjust for peNDF = F	1
3:	Af_{Conc}	adjust for peNDF = T	$\frac{100}{peNDF + 90}$
4:		adjust for peNDF = F	1
5:	kp_{Forage}	cattle	$Af_{Forage} * \left(0.38 + \left(\frac{0.022 * DMI * 1000}{FBW^{0.75}}\right) + 2 * Forage^2\right)$
6:	kp_{conc}	cattle	$Af_{Conc} * (-0.424 + 1.45 * kg_{Forage})$
7:	Kp_{Liquid}	cattle	$4.413 + \frac{0.191 * DMI * 1000}{FBW}$

#	Variable[(1)]	Description[(2)]	Equation
8:	kp_{Forage}	cattle	$2.365 + \frac{0.0214 * Forage * DMI * 1000}{FBW} + \frac{0.0734 * Concentrate * DMI * 1000}{FBW} + 0.069 * Forage * DMI$
9:	kp_{conc}	cattle	$1.169 + \frac{0.1375 * Forage * DMI * 1000}{FBW} + \frac{0.1721 * Concentrate * DMI * 1000}{FBW}$
10:	Kp_{Liquid}	cattle	$4.524 + \frac{0.0223 * Forage * DMI * 1000}{FBW} + \frac{0.2046 * Concentrate * DMI * 1000}{FBW} + 0.344 * Forage * DMI$
11:	kp_{Forage}	sheep	$1.821 * \left(\frac{NDFI * 1000}{FBW}\right)^{0.399} * Exp(0.046 * CP)$
12:	kp_{conc}	sheep	$1.572 * kp_{Forage} - 0.925$
13:	Kp_{Liquid}	sheep	$0.976 * kp_{Conc} + 3.516$
14:	kp_{Forage}	goats	$1.29 + 0.161 * \left(\frac{NDFI * 1000}{FBW}\right)^{1.503} * Exp(0.022 * FBW - 0.0375 * NDF)$
15:	kp_{conc}	goats	$1.572 * kp_{Forage} - 0.925$
16:	Kp_{Liquid}	goats	$0.976 * kp_{Conc} + 3.516$

(1) ***Concentrate*** is the fraction of dietary concentrate; ***CP*** is crude protein, %DM; ***DMI*** is dry matter intake, kg/d; ***FBW*** is full body weight, kg; ***Forage*** is the fraction of dietary forage; $\boldsymbol{kp_{Conc}}$ is fractional passage rate of concentrate, %/h; $\boldsymbol{kp_{Forage}}$ is fractional passage rate of forage, %/h; $\boldsymbol{kp_{Liquid}}$ is fractional passage rate of liquid, %/h; ***NDF*** is neutral detergent fiber, %DM; ***NDFI*** is NDF intake, kg/d; and ***peNDF*** is physically effective NDF, %DM.
(2) Equations 1 to 7 are based on Fox et al. (2004), Equations 8 to 10 are based on Seo et al. (2006), Equations 11 to 13 are based on Cannas and Van Soest (2000), and Equations 14 to 16 are based on Tedeschi et al. (2012).

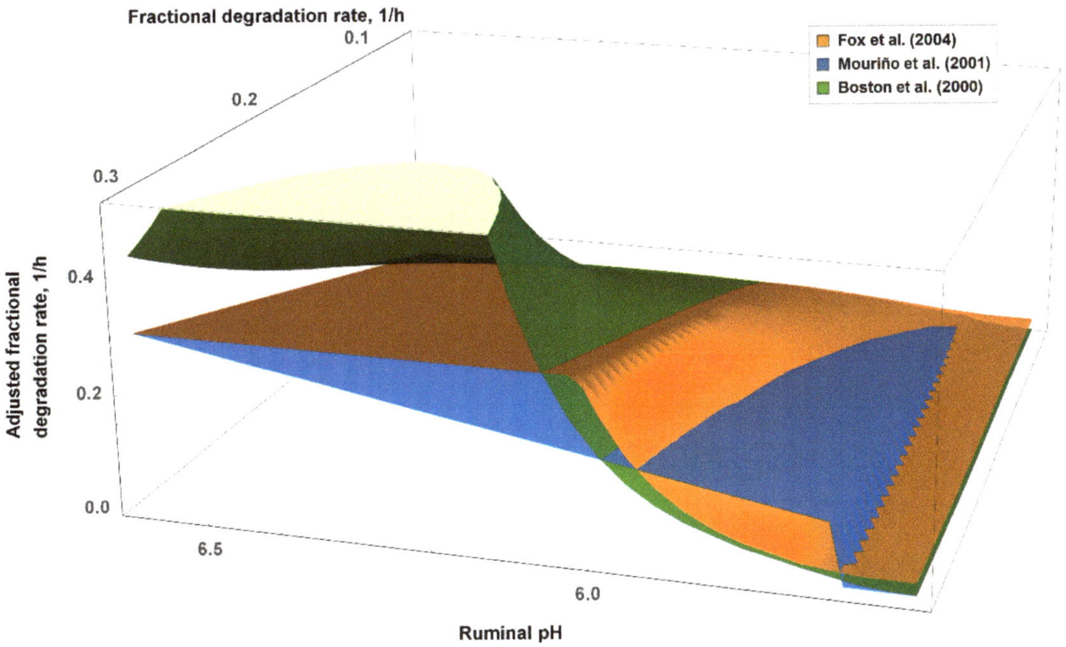

Figure 4.2. Adjusted fractional degradation rate for CHO B3 (1/h) using different approaches. When the CPM Dairy's (Boston et al., 2000) approach (green surface) is used uncapped, it shows that adjusted values (kd_{CB3}') can incorrectly become greater than original values (kd_{CB3}). The kd_{CB3} must be equal to or greater than the kd_{CB3}' (i.e., $kd_{CB3} \geq kd_{CB3}'$).

4.2.6 Bacteria yield, maximum yield, and yield improvement: calcBacteriaY(), calcBacteriaYg(), calcBacteriaYieldImprovement()

#	Variable[(1)]	Description[(2)]	Equation
1:	Yg_2'	peNDF<20	$Yg_2 * (1 - (20 - peNDF) * 0.025)$
2:		otherwise	Yg_2

#	Variable[1]	Description[2]	Equation
3:	*Yg₂'*		$Yg_2 * \left(1 - \frac{1}{1 + Exp(-100 * (0.01 * peNDF - 0.1965127))}\right) * (1 - (0.2036872 - 0.01 * peNDF) * 2.390715) + \frac{1}{1 + Exp(-100 * (0.01 * peNDF - 0.1965127))}$
4:	*Y*	kd≠0 & Yg≠0	$\frac{1}{\frac{km}{kd} + \frac{1}{Yg}}$
5:	*ratio*		$\frac{RDPep}{RDPep + RDCA4 + RDCB1 + RDCB2}$
6:	*imp*		$Min\,[1.187, 0.01 * (1 + Exp(0.404 * Ln(ratio * 100) + 1.942))]$

[1] ***imp*** is improvement of yield of nonfiber-degrading bacteria; ***kd*** is fractional degradation rate, 1/h; ***km*** is maintenance coefficient, g/(g·h); ***peNDF*** is physically effective neutral detergent fiber, %DM; ***ratio*** is the ratio between ruminally degraded peptides to ruminally degraded peptides and nonfiber carbohydrates; ***RDCA4*** is ruminally degraded carbohydrate A4 (sugars), g/d; ***RDCB1*** is ruminally degraded carbohydrate B1 (starch), g/d; ***RDCB2*** is ruminally degraded carbohydrate B2 (pectin), g/d; ***RDPB1*** is ruminally degraded protein B1, g/d; ***RDPB2*** is ruminally degraded protein B2, g/d; ***RDPB3*** is ruminally degraded protein B3, g/d; ***RDPep*** is ruminally degraded peptides, g/d; ***Y*** is the yield of bacteria, g/g; and ***Yg₂'*** is the adjusted yield of nonfiber-degrading bacteria for growth, g/g.

[2] Equations 1 and 2 are based on Fox et al. (2004) and Equation 3 is based on Boston et al. (2000). Figure 4.4 depicts these equations.

4.2.7 Bacteria peptide uptake: calcPeptideUptake()

#	Variable[1]	Description[2]	Equation
1:	*kup*	ionophore = T	$0.07 * \frac{2}{3}$
2:		ionophore = F	0.07
3:	*kLG*		$\frac{100}{100 - kp_{Liquid}}$
4:	*AmtBact* $AmtBact_{NFC}$		$\frac{NFCBact}{kp_{Forage} * \frac{24}{100}}$
5:	*PepUptake*		$AmtBact_{NFC} * kup$
6:	$PepUp_{Factor}$		$\frac{Ln\left(1 + \frac{\frac{kLG - 1}{3600} * \frac{RDPep}{24}}{\frac{PepUptake}{3600}}\right)}{\frac{Ln\left(1 + \frac{kLG - 1}{3600}\right)}{3600}}$
7:	*PepUptake'*		$Min[PepUp_{Factor} * PepUptake * 24, RDPep]$
8:		Forage≤10%	$0.0282 * (1 - 0.43)$
9:	*kup*	Forage>10% & ionophore=T	$0.0282 * (1 - 0.35)$
10:		otherwise	0.0282
11:	$AmtBact_{NFC}$		$\frac{NFCBact}{kp_{Forage} * \frac{24}{100}}$
12:	*PepUptake*		$AmtBact_{NFC} * kup$
13:	*PepUptake'*		$Min[PepUptake * 24, RDPep]$

[1] $\boldsymbol{AmtBact_{NFC}}$ is the nonfiber carbohydrate-degrading bacteria mass in the rumen, g; ***NFCBact*** is the nonfiber carbohydrate-degrading bacteria in the rumen, g/d; ***Forage*** is forage in the diet, %; ***kLG*** is growth time, h; $\boldsymbol{kp_{Forage}}$ is fractional passage rate of forage, %/h; $\boldsymbol{kp_{Liquid}}$ is fractional passage rate of liquid, %/h; ***kup*** is peptide uptake rate, g/(g·h); ***PepUptake*** is the peptide update, g/h; and $\boldsymbol{PepUp_{Factor}}$ is the peptide update adjustment factor, dimensionless.

[2] Equations 1 to 7 are based on Fox et al. (2004), and Equations 8 to 13 do not take into account the peptide update adjustment factor, and it uses a simple linear relationship between *kup* and $AmtBact_{NDF}$. Figure 4.3 depicts these equations.

Figure 4.3 compares the bacteria peptide uptake submodels. The original submodel in Figure 4.3A is based on Fox et al. (2004), and it uses an adjustment factor to scale up or down the effective peptide uptake

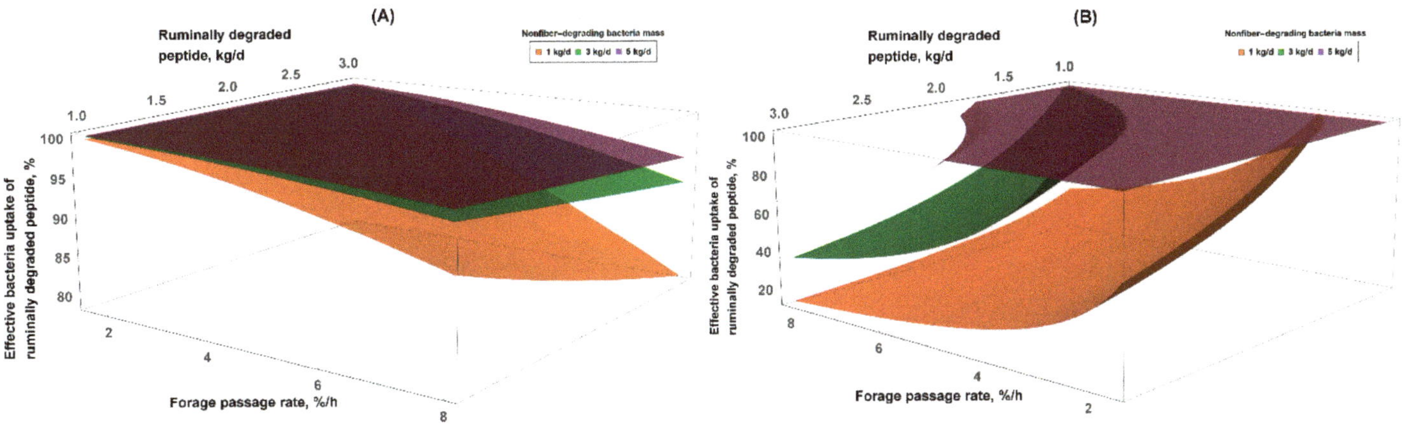

Figure 4.3. Comparison of bacteria peptide uptake models. (A) is based on Fox et al. (2004) and (B) is based on a linear relationship between nonfiber carbohydrate-degrading bacteria mass and peptide uptake rate. The liquid passage rate is a function of the forage passage rate.

rate. The adjustment factor uses the number of periods for a loan or investment equation. Although its use may be confusing, it provides a much greater effective peptide uptake rate than the submodel in Figure 4.3B that is based on a simple linear relationship between nonfiber-degrading bacteria mass and peptide uptake rate (0.0282 g/(g·h)). The effective peptide uptake rate predicted with the submodel B can go as low as 20% of the amount of ruminally degraded peptides, suggesting that the 0.0282 g/(g·h) fractional rate might be too slow or the user-inputted fractional degradation rate of protein is disconnected from the growth of the nonfiber-degrading bacteria in the rumen. Regardless of the submodel, Figure 4.3 correctly indicates that the effective peptide uptake rate is reduced when the growth rate of the nonfiber-degrading bacteria is decreased likely due to an increase in the fractional passage rate of forages.

4.2.8 Rumen submodel: calcRumen()

4.2.8.1 Carbohydrate and protein degradation, and lipid lipolyzis

#	Variable[1]	Description	Equation
1:	TFA_f		$FAC12_f + FAC14_f + FAC16_f + FAC16{:}1_f + FAC18_f + FAC18{:}1c_f + FAC18{:}1t_f + FAC18{:}2_f + FAC18{:}3_f + FAOther_f$
2:	$Klip_{Adj,f}$		$klip_f * e^{\left(-klip_{AdjFactor,f} * \frac{TFA_f}{DMI}\right)}$
3:	$Prop_f^{Glyc}$		$Glycerol_f * \left(\frac{klip_f}{klip_f + kp_{Liquid,f}}\right)$
4:	pH	peNDF-based pH	***calcRumenpH_peNDF()***
5:	$kd_{CB3,f}$	pH-adjusted kdCB3	***calcCHOB3_kgAdjustment()***
6:	Kp_f	kp_{Forage}, kp, and kp_{Liquid}	***calcPassageRate()***
7:	$RDCA1_f$	carbohydrates	$(Prop_f^{Glyc} + CA1_f) * \left(\frac{kd_{CA1,f}}{kd_{CA1,f} + kp_f}\right)$
8:	$RDCA2_f$	carbohydrates	$CA2_f * \left(\frac{kd_{CA2,f}}{kd_{CA2,f} + kp_f}\right)$
9:	$RDCA3_f$	carbohydrates	$CA3_f * \left(\frac{kd_{CA3,f}}{kd_{CA3,f} + kp_f}\right)$
10:	$RDCA4_f$	carbohydrates	$CA4_f * \left(\frac{kd_{CA4,f}}{kd_{CA4,f} + kp_f}\right)$
11:	$RDCB1_f$	carbohydrates	$CB1_f * \left(\frac{kd_{CB1,f}}{kd_{CB1,f} + kp_f}\right)$

#	Variable[(1)]	Description	Equation
12:	$RDCB2_f$	carbohydrates	$CB2_f * \left(\frac{kd_{CB2,f}}{kd_{CB2,f} + kp_f}\right)$
13:	$RDCB3_f$	carbohydrates	$CB3_f * \left(\frac{kd_{CB3,f}}{kd_{CB3,f} + kp_f}\right)$
14:	$RDPA_f$	proteins	$PA_f * \left(\frac{kd_{PA,f}}{kd_{PA,f} + kp_f}\right)$
15:	$RDPB1_f$	proteins	$PB1_f * \left(\frac{kd_{PB1}}{kd_{PB1,f} + kp_f}\right)$
16:	$RDPB2_f$	proteins	$PB2_f * \left(\frac{kd_{PB2,f}}{kd_{PB2,f} + kp_f}\right)$
17:	$RDPB3_f$	proteins	$PB3_f * \left(\frac{kd_{PB3,f}}{kd_{PB3,f} + kp_f}\right)$
18:	$RDPep_f$	proteins	$RDPB1_f + RDPB2_f + RDPB3_f$
19:	RDP_f	proteins	$RDPA_f + RDPep_f$
20:	FOM_f	organic matter	$RDCA4_f + RDCB1_f + RDCB2_f + RDCB3_f$
21:	$LFAC12_f$	fatty acids	$FAC12_f * \left(\frac{klip_{Adj,f}}{klip_{Adj,f} + kp_f}\right)$
22:	$LFAC14_f$	fatty acids	$FAC14_f * \left(\frac{klip_{Adj,f}}{klip_{Adj,f} + kp_f}\right)$
23:	$LFAC16_f$	fatty acids	$FAC16_f * \left(\frac{klip_{Adj,f}}{klip_{Adj,f} + kp_f}\right)$
24:	$LFAC16{:}1_f$	fatty acids	$FAC16{:}1_f * \left(\frac{klip_{Adj,f}}{klip_{Adj,f} + kp_f}\right)$
25:	$LFAC18_f$	fatty acids	$FAC18_f * \left(\frac{klip_{Adj,f}}{klip_{Adj,f} + kp_f}\right)$
26:	$LFAC18{:}1c_f$	fatty acids	$FAC18{:}1c_f * \left(\frac{klip_{Adj,f}}{klip_{Adj,f} + kp_f}\right)$
27:	$LFAC18{:}1t_f$	fatty acids	$FAC18{:}1t_f * \left(\frac{klip_{Adj,f}}{klip_{Adj,f} + kp_f}\right)$
28:	$LFAC18{:}2_f$	fatty acids	$FAC18{:}2_f * \left(\frac{klip_{Adj,f}}{klip_{Adj,f} + kp_f}\right)$
29:	$LFAC18{:}3_f$	fatty acids	$FAC18{:}3_f * \left(\frac{klip_{Adj,f}}{klip_{Adj,f} + kp_f}\right)$
30:	$LFAOther_f$	fatty acids	$FAOther_f * \left(\frac{klip_{Adj,f}}{klip_{Adj,f} + kp_f}\right)$

[(1)] ***CA1*** is carbohydrate fraction A1 (volatile fatty acids: acetate, propionate, and butyrate), g/d; ***CA2*** is carbohydrate fraction A2 (lactate), g/d; ***CA3*** is carbohydrate fraction A3 (other organic acids, e.g., citrate, malate, fumarate), g/d; ***CA4*** is carbohydrate fraction A4 (sugars), g/d; ***CB1*** is carbohydrate fraction B1 (starch), g/d; ***CB2*** is carbohydrate fraction B2 (pectin), g/d; ***CB3*** is carbohydrate fraction B3 (available fiber), g/d; ***DMI*** is dry matter intake, kg/d; *f* is the fth feed in the diet; ***FAC12*** is long-chain fatty acid C12 (lauric acid), g/d; ***FAC14*** is long-chain fatty acid C14 (myristic acid), g/d; ***FAC16*** is long-chain fatty acid C16 (palmitic acid), g/d; ***FAC16:1*** is long-chain fatty acid C16:1 (palmitoleic acid), g/d; ***FAC18*** is long-chain fatty acid C18 (stearic acid), g/d; ***FAC18:1c*** is long-chain fatty acid C18:1c (oleic acid), g/d; ***FAC18:1t*** is long-chain fatty acid C18:1t (elaidic and vaccenic acids), g/d; ***FAC18:2*** is long-chain fatty acid C18:2 (linoleic acid), g/d; ***FAC18:3*** is long-chain fatty acid C18:3 (linolenic acid), g/d; ***FAOther*** is other long-chain fatty acids, g/d; ***FOM*** is fermentable organic matter; g/d; ***Glycerol*** is the glycerol intake, g/d; $Kd_{CA1,CA2,CA3,CA4,CB1,CB2,CB3}$ is fractional degradation rate for CA1, CA2, CA3, CA4, CB1, CB2, and CB3, %/h; $Kd_{PA,PB1,PB2,PB3}$ is fractional degradation rate for PA, PB1, PB2, and PB3, %/h; ***klip*** is the fractional lipolisis rate, %/h; $klip_{Adj}$ is the fractional lipolisis rate adjusted for tofal fatty acids, %/h; $klip_{AdjFactor}$ is the adjustment factor for the fractional lipolisis rate; ***kp*** is frational passage rate either inputted by the user or associated with kp for concentrate or kp for forage, %/h; ***LFAC12*** is lipolyzed FAC12, g/d; ***LFAC14*** is lipolyzed FAC14, g/d; ***LFAC16*** is lipolyzed FAC16, g/d; ***LFAC16:1*** is lipolyzed FAC16:1, g/d; ***LFAC18*** is lipolyzed FAC18, g/d; ***LFAC18:1c*** is lipolyzed FAC18:1c, g/d; ***LFAC18:1t*** is lipolyzed FAC18:1t, g/d; ***LFAC18:2*** is lipolyzed FAC18:2, g/d; ***LFAC18:3*** is lipolyzed FAC18:3, g/d; ***LFAOther*** is lipolyzed FAOther, g/d; **PA** is protein fraction A, g/d; ***PB1*** is protein fraction B1, g/d; ***PB2*** is protein fraction B2, g/d; ***PB3*** is protein fraction B3, g/d; $Prop^{Glyc}$ is the propionate produced from the ruminal fermentation of lipolized glycerol, g/d; ***RDCA1*** is ruminally degraded carbohydrate fraction A1, g/d; ***RDCA2*** is ruminally degraded carbohydrate fraction A2, g/d; ***RDCA3*** is ruminally degraded carbohydrate fraction A3, g/d; ***RDCA4*** is ruminally degraded carbohydrate fraction A4, g/d; ***RDCB1*** is ruminally degraded carbohydrate fraction B1, g/d; ***RDCB2*** is ruminally degraded carbohydrate fraction B2, g/d; ***RDCB3*** is ruminally degraded carbohydrate fraction B3, g/d; ***RDP*** is ruminally degraded protein, g/d; ***RDPA*** is ruminally degraded protein fraction A, g/d; ***RDPB1*** is ruminally degraded protein fraction B1, g/d; ***RDPB2*** is ruminally degraded protein fraction B2, g/d; ***RDPB3*** is ruminally degraded protein fraction B3, g/d; ***RDPep*** is ruminally degraded peptides (RDPB1, RDPB2, and RDPB3), g/d; and ***TFA*** is total fatty acids, g/d.

4.2.8.2 Bacteria growth model

#	Variable[1]	Description	Equation
1:	$Yg_2{}'_f$	peNDF-adjusted maximum yield	***calcBacteriaYg()***
2:	*Imp*	peptide-improved bacteria yield	***calcBacteriaYieldImprovement()***
3:	$CA1Y_f$	bacterial growth	$\frac{1}{\frac{km2_f}{kd_{CA1,f}}+\frac{1}{Yg'_{2,f}}}*imp$
4:	$CA2Y_f$	bacterial growth	$\frac{1}{\frac{km2_f}{kd_{CA2,f}}+\frac{1}{Yg'_{2,f}}}*imp$
5:	$CA3Y_f$	bacterial growth	$\frac{1}{\frac{km2_f}{kd_{CA3,f}}+\frac{1}{Yg'_{2,f}}}*imp$
6:	$CA4Y_f$	bacterial growth	$\frac{1}{\frac{km2_f}{kd_{CA4,f}}+\frac{1}{Yg'_{2,f}}}*imp$
7:	$CB1Y_f$	bacterial growth	$\frac{1}{\frac{km2_f}{kd_{CB1,f}}+\frac{1}{Yg'_{2,f}}}*imp$
8:	$CB2Y_f$	bacterial growth	$\frac{1}{\frac{km2_f}{kd_{CB2,f}}+\frac{1}{Yg'_{2,f}}}*imp$
9:	$CB3Y_f$	bacterial growth	$\frac{1}{\frac{km1_f}{kd_{CB3,f}}+\frac{1}{Yg_{1,f}}}$
10:	$NFCBactA1_f$	bacterial growth	$CA1Y_f * RDCA1_f$
11:	$NFCBactA2_f$	bacterial growth	$CA2Y_f * RDCA2_f$
12:	$NFCBactA3_f$	bacterial growth	$CA3Y_f * RDCA3_f$
13:	$NFCBactA4_f$	bacterial growth	$CA4Y_f * RDCA4_f$
14:	$NFCBactB1_f$	bacterial growth	$CB1Y_f * RDCB1_f$
15:	$NFCBactB2_f$	bacterial growth	$CB2Y_f * RDCB2_f$
16:	$FCBactB3_f$	bacterial growth	$CB3Y_f * RDCB3_f$
17:	$NFCBact_f$	bacterial growth	$NFCBactA1_f + NFCBactA2_f + NFCBactA3_f + NFCBactA4_f + NFCBactB1_f + NFCBactB2_f$
18:	$FCBact_f$	bacterial growth	$FCBactB3_f$
19:	*PepUptake*	peptide uptake	***calcPeptideUpdate()***
20:	$RDPB1'_f$	peptide uptake	$PepUptake * \frac{RDPB1_f}{RDP}$
21:	$RDPB2'_f$	peptide uptake	$PepUptake * \frac{RDPB2_f}{RDP}$
22:	$RDPB3'_f$	peptide uptake	$PepUptake * \frac{RDPB3_f}{RDP}$
23:	$RDPep'_f$	peptide uptake	$RDPB1'_f + RDPB2'_f + RDPB3'_f$
24:	RDP'_f	peptide uptake	$RDPA_f + RDPep'_f$
25:	$AminoN_{NFC}$	ruminal N balance	$\left(\frac{2}{3}\right) * \left(\frac{62.5}{6.25}\right) * NFCBact$
26:	$AmmoniaN_{NFC}$	ruminal N balance	$\left(\frac{1}{3}\right) * \left(\frac{62.5}{6.25}\right) * NFCBact$
27:	$\Delta AminoN$	ruminal N balance	$\frac{PepUptake}{6.25} - AminoN_{NFC}$
28:	*SurplusN*	ruminal N balance	$Max[0, \Delta AminoN]$
29:	*RecycledN*	ruminal N balance: option 1, or	$Max\left[0{,}0.01*(121.7-12.01*CP+0.3235*CP^2)*\left(0.01*CP*\frac{DMI}{6.25}\right)\right]$
30:		ruminal N balance: option 2	$Max\left[0,(-0.1113+0.966*e^{(-0.0616*CP)})*\frac{1.192*CP*DMI-11.98}{1000}\right]$
31:	$\Delta AmmoniaN$	ruminal N balance	$\left(SurplusN+\frac{RDPA}{6.25}+RecycledN\right) - AmmoniaN_{NFC}$

#	Variable[(1)]	Description	Equation
32:	$AmmoniaN_{FC}$	ruminal N balance	$\left(\frac{62.5}{6.25}\right) * FCBact$
33:	$\Delta RuminalN$	ruminal N balance	$\left(\frac{PepUptake}{6.25} + \frac{RDPA}{6.25} + RecycledN\right) - (AminoN_{NFC} + AmmoniaN_{NFC} + AmmoniaN_{FC})$
34:	$EAFCB_f$	ΔRuminalN<0	$FCBact_f$
35:	$EANFCB_f$	ΔRuminalN<0	$NFCBact_f$
36:	EAB_f	ΔRuminalN<0	$\frac{EAFCB_f + EANFCB_f}{\sum_{f=1}^{nf}(FCBact_f + NFCBact_f)}$
37:	NAB_f	ΔRuminalN<0	$\left(\frac{PepUptake + RDPA + 6.25 * RecycledN}{0.625}\right) * EAB_f$
38:	$NABR_f$	ΔRuminalN<0	$Max[0, EAFCB_f + EANFCB_f - NAB_f]$
39:	$NAFCBR_f$	ΔRuminalN<0	$NABR_f * \left(\frac{EAFCB_f}{EAFCB_f + EANFCB_f}\right)$
40:	$NANFCBR_f$	ΔRuminalN<0	$NABR_f * \left(\frac{EANFCB_f}{EAFCB_F + EANFCB_f}\right)$
41:	$NAFCB_f$	ΔRuminalN<0	$EAFCB_f - NAFCBR_f$
42:	$NANFCB_f$	ΔRuminalN<0	$EANFCB_f - NANFCBR_f$
43:	$NARDCB3R_f$	ΔRuminalN<0	$\frac{NAFCBR_f}{CB3Y_f}$
44:	$NARDCB3_f$	ΔRuminalN<0	$RDCB3_f - NARDCB3R_f$
45:	$Bact_{Leu}$	ruminal BCAA balance	$0.625 * 0.8 * \left(\frac{7.51 * 75 + 5.9 * 25}{100}\right) * \sum_{f=1}^{nf}(0.05 * NANFCB_f + NAFCB_f)$
46:	$Bact_{Ile}$	ruminal BCAA balance	$0.625 * 0.8 * \left(\frac{5.88 * 75 + 4 * 25}{100}\right) * \sum_{f=1}^{nf}(0.05 * NANFCB_f + NAFCB_f)$
47:	$Bact_{Val}$	ruminal BCAA balance	$0.625 * 0.8 * \left(\frac{6.16 * 75 + 4.7 * 25}{100}\right) * \sum_{f=1}^{nf}(0.05 * NANFCB_f + NAFCB_f)$
48:	$RecycledBact_{Leu}$	ruminal BCAA balance	$0.625 * 0.8 * \left(\frac{7.51 * 75 + 5.9 * 25}{100}\right) * \frac{0.2 * 0.6 * (\sum_{f=1}^{nf}(NANFCB_f + NAFCB_f))}{1 - 0.2}$
49:	$RecycledBact_{Ile}$	ruminal BCAA balance	$0.625 * 0.8 * \left(\frac{5.88 * 75 + 4 * 25}{100}\right) * \frac{0.2 * 0.6 * (\sum_{f=1}^{nf}(NANFCB_f + NAFCB_f))}{1 - 0.2}$
50:	$RecycledBact_{Val}$	ruminal BCAA balance	$0.625 * 0.8 * \left(\frac{6.16 * 75 + 4.7 * 25}{100}\right) * \frac{0.2 * 0.6 * (\sum_{f=1}^{nf}(NANFCB_f + NAFCB_f))}{1 - 0.2}$
51:	$BCAA_{Leu}$	ruminal BCAA balance	$RecycledBact_{Leu} + 0.6 * Leu * \sum_{f=1}^{nf} RDPep'_f$
52:	$BCAA_{Ile}$	ruminal BCAA balance	$RecycledBact_{Ile} + 0.6 * Ile * \sum_{f=1}^{nf} RDPep'_f$
53:	$BCAA_{Val}$	ruminal BCAA balance	$RecycledBact_{Val} + 0.6 * Val * \sum_{f=1}^{nf} RDPep'_f$
54:	$\Delta BCAA_{Leu}$	ruminal BCAA balance	$Bact_{Leu} - BCAA_{Leu}$
55:	$\Delta BCAA_{Ile}$	ruminal BCAA balance	$Bact_{Ile} - BCAA_{Ile}$
56:	$\Delta BCAA_{Val}$	ruminal BCAA balance	$Bact_{Val} - BCAA_{Val}$
57:	$BCAAAFCB_{Leu}$	$\Delta BCAA_{Leu}<0$	$\frac{RecycledBact_{Leu} + 0.6 * Leu * \sum_{f=1}^{nf} RDPep'_f}{0.625 * 0.8 * (0.01 * (7.51 * 75 + 5.9 * 25))}$
58:	$BCAAAFCB_{Ile}$	$\Delta BCAA_{Ile}<0$	$\frac{RecycledBact_{Ile} + 0.6 * Ile * \sum_{f=1}^{nf} RDPep'_f}{0.625 * 0.8 * (0.01 * (5.88 * 75 + 4 * 25))}$
59:	$BCAAAFCB_{Val}$	$\Delta BCAA_{Val}<0$	$\frac{RecycledBact_{Val} + 0.6 * Val * \sum_{f=1}^{nf} RDPep'_f}{0.625 * 0.8 * (0.01 * (6.16 * 75 + 4.7 * 25))}$
60:	$BCAAAB$	ΔBCAA<0	$Min\left[BCAAAFCB_{Leu}, BCAAAFCB_{Ile}, BCAAAFCB_{Val}, \sum_{j=1}^{nf} EAFCB_f, \sum_{j=1}^{nf} NAFCB_f\right] + Min\left[\sum_{j=1}^{nf} EANFCB_f, \sum_{j=1}^{nf} NANFCB_F\right]$
61:	$BCAAAB_f$	ΔBCAA<0	$BCAAAB * EAB_f$
62:	$BCAAABR_f$	ΔBCAA<0	$EACFCB_f + EANFCB_f - BCAAAB_f$
63:	$BCAAAFCB_f$	ΔBCAA<0	$Max[0, Min[EAFCB_f, NAFCB_f] - BCAAABR_f]$

#	Variable[1]	Description	Equation
64:	$BCAAANFCB_f$	ΔBCAA<0	$If(Min[EAFCB_f, NAFCB_f] - BCAAABR_f < 0, Max[0, Min[EANFCB_f, NANFCB_f] + Min[EAFCB_f, NAFCB_f] - BCAAABR_f], Min[EANFCB_f, NANFCB_f])$
65:	$BCAAAFCBR_f$	ΔBCAA<0	$Max[0, Min[EAFCB_f, NAFCB_f] - BCAAAFCB_f]$
66:	$BCAAANFCBR_f$	ΔBCAA<0	$Max[0, Min[EANFCB_f, NANFCB_f] - BCAAANFCB_f]$
67:	$BCAAARDCB3R_f$	ΔBCAA<0	$\frac{BCAAAFCBR_f}{CB3Y_f}$
68:	$BCAAARDCB3_f$	ΔBCAA<0	$Max[0, Min[RDCB3, NARDCB3], BCAAARDCB3R]$
69:	$Bact_{NFC,f}$	bacterial mass	$Min[EANFCB_f, NANFCB_f, BCAAANFCB_f]$
70:	$Bact_{FC,f}$	bacterial mass	$Min[EAFCB_f, NAFCB_f, BCAAAFCB_f]$
71:	$RDCB3'_j$	CB3 reduction	$Min[RDCB3_f, NARDCB3_f, BCAAARDCB3_f]$
72:	$BactCP_{NFC,f}$	bacterial proteins	$Bact_{NFC,f} * 0.625$
73:	$BactCP_{FC,j}$	bacterial proteins	$Bact_{FC,f} * 0.625$
74:	$BactCP_j$	bacterial proteins	$BactCP_{NFC,f} + BactCP_{FC,f}$
75:	$BactTP_{NFC,f}$	bacterial proteins	$BactCP_{NFC,f} * 0.6$
76:	$BactTP_{FC,j}$	bacterial proteins	$BactCP_{FC,f} * 0.6$
77:	$BactTP_j$	bacterial proteins	$BactTP_{NFC,f} + BactTP_{FC,f}$
78:	$BactNA_{NFC,f}$	bacterial proteins	$BactCP_{NFC,f} * 0.15$
79:	$BactNA_{FC,j}$	bacterial proteins	$BactCP_{FC,f} * 0.15$
80:	$BactNA_j$	bacterial proteins	$BactNA_{NFC,f} + BactNA_{FC,f}$
81:	$BactCW_{NFC,f}$	bacterial proteins	$BactCP_{NFC,f} * 0.25$
82:	$BactCW_{FC,j}$	bacterial proteins	$BactCP_{FC,f} * 0.25$
83:	$BactCW_j$	bacterial proteins	$BactCW_{NFC,f} + BactCW_{FC,f}$
84:	$BactCHO_{NFC,f}$	bacterial CHO	$Bact_{NFC,f} * 0.211$
85:	$BactCHO_{FC,j}$	bacterial CHO	$Bact_{FC,f} * 0.211$
86:	$BactCHO_j$	bacterial CHO	$BactCHO_{NFC,f} + BactCHO_{FC,f}$
86:	$BactCA_{NFC,f}$	bacterial CHO	$BactCHO_{NFC,f} * 0.8$
87:	$BactCA_{FC,j}$	bacterial CHO	$BactCHO_{FC,f} * 0.8$
88:	$BactCA_j$	bacterial CHO	$BactCA_{NFC,f} + BactCA_{FC,f}$
89:	$BactCB1_{NFC,f}$	bacterial CHO	$BactCHO_{NFC,f} * 0.2$
90:	$BactCB1_{FC,j}$	bacterial CHO	$BactCHO_{FC,f} * 0.2$
91:	$BactCB1_j$	bacterial CHO	$BactCB1_{NFC,f} + BactCB1_{FC,f}$
92:	$BactFat_{NFC,f}$	bacterial fat	$Bact_{NFC,f} * 0.12$
93:	$BactFat_{FC,j}$	bacterial fat	$Bact_{FC,f} * 0.12$
94:	$BactFat_j$	bacterial fat	$BactFat_{NFC,f} + BactFat_{FC,f}$
95:	$BactAsh_{NFC,f}$	bacterial ash	$Bact_{NFC,f} * 0.044$
96:	$BactAsh_{FC,j}$	bacterial ash	$Bact_{FC,f} * 0.044$
97:	$BactAsh_j$	bacterial ash	$BactAsh_{NFC,f} + BactAsh_{FC,f}$

[1] ***$AminoN_{NFC}$*** is the amino-N uptake by the nonfiber carbohydrate-degrading bacteria, g/d; ***$AmmoniaN_{FC}$*** is the ammonia-N uptake by the fiber carbohydrate degrading bacteria, g/d; ***$AmmoniaN_{NFC}$*** is the ammonia-N uptake by the nonfiber carbohydrate degrading bacteria, g/d; ***BactCA*** is the amount of bacterial carbohydrate fraction A, g/d; ***$BactCA_{FC}$*** is the amount of fiber carbohydrate-degrading bacterial carbohydrate fraction A, g/d; ***$BactCA_{NFC}$*** is the amount of nonfiber carbohydrate-degrading bacterial carbohydrate fraction A, g/d; ***BactCB1*** is the amount of bacterial carbohydrate fraction B1, g/d; ***$BactCB1_{FC}$*** is the amount of fiber carbohydrate-degrading bacterial carbohydrate fraction B1, g/d; ***$BactCB1_{NFC}$*** is the amount of nonfiber carbohydrate-degrading bacterial carbohydrate fraction B1, g/d; ***BactCHO*** is the amount of bacterial carbohydrate, g/d; ***$BactCHO_{FC}$*** is the amount of fiber carbohydrate-degrading bacterial carbohydrate, g/d; ***$BactCHO_{NFC}$*** is the amount of nonfiber carbohydrate-degrading bacterial carbohydrate, g/d; ***BactCP*** is the amount of bacterial crude protein, g/d; ***$BactCP_{FC}$*** is the amount of fiber carbohydrate-degrading bacterial crude protein, g/d; ***$BactCP_{NFC}$*** is the amount of nonfiber carbohydrate-degrading bacterial crude protein, g/d; ***BactCW*** is the amount of bacterial cell wall, g/d; ***$BactCW_{FC}$*** is the amount of fiber carbohydrate-degrading bacterial cell wall, g/d; ***$BactCW_{NFC}$*** is the amount of nonfiber carbohydrate-degrading bacterial cell wall, g/d; ***BactFat*** is the amount of bacterial carbohydrate fat, g/d; ***$BactFat_{FC}$*** is the amount of fiber carbohydrate-degrading bacterial fat, g/d; ***$BactFat_{NFC}$*** is the amount of nonfiber carbohydrate-degrading bacterial fat, g/d; ***$Bact_{FC}$*** is the amount of fiber carbohydrate-degrading bacterial mass, g/d; ***$Bact_{Leu}$, $Bact_{Ile}$, $Bact_{Val}$*** is the total bacterial requirement of leucine, isoleucine, and valine from nonfiber carbohydrate and fiber carbohydrate-degrading bacteria, g/d; assuming 5.9%, 4.0%, and 4.7% of the bacterial cell wall true protein and 7.51%, 5.88%, and 6.16% of the bacterial noncell wall true protein, respectively, and 62.5% crude and 80% true proteins in the bacteria; ***BactNA*** is the amount of bacterial nucleic acids, g/d; ***$BactNA_{FC}$*** is the amount of fiber carbohydrate-degrading bacterial nucleic acids, g/d; ***$BactNA_{NFC}$*** is the amount of nonfiber carbohydrate-degrading bacterial nucleic acids, g/d; ***$Bact_{NFC}$*** is the amount of nonfiber carbohydrate-degrading bacterial mass, g/d; ***BactTP*** is the amount of bacterial true protein, g/d; ***$BactTP_{FC}$*** is the amount of fiber carbohydrate-degrading bacterial true protein, g/d;

$BactTP_{NFC}$ is the amount of nonfiber carbohydrate-degrading bacterial true protein, g/d; ***BCAA*** is branched-chain amino acid (i.e., leucine, isoleucine, and valine); ***BCAAAB*** is the least of energy-alowable, nitrogen-allowable, or BCAA-allowable fiber carbohydrate and nonfiber carbohydrate-degrading bacteria, g/d; ***BCAAABR*** is the BCAA-allowable bacteria reduction, g/d; ***BCAAAFCB*** is the BCAA-allowable fiber carbohydrate-degrading bacteria, g/d; ***$BCAAAFCB_{Leu}$, $BCAAAFCB_{Ile}$, $BCAAAFCB_{Val}$*** is the BCAA-allowable fiber carbohydrate-degrading bacteria given the available dietary leucine, isoleucine, and valine, respectively, g/d; ***BCAAANFCB*** is the BCAA-allowable nonfiber carbohydrate-degrading bacteria, g/d; ***BCAAARDCB3*** is the ruminally degraded carbohydrate fraction B3 adjusted for BCAA-allowable bacteria, g/d; ***BCAAARDCB3R*** is the reduction in ruminally degraded carbohydrate fraction B3 adjusted for BCAA-allowable bacteria, g/d; ***$BCAA_{Leu}$, $BCAA_{Ile}$, $BCAA_{Val}$*** is the total supply of leucine, isoleucine, and valine from ruminally recycled bacteria and dietary supply, g/d; ***CA1Y*** is the carbohydrate fraction A1 yield of bacteria, g/g; ***CA2Y*** is the carbohydrate fraction A2 yield of bacteria, g/g; ***CA3Y*** is the carbohydrate fraction A3 yield of bacteria, g/g; ***CA4Y*** is the carbohydrate fraction A4 yield of bacteria, g/g; ***CB1Y*** is the carbohydrate fraction B1 yield of bacteria, g/g; ***CB2Y*** is the carbohydrate fraction B2 yield of bacteria, g/g; ***CB3Y*** is the carbohydrate fraction B3 yield of bacteria, g/g; ***CP*** is the dietary crude protein, % DM; ***DMI*** is dry matter intake, kg/d; ***EAB*** is the proportion of energy-allowable bacteria of the fth feed, g/g; ***EAFCB*** is the energy-allowable fiber carbohydrate-degrading bacteria, g/d; ***EANFCB*** is the energy-allowable nonfiber carbohydrate-degrading bacteria, g/d; ***f*** is the fth feed in the diet; ***FCBact*** is the fiber carbohydrate-degrading bacteria, g/d; ***Ile*** is the isoleucine proportion in the dietary true protein, g/d; ***imp*** is the improvement of yield of nonfiber-degrading bacteria; ***$Kd_{CA1,CA2,CA3,CA4,CB1,CB2,CB3}$*** is the fractional degradation rate for CA1, CA2, CA3, CA4, CB1, CB2, and CB3, %/h; ***km1*** is maintenance coefficient for fiber-carbohydrate-degrading bacteria, default is 0.05 g/(g·h); ***km2*** is maintenance coefficient for nonfiber-carbohydrate-degrading bacteria, default is 0.15 g/(g·h); ***Leu*** is the leucine proportion in the dietary true protein, g/d; ***NAB*** is the nitrogen-allowable bacteria growth, g/d; ***NABR*** is the reduction of bacteria due to the negative nitrogen balance (i.e., nitrogen-allowable bacteria), g/d; ***NAFCB*** is the nitrogen-allowable fiber carbohydrate-digesting bacteria, g/d; ***NAFCBR*** is the reduction of nitrogen-allowable fiber carbohydrate-degrading bacteria, g/d; ***NANFCB*** is the nitrogen-allowable nonfiber carbohydrate-digesting bacteria, g/d; ***NANFCBR*** is the reduction of nitrogen-allowable nonfiber carbohydrate-degrading bacteria, g/d; ***NARDCB3*** is the ruminally degraded carbohydrate fraction B3 adjusted for nitrogen-allowable bacteria, g/d; ***NARDCB3R*** is the reduction in ruminally degraded carbohydrate fraction B3 adjusted for nitrogen-allowable bacteria (i.e., fiber), g/d; ***nf*** is number of feeds; ***NFCBact*** is the nonfiber carbohydrate-degrading bacteria, g/d; ***PepUptake*** is the peptide update, g/d; ***RDCB3*** is the ruminally degraded carbohydrate fraction B3, g/d; ***RDCB3'*** is the ruminally degraded carbohydrate fraction B3 adjusted for nitrogen- and BCAA-allowable bacteria, g/d; ***RDP'*** is adjusted ruminally degraded protein, g/d; ***RDPB1'*** is adjusted ruminally degraded protein fraction B1, g/d; ***RDPB2'*** is adjusted ruminally degraded protein fraction B2, g/d; ***RDPB3'*** is adjusted ruminally degraded protein fraction B3, g/d; ***RDPep'*** is adjusted ruminally degraded peptides (RDPB1', RDPB2', and RDPB3'), g/d; ***$RecycledBact_{Leu}$, $RecycledBact_{Ile}$, $RecycledBact_{Val}$*** is the amount of leucine, isoleucine, and valine from ruminally reclyced bacteria due to protozoa predation (i.e., 20%), assuming an efficiency of uptake of 60%; ***RecycledN*** is the amount of nitrogen recycled back to the rumen, g/d; ***Val*** is the valine proportion in the dietary true protein, g/d; ***Yg_1*** is the yield of fiber-carbohydrate-degrading bacteria for growth, default is 0.4 g/g; ***Yg_2'*** is the adjusted yield of nonfiber-carbohydrate -degrading bacteria for growth, default is 0.4 g/g; ***ΔAminoN*** is the balance of ruminal amino-N in the rumen, g/d; and ***ΔRuminalN*** is the ruminal nitrogen balance (a negative balance indicates there is not enough ammonia-N in the rumen to support the energy-allowable growth of fiber carbohydrate-degrading bacteria), g/d.

(2) Equation #29 is based on NRC (1985) and Equation #30 is based on Eisemann and Tedeschi (2016).

4.2.8.3 Ruminal fatty acids biohydrogenation and de novo synthesis

#	Variable(1)	Description	Equation
1:	$Kb_{C18:3,f}$	biohydrogenation	$500 * Exp\left(-0.0187884381 * \frac{LFA}{DMI}\right)$
2:	$Kb_{C18:2,f}$	biohydrogenation	87.56241579
3:	$Kb_{C18:1t,f}$	biohydrogenation	$54.4618963 * Exp\left(-0.022844773 * \frac{LFA}{DMI}\right)$
4:	$Kb_{C18:1c,f}$	biohydrogenation	27.34532619
5:	$Kb_{C16:1,f}$	biohydrogenation	$300 * Exp\left(-0.030486193 * \frac{LFA}{DMI}\right)$
6:	$LEFAC18{:}3_f$	biohydrogenation	$LFAC18{:}\,3_f * \left(\frac{kp_f}{kp_f + kb_{C18:3,f}}\right)$
7:	$LBFAC18{:}3_f$	biohydrogenation	$LFAC18{:}\,3_f - LEFC18{:}\,3_f$
8:	$LEFAC18{:}2_f$	biohydrogenation	$(LFAC18{:}\,2_f + LBFAC18{:}\,3_f) * \left(\frac{kp_f}{kp_f + kb_{C18:2,f}}\right)$
9:	$LBFAC18{:}2_f$	biohydrogenation	$(LFAC18{:}\,2_f + LBFAC18{:}\,3_f) * \left(\frac{kb_{C18:2,f}}{kp_f + kb_{C18:2,f}}\right)$
10:	$LEFAC18{:}1t_f$	biohydrogenation	$(LFAC18{:}\,1t_f + LBFAC18{:}\,2_f) * \left(\frac{kp_f}{kp_f + kb_{C18:1t,f}}\right)$
11:	$LBFAC18{:}1t_f$	biohydrogenation	$(LFAC18{:}\,1t_f + LBFAC18{:}\,2_f) * \left(\frac{kb_{C18:1t,f}}{kp_f + kb_{C18:1t,f}}\right)$

#	Variable[1]	Description	Equation
12:	*LEFAC18:1c$_f$*	biohydrogenation	$LFAC18{:}\,1c_f * \left(\frac{kp_f}{kp_f + kb_{C18:1c,f}}\right)$
13:	*LBFAC18:1c$_f$*	biohydrogenation	$LFAC18{:}\,1c_f - LEFAC18{:}\,1c_f$
14:	*LBFAC18$_f$*	biohydrogenation	$LFAC18_f + LBFAC18{:}\,1t_f + LBFAC18{:}\,1c_f$
15:	*LEFAC16:1$_f$*	biohydrogenation	$LFAC16{:}\,1_f * \left(\frac{kp_f}{kp_f + kb_{C16:1,f}}\right)$
16:	*LBFAC16:1$_f$*	biohydrogenation	$LFAC16{:}\,1_f - LEFC16{:}\,1_f$
17:	*LEFAC16$_f$*	biohydrogenation	$LFAC16_f + LBFAC16{:}\,1_f$
18:	*LEFAC14$_f$*	biohydrogenation	$LFAC14_f$
19:	*LEFAC12$_f$*	biohydrogenation	$LFAC12_f$
20:	*LEFAOther$_f$*	biohydrogenation	$LFAOther_f$
21:	*RDCHO$_f$*	*de novo* synthesis	$RDCA1_f + RDCA2_f + RDCA3_f + RDCA4_f + RDCB1_f + RDCB2_f + RDCB3'_f$
22:	*DNFAC16$_f$*	*de novo* synthesis	$5.76 * RDCHO_f * Exp\left(-2.69 * \frac{\sum_{f-1}^{nf} LEFAC16_f}{0.001 * DMI}\right)$
23:	*DNFAC16:1$_f$*	*de novo* synthesis	$0.6241 * RDCHO_f * Exp\left(-1.23 * \frac{\sum_{f-1}^{nf} LEFAC16{:}\,1_f}{0.001 * DMI}\right)$
24:	*DNFAC18$_f$*	*de novo* synthesis	$27.3 * RDCHO_f * Exp\left(-0.117 * \frac{\sum_{f-1}^{nf} LEFAC18_f}{0.001 * DMI}\right)$
25:	*DNFAOther$_f$*	*de novo* synthesis	$5.02 * RDCHO_f * Exp\left(-0.332 * \frac{\sum_{f-1}^{nf} LEFAOther_f}{0.001 * DMI}\right)$
26:	*EFAC12$_f$*	ruminal escape	$FAC12_f - LFAC12_f$
27:	*EFAC14$_f$*	ruminal escape	$FAC14_f - LFAC142_f$
28:	*EFAC16$_f$*	ruminal escape	$FAC16_f - LFAC16_f$
29:	*EFAC16:1$_f$*	ruminal escape	$FAC16{:}\,1_f - LFAC16{:}\,1_f$
30:	*EFAC18$_f$*	ruminal escape	$FAC18_f - LFAC18_f$
31:	*EFAC18:1c$_f$*	ruminal escape	$FAC18{:}\,1c_f - LFAC18{:}\,1c_f$
32:	*EFAC18:1t$_f$*	ruminal escape	$FAC18{:}\,1t_f - LFAC18{:}\,1t_f$
33:	*EFAC18:2$_f$*	ruminal escape	$FAC18{:}\,2_f - LFAC18{:}\,2_f$
34:	*EFAC18:3$_f$*	ruminal escape	$FAC18{:}\,3_f - LFAC18{:}\,3_f$
35:	*EFAOther$_f$*	ruminal escape	$FAOther_f - LFAOther_f$
36:	*EGlycerol$_f$*	ruminal escape	$Glycerol_f - Prop_f^{Glyc}$

[1] ***DMI*** is the dry matter intake, g/d; ***DNFAC16*** is *de novo* synthesis of FAC16, g/d; ***DNFAC16:1*** is *de novo* synthesis of FAC16:1, g/d; ***DNFAC18*** is *de novo* synthesis of FAC18, g/d; ***DNFAOther*** is *de novo* synthesis of FAOther, g/d; ***EFAC12*** is the escaped esterified (non-lipolized) FAC12, g/d; ***EFAC14*** is the escaped esterified (non-lipolized) FAC14, g/d; ***EFAC16*** is the escaped esterified (non-lipolized) FAC16, g/d; ***EFAC16:1*** is the escaped esterified (non-lipolized) FAC16:1, g/d; ***EFAC18*** is the escaped esterified (non-lipolized) FAC18, g/d; ***EFAC18:1c*** is the escaped esterified (non-lipolized) FAC18:1c, g/d; ***EFAC18:1t*** is the escaped esterified (non-lipolized) FAC18:1t, g/d; ***EFAC18:2*** is the escaped esterified (non-lipolized) FAC18:2, g/d; ***EFAC18:3*** is the escaped esterified (non-lipolized) FAC18:3, g/d; ***EFAOther*** is the escaped esterified (non-lipolized) FAOther, g/d; ***EGlycerol*** is the escaped glycerol, g/d; ***f*** is the fth feed in the diet; ***FAC12*** is long-chain fatty acid C12 (lauric acid), g/d; ***FAC14*** is long-chain fatty acid C14 (myristic acid), g/d; ***FAC16*** is long-chain fatty acid C16 (palmitic acid), g/d; ***FAC16:1*** is long-chain fatty acid C16:1 (palmitoleic acid), g/d; ***FAC18*** is long-chain fatty acid C18 (stearic acid), g/d; ***FAC18:1c*** is long-chain fatty acid C18:1c (oleic acid), g/d; ***FAC18:1t*** is long-chain fatty acid C18:1t (elaidic and vaccenic acids), g/d; ***FAC18:2*** is long-chain fatty acid C18:2 (linoleic acid), g/d; ***FAC18:3*** is long-chain fatty acid C18:3 (linolenic acid), g/d; ***FAOther*** is other long-chain fatty acids, g/d; ***$Kb_{C16:1}$*** is the fractional rate of biohydrogenation for long-chain fatty acid C16:1 (palmitoleic acid), %/h; ***$Kb_{C18:1c}$*** is the fractional rate of biohydrogenation for long-chain fatty acid C18:1c (oleic acid), %/h; ***$Kb_{C18:1t}$*** is the fractional rate of biohydrogenation for long-chain fatty acid C18:1t (elaidic and vaccenic acids), %/h; ***$Kb_{C18:2}$*** is the fractional rate of biohydrogenation for long-chain fatty acid C18:2 (linoleic acid), %/h; ***$Kb_{C18:3}$*** is the fractional rate of biohydrogenation for long-chain fatty acid C18:3 (linolenic acid), %/h; ***kp*** is frational passage rate either inputted by the user or associated with kp for concentrate or kp for forage, %/h; ***LBFAC16:1*** is lipolyzed biohydrogenized FAC16:1, g/d; ***LBFAC18:1c*** is lipolyzed biohydrogenized FAC18:1c, g/d; ***LBFAC18:1t*** is lipolyzed biohydrogenized FAC18:1t, g/d; ***LBFAC18:2*** is lipolyzed biohydrogenized FAC18:2, g/d; ***LBFAC18:3*** is lipolyzed biohydrogenized FAC18:3, g/d; ***LEFAC12*** is lipolyzed escaped FAC12, g/d; ***LEFAC14*** is lipolyzed escaped FAC14, g/d; ***LEFAC16*** is lipolyzed escaped FAC16, g/d; ***LEFAC16:1*** is lipolyzed escaped FAC16:1, g/d; ***LEFAC18*** is lipolyzed escaped FAC18, g/d; ***LEFAC18:1c*** is lipolyzed escaped FAC18:1c, g/d; ***LEFAC18:1t*** is lipolyzed escaped FAC18:1t, g/d; ***LEFAC18:2*** is lipolyzed escaped FAC18:2, g/d; ***LEFAC18:3*** is lipolyzed escaped FAC18:3, g/d; ***LEFAOther*** is lipolyzed escaped FAOther, g/d; ***LFA*** is the long-chain fatty acids in the diet, g/d; ***LFAC12*** is lipolyzed FAC12, g/d; ***LFAC14*** is lipolyzed FAC14, g/d; ***LFAC16*** is lipolyzed FAC16, g/d; ***LFAC16:1*** is lipolyzed FAC16:1, g/d; ***LFAC18*** is lipolyzed FAC18, g/d; ***LFAC18:1c*** is lipolyzed FAC18:1c, g/d; ***LFAC18:1t*** is lipolyzed FAC18:1t, g/d; ***LFAC18:2*** is lipolyzed FAC18:2, g/d; ***LFAC18:3*** is lipolyzed FAC18:3, g/d; ***LFAOther*** is lipolyzed FAOther, g/d; ***nf*** is the number of feeds; ***$Prop^{Glyc}$*** is the propionate produced from the ruminal fermentation of lipolized glycerol, g/d; and ***RDCHO*** is the ruminally degraded carbohydrates, g/d.

4.2.9 Ruminal volatile fatty acids: calcVFA()

#	Variable[1]	Description[2]	Equation
1:	*fracA4*	VFA	$\frac{NFCBactA4_f}{NFCBactA1_f + NFCBactA2_f + NFCBactA3_f + NFCBactA4_f + NFCBactB1_f + NFC}$
2:	*fracB1*	VFA	$\frac{NFCBactB1_f}{NFCBactA1_f + NFCBactA2_f + NFCBactA3_f + NFCBactA4_f + NFCBactB1_f + NFC}$
3:	*fracB2*	VFA	$\frac{NFCBactB2_f}{NFCBactA1_f + NFCBactA2_f + NFCBactA3_f + NFCBactA4_f + NFCBactB1_f + NFC}$
4:	$AcidA4_f$	VFA	$Max[0, (1 - 0.344) * RDCA4_f - (1 - 0.044) * NFCBactA4_f + (AmmoniaN_{NFC,f} + 6.25 * AminoN_{NFC,f}) * fracA4]$
5:	$AcidB1_f$	VFA	$Max[0, (1 - 0.344) * RDCB1_f - (1 - 0.044) * NFCBactB1_f + (AmmoniaN_{NFC,f} + 6.25 * AminoN_{NFC,f}) * fracB1]$
6:	$AcidB2_f$	VFA	$Max[0, (1 - 0.344) * RDCB2_f - (1 - 0.044) * NFCBactB2_f + (AmmoniaN_{NFC,f} + 6.25 * AminoN_{NFC,f}) * fracB2]$
7:	$AcidB3_f$	VFA	$Max[0, (1 - 0.54) * RDCB3_f - (1 - 0.044) * FCBactB3_f + AmmoniaN_{FC,f}]$
8:	$f^{A4}_{Lactate}$	VFA	$Max[0, 2.4444 - 0.3075 * pH]$
9:	$f^{B1}_{Lactate}$	VFA	$Max[0, 3.2989 - 0.4744 * pH]$
10:	$f^{B2}_{Lactate}$	VFA	0
11:	$f^{B3}_{Lactate}$	VFA	$Max[0, 2.4278 - 0.3532 * pH]$
12:	$f^{A4}_{Butyrate}$	VFA	$Max[0, 0.5733 - 0.0585 * pH]$
13:	$f^{B1}_{Butyrate}$	VFA	$Max[0, 0.7359 - 0.0921 * pH]$
14:	$f^{B2}_{Butyrate}$	VFA	$Max[0, 0.3621 - 0.0504 * pH]$
15:	$f^{B3}_{Butyrate}$	VFA	$Max[0, 5015 - 0.0631 * pH]$
16:	$f^{A4}_{A:P}$	VFA	$Max[0, -1.3209 + 0.468 * pH]$
17:	$f^{B1}_{A:P}$	VFA	$Max[0, 5.6265 - 0.627 * pH]$
18:	$f^{B2}_{A:P}$	VFA	$Max[0, 2.5186 + 0.5643 * pH]$
19:	$f^{B3}_{A:P}$	VFA	$Max[0, -0.2662 + 0.3267 * pH]$
20:	$Lact^{A4}_f$	VFA	$f^{A4}_{Lactate} * AcidA4_f$
21:	$Lact^{B1}_f$	VFA	$f^{B1}_{Lactate} * AcidB1_f$
22:	$Lact^{B2}_f$	VFA	$f^{B2}_{Lactate} * AcidB2_f$
23:	$Lact^{B3}_f$	VFA	$f^{B3}_{Lactate} * AcidB3_f$
24:	But^{A4}_f	VFA	$f^{A4}_{Butyrate} * (AcidA4_f - Lact^{A4}_f)$
25:	But^{B1}_f	VFA	$f^{B1}_{Butyrate} * (AcidB1_f - Lact^{B1}_f)$
26:	But^{B2}_f	VFA	$f^{B2}_{Butyrate} * (AcidB2_f - Lact^{B2}_f)$
27:	But^{B3}_f	VFA	$f^{B3}_{Butyrate} * (AcidB3_f - Lact^{B3}_f)$
28:	$Prop^{A4}_f$	VFA	$\frac{(1 - f^{A4}_{Butyrate}) * (AcidA4_f - Lact^{A4}_f)}{1 + f^{A4}_{A:P}}$
29:	$Prop^{B1}_f$	VFA	$\frac{(1 - f^{B1}_{Butyrate}) * (AcidB1_f - Lact^{B1}_f)}{1 + f^{B1}_{A:P}}$
30:	$Prop^{B2}_f$	VFA	$\frac{(1 - f^{B2}_{Butyrate}) * (AcidB2_f - Lact^{B2}_f)}{1 + f^{B2}_{A:P}}$
31:	$Prop^{B3}_f$	VFA	$\frac{(1 - f^{B3}_{Butyrate}) * (AcidB3_f - Lact^{B3}_f)}{1 + f^{B3}_{A:P}}$
32:	Ac^{A4}_f	VFA	$f^{A4}_{A:P} * Prop^{A4}_f$
33:	Ac^{B1}_f	VFA	$f^{B1}_{A:P} * Prop^{B1}_f$
34:	Ac^{B2}_f	VFA	$f^{B2}_{A:P} * Prop^{B2}_f$
35:	Ac^{B3}_f	VFA	$f^{B3}_{A:P} * Prop^{B3}_f$
36:	$Ac_{Ru,f}$	VFA	$Ac^{A4}_f + Ac^{B1}_f + Ac^{B2}_f + Ac^{B3}_f$
37:	$Prop_{Ru,f}$	VFA	$Prop^{Glycerol}_f + Prop^{A4}_f + Prop^{B1}_f + Prop^{B2}_f + Prop^{B3}_f$
38:	$But_{Ru,f}$	VFA	$But^{A4}_f + But^{B1}_f + But^{B2}_f + But^{B3}_f$
39:	$Lact_{Ru,f}$	VFA	$Lact^{A4}_f + Lact^{B1}_f + Lact^{B2}_f + Lact^{B3}_f$
40:	$fracP^{A4}$	CH_4	$\frac{\frac{\sum_{j=1}^{nf} Prop^{A4}_f}{74}}{\frac{\sum_{f=1}^{nf} Ac^{A4}_f}{60} + \frac{\sum_{f=1}^{nf} Prop^{A4}_f}{74} + \frac{\sum_{f=1}^{nf} But^{A4}_f}{88}}$

#	Variable[(1)]	Description[(2)]	Equation
41:	$fracP^{B1}$	CH_4	$\frac{\frac{\sum_{j=1}^{nf} Prop_f^{B1}}{74}}{\frac{\sum_{f=1}^{nf} Ac_f^{B1}}{60}+\frac{\sum_{f=1}^{nf} Prop_f^{B1}}{74}+\frac{\sum_{f=1}^{nf} But_f^{B1}}{88}}$
42:	$fracP^{B2}$	CH_4	$\frac{\frac{\sum_{j=1}^{nf} Prop_f^{B2}}{74}}{\frac{\sum_{f=1}^{nf} Ac_f^{B2}}{60}+\frac{\sum_{f=1}^{nf} Prop_f^{B2}}{74}+\frac{\sum_{f=1}^{nf} But_f^{B2}}{88}}$
43:	$fracP^{B3}$	CH_4	$\frac{\frac{\sum_{j=1}^{nf} Prop_f^{B3}}{74}}{\frac{\sum_{f=1}^{nf} Ac_f^{B3}}{60}+\frac{\sum_{f=1}^{nf} Prop_f^{B3}}{74}+\frac{\sum_{f=1}^{nf} But_f^{B3}}{88}}$
44:	$CH4Y^{A4}$	CH_4	$Max\left[0,\left(\frac{1}{2*fracP^{A4}}-\frac{3}{4}\right)*\frac{16}{74}\right]$
45:	$CH4Y^{B1}$	CH_4	$Max\left[0,\left(\frac{1}{2*fracP^{B1}}-\frac{3}{4}\right)*\frac{16}{74}\right]$
46:	$CH4Y^{B2}$	CH_4	$Max\left[0,\left(\frac{1}{2*fracP^{B2}}-\frac{3}{4}\right)*\frac{16}{74}\right]$
47:	$CH4Y^{B3}$	CH_4	$Max\left[0,\left(\frac{1}{2*fracP^{B3}}-\frac{3}{4}\right)*\frac{16}{74}\right]$
48:	$CH4_f^{A4}$	CH_4	$CH4Y^{A4}*Prop_f^{A4}$
49:	$CH4_f^{B1}$	CH_4	$CH4Y^{B1}*Prop_f^{B1}$
50:	$CH4_f^{B2}$	CH_4	$CH4Y^{B2}*Prop_f^{B2}$
51:	$CH4_f^{B3}$	CH_4	$CH4Y^{B3}*Prop_f^{B3}$
52:	$CH4_f$	CH_4	$CH4_f^{A4}+CH4_f^{B1}+CH4_f^{B2}+CH4_f^{B3}$
53:	Yg_{me}	lactate	$If[pH<5.07, 0, -1.176+0.232*pH]$
54:	m_{me}	lactate	$-2.779+0.664*pH$
55:	u_{me}	lactate	$If[pH<4.18 \; or \; pH>7.33, 0, If[pH\geq 4.18 \; and \; pH \leq 6.07, -3.631+1.255*pH-0.0925*pH^2, -6.906+2.636*pH-0.2311*pH^2]]$
56:	Y_{me}	lactate	$\frac{1}{\frac{m_{me}}{u_{me}}+\frac{1}{Yg_{me}}}$
57:	kd^L	lactate	$(u_{me}+m_{me}*Yg_{me})*24*100$
58:	f_{Lu}	lactate	$(1+10^{pH-3.86})^{-1}$
59:	ka^L	lactate	$\left(\frac{Ar}{Vr}\right)*\left(0.00405*f_{Lu}+0.00139*(1-f_{Lu})\right)*100$
60:	$Lact_{Ru+Diet,f}$	lactate	$Lact_{Ru,f}+Lact_{Diet,f}$
61:	RDL_f	lactate	$Lact_{Ru+Diet,f}*\left(\frac{kd^L}{kd^L+24*kp_{Liquid}+ka^L}\right)$
62:	$Bact_{me,f}$	lactate	RDL_F*Y_{me}
63:	$f_{Acetate}^L$	lactate	$If[4\leq pH\leq 5.65, 1.035-0.154*pH, If[5.65<pH\leq 8, -1.089+0.222*pH, 0]]$
64:	$f_{Propionate}^L$	lactate	$If[4\leq pH\leq 6, 1.568-0.206*pH, If[6<pH\leq 8, -1.408+0.29*pH, 0]]$
65:	$f_{Butyrate}^L$	lactate	$If[4.4\leq pH\leq 5.5, -1.181+0.27*pH, If[5.5<pH\leq 7, 1.316-0.184*pH, 0]]$
66:	VFA_f^L	lactate	$RDL_f*\frac{1-0.856*Bact_{me,f}}{1+f_{Acetate}^L*\frac{44}{60}}$
67:	Ac_f^L	lactate	$VFA_f^L*f_{Acetate}^L$
68:	$Prop_f^L$	lactate	$VFA_f^L*f_{Propionate}^L$
69:	But_f^L	lactate	$VFA_f^L*f_{Butyrate}^L$
70:	f_{Au}	[VFA]	$(1+10^{pH-4.76})^{-1}$
71:	f_{Pu}	[VFA]	$(1+10^{pH-4.87})^{-1}$
72:	f_{Bu}	[VFA]	$(1+10^{pH-4.81})^{-1}$
73:	ka^A	[VFA]	$\left(\frac{Ar}{Vr}\right)*\left(0.48*f_{Au}+0.12*(1-f_{Au})\right)*100$
74:	ka^P	[VFA]	$\left(\frac{Ar}{Vr}\right)*\left(0.67*f_{Pu}+0.21*(1-f_{Bu})\right)*100$
75:	Ka^B	[VFA]	$\left(\frac{Ar}{Vr}\right)*\left(1.43*f_{Bu}+0.15*(1-f_{Bu})\right)*100$
76:	$Ac_{Ru+Diet,f}$	[VFA]	$Ac_{Ru,f}+Ac_f^L+Ac_{Diet,f}$

#	Variable[(1)]	Description[(2)]	Equation
77:	$Prop_{Ru+Diet,f}$	[VFA]	$Prop_{Ru,f} + Prop_f^L + Prop_{Diet,f}$
78:	$But_{Ru+Diet,f}$	[VFA]	$But_{Ru,f} + But_f^L + But_{Diet,f}$
79:	[Lact]	[VFA]	$\frac{\sum_{f=1}^{nf} Lact_{Ru+Diet,f} * 1000}{(0.01 * kd^L + 0.01 * 24 * kp_{Liquid} + 0.01 * ka^L) * Vr * 90}$
80:	[Ac]	[VFA]	$\frac{\sum_{f=1}^{nf} Ac_{Ru+Diet,f} * 1000}{(0.01 * 24 * kp_{Liquid} + 0.01 * ka^A) * Vr * 60}$
81:	[Prop]	[VFA]	$\frac{\sum_{f=1}^{nf} Prop_{Ru+Diet,f} * 1000}{(0.01 * 24 * kp_{Liquid} + 0.01 * ka^P) * Vr * 74}$
82:	[But}	[VFA]	$\frac{\sum_{f=1}^{nf} But_{Ru+Diet,f} * 1000}{(0.01 * 24 * kp_{Liquid} + 0.01 * ka^B) * Vr * 88}$
83:	Ds	buffering	$Max[100, -177.2 + 0.01638 * (0.001 * DMI) + 4.766 * peNDF]$
84:	EatSa	buffering	$3.2 * DMI$
85:	RumSa	buffering	$255 * (0.005085 * NDF + 0.174)$
86:	RestSa	buffering	$6 * DMI * (1 - (0.005085 * NDF + 0.174))$
86:	Saliva	buffering	$Max[Ds, EatSa + RumSa + RestSa]$
87:	[Saliva]	buffering	$\frac{Saliva}{1000 * Vr * 0.01 * 24 * kp_{Liquid}}$
88:	$Saliva_{BC}$	buffering	$-33.3 + \frac{165.8}{1 + 10^{pH-6.4}}$
89:	[NDF]	buffering	$\frac{\sum_{f=1}^{nf} \left(\frac{1000 * RDCB3_f}{24 * 0.01 * kp_{Forage}} \right)}{1000 * Vr}$
90:	NDF_{pHc}	buffering	$2.388 + 0.00078 * CECNDF$
91:	NDF_{BC}	buffering	$-0.004 + 0.3 * e^{-(pH - NDF_{pHc})}$
92:	Ru_{BC}	buffering	$[Saliva] * Saliva_{BC} + [NDF] * NDF_{BC}$
93:	$Ru_{Acidity}$	buffering	$[Ac] * (1 - f_{Au}) + [Prop] * (1 - f_{Pu}) + [But] * (1 - f_{Bu}) + [Lact] * (1 - f_{Lu})$
94:	pH	buffering	$7.2 - 0.01 * ([Ac] + [Prop] + [But]) + 0.0015 * [Lact]$

(1) ***[Ac]*** is the concentration of acetate in the rumen, mM (mol/m^3); ***[But]*** is the concentration of butyrate in the rumen, mM (mol/m^3); ***[Lact]*** is the concentration of lactate in the rumen, mM (mol/m^3); ***[NDF]*** is the NDF concentration, g/L; ***[Prop]*** is the concentration of propionate in the rumen, mM (mol/m^3); ***[Saliva]*** is saliva concentration, L/L; $Ac^{A4,B1,B2,B3}$ is the amount of acetate produced from the fermentation of each carbohydrate substrate (A4, B1, B2, and B3), g/d; ***AcidA4*** is the volatile fatty acids and lactic acids produced from carbohydrate A4 (sugars), g/d; ***AcidB1*** is the volatile fatty acids and lactic acids produced from carbohydrate B1 (starch), g/d; ***AcidB2*** is the volatile fatty acids and lactic acids produced from carbohydrate B2 (pectin), g/d; ***AcidB3*** is the volatile fatty acids and lactic acids produced from carbohydrate B3 (available neutral detergent fiber) g/d; Ac^L is the acetate produced from the ruminal fermentation of lactate, g/d; Ac_{Ru} is the amount of acetate produced from the fermentation of carbohydrates, g/d; $Ac_{Ru+Diet}$ is the amount of acetate produced from the fermentation of carbohydrates plus acetate from the diet, g/d; $AminoN_{NFC}$ is the amino-N uptake by the nonfiber carbohydrate degrading bacteria, g/d; $AmmoniaN_{FC}$ is the ammonia-N uptake by the fiber carbohydrate degrading bacteria, g/d; $AmmoniaN_{NFC}$ is the ammonia-N uptake by the nonfiber carbohydrate degrading bacteria, g/d; ***Ar*** is rumen surface area, m^2; $Bact_{me}$ is the *Megasphaera elsdenii* growth rate from ruminally degraded lactate, g/d; $But^{A4,B1,B2,B3}$ is the amount of butyrate produced from the fermentation of each carbohydrate substrate (A4, B1, B2, and B3), g/d; But^L is the butyrate produced from the ruminal fermentation of lactate, g/d; But_{Ru} is the amount of butyrate produced from the fermentation of carbohydrates, g/d; $But_{Ru+Diet}$ is the amount of butyrate produced from the fermentation of carbohydrates plus butyrate from the diet, g/d; ***CECNDF*** is the cation exchange capacity of cell wall (i.e., NDF) (default is 500), mmol/kg NDF; ***CH4*** is the total methane production from the fermentation of carbohydrates, g/d; $CH4^{A4,B1,B2,B3}$ is the methane production for each carbohydrate substrate (A4, B1, B2, B3), g/d; $CH4Y^{A4,B1,B2,B3}$ is the methane yield for each carbohydrate substrate (A4, B1, B2, B3), g/g; ***DMI*** is dry matter intake, kg/d; *Ds* is empirical saliva production, L/d; ***EatSa*** is eating saliva production, L/d; ***f*** is the fth feed in the diet; $f^L_{Acetate,Propionate,Butyrate}$ is the mass fraction of ruminally degraded lactate yielding acetate, propionate, and butyrate, g/g; $f^{A4,B1,B2,B3}_{Lactate,Butyrate,A:P}$ is the mass fraction of carbohydrate substrates (A4, B1, B2, and B3) yielding lactate, butyrate, or acetate-to-propionate ratio (A:P), g/g; f_{Au} is the fraction of undissociated form of acetic acid; f_{Bu} is the fraction of undissociated form of butyric acid; f_{Lu} is the fraction of undissociated form of lactic acid; f_{Pu} is the fraction of undissociated form of propionic acid; ***fracA4*** is the proportion of nonfiber carbohydrate A4 (sugar)-degrading bacteria, g/g; ***fracB1*** is the proportion of nonfiber carbohydrate B1 (starch)-degrading bacteria, g/g; ***fracB2*** is the proportion of nonfiber carbohydrate B2 (pectin)-degrading bacteria, g/g; $fracP^{A4,B1,B2,B3}$ is the molar proportion of propionate to volatile fatty acids (i.e., acetate, propionate, and butyrate) for each carbohydrate substrate (A4, B1, B2, B3), g/g; ka^A is the fractional absorption rate of acetate, %/d; ka^B is the fractional absorption rate of butyrate, %/d; ka^L is the fractional absorption rate of lactate, %/d; ka^P is the fractional absorption rate of propionate, %/d; kd^L is fractional degradation rate of lactate, %/d; $Lact^{A4,B1,B2,B3}$ is the amount of lactate produced from the fermentation of each carbohydrate substrate (A4, B1, B2, and B3), g/d; $Lact_{Ru}$ is the amount of lactate produced from the ruminal fermentation of carbohydrates, g/d; $Lact_{Ru+Diet}$ is the amount of lactate produced from the ruminal fermentation of carbohydrates plus lactate from the diet, g/d; ***NDF*** is the concentration of neutral detergent fiber, %DM; NDF_{BC} is the buffering capacity of the cell wall (i.e., NDF), mEq/g NDF; NDF_{pHc} is the reference ruminal

pH, mmol/kg NDF; ***nf*** is number of feeds; ***NFCBactA1*** is nonfiber carbohydrate A1 (volatile fatty acids)-degrading bacteria, g/d; ***NFCBactA2*** is nonfiber carbohydrate A2 (lactate)-degrading bacteria, g/d; ***NFCBactA3*** is nonfiber carbohydrate A3 (other organic acids)-degrading bacteria, g/d; ***NFCBactA4*** is nonfiber carbohydrate A4 (sugars)-degrading bacteria, g/d; ***NFCBactB1*** is nonfiber carbohydrate B1 (starch)-degrading bacteria, g/d; ***NFCBactB2*** is nonfiber carbohydrate B2 (pectin)-degrading bacteria, g/d; ***peNDF*** is the concentration of physically effective neutral detergent fiber, % DM; ***pH*** is ruminal pH; $\boldsymbol{Prop^{A4,B1,B2,B3}}$ is the amount of propionate produced from the fermentation of each carbohydrate substrate (A4, B1, B2, and B3), g/d; $\boldsymbol{Prop^{Glyc}}$ is the propionate produced from the ruminal fermentation of lypolized glycerol, g/d; $\boldsymbol{Prop^{L}}$ is the propionate produced from the ruminal fermentation of lactate, g/d; $\boldsymbol{Prop_{Ru}}$ is the amount of propionate produced from the fermentation of glycerol and carbohydrates, g/d; $\boldsymbol{Prop_{Ru+Diet}}$ is the amount of propionate produced from the fermentation of glycerol and carbohydrates plus propionate from the diet, g/d; **RDCA4** is ruminally degraded carbohydrate A4 (sugars), g/d; **RDCB1** is ruminally degraded carbohydrate B1 (starch), g/d; **RDCB2** is ruminally degraded carbohydrate B2 (pectin), g/d; **RDCB3** is ruminally degraded carbohydrate B3 (available neutral detergent fiber), g/d; ***RDL*** is ruminally degraded lactate, g/d; ***RestSa*** is resting saliva production, L/d; $\boldsymbol{Ru_{Acidity}}$ is the total acidity in the rumen, mEq/L; ***RumSa*** is rumination saliva production, L/d; ***Saliva*** is saliva production, L/d $\boldsymbol{Saliva_{BC}}$ is the buffering capacity of the saliva, mEq/L; $\boldsymbol{VFA^{L}}$ is the volatile fatty acids produced from the ruminal fermentation of lactate, g/d; and ***Vr*** is rumen volume, m^3.

(2) Equations 1 to 39 have the calculations for volatile fatty acids, Equations 40 to 52 have the calculations for methane, Equations 53 to have the calculation for *Megasphaera elsdenii* converting lactate to volatile fatty acids. Figure 4.4 depicts the impact of ruminal pH on maintenance coefficient, maximum yield, fractional growth rate, and yield of three groups of bacteria.

In Figure 4.4, the physically effective neutral detergent fiber (peNDF) that is correlated to the ruminal pH is shown in the X-axis. The ruminal pH is not altered by peNDF when it is above 24.5 %DM. Additionally,

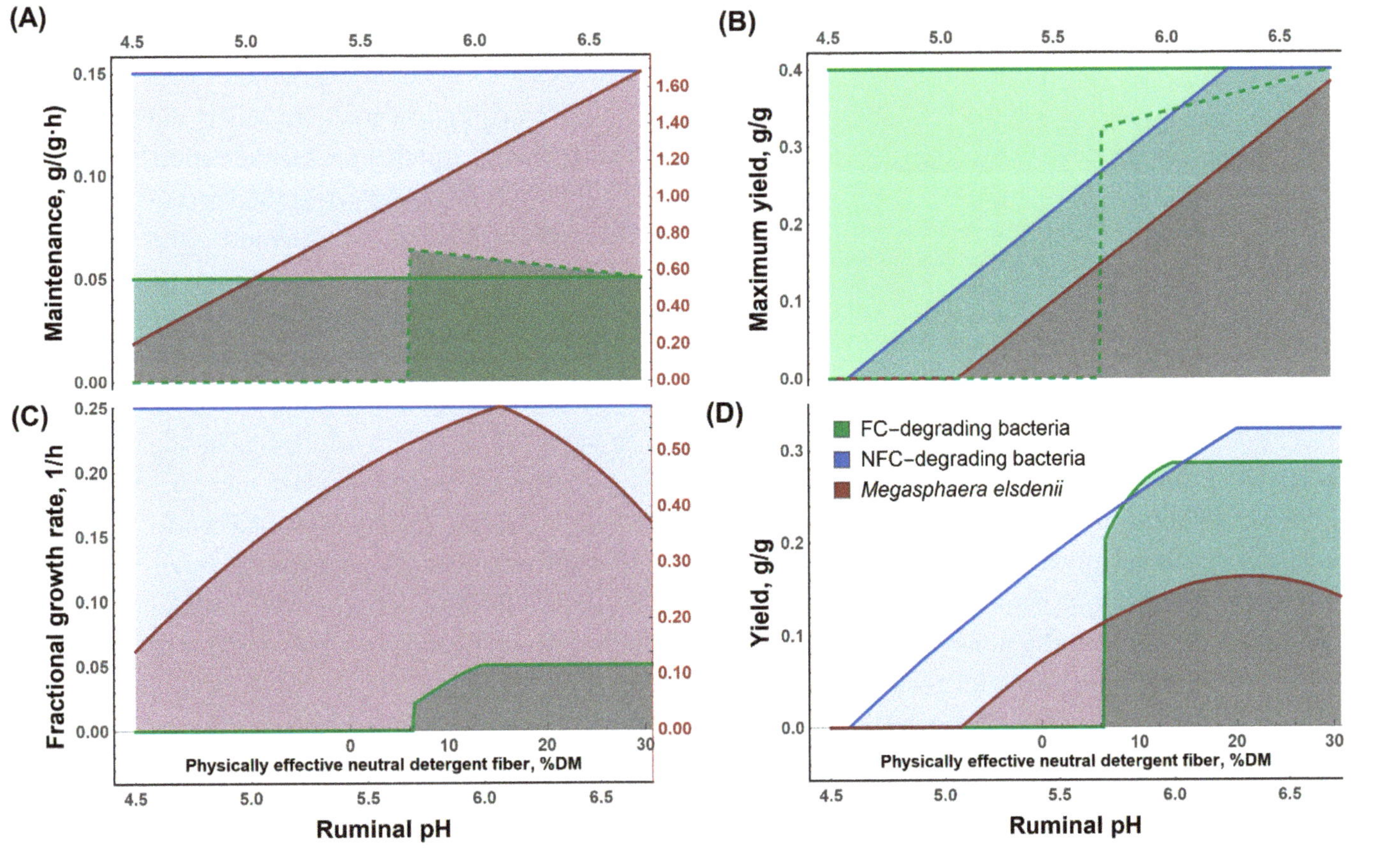

Figure 4.4. Bacteria growth submodels for fiber- and nonfiber-carbohydrate-degrading bacteria (green and blue, respectively) and *Megasphaera elsdenii* (red) showing the impact of ruminal pH on their (A) maintenance coefficient, (B) maximum yield, (C) fractional growth rate, and (D) effective yield. For panels A and C, *Megasphaera elsdenii*'s maintenance coefficient and fractional growth rate are shown in the second Y-axis. The fractional growth rate for fiber- and nonfiber-carbohydrate-degrading bacteria was assumed 5 and 25 %/h, respectively. The dashed lines represent potential impact of ruminal pH on specific coefficients (see text for additional information).

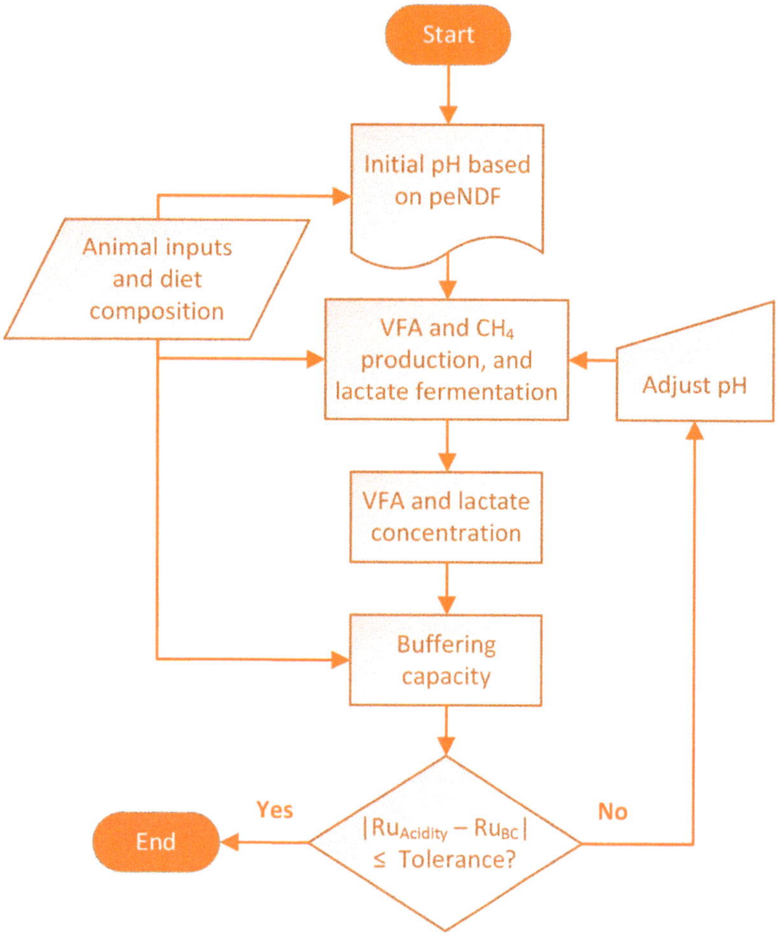

Figure 4.5. Flowchart of the optimization logic to determine ruminal pH based on the acidity and buffering capacity of the rumen.

for comparative purposes only, the calculation of the ruminal pH effects on the maintenance coefficient (m, g/(g·h)) and maximum yield (Yg, g/g) of the FC-degrading bacteria used a greater ruminal pH threshold of 6.725, as proposed initially by Pitt et al. (1996), rather than the 6.05 currently implemented in the CNCPS-based models and shown in Sections 4.2.4 and 4.3.4. The lower threshold of 5.7 for ruminal pH was used. In Figure 4.4, the dashed lines illustrate the potential impact of ruminal pH on the maintenance coefficient and the maximum yield of the FC-degrading bacteria. However, CNCPS-based models elected to alternatively adjust the fractional degradation rate of the carbohydrate B3 to reflect the impact of ruminal pH on the reduction in the ruminally degraded carbohydrate B3 and, consequently, the reduction in the FC-degrading bacteria yield. The adjustment of these three factors (m, Yg, and kd CHO B3) at the same time might result in double-accounting for the impact of the ruminal pH on the FC-degrading bacteria yield. Figure 4.4 shows the different approaches used to model bacterial growth. The resulting bacteria yield (Figure 4.4D) is the combination of the maintenance coefficient, maximum yield, and fractional growth rate. Currently, ruminal pH does not impact, directly or indirectly, the maintenance coefficient and the fractional growth rate of the nonfiber-carbohydrate-degrading bacteria. Figure 4.4D shows that NFC-degrading bacteria consistently have greater yield, and because the amount of nonfiber carbohydrate that is degraded in the rumen is usually greater than the fiber carbohydrate, a larger amount of nonfiber-carbohydrate-degrading bacteria is expected. The ruminal pH computed in Sections 4.2.8 and 4.3.8 shows an empirical regression (Eq. #94) derived by Argyle and Baldwin (1988) that uses the concentration (m*M*) of volatile fatty acids (i.e., acetate, propionate, and butyrate) and lactate in the rumen. Alternatively, the ruminal pH can be optimized to satisfy the equality $Ru_{Acidity} = Ru_{BC}$, as shown in Figure 4.5. The optimization is possible because the growth of bacteria and their impact on the ruminal degradation of carbohydrate; the production and absorption of VFA (i.e., acetate, propionate, and butyrate) from the degradation of carbohydrate; and the production, absorption, and fermentation of lactate depend on the ruminal pH. Thus, a stable ruminal pH can be reached when the rumen acidity and its buffering capacity are in [dynamic] equilibrium.

4.2.10 Duodenum submodel: calcDuodenum()

#	Variable[1]	Description	Equation
1:	$RECA1_f$	feeds' carbohydrates	$CA1_f + Prop_f^{Glyc} - RDCA1_f$
2:	$RECA2_f$	feeds' carbohydrates	$CA2_f - RDCA2_f$
3:	$RECA3_f$	feeds' carbohydrates	$CA3_f - RDCA3_f$
4:	$RECA4_f$	feeds' carbohydrates	$CA4_f - RDCA4_f$
5:	$RECB1_f$	feeds' carbohydrates	$CB1_f - RDCB1_f$
6:	$RECB2_f$	feeds' carbohydrates	$CB2_f - RDCB2_f$
7:	$RECB3_f$	feeds' carbohydrates	$CB3_f - RDCB3_f$
8:	$RECC_f$	feeds' carbohydrates	CC_f
9:	$REBCA_f$	bacteria CHO	$BactCA_f$
10:	$REBCB1_f$	bacteria CHO	$BactCB1_f$
11:	$REPA_f$	feeds' proteins	$PA_f - RDPA_f$
12:	$REPB1_f$	feeds' proteins	$PB1_f - RDPB1_f$
13:	$REPB2_f$	feeds' proteins	$PB2_f - RDPB2_f$
14:	$REPB3_f$	feeds' proteins	$PB3_f - RDPB3_f$
15:	$REPC_f$	feeds' proteins	$PC_f - RDPC_f$
16:	$RETP_j$	feeds' proteins	$REPB1_f + REPB2_j + REPB3_f$
17:	$REBCP_f$	bacteria proteins	$BactCP_f$
18:	$REBTP_j$	bacteria proteins	$BactTP_f$
19:	$REBNA_j$	bacteria proteins	$BactNA_f$
20:	$REBCW_j$	bacteria proteins	$BactCW_f$
21:	$REAA_{j,f}$	feeds' amino acids	$RETP_f * FAA_{j,f}$
22:	$REBAA_{j,f}$	bacteria amino acids	$REBTP_f * BNCWAA_j + REBCP * BCWAA_j$
23:	$REEE_f$	feeds' ether extract	EE_f
24:	$REFAC12_j$	feeds' fatty acids	$EFAC12_f + LEFAC12_f$
25:	$REFAC14_j$	feeds' fatty acids	$EFAC14_f + LEFAC14_f$
26:	$REFAC16_j$	feeds' fatty acids	$EFAC16_f + LEFAC16_f + DNFAC16_f$
27:	$REFAC16{:}1_j$	feeds' fatty acids	$EFAC16{:}1_f + LEFAC16{:}1_f + DNFAC16{:}1_f$
28:	$REFAC18_j$	feeds' fatty acids	$EFAC18_f + LEFAC18_f + DNFAC18_f$
29:	$REFAC18{:}1c_j$	feeds' fatty acids	$EFAC18{:}1c_f + LEFAC18{:}1c_f$
30:	$REFAC18{:}1t_j$	feeds' fatty acids	$EFAC18{:}1t_f + LEFAC18{:}1t_f$
31:	$REFAC18{:}2_j$	feeds' fatty acids	$EFAC18{:}2_f + LEFAC18{:}2_f$
32:	$REFAC18{:}3_j$	feeds' fatty acids	$EFAC18{:}3_f + LEFAC18{:}3_f$
33:	$REFAOther_j$	feeds' fatty acids	$EFAOther_f + LEFAOther_f + DNFAOther_f$
34:	$REGlycerol_j$	feeds' fatty acids	$EGlycerol_f$
35:	$REBFat_f$	bacteria ether extract	$BactFat_f$
36:	$REBFAC12_j$	bacteria fatty acids	$0.020667 * BactFat_f$
37:	$REBFAC14_j$	bacteria fatty acids	$0.033 * BactFat_f$
38:	$REBFAC16_j$	bacteria fatty acids	$0.305333 * BactFat_f$
39:	$REBFAC16{:}1_j$	bacteria fatty acids	$0.04 * BactFat_f$
40:	$REBFAC18_j$	bacteria fatty acids	$0.226 * BactFat_f$
41:	$REBFAC18{:}1_j$	bacteria fatty acids	$0.098667 * BactFat_f$
42:	$REBFAC18{:}2_j$	bacteria fatty acids	$0.039333 * BactFat_f$
43:	$REBFAC18{:}3_j$	bacteria fatty acids	$0.01 * BactFat_f$
44:	$REBFAOther_j$	bacteria fatty acids	$0.145 * BactFat_f$
45:	$REBAsh_f$	bacteria ash	$BactAsh_f$

[1] ***BCWAA*** is the bacteria cell wall amino acid (Met: 0.024, Lys: 0.056, Arg: 0.0382, Thr: 0.033, Leu: 0.059, Ile: 0.04, Val: 0.047, His: 0.0174, Phe: 0.042, and Trp: 0.0163) composition, g/d; ***BNCWAA*** is the bacteria noncell wall amino acid (Met: 0.0268, Lys: 0.082, Arg: 0.0696, Thr: 0.0559, Leu: 0.0751, Ile: 0.0588, Val: 0.0616, His: 0.0269, Phe: 0.0516, and Trp: 0.0163) composition, g/d; ***f*** is the jth feed; ***AA*** is the amino acids (Met, Lys, Arg, Thr, Ley, Ile, Val, His, Phe, and Trp) composition, g/d; ***j*** is the jth amino acid; ***REBAA*** is the ruminally escaped amino acid of the bacteria, g/d; ***REBAsh*** is the ruminally escaped bacterial ash, g/d; ***REBCA*** is the ruminally escaped carbohydrate fraction A of bacteria, g/d; ***REBCB1*** is the ruminally escaped carbohydrate fraction B1 of bacteria, g/d; ***REBCP*** is the ruminally escaped crude protein of bacteria, g/d; ***REBCW*** is the ruminally escaped cell wall of bacteria, g/d; ***REBFAC12*** is the ruminally escaped bacterial FAC12, g/d; ***REBFAC14*** is the ruminally escaped bacterial FAC14, g/d; ***REBFAC16*** is the ruminally escaped bacterial FAC16, g/d; ***REBFAC16:1*** is the ruminally escaped bacterial FAC16:1, g/d; ***REBFAC18*** is the

ruminally escaped bacterial FAC18, g/d; ***REBFAC18:1*** is the ruminally escaped bacterial FAC18:1, g/d; ***REBFAC18:2*** is the ruminally escaped bacterial FAC18:2, g/d; ***REBFAC18:3*** is the ruminally escaped bacterial FAC18:3, g/d; ***REBFAOther*** is the ruminally escaped bacterial FAOther, g/d; ***REBNA*** is the ruminally escaped nucleic acids of bacteria, g/d; ***REBTP*** is the ruminally escaped true protein of bacteria, g/d; ***RECA1*** is the ruminally escaped carbohydrate fraction A1, g/d; ***RECA2*** is the ruminally escaped carbohydrate fraction A2, g/d; ***RECA3*** is the ruminally escaped carbohydrate fraction A3, g/d; ***RECA4*** is the ruminally escaped carbohydrate fraction A4, g/d; ***RECB1*** is the ruminally escaped carbohydrate fraction B1, g/d; ***RECB2*** is the ruminally escaped carbohydrate fraction B2, g/d; ***RECB3*** is the ruminally escaped carbohydrate fraction B3, g/d; ***RECC*** is the ruminally escaped carbohydrate fraction C, g/d; ***REEE*** is the ruminally escaped ether extract, g/d; ***REFAA*** is the ruminally escaped amino acid of the feed, g/d; ***REFAC12*** is the ruminally escaped lipolized and non-lipolized FAC12, g/d; ***REFAC14*** is the ruminally escaped lipolized and non-lipolized FAC14, g/d; ***REFAC16*** is the ruminally escaped lipolized, non-lipolized, and *de novo* synthesized FAC16, g/d; ***REFAC16:1*** is the ruminally escaped lipolized, non-lipolized, and *de novo* synthesized FAC16:1, g/d; ***REFAC18*** is the ruminally escaped lipolized, non-lipolized, and *de novo* synthesized FAC18, g/d; ***REFAC18:1c*** is the ruminally escaped lipolized and non-lipolized FAC18:1c, g/d; ***REFAC18:1t*** is the ruminally escaped lipolized and non-lipolized FAC18:1t, g/d; ***REFAC18:2*** is the ruminally escaped lipolized and non-lipolized FAC18:2, g/d; ***REFAC18:3*** is the ruminally escaped lipolized and non-lipolized FAC18:3, g/d; ***REFAOther*** is the ruminally escaped lipolized, non-lipolized, and *de novo* synthesized FAOther, g/d; ***REGlycerol*** is the ruminally escaped glycerol, g/d; ***REPA*** is the ruminally escaped protein fraction A, g/d; ***REPB1*** is the ruminally escaped protein fraction B1, g/d; ***REPB2*** is the ruminally escaped protein fraction B2, g/d; ***REPB3*** is the ruminally escaped protein fraction B3, g/d; ***REPC*** is the ruminally escaped protein fraction C, g/d; and ***RETP*** is the ruminally escaped true protein, g/d;

4.2.11 Small and large intestine submodels: calcSI()

#	Variable[1]	Description	Equation
1:	$GCA1_f$	feeds' carbohydrates	$RECA1_f * ID_{CA1,f}$
2:	$GCA2_f$	feeds' carbohydrates	$RECA2_f * ID_{CA2,f}$
3:	$GCA3_f$	feeds' carbohydrates	$RECA3_f * ID_{CA3,f}$
4:	$GCA4_f$	feeds' carbohydrates	$RECA4_f * ID_{CA4,f}$
5:	$GCB1_f$	feeds' carbohydrates	$RECB1_f * ID_{CB1,f}$
6:	$GCB2_f$	feeds' carbohydrates	$RECB2_f * ID_{CB2,f}$
7:	$GCB3_f$	feeds' carbohydrates	$RECB3_f * ID_{CB3,f}$
8:	GCC_f	feeds' carbohydrates	$RECC_f * ID_{CC,f}$
9:	$GCHO_f$	feeds' carbohydrates	$GCA1_f + GCA2_f + GCA3_f + GCA4_f + GCB1_f + GCB2_f + GCB3_f + GCC_f$
10:	$GBCA_f$	bacteria CHO	$REBCA_f * 0.95$
11:	$GBCB1_f$	bacteria CHO	$REBCB1_f * 0.95$
12:	$GBCHO_f$	bacteria CHO	$GBCA_f + GBCB1_f$
13:	GPA_f	feeds' proteins	$REPA_f * ID_{PA,f}$
14:	$GPB1_f$	feeds' proteins	$REPB1_f * ID_{PB1,f}$
15:	$GPB2_f$	feeds' proteins	$REPB2_f * ID_{PB2,f}$
16:	$GPB3_f$	feeds' proteins	$REPB3_f * ID_{PB3,f}$
17:	GPC_f	feeds' proteins	$REPC_f * ID_{PC,f}$
18:	$GProt_f$	feeds' proteins	$GPA_f + GPB1_F + GPB2_F + GPB3_f + GPC_f$
19:	$GBTP_f$	bacteria proteins	$REBTP_f$
20:	$GBNA_f$	bacteria proteins	$REBNA_f$
21:	$GBCW_f$	bacteria proteins	0
22:	$GBProt_f$	bacteria proteins	$GBTP_f + GBNA_f + GBCW_f$
23:	$GAA_{j,f}$	feed amino acids	$ID_{AA_{j,f}} * (GPB1_f + GPB2_f + GPB3_f)$
24:	$GBAA_{j,f}$	bacteria amino acids	$GBTP_f * BNCWAA_j + GBCP * BCWAA_j$
25:	GEE_f	feeds' ether extract	$REEE_f * ID_{EE,f}$
26:	$GFAC12_j$	feeds' fatty acids	$EFAC12_f * ID_{NLFAC12,f} + LEFAC12_f * ID_{LFAC12,f}$
27:	$GFAC14_j$	feeds' fatty acids	$EFAC14_f * ID_{NLFAC14,f} + LEFAC14_f * ID_{LFAC14,f}$
28:	$GFAC16_j$	feeds' fatty acids	$EFAC16_f * ID_{NLFAC16,f} + (LEFAC16_f + DNFAC16_f) * ID_{LFAC16,f}$
29:	$GFAC16{:}1_j$	feeds' fatty acids	$EFAC16{:}1_f * ID_{NLFAC16:1,f} + (LEFAC16{:}1_f + DNFAC16{:}1_f) * ID_{LFAC16:1,f}$
30:	$GFAC18_j$	feeds' fatty acids	$EFAC18_f * ID_{NLFAC18,f} + (LEFAC18_f + DNFAC18_f) * ID_{LFAC18,f}$
31:	$GFAC18{:}1c_j$	feeds' fatty acids	$EFAC18{:}1c_f * ID_{NLFAC18:1c,f} + LEFAC18{:}1c_f * ID_{LFAC18:1c,f}$
32:	$GFAC18{:}1t_j$	feeds' fatty acids	$EFAC18{:}1t_f * ID_{NLFAC18:1t,f} + LEFAC18{:}1t_f * ID_{LFAC18:1t,f}$
33:	$GFAC18{:}2_j$	feeds' fatty acids	$EFAC18{:}2_f * ID_{NLFAC18:2,f} + LEFAC18{:}2_f * ID_{LFAC18:2,f}$
34:	$GFAC18{:}3_j$	feeds' fatty acids	$EFAC18{:}3_f * ID_{NLFAC18:3,f} + LEFAC18{:}3_f * ID_{LFAC18:3,f}$
35:	$GFAOther_j$	feeds' fatty acids	$EFAOther_f * ID_{NLFAOther,f} + (LEFAOther_f + DNFAOther_f) * ID_{LFAOther,f}$

#	Variable[(1)]	Description	Equation
36:	GFA_j	feeds' fatty acids	$GFAC12_j + GFAC14_f + GFAC16_f + GFAC16{:}1_f + GFAC18_f + GFAC18{:}1c_f + GFAC18{:}1t_f + GFAC18{:}2_f + GFAC18{:}3_f + GFAOther_j$
37:	$GGlycerol_f$	feeds' fatty acids	$EGlycerol_f * ID_{CA1,f}$
38:	$GBFat_f$	bacteria fat	$REBFat_f * 0.95$
39:	$GBFAC12_j$	bacteria fatty acids	$GBFat_f * 0.2067$
40:	$GBFAC14_j$	bacteria fatty acids	$GBFat_f * 0.033$
41:	$GBFAC16_j$	bacteria fatty acids	$GBFat_f * 0.3053$
42:	$GBFAC16{:}1_j$	bacteria fatty acids	$GBFat_f * 0.04$
43:	$GBFAC18_j$	bacteria fatty acids	$GBFat_f * 0.226$
44:	$GBFAC18{:}1_j$	bacteria fatty acids	$GBFat_f * 0.09867$
45:	$GBFAC18{:}2_j$	bacteria fatty acids	$GBFat_f * 0.0393$
46:	$GBFAC18{:}3_j$	bacteria fatty acids	$GBFat_f * 0.01$
47:	$GBFAOther_j$	bacteria fatty acids	$GBFat_f * 0.145$
48:	$GBFA_f$	bacteria fatty acids	$GBFAC12_f + GBFAC14_f + GBFAC16_f + GBFAC16{:}1_f + GBFAC18_f + GBFAC18{:}1_f + GBFAC18{:}2_f + GBFAC18{:}3_f + GBFAOther_f$
49:	$GAsh_f$	feeds' ash	$Ash_f * ID_{Ash,f}$
50:	$GBAsh_j$	bacteria ash	$REBAsh_f * 0.5$

(1) ***f*** is the jth feed; ***GAA*** is the small intestinally digested amino acids, g/d; ***GAsh*** is the small intestinally digested ash, g/d; ***GBAA*** is the small intestinally digested bacterial amino acids, g/d; ***GBAsh*** is the small intestinally digested bacterial ash, g/d; ***GBCA*** is the small intestinally digested carbohydrate fraction A of bacteria, g/d; ***GBCB1*** is the small intestinally digested carbohydrate fraction B1 of bacteria, g/d; ***GBCHO*** is the small intestinally digested carbohydrate of bacteria, g/d; ***GBCW*** is the small intestinally digested bacterial cell wall, g/d; ***GBFA*** is the small intestinally digested bacterial fatty acids, g/d; ***GBFAC12*** is the small intestinally digested bacterial FAC12, g/d; ***GBFAC14*** is the small intestinally digested bacterial FAC14, g/d; ***GBFAC16*** is the small intestinally digested bacterial FAC16, g/d; ***GBFAC16:1*** is the small intestinally digested bacterial FAC16:1, g/d; ***GBFAC18*** is the small intestinally digested bacterial FAC18, g/d; ***GBFAC18:1*** is the small intestinally digested bacterial FAC18:1, g/d; ***GBFAC18:2*** is the small intestinally digested bacterial FAC18:2, g/d; ***GBFAC18:3*** is the small intestinally digested bacterial FAC18:3, g/d; ***GBFAOther*** is the small intestinally digested bacterial FAOther, g/d; ***GBNA*** is the small intestinally digested bacterial nucleic acids, g/d; ***GBProt*** is the small intestinally digested bacterial protein, g/d; ***GBTP*** is the small intestinally digested bacterial true protein, g/d; ***GCA1*** is the small intestinally digested carbohydrate fraction A1, g/d; ***GCA2*** is the small intestinally digested carbohydrate fraction A2, g/d; ***GCA3*** is the small intestinally digested carbohydrate fraction A3, g/d; ***GCA4*** is the small intestinally digested carbohydrate fraction A4, g/d; ***GCB1*** is the small intestinally digested carbohydrate fraction B1, g/d; ***GCB2*** is the small intestinally digested carbohydrate fraction B2, g/d; ***GCB3*** is the small intestinally digested carbohydrate fraction B3, g/d; ***GCC*** is the small intestinally digested carbohydrate fraction C, g/d; ***GCHO*** is the small intestinally digested carbohydrate, g/d; ***GEE*** is the small intestinally digested ether extract, g/d; ***GFA*** is the small intestinally digested fatty acids, g/d; ***GFAC12*** is the small intestinally digested lipolized and non-lipolized FAC12, g/d; ***GFAC14*** is the small intestinally digested lipolized and non-lipolized FAC14, g/d; ***GFAC16*** is the small intestinally digested lipolized, non-lipolized, and *de novo* synthesized FAC16, g/d; ***GFAC16:1*** is the small intestinally digested lipolized, non-lipolized, and *de novo* synthesized FAC16:1, g/d; ***GFAC18*** is the small intestinally digested lipolized, non-lipolized, and *de novo* synthesized FAC18, g/d; ***GFAC18:1c*** is the small intestinally digested lipolized and non-lipolized FAC18:1c, g/d; ***GFAC18:1t*** is the small intestinally digested lipolized and non-lipolized FAC18:1t, g/d; ***GFAC18:2*** is the small intestinally digested lipolized and non-lipolized FAC18:2, g/d; ***GFAC18:3*** is the small intestinally digested lipolized and non-lipolized FAC18:3, g/d; ***GFAOther*** is the small intestinally digested lipolized, non-lipolized, and *de novo* synthesized FAOther, g/d; ***GGlycerol*** is the small intestinally digested glycerol, g/d; ***GPA*** is the small intestinally digested protein fraction A, g/d; ***GPB1*** is the small intestinally digested protein fraction B1, g/d; ***GPB2*** is the small intestinally digested protein fraction B2, g/d; ***GPB3*** is the small intestinally digested protein fraction B3, g/d; ***GPC*** is the small intestinally digested protein fraction C, g/d; ***GProt*** is the small intestinally digested protein, g/d; ID_{AA} is the intestinal digestibility of amino acids of the feeds, g/g; ID_{Ash} is the intestinal digestibility of ash (default is 0.5), g/g; ID_{CA1} is the intestinal digestibility of carbohydrate fraction A1 (default is 1), g/g; ID_{CA2} is the intestinal digestibility of carbohydrate fraction A2 (default is 1), g/g; ID_{CA3} is the intestinal digestibility of carbohydrate fraction A3 (default is 1), g/g; ID_{CA4} is the intestinal digestibility of carbohydrate fraction A4 (default is 1), g/g; ID_{CB1} is the intestinal digestibility of carbohydrate fraction B1 (default is variable, but usually above 0.75), g/g; ID_{CB2} is the intestinal digestibility of carbohydrate fraction B2 (default is variable, but usually above 0.75), g/g; ID_{CB3} is the intestinal digestibility of carbohydrate fraction B3 (default is 0.2), g/g; ID_{CC} is the intestinal digestibility of carbohydrate fraction C (default is zero), g/g; ID_{EE} is the intestinal digestibility of ether extract (default is 0.95), g/g; ID_{LFAC12} is the intestinal digestibility of lipolized FAC12 (default is 0.9539), g/g; ID_{LFAC14} is the intestinal digestibility of lipolized FAC14 (default is 0.7506), g/g; ID_{LFAC16} is the intestinal digestibility of lipolized FAC16 (default is 0.7248), g/g; $ID_{LFAC16:1}$ is the intestinal digestibility of lipolized FAC16:1 (default is 0.64), g/g; ID_{LFAC18} is the intestinal digestibility of lipolized FAC18 (default is 0.728), g/g; $ID_{LFAC18:1c}$ is the intestinal digestibility of lipolized FAC18:1c (default is 0.8925), g/g; $ID_{LFAC18:1t}$ is the intestinal digestibility of lipolized FAC18:1t (default is 0.7856), g/g; $ID_{LFAC18:2}$ is the intestinal digestibility of lipolized FAC18:2 (default is 0.83), g/g; $ID_{LFAC18:3}$ is the intestinal digestibility of lipolized FAC18:3 (default is 0.7755), g/g; $ID_{LFAOther}$ is the intestinal digestibility of lipolized FAOther (default is 0.5871), g/g; $ID_{NLFAC12}$ is the intestinal digestibility of non-lipolized FAC12 (default is 0.9539), g/g; $ID_{NLFAC14}$ is the intestinal digestibility of non-lipolized FAC14 (default is 0.4858), g/g; $ID_{NLFAC16}$ is the intestinal digestibility of non-lipolized FAC16 (default is 0.7248), g/g; $ID_{NLFAC16:1}$ is the intestinal digestibility of non-lipolized FAC16:1 (default is 0.64), g/g; $ID_{NLFAC18}$ is the intestinal digestibility of non-lipolized FAC18 (default is 0.728), g/g; $ID_{NLFAC18:1c}$ is the intestinal

digestibility of non-lipolized FAC18:1c (default is 0.6693), g/g; $\boldsymbol{ID_{NLFAC18:1t}}$ is the intestinal digestibility of non-lipolized FAC18:1t (default is 0), g/g; $\boldsymbol{ID_{NLFAC18:2}}$ is the intestinal digestibility of non-lipolized FAC18:2 (default is 0.7762), g/g; $\boldsymbol{ID_{NLFAC18:3}}$ is the intestinal digestibility of non-lipolized FAC18:3 (default is 0.7755), g/g; $\boldsymbol{ID_{NLFAOther}}$ is the intestinal digestibility of non-lipolized FAOther (default is 0.5871), g/g; $\boldsymbol{ID_{PA}}$ is the intestinal digestibility of protein fraction A (default is 1), g/g; $\boldsymbol{ID_{PB1}}$ is the intestinal digestibility of protein fraction B1 (default is 1), g/g; $\boldsymbol{ID_{PB2}}$ is the intestinal digestibility of protein fraction B2 (default is 1), g/g; $\boldsymbol{ID_{PB3}}$ is the intestinal digestibility of protein fraction B3 (default is 0.8), g/g; $\boldsymbol{ID_{PC}}$ is the intestinal digestibility of protein fraction C (default is zero), g/g; and $\boldsymbol{j}$ is the jth amino acid.

4.2.12 Fecal submodel: calcFecal()

#	Variable[1]	Description[2]	Equation
1:	$FECP_f$	feeds' proteins	$CP_f - (RDP'_f + GProt_f)$
2:	$FECHO_f$	feeds' carbohydrates	$(CHO_f + Prop_f^{Glyc}) - (RDCHO_f + GCHO_f)$
3:	$FEEE_f$	feeds' ether extract	$EE_f - GEE_f$
4:	$FEAsh_j$	feeds' ash	$Ash_f - GAsh_f$
5:	$FEGlycerol_f$	feeds' fatty acids	$(Glycerol_f - Prop_f^{Glyc}) - GGycerol_f$
6:	$FEFAC12_f$	feeds' fatty acids	$FAC12_f - GFAC12_f$
7:	$FEFAC14_f$	feeds' fatty acids	$FAC14_f - GFAC14_f$
8:	$FEFAC16_f$	feeds' fatty acids	$FAC16_f - GFAC16_f$
9:	$FEFAC16{:}1_f$	feeds' fatty acids	$FAC16{:}1_f - GFAC16{:}1_f$
10:	$FEFAC18_f$	feeds' fatty acids	$FAC18_f - GFAC18_f$
11:	$FEFAC18{:}1c_f$	feeds' fatty acids	$FAC18{:}1c_f - GFAC18{:}1c_f$
12:	$FEFAC18{:}1t_f$	feeds' fatty acids	$FAC18{:}1t_f - GFAC18{:}1t_f$
13:	$FEFAC18{:}2_f$	feeds' fatty acids	$FAC18{:}2_f - GFAC18{:}2_f$
14:	$FEFAC18{:}3_f$	feeds' fatty acids	$FAC18{:}3_f - GFAC18{:}3_f$
15:	$FEFAOther_f$	feeds' fatty acids	$FAOther_f - GFAOther_f$
16:	$FETFA_f$	feeds' fatty acids	$FEFAC12_f + FEFAC14_f + FEFAC16_f + FEFAC16{:}1_f + FEFAC18_f + FEFAC18{:}1c_f + FEFAC18{:}1t_f + FEFAC18{:}2_f + FEFAC18{:}3_f + FEFAOther_F$
17:	$FEBFAC12_f$	bacterial fatty acids	$REBFAC12_f - GBFAC12_f$
18:	$FEBFAC14_f$	bacterial fatty acids	$REBFAC14_f - GBFAC14_f$
19:	$FEBFAC16_f$	bacterial fatty acids	$REBFAC16_f - GBFAC16_f$
20:	$FEBFAC16{:}1_f$	bacterial fatty acids	$REBFAC16{:}1_f - GBFAC16{:}1_f$
21:	$FEBFAC18_f$	bacterial fatty acids	$REBFAC18_f - GBFAC18_f$
22:	$FEBFAC18{:}1_f$	bacterial fatty acids	$REBFAC18{:}1 - GBFAC18{:}1$
23:	$FEBFAC18{:}2_f$	bacterial fatty acids	$REBFAC18{:}2_f - GBFAC18{:}2_f$
24:	$FEBFAC18{:}3_f$	bacterial fatty acids	$REBFAC18{:}3_f - GBFAC18{:}3_f$
25:	$FEBFAOther_f$	bacterial fatty acids	$REBFAOther_f - GBFAOther_f$
26:	$FEENDEE_f$	option 0	$11.9 * 0.001 * DMI_f$
27:	$FEENDAsh_f$	option 0	$17 * 0.001 * DMI_f$
28:	$FEBCHO_f$	option 0	$(REBCA_f + REBCB1_f) - (GBCA_F + GBCB1_f)$
29:	$FEBCP_f$	option 0	$REBCP_f - GBProt_f$
30:	$FEBEE_f$	option 0	$REBFat_f - GBFat_f$
31:	$FEBAsh_f$	option 0	$REBAsh_f - GBFat_f$
32:	FEB_f	option 0	$FEBCHO_f + FEBCP_f + FEBEE_f + FEBAsh_f$
33:	FEC_f	option 0	$FECHO_f + FEBCHO_f$
34:	FEP_f	option 0	$FECP_F + FEBCP_f$
35:	FEF_f	option 0	$FEEE_f + FEBEE_f + FEENDEE_f$
36:	FEA_f	option 0	$FEAsh_f + FEBAsh_f + FEENDAsh_f$
37:	IDM_f	option 0	$(FEC_f + FEP_f + FEF_f + FEA_f)/0.91$
38:	IOM_f	option 0	$FEC_f + FEP_f + FEF_f$
39:	$FEENDCP_f$	option 0	$0.09 * IDM_f$
40:	FEP_f	option 0	$FECP_F + FEBCP_f + FEENDCP_f$
41:	$FEENDCP_f$	option 1	0
42:	$FEENDEE_f$	option 1	0
43:	$FEENDAsh_f$	option 1	0

#	Variable[(1)]	Description[(2)]	Equation
44:	$FEBCHO_f$	option 1	$(REBCA_f + REBCB1_f) - (GBCA_F + GBCB1_f)$
45:	$FEBCP_f$	option 1	$30 * 0.001 * DMI_f$
46:	$FEBEE_f$	option 1	$11.9 * 0.001 * DMI_f$
47:	$FEBAsh_f$	option 1	$17 * 0.001 * DMI_f$
48:	FEB_f	option 1	$FEBCHO_f + FEBCP_f + FEBEE_f + FEBAsh_f$
49:	FEC_f	option 1	$FECHO_f + FEBCHO_f$
50:	FEP_f	option 1	$FECP_F + FEBCP_f$
51:	FEF_f	option 1	$FEEE_f + FEBEE_f$
52:	FEA_f	option 1	$FEAsh_f + FEBAsh_f$
53:	IDM_f	option 1	$FEC_f + FEP_f + FEF_f + FEA_f$
54:	IOM_f	option 1	$FEC_f + FEP_f + FEF_f$
55:	$FEENDCP_f$	option 2	$0.15 * 30 * 0.001 * DMI_f$
56:	$FEENDEE_f$	option 2	$11.9 * 0.001 * DMI_f$
57:	$FEENDAsh_f$	option 2	$17 * 0.001 * DMI_f$
58:	$FEBCHO_f$	option 2	$(REBCA_f + REBCB1_f) - (GBCA_F + GBCB1_f)$
59:	$FEBCP_f$	option 2	$REBCP_f - GBProt_f$
60:	$FEBEE_f$	option 2	$REBFat_f - GBFat_f$
61:	$FEBAsh_f$	option 2	$REBAsh_f - GBFat_f$
62:	FEB_f	option 2	$FEBCHO_f + FEBCP_f + FEBEE_f + FEBAsh_f$
63:	FEC_f	option 2	$FECHO_f + FEBCHO_f$
64:	FEP_f	option 2	$FECP_F + FEBCP_f + FEENDCP_f$
65:	FEF_f	option 2	$FEEE_f + FEBEE_f + FEENDEE_f$
66:	FEA_f	option 2	$FEAsh_f + FEBAsh_f + FEENDAsh_f$
67:	IDM_f	option 2	$FEC_f + FEP_f + FEF_f + FEA_f$
68:	IOM_f	option 2	$FEC_f + FEP_f + FEF_f$
69:	$FEMCP_f$	metabolic matter	$FEENDCP_f + FEBCP_f$
70:	$FEMCHO_f$	metabolic matter	$FEBCHO_f$
71:	$FEMFat_f$	metabolic matter	$FEENDEE_f + FEBEE_f$
72:	$FEMAsh_f$	metabolic matter	$FEENDAsh_f + FEBAsh_f$
73:	FEM_f	metabolic matter	$FEMCP_f + FEMCHO_f + FEMFat_f + FEMAsh_f$

[(1)] ***f*** is the jth feed; ***FEA*** is fecal ash from bacteria and feeds, g/d; ***FEAsh*** is the fecal ash, g/d; ***FEB*** is the fecal bacterial mass, g/d; ***FEBAsh*** is the fecal bacterial ash, g/d; ***FEBCHO*** is the fecal bacterial carbohydrate, g/d; ***FEBCP*** is the fecal bacterial crude protein, g/d; ***FEBEE*** is the fecal bacterial ether extract, g/;d ***FEBFAC12*** is the fecal bacterial fatty acid FAC12, g/d; ***FEBFAC14*** is the fecal bacterial fatty acid FAC14, g/d; ***FEBFAC16*** is the fecal bacterial fatty acid FAC16, g/d; ***FEBFAC16:1*** is the fecal bacterial fatty acid FAC16:1, g/d; ***FEBFAC18*** is the fecal bacterial fatty acid FAC18, g/d; ***FEBFAC18:1*** is the fecal bacterial fatty acid FAC18:1t, g/d; ***FEBFAC18:2*** is the fecal bacterial fatty acid FAC18:2, g/d; ***FEBFAC18:3*** is the fecal bacterial fatty acid FAC18:3, g/d; ***FEBFAOther*** is the fecal bacterial fatty acid FAOther, g/d; ***FEC*** is fecal carbohydrate from bacteria and feeds, g/d; ***FECHO*** is the fecal carbohydrate, g/d; ***FECP*** is the fecal crude protein, g/d; ***FEEE*** is the fecal ether extract, g/d; ***FEENDAsh*** is the fecal endogenous ash, g/d; ***FEENDCP*** is the fecal endogenous crude protein, g/d; ***FEENDEE*** is the fecal endogenous ether extract (i.e., fat), g/d; ***FEF*** is fecal fat from bacteria and feeds, g/d; ***FEFAC12*** is the fecal fatty acid FAC12, g/d; ***FEFAC14*** is the fecal fatty acid FAC14, g/d; ***FEFAC16*** is the fecal fatty acid FAC16, g/d; ***FEFAC16:1*** is the fecal fatty acid FAC16:1, g/d; ***FEFAC18*** is the fecal fatty acid FAC18, g/d; ***FEFAC18:1c*** is the fecal fatty acid FAC18:1c, g/d; ***FEFAC18:1t*** is the fecal fatty acid FAC18:1t, g/d; ***FEFAC18:2*** is the fecal fatty acid FAC18:2, g/d; ***FEFAC18:3*** is the fecal fatty acid FAC18:3, g/d; ***FEFAOther*** is the fecal fatty acid FAOther, g/d; ***FEGlycerol*** is the fecal glycerol, g/d; ***FEM*** is fecal metabolic (endogenous and bacterial matter), g/d; ***FEMAsh*** is fecal metabolic ash, g/d; ***FEMCHO*** is fecal metabolic carbohydrate, g/d; ***FEMCP*** is fecal metabolic crude protein, g/d; ***FEMFat*** is fecal metabolic fat, g/d; ***FEP*** is fecal protein from bacteria and feeds, g/d; ***FETFA*** is the fecal total fatty acids, g/d; ***IDM*** is indigestible dry matter, g/d; and ***IOM*** is indigestible organic matter, g/d.

[(2)] Equations 26 to 40 (option 0) are based on Fox et al. (2004), Equations 41 to 54 (option 1) are based on Cannas et al. (2004), and Equations 55 to 68 (option 2) are based on Tedeschi et al. (2010).

4.2.13 Digestibility: calcDIG()

#	Variable[1]	Description	Equation
1:	$aDDM_f$	apparent digestibility	$DMI_f - IDM_f$
2:	$aDMD_f$	apparent digestibility	$\frac{aDDM_f}{DMI_f}$
3:	$aDMI_f$	apparent digestibility	$OMI_f - IOM_f$
4:	$aOMD_f$	apparent digestibility	$\frac{aDMI_f}{OMI_f}$
5:	$tDDM_f$	true digestibility	$DMI_f - IDM_f + FEM_f$
6:	$tDMD_f$	true digestibility	$\frac{tDDM_f}{DMI_f}$
7:	$tDOM_f$	true digestibility	$OMI_f - IOM_f + (FEM_f - FEMAsh_f)$
8:	$tOMD_f$	true digestibility	$\frac{tDOM_f}{OMI_f}$

[1] ***aDDM*** is the apparent digestible dry matter, g/d; ***aDMD*** is the apparent dry matter digestibility, g/d; ***aDOM*** is the apparent digestible organic matter, g/d; ***aOMD*** is the apparent organic matter digestibility, g/d; ***tDDM*** is the true digestible dry matter, g/d; ***tDMD*** is the true dry matter digestibility, g/d; ***tDOM*** is the true digestible organic matter, g/d; and ***tOMD*** is the true organic matter digestibility, g/d.

4.2.14 Total digestible nutrients, and gross, digestible, and metabolizable energies: calcTDN()

#	Variable[1]	Description[2]	Equation
1:	GE_f		$9.4 * EE_f + 5.65 * CP_f + 4.1 * (NFC_f + FC_f)$
2:	$aTDProt_f$		$CP_f - FEP_j$
3:	$aTDEE_f$	option 0	$2.25 * (EE_f - FEF_f)$
4:	$aTDCHO_f$	option 0	$CHO_f - FEC_f$
5:	$aTDEE_f$	option 1 without bacteria fatty acids	$2.25 * GFA_f$
6:	$aTDEE_f$	option 1 with bacteria fatty acids	$2.25 * (GFA_f + GBFA_f)$
7:	$aTDCHO_f$	option 1	$(CHO_f + Glycerol_f) - FEC_f - 2.25 * (DNFAC16_f + DNFAC16{:}1_f + DNFAC18_f + DNFAOther_f)$
8:	$aTDEE_f$	option 2 without bacteria fatty acids	$2.25 * (GFA_f - FEMFat_f)$
9:	$aTDEE_f$	option 2 with bacteria fatty acids	$2.25 * (GFA_f + GBFA_f - FEMFat_f)$
10:	$aTDCHO_f$	option 2	$(CHO_f + Glycerol_f) - FEC_f - 2.25 * (DNFAC16_f + DNFAC16{:}1_f + DNFAC18_f + DNFAOther_f)$
11:	$aTDN_f$		$aTDProt_f + aTDEE_f + aTDCHO_f$
12:	$tTDProt_f$		$CP_f - FEP_j + FEMCP_f$
13:	$tTDEE_f$	option 0	$2.25 * (EE_f - FEF_f + FEMFat_f)$
14:	$tTDCHO_f$	option 0	$CHO_f - FEC_f + FEMCHO_f$
15:	$tTDEE_f$	option 1 or 2 without bacteria fatty acids	$2.25 * GFA_f$
16:	$tTDEE_f$	option 1 or 2 with bacteria fatty acids	$2.25 * (GFA_f + GBFA_f)$
17:	$tTDCHO_f$	option 1 or 2	$(CHO_f + Glycerol_f) - FEC_f + FEMCHO_f - 2.25 * (DNFAC16_f + DNFAC16{:}1_f + DNFAC18_f + DNFAOther_f)$
18:	$tTDN_f$		$tTDProt_f + tTDEE_f + tTDCHO_f$
19:	$DEProt_f$		$4.409 * aTDProt_f$
20:	$DECHO_f$		$4.409 * aTDCHO_f$
21:	$DEEE_f$		$4.409 * aTDEE_f$
22:	DE_f		$DEProt_f + DECHO_f + DEEE_f$

#	Variable[(1)]	Description[(2)]	Equation
23:	$[ME]_f$	lactating or dry dairy	$If\left[[EE]_f < 3, 1.01 * \frac{DE_f}{DMI_f} - 0.45, 1.01 * \frac{DE_f}{DMI_f} - 0.45 + 0.0046 * ([EE]_f - 3)\right] * If[\text{Ionophore=True \& Adjust ME=True}, 1.023, 1]$
24:		otherwise	$0.82 * \frac{DE_f}{DMI_f} * If[\text{Ionophore=True \& Adjust ME=True}, 1.023, 1]$
25:	ME_f		$DMI_f * [ME]_f$
26:	$[NEm]_f$	lactating dairy	$0.644 * [ME]_f$
27:		otherwise	$(1.37 * [ME]_f - 0.138 * [ME]_f^2 + 0.0105 * [ME]_f^3 - 1.12) * If[\text{Ionophore=True \& Adjust ME=False}, 1.12, 1]$
28:	$[NEg]_f$		$1.42 * [ME]_f - 0.174 * [ME]_f^2 + 0.0122 * [ME]_f^3 - 1.65$
29:	$[NEl]_f$		$0.644 * [ME]_f$
30:	NEm_f		$DMI_f * [NEm]_f$
31:	NEg_f		$DMI_f * [NEg]_f$
32:	NEl_f		$DMI_f * [NEl]_f$
33:	k_m		$\frac{\sum_{f=1}^{nf} NEm_f}{\sum_{f=1}^{nf} ME_f}$
34:	k_g		$\frac{\sum_{f=1}^{nf} NEg_f}{\sum_{f=1}^{nf} ME_f}$
35:	k_l		$\frac{\sum_{f=1}^{nf} NEl_f}{\sum_{f=1}^{nf} ME_f}$

(1) ***[ME]*** is the dietary content of metabolizable energy, Mcal/kg; ***[NEg]*** is the dietary content of net energy for growth (also called ***NEga***), Mcal/kg; ***[NEl]*** is the dietary content of net energy for lactation (also called ***NEla***), Mcal/kg; ***[NEm]*** is the dietary content of net energy for maintenance (also called ***NEma***), Mcal/kg; ***aTDCHO*** is the apparent total digestible carbohydrate, g/d; ***aTDEE*** is the apparent total digestible ether extract, g/d; ***aTDN*** is apparent total digestible nutrients, g/d; ***aTDProt*** is the apparent total digestible protein, g/d; ***DECHO*** is the digestible energy from carbohydrates, Mcal/d; ***DEEE*** is the digestible energy from ether extract, Mcal/d; ***DEProt*** is the digestible energy from proteins, Mcal/d; ***f*** is the jth feed; ***GE*** is the gross energy, Mcal/d; k_g is the partial efficiency of utilization of metabolizable energy for net energy for growth, dimensionless; k_l is the partial efficiency of utilization of metabolizable energy for net energy for lactation, dimensionless; k_m is the partial efficiency of utilization of metabolizable energy for net energy for maintenance, dimensionless; ***ME*** is the metabolizable energy, Mcal/d; ***tTDCHO*** is the true total digestible carbohydrate, g/d; ***tTDEE*** is the true total digestible ether extract, g/d; ***tTDN*** is true total digestible nutrients, g/d; and ***tTDProt*** is the true total digestible protein, g/d.

4.2.15 Metabolizable protein: calcMP()

#	Variable[(1)]	Description	Equation
1:	$MP_{Bact,f}$		$GBProt_f - GBNA_f$
2:	$MP_{Feed,f}$		$GProt_f$
3:	MP_f		$MP_{Bact,f} + MP_{Feed,f}$

(1) ***f*** is the fth feed; ***MP*** is the metabolizable protein, g/d; MP_{Bact} is the metabolizable protein from bacteria, g/d; and MP_{Feed} is the metabolizable protein from feed, g/d.

4.3 Code

4.3.1 Carbohydrate and protein fractionation, fatty acids, minerals, and plant defensive compounds

```
getBasicChemistry2 <- function(fds = feeds3, genRPT = TRUE)
{
  # CHO (DM)
  anim.fd.acetate.conc <<- as.numeric(fds[, "Acetic_DM"])
  anim.fd.propionate.conc <<- as.numeric(fds[, "Propionic_DM"])
  anim.fd.butyrate.conc <<- as.numeric(fds[, "Butyric_DM"])
  anim.fd.lactate.conc <<- as.numeric(fds[, "Lactic_DM"])
  anim.fd.otherOA.conc <<- as.numeric(fds[, "OtherOA_DM"])
  anim.fd.sugars.conc <<- as.numeric(fds[, "Sugars_DM"])
  anim.fd.starch.conc <<- as.numeric(fds[, "Starch_DM"])
  anim.fd.SF.conc <<- as.numeric(fds[, "SF_DM"])
  anim.fd.NDF.conc <<- as.numeric(fds[, "AdjNDF_DM"])
  anim.fd.UnAdjNDF.conc <<- as.numeric(fds[, "NDF_DM"])
  anim.fd.ADF.conc <<- as.numeric(fds[, "ADF_DM"])
  anim.fd.lignin.conc <<- as.numeric(fds[, "Lignin_DM"])
  anim.fd.peNDF.conc <<- as.numeric(fds[, "peNDF_DM"])
  anim.fd.CHO.conc <<- as.numeric(fds[, "CHO_DM"])
  anim.fd.NFC.conc <<- as.numeric(fds[, "NFC_DM"])
  anim.fd.acetate.rate <<- anim.fd.acetate.conc * anim.fd.DMI.rate/100
  anim.fd.propionate.rate <<- anim.fd.propionate.conc * anim.fd.DMI.rate/100
  anim.fd.butyrate.rate <<- anim.fd.butyrate.conc * anim.fd.DMI.rate/100
  anim.fd.lactate.rate <<- anim.fd.lactate.conc * anim.fd.DMI.rate/100
  anim.fd.otherOA.rate <<- anim.fd.otherOA.conc * anim.fd.DMI.rate/100
  anim.fd.sugars.rate <<- anim.fd.sugars.conc * anim.fd.DMI.rate/100
  anim.fd.starch.rate <<- anim.fd.starch.conc * anim.fd.DMI.rate/100
  anim.fd.SF.rate <<- anim.fd.SF.conc * anim.fd.DMI.rate/100
  anim.fd.NDF.rate <<- anim.fd.NDF.conc * anim.fd.DMI.rate/100
  anim.fd.UnAdjNDF.rate <<- anim.fd.UnAdjNDF.conc * anim.fd.DMI.rate/100
  anim.fd.ADF.rate <<- anim.fd.ADF.conc * anim.fd.DMI.rate/100
  anim.fd.lignin.rate <<- anim.fd.lignin.conc * anim.fd.DMI.rate/100
  anim.fd.peNDF.rate <<- anim.fd.peNDF.conc * anim.fd.DMI.rate/100
  anim.fd.CHO.rate <<- anim.fd.CHO.conc * anim.fd.DMI.rate/100
  anim.fd.NFC.rate <<- anim.fd.NFC.conc * anim.fd.DMI.rate/100
  anim.fd.FC.rate <<- anim.fd.CHO.rate - anim.fd.NFC.rate
  anim.diet.acetate.rate <<- sum(anim.fd.acetate.rate)
  anim.diet.propionate.rate <<- sum(anim.fd.propionate.rate)
  anim.diet.butyrate.rate <<- sum(anim.fd.butyrate.rate)
  anim.diet.lactate.rate <<- sum(anim.fd.lactate.rate)
  anim.diet.otherOA.rate <<- sum(anim.fd.otherOA.rate)
  anim.diet.sugars.rate <<- sum(anim.fd.sugars.rate)
  anim.diet.starch.rate <<- sum(anim.fd.starch.rate)
  anim.diet.SF.rate <<- sum(anim.fd.SF.rate)
  anim.diet.NDF.rate <<- sum(anim.fd.NDF.rate)
```

```
    anim.diet.UnAdjNDF.rate <<- sum(anim.fd.UnAdjNDF.rate)
    anim.diet.ADF.rate <<- sum(anim.fd.ADF.rate)
    anim.diet.lignin.rate <<- sum(anim.fd.lignin.rate)
    anim.diet.peNDF.rate <<- sum(anim.fd.peNDF.rate)
    anim.diet.CHO.rate <<- sum(anim.fd.CHO.rate)
    anim.diet.NFC.rate <<- sum(anim.fd.NFC.rate)
    anim.diet.FC.rate <<- anim.diet.CHO.rate - anim.diet.NFC.rate
    if (genRPT)
    {
      rptCHOComposition_DM <- fds["FeedName.x"]
      names(rptCHOComposition_DM) <- "FeedName"
      rptCHOComposition_DM["Acetate"] <- anim.fd.acetate.conc
      rptCHOComposition_DM["Propionate"] <- anim.fd.propionate.conc
      rptCHOComposition_DM["Butyrate"] <- anim.fd.butyrate.conc
      rptCHOComposition_DM["Lactate"] <- anim.fd.lactate.conc
      rptCHOComposition_DM["OtherOA"] <- anim.fd.otherOA.conc
      rptCHOComposition_DM["Sugars"] <- anim.fd.sugars.conc
      rptCHOComposition_DM["Starch"] <- anim.fd.starch.conc
      rptCHOComposition_DM["SF"] <- anim.fd.SF.conc
      rptCHOComposition_DM["NFC"] <- anim.fd.NFC.conc
      rptCHOComposition_DM["NDF"] <- anim.fd.NDF.conc
      rptCHOComposition_DM["ADF"] <- anim.fd.ADF.conc
      rptCHOComposition_DM["Lignin(1), %NDF"] <- isz(anim.fd.lignin.rate * 100, anim.fd.UnAdjNDF.rate)
      rptCHOComposition_DM["Lignin(2), %NDF"] <- isz(anim.fd.lignin.rate * 100, anim.fd.NDF.rate)
      rptCHOComposition_DM["peNDF, %NDF"] <- isz(anim.fd.peNDF.rate * 100, anim.fd.NDF.rate)
      rptCHOComposition_DM2 <- data.frame(FeedName = "Ration")
      rptCHOComposition_DM2["Acetate"] <- isz(anim.diet.acetate.rate * 100, anim.diet.DMI.rate)
      rptCHOComposition_DM2["Propionate"] <- isz(anim.diet.propionate.rate * 100, anim.diet.DMI.rate)
      rptCHOComposition_DM2["Butyrate"] <- isz(anim.diet.butyrate.rate * 100, anim.diet.DMI.rate)
      rptCHOComposition_DM2["Lactate"] <- isz(anim.diet.lactate.rate * 100, anim.diet.DMI.rate)
      rptCHOComposition_DM2["OtherOA"] <- isz(anim.diet.otherOA.rate * 100, anim.diet.DMI.rate)
      rptCHOComposition_DM2["Sugars"] <- isz(anim.diet.sugars.rate * 100, anim.diet.DMI.rate)
      rptCHOComposition_DM2["Starch"] <- isz(anim.diet.starch.rate * 100, anim.diet.DMI.rate)
      rptCHOComposition_DM2["SF"] <- isz(anim.diet.SF.rate * 100, anim.diet.DMI.rate)
      rptCHOComposition_DM2["NFC"] <- isz(anim.diet.NFC.rate * 100, anim.diet.DMI.rate)
      rptCHOComposition_DM2["NDF"] <- isz(anim.diet.NDF.rate * 100, anim.diet.DMI.rate)
      rptCHOComposition_DM2["ADF"] <- isz(anim.diet.ADF.rate * 100, anim.diet.DMI.rate)
      rptCHOComposition_DM2["Lignin(1), %NDF"] <- isz(anim.diet.lignin.rate * 100, anim.diet.UnAdjNDF.rate)
      rptCHOComposition_DM2["Lignin(2), %NDF"] <- isz(anim.diet.lignin.rate * 100, anim.diet.NDF.rate)
      rptCHOComposition_DM2["peNDF, %NDF"] <- isz(anim.diet.peNDF.rate * 100, anim.diet.NDF.rate)
      rptCHOComposition_DM <- rbind(rptCHOComposition_DM, rptCHOComposition_DM2)
      footnote <- paste("(1) User-entered NDF\n", "(2) RNS-adjusted NDF (RNS uses this value)\nWhen sodium sulfite is used, NDF
  and adjusted NDF values are identical", sep = "")
      report(rptCHOComposition_DM, "Carbohydrate Composition, %DM", "", footnote, 3, 3, 1, 8, FALSE, FALSE, FALSE, FALSE, FALSE,
  FALSE, TRUE)
      rptCHOComposition_CHO <- fds["FeedName.x"]
      names(rptCHOComposition_CHO) <- "FeedName"
      rptCHOComposition_CHO["Acetate"] <- isz(anim.fd.acetate.conc * 100, anim.fd.CHO.conc)
      rptCHOComposition_CHO["Propionate"] <- isz(anim.fd.propionate.conc * 100, anim.fd.CHO.conc)
      rptCHOComposition_CHO["Butyrate"] <- isz(anim.fd.butyrate.conc * 100, anim.fd.CHO.conc)
      rptCHOComposition_CHO["Lactate"] <- isz(anim.fd.lactate.conc * 100, anim.fd.CHO.conc)
```

```
	rptCHOComposition_CHO["OtherOA"] <- isz(anim.fd.otherOA.conc * 100, anim.fd.CHO.conc)
	rptCHOComposition_CHO["Sugars"] <- isz(anim.fd.sugars.conc * 100, anim.fd.CHO.conc)
	rptCHOComposition_CHO["Starch"] <- isz(anim.fd.starch.conc * 100, anim.fd.CHO.conc)
	rptCHOComposition_CHO["SF"] <- isz(anim.fd.SF.conc * 100, anim.fd.CHO.conc)
	rptCHOComposition_CHO["NFC"] <- isz(anim.fd.NFC.conc * 100, anim.fd.CHO.conc)
	rptCHOComposition_CHO["NDF"] <- isz(anim.fd.NDF.conc * 100, anim.fd.CHO.conc)
	rptCHOComposition_CHO["ADF"] <- isz(anim.fd.ADF.conc * 100, anim.fd.CHO.conc)
	rptCHOComposition_CHO["Lignin"] <- isz(anim.fd.lignin.conc * 100, anim.fd.CHO.conc)
	rptCHOComposition_CHO["peNDF"] <- isz(anim.fd.peNDF.conc * 100, anim.fd.CHO.conc)
	rptCHOComposition_CHO2 <- data.frame(FeedName = "Ration")
	rptCHOComposition_CHO2["Acetate"] <- isz(anim.diet.acetate.rate * 100, anim.diet.CHO.rate)
	rptCHOComposition_CHO2["Propionate"] <- isz(anim.diet.propionate.rate * 100, anim.diet.CHO.rate)
	rptCHOComposition_CHO2["Butyrate"] <- isz(anim.diet.butyrate.rate * 100, anim.diet.CHO.rate)
	rptCHOComposition_CHO2["Lactate"] <- isz(anim.diet.lactate.rate * 100, anim.diet.CHO.rate)
	rptCHOComposition_CHO2["OtherOA"] <- isz(anim.diet.otherOA.rate * 100, anim.diet.CHO.rate)
	rptCHOComposition_CHO2["Sugars"] <- isz(anim.diet.sugars.rate * 100, anim.diet.CHO.rate)
	rptCHOComposition_CHO2["Starch"] <- isz(anim.diet.starch.rate * 100, anim.diet.CHO.rate)
	rptCHOComposition_CHO2["SF"] <- isz(anim.diet.SF.rate * 100, anim.diet.CHO.rate)
	rptCHOComposition_CHO2["NFC"] <- isz(anim.diet.NFC.rate * 100, anim.diet.CHO.rate)
	rptCHOComposition_CHO2["NDF"] <- isz(anim.diet.NDF.rate * 100, anim.diet.CHO.rate)
	rptCHOComposition_CHO2["ADF"] <- isz(anim.diet.ADF.rate * 100, anim.diet.CHO.rate)
	rptCHOComposition_CHO2["Lignin"] <- isz(anim.diet.lignin.rate * 100, anim.diet.CHO.rate)
	rptCHOComposition_CHO2["peNDF"] <- isz(anim.diet.peNDF.rate * 100, anim.diet.CHO.rate)
	rptCHOComposition_CHO <- rbind(rptCHOComposition_CHO, rptCHOComposition_CHO2)
	report(rptCHOComposition_CHO, "Carbohydrate Composition, %CHO", "", "", 3, 3, 1, 8, FALSE, FALSE, FALSE, FALSE, FALSE,
FALSE, TRUE)
	rptCHOComposition_DMI <- fds["FeedName.x"]
	names(rptCHOComposition_DMI) <- "FeedName"
	rptCHOComposition_DMI["Acetate"] <- anim.fd.acetate.rate
	rptCHOComposition_DMI["Propionate"] <- anim.fd.propionate.rate
	rptCHOComposition_DMI["Butyrate"] <- anim.fd.butyrate.rate
	rptCHOComposition_DMI["Lactate"] <- anim.fd.lactate.rate
	rptCHOComposition_DMI["OtherOA"] <- anim.fd.otherOA.rate
	rptCHOComposition_DMI["Sugars"] <- anim.fd.sugars.rate
	rptCHOComposition_DMI["Starch"] <- anim.fd.starch.rate
	rptCHOComposition_DMI["SF"] <- anim.fd.SF.rate
	rptCHOComposition_DMI["NFC"] <- anim.fd.NFC.rate
	rptCHOComposition_DMI["NDF"] <- anim.fd.NDF.rate
	rptCHOComposition_DMI["ADF"] <- anim.fd.ADF.rate
	rptCHOComposition_DMI["Lignin"] <- anim.fd.lignin.rate
	rptCHOComposition_DMI["peNDF"] <- anim.fd.peNDF.rate
	rptCHOComposition_DMI2 <- data.frame(FeedName = "Ration")
	rptCHOComposition_DMI2["Acetate"] <- anim.diet.acetate.rate
	rptCHOComposition_DMI2["Propionate"] <- anim.diet.propionate.rate
	rptCHOComposition_DMI2["Butyrate"] <- anim.diet.butyrate.rate
	rptCHOComposition_DMI2["Lactate"] <- anim.diet.lactate.rate
	rptCHOComposition_DMI2["OtherOA"] <- anim.diet.otherOA.rate
	rptCHOComposition_DMI2["Sugars"] <- anim.diet.sugars.rate
	rptCHOComposition_DMI2["Starch"] <- anim.diet.starch.rate
	rptCHOComposition_DMI2["SF"] <- anim.diet.SF.rate
	rptCHOComposition_DMI2["NFC"] <- anim.diet.NFC.rate
```

```
      rptCHOComposition_DMI2["NDF"] <- anim.diet.NDF.rate
      rptCHOComposition_DMI2["ADF"] <- anim.diet.ADF.rate
      rptCHOComposition_DMI2["Lignin"] <- anim.diet.lignin.rate
      rptCHOComposition_DMI2["peNDF"] <- anim.diet.peNDF.rate
      rptCHOComposition_DMI <- rbind(rptCHOComposition_DMI, rptCHOComposition_DMI2)
      report(rptCHOComposition_DMI, "Carbohydrate Intake, kg/d", "", "", 3, 3, 1, 8, FALSE, FALSE, FALSE, FALSE, FALSE, FALSE,
TRUE)
    }
    # Protein
    anim.fd.CP.conc <<- as.numeric(fds[, "CP_DM"])
    anim.fd.SP.conc <<- as.numeric(fds[, "SP_DM"])
    anim.fd.NPN.conc <<- as.numeric(fds[, "NPN_DM"])
    anim.fd.NDIP.conc <<- as.numeric(fds[, "NDIP_DM"])
    anim.fd.ADIP.conc <<- as.numeric(fds[, "ADIP_DM"])
    anim.fd.Leu_CP.conc <<- as.numeric(fds[, "Leu_CP"])
    anim.fd.Ile_CP.conc <<- as.numeric(fds[, "Ile_CP"])
    anim.fd.Val_CP.conc <<- as.numeric(fds[, "Val_CP"])
    anim.fd.CP.rate <<- anim.fd.CP.conc * anim.fd.DMI.rate/100
    anim.fd.SP.rate <<- anim.fd.SP.conc * anim.fd.DMI.rate/100
    anim.fd.NPN.rate <<- anim.fd.NPN.conc * anim.fd.DMI.rate/100
    anim.fd.NDIP.rate <<- anim.fd.NDIP.conc * anim.fd.DMI.rate/100
    anim.fd.ADIP.rate <<- anim.fd.ADIP.conc * anim.fd.DMI.rate/100
    anim.fd.Leu.rate <<- anim.fd.Leu_CP.conc * anim.fd.CP.rate/100
    anim.fd.Ile.rate <<- anim.fd.Ile_CP.conc * anim.fd.CP.rate/100
    anim.fd.Val.rate <<- anim.fd.Val_CP.conc * anim.fd.CP.rate/100
    anim.diet.CP.rate <<- sum(anim.fd.CP.rate)
    anim.diet.SP.rate <<- sum(anim.fd.SP.rate)
    anim.diet.NPN.rate <<- sum(anim.fd.NPN.rate)
    anim.diet.NDIP.rate <<- sum(anim.fd.NDIP.rate)
    anim.diet.ADIP.rate <<- sum(anim.fd.ADIP.rate)
    anim.diet.Leu.rate <<- sum(anim.fd.Leu.rate)
    anim.diet.Ile.rate <<- sum(anim.fd.Ile.rate)
    anim.diet.Val.rate <<- sum(anim.fd.Val.rate)
    if (genRPT)
    {
      rptProtComposition_DM <- fds["FeedName.x"]
      names(rptProtComposition_DM) <- "FeedName"
      rptProtComposition_DM["CP, %DM"] <- anim.fd.CP.conc
      rptProtComposition_DM["SP, %DM"] <- anim.fd.SP.conc
      rptProtComposition_DM["NPN, %DM"] <- anim.fd.NPN.conc
      rptProtComposition_DM["NDIP, %DM"] <- anim.fd.NDIP.conc
      rptProtComposition_DM["ADIP, %DM"] <- anim.fd.ADIP.conc
      rptProtComposition_DM["Leu, %DM"] <- anim.fd.Leu_CP.conc * anim.fd.CP.conc/100
      rptProtComposition_DM["Ile, %DM"] <- anim.fd.Ile_CP.conc * anim.fd.CP.conc/100
      rptProtComposition_DM["Val, %DM"] <- anim.fd.Val_CP.conc * anim.fd.CP.conc/100
      rptProtComposition_DM2 <- data.frame(FeedName = "Ration")
      rptProtComposition_DM2["CP, %DM"] <- isz(anim.diet.CP.rate * 100, anim.diet.DMI.rate)
      rptProtComposition_DM2["SP, %DM"] <- isz(anim.diet.SP.rate * 100, anim.diet.DMI.rate)
      rptProtComposition_DM2["NPN, %DM"] <- isz(anim.diet.NPN.rate * 100, anim.diet.DMI.rate)
      rptProtComposition_DM2["NDIP, %DM"] <- isz(anim.diet.NDIP.rate * 100, anim.diet.DMI.rate)
      rptProtComposition_DM2["ADIP, %DM"] <- isz(anim.diet.ADIP.rate * 100, anim.diet.DMI.rate)
```

```
    rptProtComposition_DM2["Leu, %DM"] <- isz(anim.diet.Leu.rate * 100, anim.diet.DMI.rate)
    rptProtComposition_DM2["Ile, %DM"] <- isz(anim.diet.Ile.rate * 100, anim.diet.DMI.rate)
    rptProtComposition_DM2["Val, %DM"] <- isz(anim.diet.Val.rate * 100, anim.diet.DMI.rate)
    rptProtComposition_DM <- rbind(rptProtComposition_DM, rptProtComposition_DM2)
    report(rptProtComposition_DM, "Protein Composition, %DM or %CP or %SP", "", "", 3, 3, 1, 8, FALSE, FALSE, FALSE, FALSE,
FALSE, FALSE, FALSE, 0, TRUE, "=", TRUE, "-", TRUE)
    rptProtComposition_DM <- fds["FeedName.x"]
    names(rptProtComposition_DM) <- "FeedName"
    rptProtComposition_DM["SP, %CP"] <- isz(anim.fd.SP.rate * 100, anim.fd.CP.rate)
    rptProtComposition_DM["NPN, %CP"] <- isz(anim.fd.NPN.rate * 100, anim.fd.CP.rate)
    rptProtComposition_DM["NPN, %SP"] <- isz(anim.fd.NPN.rate * 100, anim.fd.SP.rate)
    rptProtComposition_DM["NDIP, %CP"] <- isz(anim.fd.NDIP.rate * 100, anim.fd.CP.rate)
    rptProtComposition_DM["ADIP, %CP"] <- isz(anim.fd.ADIP.rate * 100, anim.fd.CP.rate)
    rptProtComposition_DM["Leu, %CP"] <- anim.fd.Leu_CP.conc
    rptProtComposition_DM["Ile, %CP"] <- anim.fd.Ile_CP.conc
    rptProtComposition_DM["Val, %CP"] <- anim.fd.Val_CP.conc
    rptProtComposition_DM2 <- data.frame(FeedName = "Ration")
    rptProtComposition_DM2["SP, %CP"] <- isz(anim.diet.SP.rate * 100, anim.diet.CP.rate)
    rptProtComposition_DM2["NPN, %CP"] <- isz(anim.diet.NPN.rate * 100, anim.diet.CP.rate)
    rptProtComposition_DM2["NPN, %SP"] <- isz(anim.diet.NPN.rate * 100, anim.diet.SP.rate)
    rptProtComposition_DM2["NDIP, %CP"] <- isz(anim.diet.NDIP.rate * 100, anim.diet.CP.rate)
    rptProtComposition_DM2["ADIP, %CP"] <- isz(anim.diet.ADIP.rate * 100, anim.diet.CP.rate)
    rptProtComposition_DM2["Leu, %CP"] <- isz(anim.diet.Leu.rate * 100, anim.diet.CP.rate)
    rptProtComposition_DM2["Ile, %CP"] <- isz(anim.diet.Ile.rate * 100, anim.diet.CP.rate)
    rptProtComposition_DM2["Val, %CP"] <- isz(anim.diet.Val.rate * 100, anim.diet.CP.rate)
    rptProtComposition_DM <- rbind(rptProtComposition_DM, rptProtComposition_DM2)
    report(rptProtComposition_DM, "\n", "", "", 3, 3, 1, 8, FALSE, FALSE, FALSE, FALSE, FALSE, FALSE, FALSE, 0, FALSE, "=",
TRUE, "=", FALSE)
    rptProtComposition_DMI <- fds["FeedName.x"]
    names(rptProtComposition_DMI) <- "FeedName"
    rptProtComposition_DMI["CP"] <- anim.fd.CP.rate
    rptProtComposition_DMI["SP"] <- anim.fd.SP.rate
    rptProtComposition_DMI["NPN"] <- anim.fd.NPN.rate
    rptProtComposition_DMI["NDIP"] <- anim.fd.NDIP.rate
    rptProtComposition_DMI["ADIP"] <- anim.fd.ADIP.rate
    rptProtComposition_DMI["Leu"] <- anim.fd.Leu.rate
    rptProtComposition_DMI["Ile"] <- anim.fd.Ile.rate
    rptProtComposition_DMI["Val"] <- anim.fd.Val.rate
    rptProtComposition_DMI2 <- data.frame(FeedName = "Ration")
    rptProtComposition_DMI2["CP"] <- anim.diet.CP.rate
    rptProtComposition_DMI2["SP"] <- anim.diet.SP.rate
    rptProtComposition_DMI2["NPN"] <- anim.diet.NPN.rate
    rptProtComposition_DMI2["NDIP"] <- anim.diet.NDIP.rate
    rptProtComposition_DMI2["ADIP"] <- anim.diet.ADIP.rate
    rptProtComposition_DMI2["Leu"] <- anim.diet.Leu.rate
    rptProtComposition_DMI2["Ile"] <- anim.diet.Ile.rate
    rptProtComposition_DMI2["Val"] <- anim.diet.Val.rate
    rptProtComposition_DMI <- rbind(rptProtComposition_DMI, rptProtComposition_DMI2)
    report(rptProtComposition_DMI, "\nProtein Intake, kg/d", "", "", 3, 3, 1, 8, FALSE, FALSE, FALSE, FALSE, FALSE, FALSE,
TRUE)
  }
```

```
# Esterified fatty acids (FA)
anim.fd.EE.conc <<- as.numeric(fds[, "EE_DM"])
anim.fd.TFA.conc <<- as.numeric(fds[, "TFA_DM"])
anim.fd.Glycerol.conc <<- as.numeric(fds[, "Glycerol_DM"])
anim.fd.Pigment.conc <<- as.numeric(fds[, "Pigment_DM"])
anim.fd.FAC12.conc <<- as.numeric(fds[, "C12_0_DM"])
anim.fd.FAC14.conc <<- as.numeric(fds[, "C14_0_DM"])
anim.fd.FAC16.conc <<- as.numeric(fds[, "C16_0_DM"])
anim.fd.FAC16_1.conc <<- as.numeric(fds[, "C16_1_DM"])
anim.fd.FAC18.conc <<- as.numeric(fds[, "C18_0_DM"])
anim.fd.FAC18_1c.conc <<- as.numeric(fds[, "C18_1c_DM"])
anim.fd.FAC18_1t.conc <<- as.numeric(fds[, "C18_1t_DM"])
anim.fd.FAC18_2.conc <<- as.numeric(fds[, "C18_2_DM"])
anim.fd.FAC18_3.conc <<- as.numeric(fds[, "C18_3_DM"])
anim.fd.FAOther.conc <<- as.numeric(fds[, "OtherLipids_DM"])
anim.fd.EE.rate <<- anim.fd.EE.conc * anim.fd.DMI.rate/100
anim.fd.TFA.rate <<- anim.fd.TFA.conc * anim.fd.DMI.rate/100
anim.fd.Glycerol.rate <<- anim.fd.Glycerol.conc * anim.fd.DMI.rate/100
anim.fd.Pigment.rate <<- anim.fd.Pigment.conc * anim.fd.DMI.rate/100
anim.fd.FAC12.rate <<- anim.fd.FAC12.conc * anim.fd.DMI.rate/100
anim.fd.FAC14.rate <<- anim.fd.FAC14.conc * anim.fd.DMI.rate/100
anim.fd.FAC16.rate <<- anim.fd.FAC16.conc * anim.fd.DMI.rate/100
anim.fd.FAC16_1.rate <<- anim.fd.FAC16_1.conc * anim.fd.DMI.rate/100
anim.fd.FAC18.rate <<- anim.fd.FAC18.conc * anim.fd.DMI.rate/100
anim.fd.FAC18_1c.rate <<- anim.fd.FAC18_1c.conc * anim.fd.DMI.rate/100
anim.fd.FAC18_1t.rate <<- anim.fd.FAC18_1t.conc * anim.fd.DMI.rate/100
anim.fd.FAC18_2.rate <<- anim.fd.FAC18_2.conc * anim.fd.DMI.rate/100
anim.fd.FAC18_3.rate <<- anim.fd.FAC18_3.conc * anim.fd.DMI.rate/100
anim.fd.FAOther.rate <<- anim.fd.FAOther.conc * anim.fd.DMI.rate/100
anim.diet.EE.rate <<- sum(anim.fd.EE.rate)
anim.diet.TFA.rate <<- sum(anim.fd.TFA.rate)
anim.diet.Glycerol.rate <<- sum(anim.fd.Glycerol.rate)
anim.diet.Pigment.rate <<- sum(anim.fd.Pigment.rate)
anim.diet.FAC12.rate <<- sum(anim.fd.FAC12.rate)
anim.diet.FAC14.rate <<- sum(anim.fd.FAC14.rate)
anim.diet.FAC16.rate <<- sum(anim.fd.FAC16.rate)
anim.diet.FAC16_1.rate <<- sum(anim.fd.FAC16_1.rate)
anim.diet.FAC18.rate <<- sum(anim.fd.FAC18.rate)
anim.diet.FAC18_1c.rate <<- sum(anim.fd.FAC18_1c.rate)
anim.diet.FAC18_1t.rate <<- sum(anim.fd.FAC18_1t.rate)
anim.diet.FAC18_2.rate <<- sum(anim.fd.FAC18_2.rate)
anim.diet.FAC18_3.rate <<- sum(anim.fd.FAC18_3.rate)
anim.diet.FAOther.rate <<- sum(anim.fd.FAOther.rate)
if (genRPT)
{
  rptFAComposition_DM <- fds["FeedName.x"]
  names(rptFAComposition_DM) <- "FeedName"
  rptFAComposition_DM["C12:0"] <- fds["C12_0_DM"]
  rptFAComposition_DM["C14:0"] <- fds["C14_0_DM"]
  rptFAComposition_DM["C16:0"] <- fds["C16_0_DM"]
  rptFAComposition_DM["C16:1"] <- fds["C16_1_DM"]
```

```
    rptFACompositioin_DM["C18:0"] <- fds["C18_0_DM"]
    rptFAComposition_DM["C18:1c"] <- fds["C18_1c_DM"]
    rptFAComposition_DM["C18:1t"] <- fds["C18_1t_DM"]
    rptFAComposition_DM["C18:2"] <- fds["C18_2_DM"]
    rptFAComposition_DM["C18:3"] <- fds["C18_3_DM"]
    rptFAComposition_DM["Other FA"] <- fds["OtherLipids_DM"]
    rptFAComposition_DM2 <- data.frame(FeedName = "Ration")
    rptFAComposition_DM2["C12:0"] <- isz(anim.diet.FAC12.rate * 100, anim.diet.DMI.rate)
    rptFAComposition_DM2["C14:0"] <- isz(anim.diet.FAC14.rate * 100, anim.diet.DMI.rate)
    rptFAComposition_DM2["C16:0"] <- isz(anim.diet.FAC16.rate * 100, anim.diet.DMI.rate)
    rptFAComposition_DM2["C16:1"] <- isz(anim.diet.FAC16_1.rate * 100, anim.diet.DMI.rate)
    rptFAComposition_DM2["C18:0"] <- isz(anim.diet.FAC18.rate * 100, anim.diet.DMI.rate)
    rptFAComposition_DM2["C18:1c"] <- isz(anim.diet.FAC18_1c.rate * 100, anim.diet.DMI.rate)
    rptFAComposition_DM2["C18:1t"] <- isz(anim.diet.FAC18_1t.rate * 100, anim.diet.DMI.rate)
    rptFAComposition_DM2["C18:2"] <- isz(anim.diet.FAC18_2.rate * 100, anim.diet.DMI.rate)
    rptFAComposition_DM2["C18:3"] <- isz(anim.diet.FAC18_3.rate * 100, anim.diet.DMI.rate)
    rptFAComposition_DM2["Other FA"] <- isz(anim.diet.FAOther.rate * 100, anim.diet.DMI.rate)
    rptFAComposition_DM <- rbind(rptFAComposition_DM, rptFAComposition_DM2)
    report(rptFAComposition_DM, "Esterified Fatty Acid Composition, %DM", "", "", 3, 3, 1, 7, FALSE, FALSE, TRUE, FALSE,
FALSE, FALSE, TRUE)
    rptFAComposition_EE <- fds["FeedName.x"]
    names(rptFAComposition_EE) <- "FeedName"
    rptFAComposition_EE["C12:0"] <- fds["C12_0_EE"]
    rptFAComposition_EE["C14:0"] <- fds["C14_0_EE"]
    rptFAComposition_EE["C16:0"] <- fds["C16_0_EE"]
    rptFAComposition_EE["C16:1"] <- fds["C16_1_EE"]
    rptFAComposition_EE["C18:0"] <- fds["C18_0_EE"]
    rptFAComposition_EE["C18:1c"] <- fds["C18_1c_EE"]
    rptFAComposition_EE["C18:1t"] <- fds["C18_1t_EE"]
    rptFAComposition_EE["C18:2"] <- fds["C18_2_EE"]
    rptFAComposition_EE["C18:3"] <- fds["C18_3_EE"]
    rptFAComposition_EE["Other FA"] <- fds["OtherLipids_EE"]
    rptFAComposition_EE2 <- data.frame(FeedName = "Ration")
    rptFAComposition_EE2["C12:0"] <- isz(anim.diet.FAC12.rate * 100, anim.diet.EE.rate)
    rptFAComposition_EE2["C14:0"] <- isz(anim.diet.FAC14.rate * 100, anim.diet.EE.rate)
    rptFAComposition_EE2["C16:0"] <- isz(anim.diet.FAC16.rate * 100, anim.diet.EE.rate)
    rptFAComposition_EE2["C16:1"] <- isz(anim.diet.FAC16_1.rate * 100, anim.diet.EE.rate)
    rptFAComposition_EE2["C18:0"] <- isz(anim.diet.FAC18.rate * 100, anim.diet.EE.rate)
    rptFAComposition_EE2["C18:1c"] <- isz(anim.diet.FAC18_1c.rate * 100, anim.diet.EE.rate)
    rptFAComposition_EE2["C18:1t"] <- isz(anim.diet.FAC18_1t.rate * 100, anim.diet.EE.rate)
    rptFAComposition_EE2["C18:2"] <- isz(anim.diet.FAC18_2.rate * 100, anim.diet.EE.rate)
    rptFAComposition_EE2["C18:3"] <- isz(anim.diet.FAC18_3.rate * 100, anim.diet.EE.rate)
    rptFAComposition_EE2["Other FA"] <- isz(anim.diet.FAOther.rate * 100, anim.diet.EE.rate)
    rptFAComposition_EE <- rbind(rptFAComposition_EE, rptFAComposition_EE2)
    report(rptFAComposition_EE, "Esterified Fatty Acid Composition, %EE", "", "", 3, 3, 1, 7, FALSE, FALSE, TRUE, FALSE,
FALSE, FALSE, TRUE)
    rptFAComposition_TFA <- fds["FeedName.x"]
    names(rptFAComposition_TFA) <- "FeedName"
    rptFAComposition_TFA["C12:0"] <- fds["C12_0_TFA"]
    rptFAComposition_TFA["C14:0"] <- fds["C14_0_TFA"]
    rptFAComposition_TFA["C16:0"] <- fds["C16_0_TFA"]
```

```
    rptFACompositon_TFA["C16:1"] <- fds["C16_1_TFA"]
    rptFAComposition_TFA["C18:0"] <- fds["C18_0_TFA"]
    rptFAComposition_TFA["C18:1c"] <- fds["C18_1c_TFA"]
    rptFAComposition_TFA["C18:1t"] <- fds["C18_1t_TFA"]
    rptFAComposition_TFA["C18:2"] <- fds["C18_2_TFA"]
    rptFAComposition_TFA["C18:3"] <- fds["C18_3_TFA"]
    rptFAComposition_TFA["Other FA"] <- fds["OtherLipids_TFA"]
    rptFAComposition_TFA2 <- fds["FeedName.x"]
    names(rptFAComposition_TFA2) <- "FeedName"
    rptFAComposition_TFA2 <- data.frame(FeedName = "Ration")
    rptFAComposition_TFA2["C12:0"] <- isz(anim.diet.FAC12.rate * 100, anim.diet.TFA.rate)
    rptFAComposition_TFA2["C14:0"] <- isz(anim.diet.FAC14.rate * 100, anim.diet.TFA.rate)
    rptFAComposition_TFA2["C16:0"] <- isz(anim.diet.FAC16.rate * 100, anim.diet.TFA.rate)
    rptFAComposition_TFA2["C16:1"] <- isz(anim.diet.FAC16_1.rate * 100, anim.diet.TFA.rate)
    rptFAComposition_TFA2["C18:0"] <- isz(anim.diet.FAC18.rate * 100, anim.diet.TFA.rate)
    rptFAComposition_TFA2["C18:1c"] <- isz(anim.diet.FAC18_1c.rate * 100, anim.diet.TFA.rate)
    rptFAComposition_TFA2["C18:1t"] <- isz(anim.diet.FAC18_1t.rate * 100, anim.diet.TFA.rate)
    rptFAComposition_TFA2["C18:2"] <- isz(anim.diet.FAC18_2.rate * 100, anim.diet.TFA.rate)
    rptFAComposition_TFA2["C18:3"] <- isz(anim.diet.FAC18_3.rate * 100, anim.diet.TFA.rate)
    rptFAComposition_TFA2["Other FA"] <- isz(anim.diet.FAOther.rate * 100, anim.diet.TFA.rate)
    rptFAComposition_TFA <- rbind(rptFAComposition_TFA, rptFAComposition_TFA2)
    report(rptFAComposition_TFA, "Esterified Fatty Acid Composition, %TFA", "", "", 3, 3, 1, 7, FALSE, FALSE, TRUE, FALSE, FALSE, FALSE, TRUE)
    rptFAComposition_DMI <- fds["FeedName.x"]
    names(rptFAComposition_DMI) <- "FeedName"
    rptFAComposition_DMI["C12:0"] <- anim.fd.FAC12.rate
    rptFAComposition_DMI["C14:0"] <- anim.fd.FAC14.rate
    rptFAComposition_DMI["C16:0"] <- anim.fd.FAC16.rate
    rptFAComposition_DMI["C16:1"] <- anim.fd.FAC16_1.rate
    rptFAComposition_DMI["C18:0"] <- anim.fd.FAC18.rate
    rptFAComposition_DMI["C18:1c"] <- anim.fd.FAC18_1c.rate
    rptFAComposition_DMI["C18:1t"] <- anim.fd.FAC18_1t.rate
    rptFAComposition_DMI["C18:2"] <- anim.fd.FAC18_2.rate
    rptFAComposition_DMI["C18:3"] <- anim.fd.FAC18_3.rate
    rptFAComposition_DMI["Other FA"] <- anim.fd.FAOther.rate
    rptFAComposition_DMI2 <- data.frame(FeedName = "Ration")
    rptFAComposition_DMI2["C12:0"] <- anim.diet.FAC12.rate
    rptFAComposition_DMI2["C14:0"] <- anim.diet.FAC14.rate
    rptFAComposition_DMI2["C16:0"] <- anim.diet.FAC16.rate
    rptFAComposition_DMI2["C16:1"] <- anim.diet.FAC16_1.rate
    rptFAComposition_DMI2["C18:0"] <- anim.diet.FAC18.rate
    rptFAComposition_DMI2["C18:1c"] <- anim.diet.FAC18_1c.rate
    rptFAComposition_DMI2["C18:1t"] <- anim.diet.FAC18_1t.rate
    rptFAComposition_DMI2["C18:2"] <- anim.diet.FAC18_2.rate
    rptFAComposition_DMI2["C18:3"] <- anim.diet.FAC18_3.rate
    rptFAComposition_DMI2["Other FA"] <- anim.diet.FAOther.rate
    rptFAComposition_DMI <- rbind(rptFAComposition_DMI, rptFAComposition_DMI2)
    description <- paste("Dietary glycerol, g/d : ", formatC(anim.diet.Glycerol.rate * 1000, digits = 3, width = 8), "\n",
                         "Dietary pigments, g/d : ", formatC(anim.diet.Pigment.rate * 1000, digits = 3, width = 8), "\n", sep = "")
```

```
        report(rptFAComposition_DMI, "Esterified Fatty Acid Intake, g/d", description, "", 2, 2, 1000, 7, FALSE, FALSE, TRUE, FALSE, TRUE, FALSE, TRUE)
        # Glycerol and Pigments
        rptFAComposition_DM <- fds["FeedName.x"]
        names(rptFAComposition_DM) <- "FeedName"
        rptFAComposition_DM["Glycerol, %DM"] <- fds["Glycerol_DM"]
        rptFAComposition_DM["Pigment, %DM"] <- fds["Pigment_DM"]
        rptFAComposition_DM["Glycerol, %EE"] <- fds["Glycerol_EE"]
        rptFAComposition_DM["Pigment, %EE"] <- fds["Pigment_EE"]
        rptFAComposition_DM["Glycerol, g/d"] <- anim.fd.Glycerol.rate * 1000
        rptFAComposition_DM["Pigment, g/d"] <- anim.fd.Pigment.rate * 1000
        rptFAComposition_DM2 <- data.frame(FeedName = "Ration")
        rptFAComposition_DM2["Glycerol, %DM"] <- isz(anim.diet.Glycerol.rate * 100, anim.diet.DMI.rate)
        rptFAComposition_DM2["Pigment, %DM"] <- isz(anim.diet.Pigment.rate * 100, anim.diet.DMI.rate)
        rptFAComposition_DM2["Glycerol, %EE"] <- isz(anim.diet.Glycerol.rate * 100, anim.diet.EE.rate)
        rptFAComposition_DM2["Pigment, %EE"] <- isz(anim.diet.Pigment.rate * 100, anim.diet.EE.rate)
        rptFAComposition_DM2["Glycerol, g/d"] <- anim.diet.Glycerol.rate * 1000
        rptFAComposition_DM2["Pigment, g/d"] <- anim.diet.Pigment.rate * 1000
        rptFAComposition_DM <- rbind(rptFAComposition_DM, rptFAComposition_DM2)
        report(rptFAComposition_DM, "Glycerol and Pigment Composition", "", "", 2, 2, 1, 4, FALSE, FALSE, FALSE, FALSE, TRUE, FALSE, TRUE)
    }
    # Minerals and vitamins
    anim.fd.ash.conc <<- as.numeric(fds[, "Ash_DM"])
    anim.fd.Ca.conc <<- as.numeric(fds[, "Ca_DM"])
    anim.fd.P.conc <<- as.numeric(fds[, "P_DM"])
    anim.fd.Mg.conc <<- as.numeric(fds[, "Mg_DM"])
    anim.fd.K.conc <<- as.numeric(fds[, "K_DM"])
    anim.fd.S.conc <<- as.numeric(fds[, "S_DM"])
    anim.fd.Cl.conc <<- as.numeric(fds[, "Cl_DM"])
    anim.fd.Na.conc <<- as.numeric(fds[, "Na_DM"])
    anim.fd.Fe_ppm.conc <<- as.numeric(fds[, "Fe_ppmDM"])
    anim.fd.Zn_ppm.conc <<- as.numeric(fds[, "Zn_ppmDM"])
    anim.fd.Cu_ppm.conc <<- as.numeric(fds[, "Cu_ppmDM"])
    anim.fd.Mn_ppm.conc <<- as.numeric(fds[, "Mn_ppmDM"])
    anim.fd.Se_ppm.conc <<- as.numeric(fds[, "Se_ppmDM"])
    anim.fd.Co_ppm.conc <<- as.numeric(fds[, "Co_ppmDM"])
    anim.fd.I_ppm.conc <<- as.numeric(fds[, "I_ppmDM"])
    anim.fd.Cr_ppm.conc <<- as.numeric(fds[, "Cr_ppmDM"])
    anim.fd.VitA.conc <<- as.numeric(fds[, "VitA_kIU"])
    anim.fd.VitD.conc <<- as.numeric(fds[, "VitD_kIU"])
    anim.fd.VitE.conc <<- as.numeric(fds[, "VitE_IU"])
    anim.fd.ash.rate <<- anim.fd.ash.conc * anim.fd.DMI.rate/100
    anim.fd.Ca.rate <<- anim.fd.Ca.conc * anim.fd.DMI.rate/100
    anim.fd.P.rate <<- anim.fd.P.conc * anim.fd.DMI.rate/100
    anim.fd.Mg.rate <<- anim.fd.Mg.conc * anim.fd.DMI.rate/100
    anim.fd.K.rate <<- anim.fd.K.conc * anim.fd.DMI.rate/100
    anim.fd.S.rate <<- anim.fd.S.conc * anim.fd.DMI.rate/100
    anim.fd.Cl.rate <<- anim.fd.Cl.conc * anim.fd.DMI.rate/100
    anim.fd.Na.rate <<- anim.fd.Na.conc * anim.fd.DMI.rate/100
    anim.fd.Fe.rate <<- anim.fd.Fe_ppm.conc * anim.fd.DMI.rate/1e+06
```

```
anim.fd.Zn.rate <<- anim.fd.Zn_ppm.conc * anim.fd.DMI.rate/1e+06
anim.fd.Cu.rate <<- anim.fd.Cu_ppm.conc * anim.fd.DMI.rate/1e+06
anim.fd.Mn.rate <<- anim.fd.Mn_ppm.conc * anim.fd.DMI.rate/1e+06
anim.fd.Se.rate <<- anim.fd.Se_ppm.conc * anim.fd.DMI.rate/1e+06
anim.fd.Co.rate <<- anim.fd.Co_ppm.conc * anim.fd.DMI.rate/1e+06
anim.fd.I.rate <<- anim.fd.I_ppm.conc * anim.fd.DMI.rate/1e+06
anim.fd.Cr.rate <<- anim.fd.Cr_ppm.conc * anim.fd.DMI.rate/1e+06
anim.fd.VitA.rate <<- anim.fd.VitA.conc * anim.fd.DMI.rate
anim.fd.VitD.rate <<- anim.fd.VitD.conc * anim.fd.DMI.rate
anim.fd.VitE.rate <<- anim.fd.VitE.conc * anim.fd.DMI.rate
anim.diet.ash.rate <<- sum(anim.fd.ash.rate)
anim.diet.Ca.rate <<- sum(anim.fd.Ca.rate)
anim.diet.P.rate <<- sum(anim.fd.P.rate)
anim.diet.Mg.rate <<- sum(anim.fd.Mg.rate)
anim.diet.K.rate <<- sum(anim.fd.K.rate)
anim.diet.S.rate <<- sum(anim.fd.S.rate)
anim.diet.Cl.rate <<- sum(anim.fd.Cl.rate)
anim.diet.Na.rate <<- sum(anim.fd.Na.rate)
anim.diet.Fe.rate <<- sum(anim.fd.Fe.rate)
anim.diet.Zn.rate <<- sum(anim.fd.Zn.rate)
anim.diet.Cu.rate <<- sum(anim.fd.Cu.rate)
anim.diet.Mn.rate <<- sum(anim.fd.Mn.rate)
anim.diet.Se.rate <<- sum(anim.fd.Se.rate)
anim.diet.Co.rate <<- sum(anim.fd.Co.rate)
anim.diet.I.rate <<- sum(anim.fd.I.rate)
anim.diet.Mo.rate <<- 0
anim.diet.Cr.rate <<- sum(anim.fd.Cr.rate)
anim.diet.VitA.rate <<- sum(anim.fd.VitA.rate)
anim.diet.VitD.rate <<- sum(anim.fd.VitD.rate)
anim.diet.VitE.rate <<- sum(anim.fd.VitE.rate)
if (genRPT)
{
  rptMinerals_DM <- fds["FeedName.x"]
  names(rptMinerals_DM) <- "FeedName"
  rptMinerals_DM["Ash, %DM"] <- fds[, "Ash_DM"]
  rptMinerals_DM["Ca, %DM"] <- fds[, "Ca_DM"]
  rptMinerals_DM["P, %DM"] <- fds[, "P_DM"]
  rptMinerals_DM["Mg, %DM"] <- fds[, "Mg_DM"]
  rptMinerals_DM["K, %DM"] <- fds[, "K_DM"]
  rptMinerals_DM["S, %DM"] <- fds[, "S_DM"]
  rptMinerals_DM["Cl, %DM"] <- fds[, "Cl_DM"]
  rptMinerals_DM["Na, %DM"] <- fds[, "Na_DM"]
  rptMinerals_DM["Fe, ppm"] <- fds[, "Fe_ppmDM"]
  rptMinerals_DM["Zn, ppm"] <- fds[, "Zn_ppmDM"]
  rptMinerals_DM["Cu, ppm"] <- fds[, "Cu_ppmDM"]
  rptMinerals_DM["Mn, ppm"] <- fds[, "Mn_ppmDM"]
  rptMinerals_DM["Se, ppm"] <- fds[, "Se_ppmDM"]
  rptMinerals_DM["Co, ppm"] <- fds[, "Co_ppmDM"]
  rptMinerals_DM["I, ppm"] <- fds[, "I_ppmDM"]
  rptMinerals_DM["Cr, ppm"] <- fds[, "Cr_ppmDM"]
  rptMinerals_DM2 <- data.frame(FeedName = "Ration")
```

```
    rptMinerals_DM2["Ash, %DM"] <- isz(anim.diet.ash.rate * 100, anim.diet.DMI.rate)
    rptMinerals_DM2["Ca, %DM"] <- isz(anim.diet.Ca.rate * 100, anim.diet.DMI.rate)
    rptMinerals_DM2["P, %DM"] <- isz(anim.diet.P.rate * 100, anim.diet.DMI.rate)
    rptMinerals_DM2["Mg, %DM"] <- isz(anim.diet.Mg.rate * 100, anim.diet.DMI.rate)
    rptMinerals_DM2["K, %DM"] <- isz(anim.diet.K.rate * 100, anim.diet.DMI.rate)
    rptMinerals_DM2["S, %DM"] <- isz(anim.diet.S.rate * 100, anim.diet.DMI.rate)
    rptMinerals_DM2["Cl, %DM"] <- isz(anim.diet.Cl.rate * 100, anim.diet.DMI.rate)
    rptMinerals_DM2["Na, %DM"] <- isz(anim.diet.Na.rate * 100, anim.diet.DMI.rate)
    rptMinerals_DM2["Fe, ppm"] <- isz(anim.diet.Fe.rate * 1e+06, anim.diet.DMI.rate)
    rptMinerals_DM2["Zn, ppm"] <- isz(anim.diet.Zn.rate * 1e+06, anim.diet.DMI.rate)
    rptMinerals_DM2["Cu, ppm"] <- isz(anim.diet.Cu.rate * 1e+06, anim.diet.DMI.rate)
    rptMinerals_DM2["Mn, ppm"] <- isz(anim.diet.Mn.rate * 1e+06, anim.diet.DMI.rate)
    rptMinerals_DM2["Se, ppm"] <- isz(anim.diet.Se.rate * 1e+06, anim.diet.DMI.rate)
    rptMinerals_DM2["Co, ppm"] <- isz(anim.diet.Co.rate * 1e+06, anim.diet.DMI.rate)
    rptMinerals_DM2["I, ppm"] <- isz(anim.diet.I.rate * 1e+06, anim.diet.DMI.rate)
    rptMinerals_DM2["Cr, ppm"] <- isz(anim.diet.Cr.rate * 1e+06, anim.diet.DMI.rate)
    rptMinerals_DM <- rbind(rptMinerals_DM, rptMinerals_DM2)
    report(rptMinerals_DM, "Macromineral and Micromineral Composition, %DM or ppm", "", "", 3, 3, 1, 8, FALSE, FALSE, FALSE,
FALSE, FALSE, FALSE, TRUE)
    rptMinerals_Ash <- fds["FeedName.x"]
    names(rptMinerals_Ash) <- "FeedName"
    rptMinerals_Ash["Ca"] <- fds[, "Ca_Ash"]
    rptMinerals_Ash["P"] <- fds[, "P_Ash"]
    rptMinerals_Ash["Mg"] <- fds[, "Mg_Ash"]
    rptMinerals_Ash["K"] <- fds[, "K_Ash"]
    rptMinerals_Ash["S"] <- fds[, "S_Ash"]
    rptMinerals_Ash["Cl"] <- fds[, "Cl_Ash"]
    rptMinerals_Ash["Na"] <- fds[, "Na_Ash"]
    rptMinerals_Ash["Fe"] <- fds[, "Fe_Ash"]
    rptMinerals_Ash["Zn"] <- fds[, "Zn_Ash"]
    rptMinerals_Ash["Cu"] <- fds[, "Cu_Ash"]
    rptMinerals_Ash["Mn"] <- fds[, "Mn_Ash"]
    rptMinerals_Ash["Se"] <- fds[, "Se_Ash"]
    rptMinerals_Ash["Co"] <- fds[, "Co_Ash"]
    rptMinerals_Ash["I"] <- fds[, "I_Ash"]
    rptMinerals_Ash["Cr"] <- fds[, "Cr_Ash"]
    rptMinerals_Ash2 <- data.frame(FeedName = "Ration")
    rptMinerals_Ash2["Ca"] <- isz(anim.diet.Ca.rate * 100, anim.diet.ash.rate)
    rptMinerals_Ash2["P"] <- isz(anim.diet.P.rate * 100, anim.diet.ash.rate)
    rptMinerals_Ash2["Mg"] <- isz(anim.diet.Mg.rate * 100, anim.diet.ash.rate)
    rptMinerals_Ash2["K"] <- isz(anim.diet.K.rate * 100, anim.diet.ash.rate)
    rptMinerals_Ash2["S"] <- isz(anim.diet.S.rate * 100, anim.diet.ash.rate)
    rptMinerals_Ash2["Cl"] <- isz(anim.diet.Cl.rate * 100, anim.diet.ash.rate)
    rptMinerals_Ash2["Na"] <- isz(anim.diet.Na.rate * 100, anim.diet.ash.rate)
    rptMinerals_Ash2["Fe"] <- isz(anim.diet.Fe.rate * 100, anim.diet.ash.rate)
    rptMinerals_Ash2["Zn"] <- isz(anim.diet.Zn.rate * 100, anim.diet.ash.rate)
    rptMinerals_Ash2["Cu"] <- isz(anim.diet.Cu.rate * 100, anim.diet.ash.rate)
    rptMinerals_Ash2["Mn"] <- isz(anim.diet.Mn.rate * 100, anim.diet.ash.rate)
    rptMinerals_Ash2["Se"] <- isz(anim.diet.Se.rate * 100, anim.diet.ash.rate)
    rptMinerals_Ash2["Co"] <- isz(anim.diet.Co.rate * 100, anim.diet.ash.rate)
    rptMinerals_Ash2["I"] <- isz(anim.diet.I.rate * 100, anim.diet.ash.rate)
```

```
    rptMinerals_Ash2["Cr"] <- isz(anim.diet.Cr.rate * 100, anim.diet.ash.rate)
    rptMinerals_Ash <- rbind(rptMinerals_Ash, rptMinerals_Ash2)
    description <- paste("Least % of ash accounted for by the sum of macromineral and microminerals of feeds    : ", formatC(min(rowSums(rptMinerals_Ash[2:length(rptMinerals_Ash)])), format = "f", digits = 3, width = 7), "% \n",
                         "Greatest % of ash accounted for by the sum of macromineral and microminerals of feeds: ", formatC(max(rowSums(rptMinerals_Ash[2:length(rptMinerals_Ash)])), format = "f", digits = 3, width = 7), "% \n",
                         "% of ash accounted for by the sum of macromineral and microminerals of the ration     : ", formatC(rowSums(rptMinerals_Ash[nrow(rptMinerals_Ash), 2:length(rptMinerals_Ash)]), format = "f", digits = 3, width = 7), "% \n\n", sep = "")
    report(rptMinerals_Ash, "Macromineral and Micromineral Composition, %Ash", description, "", 3, 3, 1, 8, FALSE, FALSE, TRUE, FALSE, FALSE, FALSE, TRUE)
    rptMinerals_DMI <- fds["FeedName.x"]
    names(rptMinerals_DMI) <- "FeedName"
    rptMinerals_DMI["Ash"] <- anim.fd.ash.rate
    rptMinerals_DMI["Ca"] <- anim.fd.Ca.rate
    rptMinerals_DMI["P"] <- anim.fd.P.rate
    rptMinerals_DMI["Mg"] <- anim.fd.Mg.rate
    rptMinerals_DMI["K"] <- anim.fd.K.rate
    rptMinerals_DMI["S"] <- anim.fd.S.rate
    rptMinerals_DMI["Cl"] <- anim.fd.Cl.rate
    rptMinerals_DMI["Na"] <- anim.fd.Na.rate
    rptMinerals_DMI["Fe"] <- anim.fd.Fe.rate
    rptMinerals_DMI["Zn"] <- anim.fd.Zn.rate
    rptMinerals_DMI["Cu"] <- anim.fd.Cu.rate
    rptMinerals_DMI["Mn"] <- anim.fd.Mn.rate
    rptMinerals_DMI["Se"] <- anim.fd.Se.rate
    rptMinerals_DMI["Co"] <- anim.fd.Co.rate
    rptMinerals_DMI["I"] <- anim.fd.I.rate
    rptMinerals_DMI["Cr"] <- anim.fd.Cr.rate
    rptMinerals_DMI["VitA, kIU"] <- anim.fd.VitA.rate
    rptMinerals_DMI["VitD, kIU"] <- anim.fd.VitD.rate
    rptMinerals_DMI["VitE, IU"] <- anim.fd.VitE.rate
    rptMinerals_DMI2 <- data.frame(FeedName = "Ration")
    rptMinerals_DMI2["Ash"] <- anim.diet.ash.rate
    rptMinerals_DMI2["Ca"] <- anim.diet.Ca.rate
    rptMinerals_DMI2["P"] <- anim.diet.P.rate
    rptMinerals_DMI2["Mg"] <- anim.diet.Mg.rate
    rptMinerals_DMI2["K"] <- anim.diet.K.rate
    rptMinerals_DMI2["S"] <- anim.diet.S.rate
    rptMinerals_DMI2["Cl"] <- anim.diet.Cl.rate
    rptMinerals_DMI2["Na"] <- anim.diet.Na.rate
    rptMinerals_DMI2["Fe"] <- anim.diet.Fe.rate
    rptMinerals_DMI2["Zn"] <- anim.diet.Zn.rate
    rptMinerals_DMI2["Cu"] <- anim.diet.Cu.rate
    rptMinerals_DMI2["Mn"] <- anim.diet.Mn.rate
    rptMinerals_DMI2["Se"] <- anim.diet.Se.rate
    rptMinerals_DMI2["Co"] <- anim.diet.Co.rate
    rptMinerals_DMI2["I"] <- anim.diet.I.rate
    rptMinerals_DMI2["Cr"] <- anim.diet.Cr.rate
    rptMinerals_DMI2["VitA, kIU"] <- anim.diet.VitA.rate
    rptMinerals_DMI2["VitD, kIU"] <- anim.diet.VitD.rate
```

```
      rptMinerals_DMI2["VitE, IU"] <- anim.diet.VitE.rate
      rptMinerals_DMI <- rbind(rptMinerals_DMI, rptMinerals_DMI2)
      report(rptMinerals_DMI, "Macromineral and Micromineral (g/d) and Vitamin (IU/d) Intake", "", "", 3, 3, 1000, 8, FALSE,
  FALSE, FALSE, FALSE, FALSE, FALSE, TRUE)
    }
    # Plant defensive compounds (PDC)
    anim.fd.TCT.conc <<- as.numeric(fds[, "TCT_DM"])
    anim.fd.SCT.conc <<- as.numeric(fds[, "SCT_DM"])
    anim.fd.PCT.conc <<- as.numeric(fds[, "PCT_DM"])
    anim.fd.FCT.conc <<- as.numeric(fds[, "FCT_DM"])
    anim.fd.Alkaloids.conc <<- as.numeric(fds[, "Alkaloids_DM"])
    anim.fd.Terpenoids.conc <<- as.numeric(fds[, "Terpenoids_DM"])
    anim.fd.ODC.conc <<- as.numeric(fds[, "ODC_DM"])
    anim.fd.TCT.rate <<- anim.fd.TCT.conc * anim.fd.DMI.rate/100
    anim.fd.SCT.rate <<- anim.fd.SCT.conc * anim.fd.DMI.rate/100
    anim.fd.PCT.rate <<- anim.fd.PCT.conc * anim.fd.DMI.rate/100
    anim.fd.FCT.rate <<- anim.fd.FCT.conc * anim.fd.DMI.rate/100
    anim.fd.Alkaloids.rate <<- anim.fd.Alkaloids.conc * anim.fd.DMI.rate/100
    anim.fd.Terpenoids.rate <<- anim.fd.Terpenoids.conc * anim.fd.DMI.rate/100
    anim.fd.ODC.rate <<- anim.fd.ODC.conc * anim.fd.DMI.rate/100
    anim.fd.TDC.rate <<- anim.fd.TCT.rate + anim.fd.Alkaloids.rate + anim.fd.Terpenoids.rate + anim.fd.ODC.rate
    anim.diet.TCT.rate <<- sum(anim.fd.TCT.rate)
    anim.diet.SCT.rate <<- sum(anim.fd.SCT.rate)
    anim.diet.PCT.rate <<- sum(anim.fd.PCT.rate)
    anim.diet.FCT.rate <<- sum(anim.fd.FCT.rate)
    anim.diet.Alkaloids.rate <<- sum(anim.fd.Alkaloids.rate)
    anim.diet.Terpenoids.rate <<- sum(anim.fd.Terpenoids.rate)
    anim.diet.ODC.rate <<- sum(anim.fd.ODC.rate)
    anim.diet.TDC.rate <<- sum(anim.fd.TDC.rate)
    if (genRPT)
    {
      rptPDC_DM <- fds["FeedName.x"]
      names(rptPDC_DM) <- "FeedName"
      rptPDC_DM["TCT"] <- fds[, "TCT_DM"]
      rptPDC_DM["SCT"] <- fds[, "SCT_DM"]
      rptPDC_DM["PCT"] <- fds[, "PCT_DM"]
      rptPDC_DM["FCT"] <- fds[, "FCT_DM"]
      rptPDC_DM["Alkaloids"] <- fds[, "Alkaloids_DM"]
      rptPDC_DM["Terpenoids"] <- fds[, "Terpenoids_DM"]
      rptPDC_DM["ODC"] <- fds[, "ODC_DM"]
      rptPDC_DM2 <- data.frame(FeedName = "Ration")
      rptPDC_DM2["TCT"] <- isz(anim.diet.TCT.rate * 100, anim.diet.DMI.rate)
      rptPDC_DM2["SCT"] <- isz(anim.diet.SCT.rate * 100, anim.diet.DMI.rate)
      rptPDC_DM2["PCT"] <- isz(anim.diet.PCT.rate * 100, anim.diet.DMI.rate)
      rptPDC_DM2["FCT"] <- isz(anim.diet.FCT.rate * 100, anim.diet.DMI.rate)
      rptPDC_DM2["Alkaloids"] <- isz(anim.diet.Alkaloids.rate * 100, anim.diet.DMI.rate)
      rptPDC_DM2["Terpenoids"] <- isz(anim.diet.Terpenoids.rate * 100, anim.diet.DMI.rate)
      rptPDC_DM2["ODC"] <- isz(anim.diet.ODC.rate * 100, anim.diet.DMI.rate)
      rptPDC_DM <- rbind(rptPDC_DM, rptPDC_DM2)
      report(rptPDC_DM, "Plant Defensive Compounds Composition, %DM", "", "", 3, 3, 1, 8, FALSE, FALSE, FALSE, FALSE, FALSE,
  FALSE, FALSE)
```

```
    rptPDC_DC <- fds["FeedName.x"]
    names(rptPDC_DC) <- "FeedName"
    rptPDC_DC["TCT"] <- isz(anim.fd.TCT.rate * 100, anim.fd.TDC.rate)
    rptPDC_DC["SCT"] <- isz(anim.fd.SCT.rate * 100, anim.fd.TDC.rate)
    rptPDC_DC["PCT"] <- isz(anim.fd.PCT.rate * 100, anim.fd.TDC.rate)
    rptPDC_DC["FCT"] <- isz(anim.fd.FCT.rate * 100, anim.fd.TDC.rate)
    rptPDC_DC["Alkaloids"] <- isz(anim.fd.Alkaloids.rate * 100, anim.fd.TDC.rate)
    rptPDC_DC["Terpenoids"] <- isz(anim.fd.Terpenoids.rate * 100, anim.fd.TDC.rate)
    rptPDC_DC["ODC"] <- isz(anim.fd.ODC.rate * 100, anim.fd.TDC.rate)
    rptPDC_DC2 <- data.frame(FeedName = "Ration")
    rptPDC_DC2["TCT"] <- isz(anim.diet.TCT.rate * 100, anim.diet.TDC.rate)
    rptPDC_DC2["SCT"] <- isz(anim.diet.SCT.rate * 100, anim.diet.TDC.rate)
    rptPDC_DC2["PCT"] <- isz(anim.diet.PCT.rate * 100, anim.diet.TDC.rate)
    rptPDC_DC2["FCT"] <- isz(anim.diet.FCT.rate * 100, anim.diet.TDC.rate)
    rptPDC_DC2["Alkaloids"] <- isz(anim.diet.Alkaloids.rate * 100, anim.diet.TDC.rate)
    rptPDC_DC2["Terpenoids"] <- isz(anim.diet.Terpenoids.rate * 100, anim.diet.TDC.rate)
    rptPDC_DC2["ODC"] <- isz(anim.diet.ODC.rate * 100, anim.diet.TDC.rate)
    rptPDC_DC <- rbind(rptPDC_DC, rptPDC_DC2)
    report(rptPDC_DC, "\nPlant Defensive Compounds Composition, %DC", "", "", 3, 3, 1, 8, FALSE, FALSE, FALSE, FALSE, FALSE,
  FALSE, FALSE)
    rptPDC_DMI <- fds["FeedName.x"]
    names(rptPDC_DMI) <- "FeedName"
    rptPDC_DMI["TCT"] <- anim.fd.TCT.rate
    rptPDC_DMI["SCT"] <- anim.fd.SCT.rate
    rptPDC_DMI["PCT"] <- anim.fd.PCT.rate
    rptPDC_DMI["FCT"] <- anim.fd.FCT.rate
    rptPDC_DMI["Alkaloids"] <- anim.fd.Alkaloids.rate
    rptPDC_DMI["Terpenoids"] <- anim.fd.Terpenoids.rate
    rptPDC_DMI["ODC"] <- anim.fd.ODC.rate
    rptPDC_DMI2 <- data.frame(FeedName = "Ration")
    rptPDC_DMI2["TCT"] <- anim.diet.TCT.rate
    rptPDC_DMI2["SCT"] <- anim.diet.SCT.rate
    rptPDC_DMI2["PCT"] <- anim.diet.PCT.rate
    rptPDC_DMI2["FCT"] <- anim.diet.FCT.rate
    rptPDC_DMI2["Alkaloids"] <- anim.diet.Alkaloids.rate
    rptPDC_DMI2["Terpenoids"] <- anim.diet.Terpenoids.rate
    rptPDC_DMI2["ODC"] <- anim.diet.ODC.rate
    rptPDC_DMI <- rbind(rptPDC_DMI, rptPDC_DMI2)
    report(rptPDC_DMI, "\nPlant Defensive Compounds Intake, g/d", "", "", 3, 3, 1000, 8, FALSE, FALSE, FALSE, FALSE, FALSE,
  FALSE, TRUE)
  }
  # ++++++++++++++++
  # Organic matter
  # ++++++++++++++++
  anim.fd.OMI.rate <<- anim.fd.CP.rate + anim.fd.CHO.rate + anim.fd.EE.rate
  anim.diet.OMI.rate <<- sum(anim.fd.OMI.rate)
  # ++++++++++++++++++++++++++++++
  # Fractions of Protein (Prot)
  # ++++++++++++++++++++++++++++++
  anim.fd.ProtA_CP.conc <<- as.numeric(fds[, "Prot_A_CP"])
  anim.fd.ProtB1_CP.conc <<- as.numeric(fds[, "Prot_B1_CP"])
```

```
    anim.fd.ProtB2_CP.conc <<- as.numeric(fds[, "Prot_B2_CP"])
    anim.fd.ProtB3_CP.conc <<- as.numeric(fds[, "Prot_B3_CP"])
    anim.fd.ProtC_CP.conc <<- as.numeric(fds[, "Prot_C_CP"])
    anim.fd.ProtA.rate <<- anim.fd.ProtA_CP.conc * anim.fd.CP.rate/100
    anim.fd.ProtB1.rate <<- anim.fd.ProtB1_CP.conc * anim.fd.CP.rate/100
    anim.fd.ProtB2.rate <<- anim.fd.ProtB2_CP.conc * anim.fd.CP.rate/100
    anim.fd.ProtB3.rate <<- anim.fd.ProtB3_CP.conc * anim.fd.CP.rate/100
    anim.fd.ProtC.rate <<- anim.fd.ProtC_CP.conc * anim.fd.CP.rate/100
    anim.diet.ProtA.rate <<- sum(anim.fd.ProtA.rate)
    anim.diet.ProtB1.rate <<- sum(anim.fd.ProtB1.rate)
    anim.diet.ProtB2.rate <<- sum(anim.fd.ProtB2.rate)
    anim.diet.ProtB3.rate <<- sum(anim.fd.ProtB3.rate)
    anim.diet.ProtC.rate <<- sum(anim.fd.ProtC.rate)
    if (genRPT)
    {
      rptProtFraction_DM <- fds["FeedName.x"]
      names(rptProtFraction_DM) <- "FeedName"
      rptProtFraction_DM["Prot A"] <- fds["Prot_A_DM"]
      rptProtFraction_DM["Prot B1"] <- fds["Prot_B1_DM"]
      rptProtFraction_DM["Prot B2"] <- fds["Prot_B2_DM"]
      rptProtFraction_DM["Prot B3"] <- fds["Prot_B3_DM"]
      rptProtFraction_DM["Prot C"] <- fds["Prot_C_DM"]
      report(rptProtFraction_DM, "Protein Fractionation, %DM", "", "", 3, 3, 1, 8, FALSE, FALSE, TRUE, FALSE, FALSE, FALSE, FALSE)
      rptProtFraction_CP <- fds["FeedName.x"]
      names(rptProtFraction_CP) <- "FeedName"
      rptProtFraction_CP["Prot A"] <- fds["Prot_A_CP"]
      rptProtFraction_CP["Prot B1"] <- fds["Prot_B1_CP"]
      rptProtFraction_CP["Prot B2"] <- fds["Prot_B2_CP"]
      rptProtFraction_CP["Prot B3"] <- fds["Prot_B3_CP"]
      rptProtFraction_CP["Prot C"] <- fds["Prot_C_CP"]
      report(rptProtFraction_CP, "\nProtein Fractionation, %CP", "", "", 3, 3, 1, 8, FALSE, FALSE, TRUE, FALSE, FALSE, FALSE, FALSE)
      rptProtFraction_DMI <- fds["FeedName.x"]
      names(rptProtFraction_DMI) <- "FeedName"
      rptProtFraction_DMI["Prot A"] <- anim.fd.ProtA.rate
      rptProtFraction_DMI["Prot B1"] <- anim.fd.ProtB1.rate
      rptProtFraction_DMI["Prot B2"] <- anim.fd.ProtB2.rate
      rptProtFraction_DMI["Prot B3"] <- anim.fd.ProtB3.rate
      rptProtFraction_DMI["Prot C"] <- anim.fd.ProtC.rate
      report(rptProtFraction_DMI, "\nProtein Fraction Intake, kg/d", "", "", 3, 3, 1, 8, TRUE, FALSE, TRUE, FALSE, TRUE, FALSE, TRUE)
    }
    # +++++++++++++++++++++++++++++++++++
    # Fractions of carbohydrate (CHO)
    # +++++++++++++++++++++++++++++++++++
    anim.fd.CHOA1.conc <<- as.numeric(fds[, "CHO_A1_CHO"])
    anim.fd.CHOA2.conc <<- as.numeric(fds[, "CHO_A2_CHO"])
    anim.fd.CHOA3.conc <<- as.numeric(fds[, "CHO_A3_CHO"])
    anim.fd.CHOA4.conc <<- as.numeric(fds[, "CHO_A4_CHO"])
    anim.fd.CHOB1.conc <<- as.numeric(fds[, "CHO_B1_CHO"])
```

```
    anim.fd.CHOB2.conc <<- as.numeric(fds[, "CHO_B2_CHO"])
    anim.fd.CHOB3.conc <<- as.numeric(fds[, "CHO_B3_CHO"])
    anim.fd.CHOC.conc <<- as.numeric(fds[, "CHO_C_CHO"])
    anim.fd.CHOA1.rate <<- anim.fd.CHOA1.conc * anim.fd.CHO.rate/100
    anim.fd.CHOA2.rate <<- anim.fd.CHOA2.conc * anim.fd.CHO.rate/100
    anim.fd.CHOA3.rate <<- anim.fd.CHOA3.conc * anim.fd.CHO.rate/100
    anim.fd.CHOA4.rate <<- anim.fd.CHOA4.conc * anim.fd.CHO.rate/100
    anim.fd.CHOB1.rate <<- anim.fd.CHOB1.conc * anim.fd.CHO.rate/100
    anim.fd.CHOB2.rate <<- anim.fd.CHOB2.conc * anim.fd.CHO.rate/100
    anim.fd.CHOB3.rate <<- anim.fd.CHOB3.conc * anim.fd.CHO.rate/100
    anim.fd.CHOC.rate <<- anim.fd.CHOC.conc * anim.fd.CHO.rate/100
    anim.diet.CHOA1.rate <<- sum(anim.fd.CHOA1.rate)
    anim.diet.CHOA2.rate <<- sum(anim.fd.CHOA2.rate)
    anim.diet.CHOA3.rate <<- sum(anim.fd.CHOA3.rate)
    anim.diet.CHOA4.rate <<- sum(anim.fd.CHOA4.rate)
    anim.diet.CHOB1.rate <<- sum(anim.fd.CHOB1.rate)
    anim.diet.CHOB2.rate <<- sum(anim.fd.CHOB2.rate)
    anim.diet.CHOB3.rate <<- sum(anim.fd.CHOB3.rate)
    anim.diet.CHOC.rate <<- sum(anim.fd.CHOC.rate)
    if (genRPT)
    {
      rptCHOFraction_DM <- fds["FeedName.x"]
      names(rptCHOFraction_DM) <- "FeedName"
      rptCHOFraction_DM["CHO A1"] <- fds["CHO_A1_DM"]
      rptCHOFraction_DM["CHO A2"] <- fds["CHO_A2_DM"]
      rptCHOFraction_DM["CHO A3"] <- fds["CHO_A3_DM"]
      rptCHOFraction_DM["CHO A4"] <- fds["CHO_A4_DM"]
      rptCHOFraction_DM["CHO B1"] <- fds["CHO_B1_DM"]
      rptCHOFraction_DM["CHO B2"] <- fds["CHO_B2_DM"]
      rptCHOFraction_DM["CHO B3"] <- fds["CHO_B3_DM"]
      rptCHOFraction_DM["CHO C"] <- fds["CHO_C_DM"]
      report(rptCHOFraction_DM, "Carbohydrate Fractionation, %DM", "", "", 3, 3, 1, 9, FALSE, FALSE, TRUE, FALSE, FALSE, FALSE,
  FALSE)
      rptCHOFraction_CHO <- fds["FeedName.x"]
      names(rptCHOFraction_CHO) <- "FeedName"
      rptCHOFraction_CHO["CHO A1"] <- fds["CHO_A1_CHO"]
      rptCHOFraction_CHO["CHO A2"] <- fds["CHO_A2_CHO"]
      rptCHOFraction_CHO["CHO A3"] <- fds["CHO_A3_CHO"]
      rptCHOFraction_CHO["CHO A4"] <- fds["CHO_A4_CHO"]
      rptCHOFraction_CHO["CHO B1"] <- fds["CHO_B1_CHO"]
      rptCHOFraction_CHO["CHO B2"] <- fds["CHO_B2_CHO"]
      rptCHOFraction_CHO["CHO B3"] <- fds["CHO_B3_CHO"]
      rptCHOFraction_CHO["CHO C"] <- fds["CHO_C_CHO"]
      report(rptCHOFraction_CHO, "\nCarbohydrate Fractionation, %CHO", "", "", 3, 3, 1, 9, FALSE, FALSE, TRUE, FALSE, FALSE,
  FALSE, FALSE)
      rptCHOFraction_DMI <- fds["FeedName.x"]
      names(rptCHOFraction_DMI) <- "FeedName"
      rptCHOFraction_DMI["CHO A1"] <- anim.fd.CHOA1.rate
      rptCHOFraction_DMI["CHO A2"] <- anim.fd.CHOA2.rate
      rptCHOFraction_DMI["CHO A3"] <- anim.fd.CHOA3.rate
      rptCHOFraction_DMI["CHO A4"] <- anim.fd.CHOA4.rate
```

```
    rptCHOFraction_DMI["CHO B1"] <- anim.fd.CHOB1.rate
    rptCHOFraction_DMI["CHO B2"] <- anim.fd.CHOB2.rate
    rptCHOFraction_DMI["CHO B3"] <- anim.fd.CHOB3.rate
    rptCHOFraction_DMI["CHO C"] <- anim.fd.CHOC.rate
    report(rptCHOFraction_DMI, "\nCarbohydrate Fraction Intake, kg/d", "", "", 3, 3, 1, 9, TRUE, FALSE, TRUE, FALSE, TRUE,
FALSE, TRUE)
  }
}
```

4.3.2 Rumen volume and area

```
calcRumenVolume <- function(anim.FBW)
{
  Vr <- (0.0888 * (anim.FBW)^1.034)  # liters
  return(Vr)
}

calcRumenArea <- function(NDF)
{
  if (!exists("rum.volume")) Vr <- calcRumenVolume(anim.FBW)/1000 else Vr <- rum.volume/1000
  r.NDF.Ar <- ifelse(NDF > 32, 1, 3 - 0.062 * NDF)
  Ar <- 4.836 * (Vr^(2/3)) * r.NDF.Ar
}
```

4.3.3 Empirical ruminal pH

```
calcRumenpH_peNDF <- function(flag_ph, anim.diet.peNDF.conc)
{
  if (flag_ph == 0)
  {
    # Fox et al. (2004; Anim. Feed Sci. Technol. 112:29-78)
    rum.pH_peNDF <<- ifelse(anim.diet.peNDF.conc >= 24.5, 6.46, 5.425 + 0.04229 * anim.diet.peNDF.conc)
  } else
  {
    # Boston et al. (2000; Modelling Nutrient Utilization in Farm Animals 361-377)
    anim.diet.peNDF.frac <- anim.diet.peNDF.conc/100
    gtemp <- 1/(1 + exp(-282.77726 * (anim.diet.peNDF.frac - 0.2429614)))
    rum.pH_peNDF <<- ((1 - gtemp) * (5.418454 + 4.26014 * anim.diet.peNDF.frac) + (gtemp * 6.459806))
  }
  return(rum.pH_peNDF)
}
```

4.3.4 Carbohydrate B3 kd adjustment for ruminal pH

```
calcCHOB3_kdAdjustment <- function(flag_CHOB3_kd, Parm_rum.bact.km1, Parm_rum.bact.Yg1, rum.fd.CHOB3_kd.fracprate, rum.pH,
FCBacteriaParms)
{
  FCBacteriaParms["CHOB3 kd"] <- rum.fd.CHOB3_kd.fracprate
  FCBacteriaParms["CHOB3 Y"] <- 0
  FCBacteriaParms["CHOB3 Yg'"] <- 0
  FCBacteriaParms["CHOB3 RelY"] <- 0
  FCBacteriaParms["CHOB3 Y'"] <- 0
  FCBacteriaParms["CHOB3 kd'"] <- 0
  # Fox et al. (2004; Anim. Feed Sci. Technol. 112:29-78)
  if (flag_CHOB3_kd == 0)
  {
    if (rum.pH<=5.7)
    {
      return(FCBacteriaParms)
    } else
    {
      if (rum.pH < 6.05)
      {
        rum.fd.CHOB3_kd.fracrate <- rum.fd.CHOB3_kd.fracprate/100
        Y1 <- ifelse((rum.fd.CHOB3_kd.fracrate - Parm_rum.bact.km1 * Parm_rum.bact.Yg1) > 0 &
                       (Parm_rum.bact.km1/(rum.fd.CHOB3_kd.fracrate - Parm_rum.bact.km1 * Parm_rum.bact.Yg1)
                       + 1/Parm_rum.bact.Yg1) > 0, 1/(Parm_rum.bact.km1/(rum.fd.CHOB3_kd.fracrate -
                       Parm_rum.bact.km1 * Parm_rum.bact.Yg1) + 1/Parm_rum.bact.Yg1), 0)
        km1_prime <- 0.1409 - 0.0135 * rum.pH
        Yg1_prime <- 0.0752 * rum.pH - 0.1058
        RelY <- (1 - exp(-5.624 * (rum.pH - 5.7)^0.909))/0.9968
        Y1_prime <- RelY * Y1
        CHOB3_kd_prime <- ((km1_prime * Y1_prime * Yg1_prime)/(Yg1_prime - Y1_prime) + km1_prime * Yg1_prime) * 100
        CHOB3_kd_prime <- pmin(CHOB3_kd_prime, rum.fd.CHOB3_kd.fracprate)
        FCBacteriaParms["CHOB3 Y"] <- as.numeric(formatC(Y1, format = "f"))
        FCBacteriaParms["CHOB3 Yg'"] <- as.numeric(formatC(Yg1_prime, format = "f"))
        FCBacteriaParms["CHOB3 RelY"] <- as.numeric(formatC(RelY, format = "f"))
        FCBacteriaParms["CHOB3 Y'"] <- as.numeric(formatC(Y1_prime, format = "f"))
        FCBacteriaParms["CHOB3 kd'"] <- as.numeric(formatC(CHOB3_kd_prime, format = "f"))
        return(FCBacteriaParms)
      } else
      {
        rum.fd.CHOB3_kd.fracrate <- rum.fd.CHOB3_kd.fracprate/100
        Y1 <- ifelse((rum.fd.CHOB3_kd.fracrate - Parm_rum.bact.km1 * Parm_rum.bact.Yg1) > 0 &
                       (Parm_rum.bact.km1/(rum.fd.CHOB3_kd.fracrate - Parm_rum.bact.km1 * Parm_rum.bact.Yg1)
                       + 1/Parm_rum.bact.Yg1) > 0, 1/(Parm_rum.bact.km1/(rum.fd.CHOB3_kd.fracrate -
                       Parm_rum.bact.km1 * Parm_rum.bact.Yg1) + 1/Parm_rum.bact.Yg1), 0)
        km1_prime <- Parm_rum.bact.km1
        Yg1_prime <- Parm_rum.bact.Yg1
        RelY <- 1
        Y1_prime <- RelY * Y1
        CHOB3_kd_prime <- rum.fd.CHOB3_kd.fracprate
```

```
          FCBacteriaParms["CHOB3 Y"] <- as.numeric(formatC(Y1, format = "f"))
          FCBacteriaParms["CHOB3 Yg'"] <- as.numeric(formatC(Yg1_prime, format = "f"))
          FCBacteriaParms["CHOB3 RelY"] <- as.numeric(formatC(RelY, format = "f"))
          FCBacteriaParms["CHOB3 Y'"] <- as.numeric(formatC(Y1_prime, format = "f"))
          FCBacteriaParms["CHOB3 kd'"] <- as.numeric(formatC(CHOB3_kd_prime, format = "f"))
          return(FCBacteriaParms)
        }
      }
    }
    if (flag_CHOB3_kd == 1)
    {
      # New RNS submodel
      if (rum.pH > 5.4)
      {
        if (rum.pH > 6.6)
        {
          AdjCHOB3 <- 1
        } else
        {
          AdjCHOB3 <- (1 - 0.7282 * (6.6 - rum.pH))
        }
        FCBacteriaParms["CHOB3 kd'"] <- pmin(rum.fd.CHOB3_kd.fracprate, rum.fd.CHOB3_kd.fracprate * AdjCHOB3)
        return(FCBacteriaParms)
      }
    }
    if (flag_CHOB3_kd == 2)
    {
      # Boston et al. (2000; Modelling Nutrient Utilization in Farm Animals 361-377)
      rum.fd.CHOB3_kd.fracrate <- rum.fd.CHOB3_kd.fracprate/100
      mPrime <- 0.1409 - 0.0135 * rum.pH
      YgPrime <- 0.0752 * rum.pH - 0.1058
      FCBacteriaParms["CHOB3 Yg'"] <- as.numeric(formatC(YgPrime, format = "f"))
      tmp <- exp(-5.624 * (rum.pH - 5.7))
      ytemp <- (1 - tmp)/0.9968
      tmp <- exp(-8.9094 * (rum.pH - 5.5832))
      if (tmp != -1)
      {
        gtemp <- 1/(1 + tmp)
      } else
      {
        gtemp <- 1
      }
      tmp <- exp(-20 * (rum.pH - 5.6988))
      if (tmp != -1)
      {
        htemp <- 1/(1 + tmp)
      } else
      {
        htemp <- 1
      }
      RelY <- htemp * ((1 - gtemp) + (ytemp * gtemp))
```

```
        FCBacteriaParms["CHOB3 RelY"] <- as.numeric(formatC(RelY, format = "f"))
        temp <- as.numeric(formatC((Parm_rum.bact.km1/(rum.fd.CHOB3_kd.fracrate - Parm_rum.bact.km1 * Parm_rum.bact.Yg1) +
    1/Parm_rum.bact.Yg1), format = "f"))
        FCBacteriaParms["CHOB3 Y"] <- ifelse(temp != 0, as.numeric(formatC(1/temp, format = "f")), 0)
        YPrime <- ifelse(temp != 0, RelY * (1/temp), 0)
        FCBacteriaParms["CHOB3 Y'"] <- as.numeric(formatC(YPrime, format = "f"))
        x <- ((mPrime * YPrime * YgPrime)/(YgPrime - YPrime) + mPrime * YgPrime) * 100
        gtemp <- exp(-35 * (rum.pH - 5.6992))
        gtemp <- 1/(1 + gtemp)
        CHOB3_kd_prime <- pmin(x * gtemp, rum.fd.CHOB3_kd.fracprate)
        FCBacteriaParms["CHOB3 kd'"] <- as.numeric(formatC(CHOB3_kd_prime, format = "f"))
        return(FCBacteriaParms)
      }
    }
```

4.3.5 Ruminal passage rate

```
calcPassageRate <- function(flag_kp_cattle, flag_adjust_kp_for_pendf, fd, anim.diet.DMI.rate, anim.FBW, anim.SBW, anim.diet.Forage.frac, anim.diet.Concentrate.frac)
{
  DMI <- anim.diet.DMI.rate

  if (anim.species == "Cattle")
  {
    if (flag_kp_cattle == 0)
    {
      # Fox et al. (2004; Anim. Feed Sci. Technol. 112:29-78)
      kp_forage <- 0.38 + (0.022 * DMI * 1000/(anim.FBW^0.75)) + 2 * anim.diet.Forage.frac^2
      kp_concentrate <- -0.424 + 1.45 * kp_forage
      kp_liquid <- 4.413 + 0.191 * DMI * 1000/anim.FBW
      if (flag_adjust_kp_for_pendf == TRUE)
      {
        Adjusted_kp_forage <- kp_forage * (100/(as.numeric(fd[, "NDF_DM"]) * as.numeric(fd[, "peNDF_NDF"])/100 + 70))
        Adjusted_kp_concentrate <- kp_concentrate * (100/(as.numeric(fd[, "NDF_DM"]) * as.numeric(fd[, "peNDF_NDF"])/100 + 90))
      } else
      {
        Adjusted_kp_forage <- kp_forage
        Adjusted_kp_concentrate <- kp_concentrate
      }
    } else
    {
      if (flag_kp_cattle == 1)
      {
        # Seo et al. (2006; Anim. Feed Sci. Technol. 128:67-83)
        FpBW <- anim.diet.Forage.frac * DMI * 1000/anim.FBW
        CpBW <- anim.diet.Concentrate.frac * DMI * 1000/anim.FBW
        FDMI <- anim.diet.Forage.frac * DMI
        kp_forage <- 2.365 + 0.0214 * FpBW + 0.0734 * CpBW + 0.069 * FDMI
        kp_concentrate <- 1.169 + 0.1375 * FpBW + 0.1721 * CpBW
        kp_liquid <- 4.524 + 0.0223 * FpBW + 0.2046 * CpBW + 0.344 * FDMI
        # No adjustments for peNDF
        Adjusted_kp_forage <- kp_forage
        Adjusted_kp_concentrate <- kp_concentrate
      }
    }
  } else
  {
    if (anim.species == "Sheep")
    {
      # Cannas and Van Soest (2000; Modelling Nutrient Utilization in Farm Animals: 49-62)
      NDFI <- anim.diet.NDF.rate * 100/anim.FBW
      anim.diet.CP.conc <- anim.diet.CP.rate * 100/DMI
      kp_forage <- 1.821 * (NDFI^0.399) * exp(0.046 * anim.diet.CP.conc)
      kp_concentrate <- 1.572 * kp_forage - 0.925
```

```
        kp_liquid <- 0.976 * kp_concentrate + 3.516
        # No adjustments for peNDF
        Adjusted_kp_forage <- kp_forage
        Adjusted_kp_concentrate <- kp_concentrate
      } else
      {
        if (anim.species == "Goats")
        {
          # Tedeschi et al. (2012; J. Agric. Sci. 150:95-107)
          NDFI <- anim.diet.NDF.rate * 1000/anim.FBW
          anim.diet.NDF.conc <- anim.diet.NDF.rate * 100/DMI
          kp_forage <- 1.29 + 0.161 * (NDFI^1.503) * exp(0.022 * anim.FBW - 0.0375 * anim.diet.NDF.conc)
          kp_concentrate <- 1.572 * kp_forage - 0.925
          kp_liquid <- 0.976 * kp_concentrate + 3.516
          # No adjustments for peNDF
          Adjusted_kp_forage <- kp_forage
          Adjusted_kp_concentrate <- kp_concentrate
        }
      }
    }
    feed_kp <- ifelse(as.numeric(fd[, "Forage"]) > 0, Adjusted_kp_forage, Adjusted_kp_concentrate)
    return(c(kp_forage, kp_concentrate, kp_liquid, feed_kp))
  }
```

4.3.6 Bacteria yield, maximum yield, and yield improvement

```
calcBacteriaYg <- function(flag_yg, Parm_rum.bact.Yg2, anim.diet.peNDF.conc)
{
  if (flag_yg == 0)
  {
    # Fox et al. (2004; Anim. Feed Sci. Technol. 112:29-78)
    if (anim.diet.peNDF.conc < 20)
    {
      YgAdjusted <- Parm_rum.bact.Yg2 * (1 - ((20 - anim.diet.peNDF.conc) * 0.025))
      return(YgAdjusted)
    } else
    {
      return(Parm_rum.bact.Yg2)
    }
  } else
  {
    # Boston et al. (2000; Modelling Nutrient Utilization in Farm Animals 361-377)
    a <- anim.diet.peNDF.conc/100
    g <- -100 * (a - 0.1965127)
    g <- 1/(1 + exp(g))
    d <- (1 - g) * (1 - (0.2036872 - a) * 2.390715) + g
    YgAdjusted <- d * Parm_rum.bact.Yg2
    return(YgAdjusted)
  }
}

calcBacteriaY <- function(km, Yg, kd)
{
  y <- ifelse(kd != 0 & Yg != 0, 1/((km/(kd/100)) + (1/Yg)), 0)
  return(y)
}

calcBacteriaYieldImprovement <- function(rum.diet.DPep.rate, rum.diet.DCHOA4.rate, rum.diet.DCHOB1.rate, rum.diet.DCHOB2.rate)
{
  rum.degraded.PeptideCHO <- rum.diet.DPep.rate + rum.diet.DCHOA4.rate + rum.diet.DCHOB1.rate + rum.diet.DCHOB2.rate
  PeptideTONFCHORatio <- ifelse(rum.degraded.PeptideCHO > 0, rum.diet.DPep.rate/rum.degraded.PeptideCHO, 0)
  value <- min(1.187, 1 + (exp(0.404 * log(PeptideTONFCHORatio * 100) + 1.942))/100)
  return(value)
}

```

4.3.7 Bacteria peptide uptake

```
calcPeptideUptake <- function(flag_peptide, Parm_rum.bact.PepUp, rum.kp_forage.fracprate, rum.kp_liquid.fracprate,
rum.diet.bact.NFC.rate,
                                rum.diet.DPep.rate, anim.diet.Concentrate.frac)
{
  # (kg/d)/(1/h*h/d) ==> kg NFC bacteria
  rum.bact.NFC.amt <- ifelse(rum.kp_forage.fracprate != 0, rum.diet.bact.NFC.rate/((rum.kp_forage.fracprate/100) * 24), 0)
  if (flag_peptide == 0)
  {
    # Fox et al. (2004; Anim. Feed Sci. Technol. 112:29-78)
    # CNCPS v3.x started using the NPER function of VBA to compute 'time to disappearance, h'
    # Time to disappearance = NPER(((LiqGrowth - 1) / 3600), -1 * (NSC_Bact_Peptide_Uptake / 3600), 0, HourlyRDPEP) / 3600
    # rum.diet.DPepUptake.factor = NPER(((rum.bact.kLG.time - 1) / 3600), -1 * (rum.diet.DPepUptake.rate / 3600), 0,
rum.diet.DPep.rate_h) / 3600
    rum.bact.kup.rate <- ifelse(anim.diet.ionophore == TRUE, 2/3, 1) * 0.07 # kg peptide/kg bacteria/h
    # survival fractional rate was assumed to be 100 - rum.kp_liquid.fracprate, %/h
    rum.bact.kLG.time <- ifelse(rum.kp_liquid.fracprate != 100, 100/(100 - rum.kp_liquid.fracprate), 0)  # h
    rum.diet.DPepUptake.rate <- rum.bact.NFC.amt * rum.bact.kup.rate  # kg/h
    rum.diet.DPep.rate_h <- rum.diet.DPep.rate/24  # kg/h
    rum.diet.DPepUptake.factor <- ifelse(rum.diet.DPepUptake.rate > 0 & ((rum.bact.kLG.time - 1)/3600) != -1,
                                 log(1 + (((rum.bact.kLG.time - 1)/3600) *
rum.diet.DPep.rate_h)/(rum.diet.DPepUptake.rate/3600))/
                                 (log(1 + ((rum.bact.kLG.time - 1)/3600)))/3600, 0)
    value <- min(rum.diet.DPepUptake.factor * rum.diet.DPepUptake.rate, rum.diet.DPep.rate_h) * 24  # kg/d
    return(value)
  } else
  {
    # New RNS submodel
    rum.bact.kup.rate <- Parm_rum.bact.PepUp  # g peptide/g bacteria/h
    if (anim.diet.Concentrate.frac > 0.9)
    {
      rum.bact.kup.rate <- rum.bact.kup.rate * (1 - 0.43)
    } else
    {
      if (anim.diet.ionophore == TRUE)
        rum.bact.kup.rate <- rum.bact.kup.rate * (1 - 0.35)
    }
    rum.diet.DPepUptake.rate_h <- rum.bact.NFC.amt * rum.bact.kup.rate  # kg/h
    rum.diet.DPepUptake.rate <- min(rum.diet.DPepUptake.rate_h * 24, rum.diet.DPep.rate)  # kg/d
    return(rum.diet.DPepUptake.rate)
  }
}
```

4.3.8 Rumen submodel

```
calcRumen <- function(fds = feeds3, genRPT = TRUE)
{
  anim.fd.Forage.conc <<- as.numeric(fds[, "Forage"])
  anim.diet.Forage.frac <<- sum(anim.fd.Forage.conc * anim.fd.DMI.rate/100)/anim.diet.DMI.rate
  anim.diet.Concentrate.frac <<- 1 - anim.diet.Forage.frac
  anim.diet.peNDF.conc <<- anim.diet.peNDF.rate * 100/anim.diet.DMI.rate
  rum.volume <<- calcRumenVolume(anim.FBW)
  # +++++++++++++++++++
  # Degradation rates
  # +++++++++++++++++++
  rum.fd.CHOA1_kd.fracprate <<- as.numeric(fds[, "CHO_A1_kd"])
  rum.fd.CHOA2_kd.fracprate <<- as.numeric(fds[, "CHO_A2_kd"])
  rum.fd.CHOA3_kd.fracprate <<- as.numeric(fds[, "CHO_A3_kd"])
  rum.fd.CHOA4_kd.fracprate <<- as.numeric(fds[, "CHO_A4_kd"])
  rum.fd.CHOB1_kd.fracprate <<- as.numeric(fds[, "CHO_B1_kd"])
  rum.fd.CHOB2_kd.fracprate <<- as.numeric(fds[, "CHO_B2_kd"])
  rum.fd.CHOB3_kd.fracprate <<- as.numeric(fds[, "CHO_B3_kd"])
  rum.fd.CHOBC_kd.fracprate <<- 0
  rum.fd.ProtA_kd.fracprate <<- as.numeric(fds[, "Prot_A_kd"])
  rum.fd.ProtB1_kd.fracprate <<- as.numeric(fds[, "Prot_B1_kd"])
  rum.fd.ProtB2_kd.fracprate <<- as.numeric(fds[, "Prot_B2_kd"])
  rum.fd.ProtB3_kd.fracprate <<- as.numeric(fds[, "Prot_B3_kd"])
  rum.fd.ProtC_kd.fracprate <<- 0
  rum.fd.FA_klip.fracprate <<- as.numeric(fds[, "LipolysisRate"])
  rum.fd.FA_Adjklip.fracprate <<- rum.fd.FA_klip.fracprate * exp(-as.numeric(fds[, "AdjFactor"]) * (anim.fd.TFA.rate/anim.diet.DMI.rate))
  FCBacteriaParms <- fds["FeedName.x"]
  names(FCBacteriaParms) <- "FeedName"
  # +++++++++++++# Ruminal pH # +++++++++++++#
  rum.pH <<- calcRumenpH_peNDF(flag_ph, anim.diet.peNDF.conc)
  rum.pH_peNDF <<- rum.pH
  # ++++++++++++++++++++++++++++++++++++++++++++++++++++
  # Adjustment of available NDF (CHO B3) for ruminal pH
  # ++++++++++++++++++++++++++++++++++++++++++++++++++++
  FCBacteriaParms <- calcCHOB3_kdAdjustment(flag_CHOB3_kd, Parm_rum.bact.km1, Parm_rum.bact.Yg1, rum.fd.CHOB3_kd.fracprate, rum.pH, FCBacteriaParms)
  rum.fd.CHOB3_kd.fracprate_original <<- rum.fd.CHOB3_kd.fracprate
  rum.fd.CHOB3_kd.fracprate <<- pmin(pmax(as.numeric(FCBacteriaParms[, "CHOB3_kd'"]), 0), pmax(rum.fd.CHOB3_kd.fracprate, 0))
  # +++++++++++++++++++
  # Passage rate, %/h
  # +++++++++++++++++++
  kp <- calcPassageRate(flag_kp_cattle, flag_adjust_kp_for_pendf, fds, anim.diet.DMI.rate, anim.FBW, anim.SBW, anim.diet.Forage.frac, anim.diet.Concentrate.frac)
  rum.kp_forage.fracprate <<- kp[1]
  rum.kp_concentrate.fracprate <<- kp[2]
  rum.kp_liquid.fracprate <<- kp[3]
  rum.fd.kp.fracprate <<- kp[4:length(kp)]
  # rum.fd.CHOA1_kp.fracprate<<-ifelse(fds[,'CHO_A1_Kp_Opt']=='A', rum.fd.kp.fracprate,as.numeric(fds[,'CHO_A1_Kp']))
```

```
    # rum.fd.CHOA2_kp.fracprate<<-ifelse(fds[,'CHO_A2_Kp_Opt']=='A', rum.fd.kp.fracprate,as.numeric(fds[,'CHO_A2_Kp']))
    # rum.fd.CHOA3_kp.fracprate<<-ifelse(fds[,'CHO_A3_Kp_Opt']=='A',rum.fd.kp.fracprate,as.numeric(fds[,'CHO_A3_Kp']))
    # rum.fd.CHOA4_kp.fracprate<<-ifelse(fds[,'CHO_A4_Kp_Opt']=='A',rum.fd.kp.fracprate,as.numeric(fds[,'CHO_A4_Kp']))
    rum.fd.CHOA1_kp.fracprate <<- ifelse(fds[, "CHO_A1_Kp_Opt"] == "A", rum.kp_liquid.fracprate, as.numeric(fds[, "CHO_A1_Kp"]))
    rum.fd.CHOA2_kp.fracprate <<- ifelse(fds[, "CHO_A2_Kp_Opt"] == "A", rum.kp_liquid.fracprate, as.numeric(fds[, "CHO_A2_Kp"]))
    rum.fd.CHOA3_kp.fracprate <<- ifelse(fds[, "CHO_A3_Kp_Opt"] == "A", rum.kp_liquid.fracprate, as.numeric(fds[, "CHO_A3_Kp"]))
    rum.fd.CHOA4_kp.fracprate <<- ifelse(fds[, "CHO_A4_Kp_Opt"] == "A", rum.kp_liquid.fracprate, as.numeric(fds[, "CHO_A4_Kp"]))
    rum.fd.CHOB1_kp.fracprate <<- ifelse(fds[, "CHO_B1_Kp_Opt"] == "A", rum.fd.kp.fracprate, as.numeric(fds[, "CHO_B1_Kp"]))
    rum.fd.CHOB2_kp.fracprate <<- ifelse(fds[, "CHO_B2_Kp_Opt"] == "A", rum.fd.kp.fracprate, as.numeric(fds[, "CHO_B2_Kp"]))
    rum.fd.CHOB3_kp.fracprate <<- ifelse(fds[, "CHO_B3_Kp_Opt"] == "A", rum.fd.kp.fracprate, as.numeric(fds[, "CHO_B3_Kp"]))
    rum.fd.CHOC_kp.fracprate <<- ifelse(fds[, "CHO_C_Kp_Opt"] == "A", rum.fd.kp.fracprate, as.numeric(fds[, "CHO_C_Kp"]))
    # rum.fd.ProtA_kp.fracprate<<-ifelse(fds[,'Prot_A_Kp_Opt']=='A',rum.fd.kp.fracprate,as.numeric(fds[,'Prot_A_Kp']))
    # rum.fd.ProtB1_kp.fracprate<<-ifelse(fds[,'Prot_B1_Kp_Opt']=='A',rum.fd.kp.fracprate,as.numeric(fds[,'Prot_B1_Kp']))
    rum.fd.ProtA_kp.fracprate <<- ifelse(fds[, "Prot_A_Kp_Opt"] == "A", rum.kp_liquid.fracprate, as.numeric(fds[, "Prot_A_Kp"]))
    rum.fd.ProtB1_kp.fracprate <<- ifelse(fds[, "Prot_B1_Kp_Opt"] == "A", rum.kp_liquid.fracprate, as.numeric(fds[,
  "Prot_B1_Kp"]))
    rum.fd.ProtB2_kp.fracprate <<- ifelse(fds[, "Prot_B2_Kp_Opt"] == "A", rum.fd.kp.fracprate, as.numeric(fds[, "Prot_B2_Kp"]))
    rum.fd.ProtB3_kp.fracprate <<- ifelse(fds[, "Prot_B3_Kp_Opt"] == "A", rum.fd.kp.fracprate, as.numeric(fds[, "Prot_B3_Kp"]))
    rum.fd.ProtC_kp.fracprate <<- ifelse(fds[, "Prot_C_Kp_Opt"] == "A", rum.fd.kp.fracprate, as.numeric(fds[, "Prot_C_Kp"]))
    # rum.fd.Glycerol_kp.fracprate<<-rum.fd.kp.fracprate
    rum.fd.Glycerol_kp.fracprate <<- rum.kp_liquid.fracprate
    rum.fd.FAC12_kp.fracprate <<- ifelse(fds[, "C120_Kp_Opt"] == "A", rum.fd.kp.fracprate, as.numeric(fds[, "C120_Kp"]))
    rum.fd.FAC14_kp.fracprate <<- ifelse(fds[, "C140_Kp_Opt"] == "A", rum.fd.kp.fracprate, as.numeric(fds[, "C140_Kp"]))
    rum.fd.FAC16_kp.fracprate <<- ifelse(fds[, "C160_Kp_Opt"] == "A", rum.fd.kp.fracprate, as.numeric(fds[, "C160_Kp"]))
    rum.fd.FAC16_1_kp.fracprate <<- ifelse(fds[, "C161_Kp_Opt"] == "A", rum.fd.kp.fracprate, as.numeric(fds[, "C161_Kp"]))
    rum.fd.FAC18_kp.fracprate <<- ifelse(fds[, "C180_Kp_Opt"] == "A", rum.fd.kp.fracprate, as.numeric(fds[, "C180_Kp"]))
    rum.fd.FAC18_1c_kp.fracprate <<- ifelse(fds[, "C181c_Kp_Opt"] == "A", rum.fd.kp.fracprate, as.numeric(fds[, "C181c_Kp"]))
    rum.fd.FAC18_1t_kp.fracprate <<- ifelse(fds[, "C181t_Kp_Opt"] == "A", rum.fd.kp.fracprate, as.numeric(fds[, "C181t_Kp"]))
    rum.fd.FAC18_2_kp.fracprate <<- ifelse(fds[, "C182_Kp_Opt"] == "A", rum.fd.kp.fracprate, as.numeric(fds[, "C182_Kp"]))
    rum.fd.FAC18_3_kp.fracprate <<- ifelse(fds[, "C183_Kp_Opt"] == "A", rum.fd.kp.fracprate, as.numeric(fds[, "C183_Kp"]))
    rum.fd.FAOther_kp.fracprate <<- ifelse(fds[, "Other_Kp_Opt"] == "A", rum.fd.kp.fracprate, as.numeric(fds[, "Other_Kp"]))
    if (genRPT)
    {
      kdANDkp <- fds["FeedName.x"]
      names(kdANDkp) <- "FeedName"
      kdANDkp["CHOA1 kd"] <- rum.fd.CHOA1_kd.fracprate
      kdANDkp["CHOA2 kd"] <- rum.fd.CHOA2_kd.fracprate
      kdANDkp["CHOA3 kd"] <- rum.fd.CHOA3_kd.fracprate
      kdANDkp["CHOA4 kd"] <- rum.fd.CHOA4_kd.fracprate
      kdANDkp["CHOB1 kd"] <- rum.fd.CHOB1_kd.fracprate
      kdANDkp["CHOB2 kd"] <- rum.fd.CHOB2_kd.fracprate
      kdANDkp["CHOB3 kd"] <- rum.fd.CHOB3_kd.fracprate_original
      kdANDkp["CHOB3 kd'"] <- rum.fd.CHOB3_kd.fracprate
      kdANDkp["ProtA kd"] <- rum.fd.ProtA_kd.fracprate
      kdANDkp["ProtB1 kd"] <- rum.fd.ProtB1_kd.fracprate
      kdANDkp["ProtB2 kd"] <- rum.fd.ProtB2_kd.fracprate
      kdANDkp["ProtB3 kd"] <- rum.fd.ProtB3_kd.fracprate
      kdANDkp["FA kd"] <- rum.fd.FA_klip.fracprate
      kdANDkp["FA kd'"] <- rum.fd.FA_Adjklip.fracprate
      kdANDkp["Auto kp"] <- rum.fd.kp.fracprate
      kdANDkp["CHOA1 kp"] <- rum.fd.CHOA1_kp.fracprate
```

```
    kdANDkp["CHOA2 kp"] <- rum.fd.CHOA2_kp.fracprate
    kdANDkp["CHOA3 kp"] <- rum.fd.CHOA3_kp.fracprate
    kdANDkp["CHOA4 kp"] <- rum.fd.CHOA4_kp.fracprate
    kdANDkp["CHOB1 kp"] <- rum.fd.CHOB1_kp.fracprate
    kdANDkp["CHOB2 kp"] <- rum.fd.CHOB2_kp.fracprate
    kdANDkp["CHOB3 kp"] <- rum.fd.CHOB3_kp.fracprate
    kdANDkp["CHOC kp"] <- rum.fd.CHOC_kp.fracprate
    kdANDkp["ProtA kp"] <- rum.fd.ProtA_kp.fracprate
    kdANDkp["ProtB1 kp"] <- rum.fd.ProtB1_kp.fracprate
    kdANDkp["ProtB2 kp"] <- rum.fd.ProtB2_kp.fracprate
    kdANDkp["ProtB3 kp"] <- rum.fd.ProtB3_kp.fracprate
    kdANDkp["ProtC kp"] <- rum.fd.ProtC_kp.fracprate
    kdANDkp["Gly kp"] <- rum.fd.Glycerol_kp.fracprate
    kdANDkp["C12:0 kp"] <- rum.fd.FAC12_kp.fracprate
    kdANDkp["C14:0 kp"] <- rum.fd.FAC14_kp.fracprate
    kdANDkp["c16:0 kp"] <- rum.fd.FAC16_kp.fracprate
    kdANDkp["C16:1 kp"] <- rum.fd.FAC16_1_kp.fracprate
    kdANDkp["C18:0 kp"] <- rum.fd.FAC18_kp.fracprate
    kdANDkp["C18:1c kp"] <- rum.fd.FAC18_1c_kp.fracprate
    kdANDkp["C18:1t kp"] <- rum.fd.FAC18_1t_kp.fracprate
    kdANDkp["C18:2 kp"] <- rum.fd.FAC18_2_kp.fracprate
    kdANDkp["C18:3 kp"] <- rum.fd.FAC18_3_kp.fracprate
    kdANDkp["Other FA kp"] <- rum.fd.FAOther_kp.fracprate
    description <- paste("Forage kp, %/h       : ", formatC(rum.kp_forage.fracprate, format = "f", digits = 3, width = 8), "\nConcentrate kp, %/h : ",
                           formatC(rum.kp_concentrate.fracprate, format = "f", digits = 3, width = 8), "\nLiquid kp, %/h      : ",
                           formatC(rum.kp_liquid.fracprate, format = "f", digits = 3, width = 8), "\n", sep = "")
    if (flag_ph == 0) footnote <- "Algorithm for ruminal pH: CNCPS v. 5; Fox et al. (2004)"
    if (flag_ph == 1) footnote <- "Algorithm for ruminal pH: CPM Dairy v. 1.08; Boston et al. (2000)"
    if (flag_CHOB3_kd == 0) footnote <- paste(footnote, "\nAlgorithm for CHO B3 adjustment due to ruminal pH: CNCPS v. 5; Fox et al. (2004)", sep = "")
    if (flag_CHOB3_kd == 1) footnote <- paste(footnote, "\nAlgorithm for CHO B3 adjustment due to ruminal pH: RNS v. 1.0", sep = "")
    if (flag_CHOB3_kd == 2) footnote <- paste(footnote, "\nAlgorithm for CHO B3 adjustment due to ruminal pH: CPM Dairy v. 1.08; Boston et al. (2000)", sep = "")
    if (flag_kp_cattle == 0) footnote <- paste(footnote, "\nAlgorithm for fractional passage rate: CNCPS v. 5; Fox et al. (2004)", sep = "")
    if (flag_kp_cattle == 1) footnote <- paste(footnote, "\nAlgorithm for fractional passage rate: CPM Dairy v. 1.08; Boston et al. (2000)", sep = "")
    footnote <- paste(footnote, "\nGly = glycerol", sep="")
    report(kdANDkp, "Fractional Rates of Degradation (kd) and Passage (kp)", description, footnote, 3, 3, 1, 8, FALSE, FALSE, FALSE, FALSE, FALSE, FALSE, TRUE, 3)
  }
  # +++++++++++++++++++++++++++++
  # Ruminally degraded nutrients
  # +++++++++++++++++++++++++++++
  # D = Degraded L = Lipolyzed B = Biohydrogenized
  rum.fd.LGlycerol.rate <<- ifelse((rum.fd.FA_klip.fracprate + rum.fd.Glycerol_kp.fracprate) > 0, anim.fd.Glycerol.rate * (rum.fd.FA_klip.fracprate/(rum.fd.FA_klip.fracprate + rum.fd.Glycerol_kp.fracprate)), 0)
  rum.fd.LGlycerol.propionate.rate <<- rum.fd.LGlycerol.rate
```

```
    rum.fd.DCHOA1.rate <<- ifelse((rum.fd.CHOA1_kd.fracprate + rum.fd.CHOA1_kp.fracprate) > 0, rum.fd.LGlycerol.propionate.rate
  + anim.fd.CHOA1.rate * (rum.fd.CHOA1_kd.fracprate/(rum.fd.CHOA1_kd.fracprate + rum.fd.CHOA1_kp.fracprate)), 0)
    rum.fd.DCHOA2.rate <<- ifelse((rum.fd.CHOA2_kd.fracprate + rum.fd.CHOA2_kp.fracprate) > 0, anim.fd.CHOA2.rate *
  (rum.fd.CHOA2_kd.fracprate/(rum.fd.CHOA2_kd.fracprate + rum.fd.CHOA2_kp.fracprate)), 0)
    rum.fd.DCHOA3.rate <<- ifelse((rum.fd.CHOA3_kd.fracprate + rum.fd.CHOA3_kp.fracprate) > 0, anim.fd.CHOA3.rate *
  (rum.fd.CHOA3_kd.fracprate/(rum.fd.CHOA3_kd.fracprate + rum.fd.CHOA3_kp.fracprate)), 0)
    rum.fd.DCHOA4.rate <<- ifelse((rum.fd.CHOA4_kd.fracprate + rum.fd.CHOA4_kp.fracprate) > 0, anim.fd.CHOA4.rate *
  (rum.fd.CHOA4_kd.fracprate/(rum.fd.CHOA4_kd.fracprate + rum.fd.CHOA4_kp.fracprate)), 0)
    rum.fd.DCHOB1.rate <<- ifelse((rum.fd.CHOB1_kd.fracprate + rum.fd.CHOB1_kp.fracprate) > 0, anim.fd.CHOB1.rate *
  (rum.fd.CHOB1_kd.fracprate/(rum.fd.CHOB1_kd.fracprate + rum.fd.CHOB1_kp.fracprate)), 0)
    rum.fd.DCHOB2.rate <<- ifelse((rum.fd.CHOB2_kd.fracprate + rum.fd.CHOB2_kp.fracprate) > 0, anim.fd.CHOB2.rate *
  (rum.fd.CHOB2_kd.fracprate/(rum.fd.CHOB2_kd.fracprate + rum.fd.CHOB2_kp.fracprate)), 0)
    rum.fd.DCHOB3.rate <<- ifelse((rum.fd.CHOB3_kd.fracprate + rum.fd.CHOB3_kp.fracprate) > 0, anim.fd.CHOB3.rate *
  (rum.fd.CHOB3_kd.fracprate/(rum.fd.CHOB3_kd.fracprate + rum.fd.CHOB3_kp.fracprate)), 0)
    rum.fd.DCHOC.rate <<- ifelse((0 + rum.fd.CHOC_kp.fracprate) > 0, anim.fd.CHOC.rate * (0/(0 + rum.fd.CHOC_kp.fracprate)), 0)
    rum.fd.DCHO.rate <<- rum.fd.DCHOA1.rate + rum.fd.DCHOA2.rate + rum.fd.DCHOA3.rate + rum.fd.DCHOA4.rate + rum.fd.DCHOB1.rate
  + rum.fd.DCHOB2.rate + rum.fd.DCHOB3.rate + rum.fd.DCHOC.rate
    rum.diet.LGlycerol.rate <<- sum(rum.fd.LGlycerol.rate)
    rum.diet.DCHOA1.rate <<- sum(rum.fd.DCHOA1.rate)
    rum.diet.DCHOA2.rate <<- sum(rum.fd.DCHOA2.rate)
    rum.diet.DCHOA3.rate <<- sum(rum.fd.DCHOA3.rate)
    rum.diet.DCHOA4.rate <<- sum(rum.fd.DCHOA4.rate)
    rum.diet.DCHOB1.rate <<- sum(rum.fd.DCHOB1.rate)
    rum.diet.DCHOB2.rate <<- sum(rum.fd.DCHOB2.rate)
    rum.diet.DCHOB3.rate <<- sum(rum.fd.DCHOB3.rate)
    rum.diet.DCHOC.rate <<- sum(rum.fd.DCHOC.rate)
    rum.diet.DCHO.rate <<- sum(rum.fd.DCHO.rate)
    if (genRPT)
    {
      rptRDCHO_DMI <- fds["FeedName.x"]
      names(rptRDCHO_DMI) <- "FeedName"
      rptRDCHO_DMI["CHO A1"] <- rum.fd.DCHOA1.rate
      rptRDCHO_DMI["CHO A2"] <- rum.fd.DCHOA2.rate
      rptRDCHO_DMI["CHO A3"] <- rum.fd.DCHOA3.rate
      rptRDCHO_DMI["CHO A4"] <- rum.fd.DCHOA4.rate
      rptRDCHO_DMI["CHO B1"] <- rum.fd.DCHOB1.rate
      rptRDCHO_DMI["CHO B2"] <- rum.fd.DCHOB2.rate
      rptRDCHO_DMI["CHO B3"] <- rum.fd.DCHOB3.rate
      report(rptRDCHO_DMI, "Ruminally Degraded Carbohydrate Intake, kg/d", "", "", 3, 3, 1, 8, TRUE, FALSE, TRUE, FALSE, TRUE,
  FALSE, FALSE)
    }
    # Carbohydrate fermentability
    rum.fd.DTrueCHO.rate <<- rum.fd.DCHOA4.rate + rum.fd.DCHOB1.rate + rum.fd.DCHOB2.rate + rum.fd.DCHOB3.rate
    rum.diet.DTrueCHO.rate <<- sum(rum.fd.DTrueCHO.rate)
    if (genRPT)
    {
      rptCHOFermentFd_DMI <- fds["FeedName.x"]
      names(rptCHOFermentFd_DMI) <- "FeedName"
      rptCHOFermentFd_DMI["Sugar, kg/d"] <- rum.fd.DCHOA4.rate
      rptCHOFermentFd_DMI["Sugar, %A4"] <- ifelse(anim.fd.CHOA4.rate > 0, rum.fd.DCHOA4.rate * 100/anim.fd.CHOA4.rate, 0)
      rptCHOFermentFd_DMI["Starch, kg/d"] <- rum.fd.DCHOB1.rate
```

```
    rptCHOFermentFd_DMI["Starch, %B1"] <- ifelse(anim.fd.CHOB1.rate > 0, rum.fd.DCHOB1.rate * 100/anim.fd.CHOB1.rate, 0)
    rptCHOFermentFd_DMI["SF, kg/d"] <- rum.fd.DCHOB2.rate
    rptCHOFermentFd_DMI["SF, %B2"] <- ifelse(anim.fd.CHOB2.rate > 0, rum.fd.DCHOB2.rate * 100/anim.fd.CHOB2.rate, 0)
    rptCHOFermentFd_DMI["NDF, kg/d"] <- rum.fd.DCHOB3.rate
    rptCHOFermentFd_DMI["NDF, %"] <- ifelse(anim.fd.CHOB3.rate > 0, rum.fd.DCHOB3.rate * 100/anim.fd.NDF.rate, 0)
    rptCHOFermentFd_DMI["CHO, kg/d"] <- rum.fd.DTrueCHO.rate
    rptCHOFermentFd_DMI["CHO, %DM"] <- ifelse(anim.fd.DMI.rate > 0, rum.fd.DTrueCHO.rate * 100/anim.fd.DMI.rate, 0)
    rptCHOFermentFd_DMI["RFC-Fill"] <- ifelse((anim.fd.CHOB3.rate - rum.fd.DCHOB3.rate) > 0, (rum.fd.DCHOB3.rate + anim.fd.CHOB1.rate)/(anim.fd.CHOB3.rate - rum.fd.DCHOB3.rate), 0)
    rptCHOFermentDiet_DMI <- data.frame(FeedName = "Ration")
    rptCHOFermentDiet_DMI["Sugar, kg/d"] <- rum.diet.DCHOA4.rate
    rptCHOFermentDiet_DMI["Sugar, %A4"] <- ifelse(anim.diet.CHOA4.rate > 0, rum.diet.DCHOA4.rate * 100/anim.diet.CHOA4.rate, 0)
    rptCHOFermentDiet_DMI["Starch, kg/d"] <- rum.diet.DCHOB1.rate
    rptCHOFermentDiet_DMI["Starch, %B1"] <- ifelse(anim.diet.CHOB1.rate > 0, rum.diet.DCHOB1.rate * 100/anim.diet.CHOB1.rate, 0)
    rptCHOFermentDiet_DMI["SF, kg/d"] <- rum.diet.DCHOB2.rate
    rptCHOFermentDiet_DMI["SF, %B2"] <- ifelse(anim.diet.CHOB2.rate > 0, rum.diet.DCHOB2.rate * 100/anim.diet.CHOB2.rate, 0)
    rptCHOFermentDiet_DMI["NDF, kg/d"] <- rum.diet.DCHOB3.rate
    rptCHOFermentDiet_DMI["NDF, %"] <- ifelse(anim.diet.CHOB3.rate > 0, rum.diet.DCHOB3.rate * 100/anim.diet.NDF.rate, 0)
    rptCHOFermentDiet_DMI["CHO, kg/d"] <- rum.diet.DTrueCHO.rate
    rptCHOFermentDiet_DMI["CHO, %DM"] <- ifelse(anim.diet.DMI.rate > 0, rum.diet.DTrueCHO.rate * 100/anim.diet.DMI.rate, 0)
    rptCHOFermentDiet_DMI["RFC-Fill"] <- ifelse((anim.diet.CHOB3.rate - rum.diet.DCHOB3.rate) > 0, (rum.diet.DCHOB3.rate + anim.diet.CHOB1.rate)/(anim.diet.CHOB3.rate - rum.diet.DCHOB3.rate), 0)
    rptCHOFerment_DMI <- rbind(rptCHOFermentFd_DMI, rptCHOFermentDiet_DMI)
    description <- paste("Sugar fermentability, % DM            : ",
                         formatC(ifelse(anim.diet.CHOA4.rate > 0, rum.diet.DCHOA4.rate * 100/anim.diet.DMI.rate, 0), format = "f", digits = 3, width = 8), "\nStarch fermentability, % DM         : ",
                         formatC(ifelse(anim.diet.CHOB1.rate > 0, rum.diet.DCHOB1.rate * 100/anim.diet.DMI.rate, 0), format = "f", digits = 3, width = 8), "\nSoluble fiber fermentability, % DM : ",
                         formatC(ifelse(anim.diet.CHOB2.rate > 0, rum.diet.DCHOB2.rate * 100/anim.diet.DMI.rate, 0), format = "f", digits = 3, width = 8), "\nFiber fermentability, % DM          : ",
                         formatC(ifelse(anim.diet.CHOB3.rate > 0, rum.diet.DCHOB3.rate * 100/anim.diet.DMI.rate, 0), format = "f", digits = 3, width = 8), "\nCarbohydrate fermentability, % DM  : ",
                         formatC(ifelse(anim.diet.DMI.rate > 0, rum.diet.DTrueCHO.rate * 100/anim.diet.DMI.rate, 0), format = "f", digits = 3, width = 8), "\n", sep = "")
    footnote <- "RFC-Fill is rumen fermentable CHO (degraded NDF + starch) divided by gut fill (undegraded NDF).\nFor corn silage, the mean is 3.5, SD is 0.73, and CV is 20.8% (Jones and Siciliano-Jones, 2015)."
    # Jones, L. R., and J. Siciliano Jones. 2015. Index useful for ranking silage samples. Feedstuffs. 87 (30):17-19.
    report(rptCHOFerment_DMI, "\nCarbohydrate Fermentability", description, footnote, 3, 3, 1, 6, FALSE, FALSE, FALSE, FALSE, TRUE, FALSE, TRUE)
  }
  rum.fd.DProtA.rate <<- ifelse((rum.fd.ProtA_kd.fracprate + rum.fd.ProtA_kp.fracprate) > 0, anim.fd.ProtA.rate * (rum.fd.ProtA_kd.fracprate/(rum.fd.ProtA_kd.fracprate + rum.fd.ProtA_kp.fracprate)), 0)
  rum.fd.DProtB1.rate <<- ifelse((rum.fd.ProtB1_kd.fracprate + rum.fd.ProtB1_kp.fracprate) > 0, anim.fd.ProtB1.rate * (rum.fd.ProtB1_kd.fracprate/(rum.fd.ProtB1_kd.fracprate + rum.fd.ProtB1_kp.fracprate)), 0)
  rum.fd.DProtB2.rate <<- ifelse((rum.fd.ProtB2_kd.fracprate + rum.fd.ProtB2_kp.fracprate) > 0, anim.fd.ProtB2.rate * (rum.fd.ProtB2_kd.fracprate/(rum.fd.ProtB2_kd.fracprate + rum.fd.ProtB2_kp.fracprate)), 0)
  rum.fd.DProtB3.rate <<- ifelse((rum.fd.ProtB3_kd.fracprate + rum.fd.ProtB3_kp.fracprate) > 0, anim.fd.ProtB3.rate * (rum.fd.ProtB3_kd.fracprate/(rum.fd.ProtB3_kd.fracprate + rum.fd.ProtB3_kp.fracprate)), 0)
```

```
    rum.fd.DProtC.rate <<- ifelse((0 + rum.fd.ProtC_kp.fracprate) > 0, anim.fd.ProtC.rate * (0/(0 + rum.fd.ProtC_kp.fracprate)),
  0)
    rum.fd.DPep.rate <<- rum.fd.DProtB1.rate + rum.fd.DProtB2.rate + rum.fd.DProtB3.rate
    rum.fd.RDP.rate <<- rum.fd.DProt.rate <<- rum.fd.DProtA.rate + rum.fd.DPep.rate + rum.fd.DProtC.rate
    rum.diet.DProtA.rate <<- sum(rum.fd.DProtA.rate)
    rum.diet.DProtB1.rate <<- sum(rum.fd.DProtB1.rate)
    rum.diet.DProtB2.rate <<- sum(rum.fd.DProtB2.rate)
    rum.diet.DProtB3.rate <<- sum(rum.fd.DProtB3.rate)
    rum.diet.DProtC.rate <<- sum(rum.fd.DProtC.rate)
    rum.diet.DPep.rate <<- sum(rum.fd.DPep.rate)
    rum.diet.DProt.rate <<- sum(rum.fd.DProt.rate)
    rum.diet.RDP.rate <<- sum(rum.fd.RDP.rate)
    # Fermentable organic matter (CHO and Protein)
    rum.fd.FOM.rate <<- rum.fd.DTrueCHO.rate + rum.fd.RDP.rate
    rum.diet.FOM.rate <<- sum(rum.fd.FOM.rate)
    anim.diet.FOMI.rate <<- rum.diet.FOM.rate
    if (genRPT)
    {
      rptRDProt_DMI <- fds["FeedName.x"]
      names(rptRDProt_DMI) <- "FeedName"
      rptRDProt_DMI["Prot A"] <- rum.fd.DProtA.rate
      rptRDProt_DMI["Prot B1"] <- rum.fd.DProtB1.rate
      rptRDProt_DMI["Prot B2"] <- rum.fd.DProtB2.rate
      rptRDProt_DMI["Prot B3"] <- rum.fd.DProtB3.rate
      description <- paste("Dry Matter Intake (DMI), kg/d                    : ", formatC(ifelse(anim.diet.DMI.rate > 0,
  anim.diet.DMI.rate, 0), format = "f", digits = 3, width = 8), "\n",
                           "Organic Matter Intake (OMI), kg/d                : ", formatC(ifelse(anim.diet.OMI.rate > 0,
  anim.diet.OMI.rate, 0), format = "f", digits = 3, width = 8), "\n",
                           "   Organic matter, % DM                          : ", formatC(ifelse(anim.diet.DMI.rate > 0,
  anim.diet.OMI.rate*100/anim.diet.DMI.rate, 0), format = "f", digits = 3, width = 8), "\n",
                           "Fermentable Organic Matter Intake (FOMI), kg/d : ", formatC(ifelse(anim.diet.FOMI.rate > 0,
  anim.diet.FOMI.rate, 0), format = "f", digits = 3, width = 8), "\n",
                           "   Fementable oganic matter, % OM                : ", formatC(ifelse(anim.diet.OMI.rate > 0,
  anim.diet.FOMI.rate*100/anim.diet.OMI.rate, 0), format = "f", digits = 3, width = 8), "\n",
                           "   Fementable oganic matter, % DM                : ", formatC(ifelse(anim.diet.DMI.rate > 0,
  anim.diet.FOMI.rate*100/anim.diet.DMI.rate, 0), format = "f", digits = 3, width = 8), "\n", sep = "")
      report(rptRDProt_DMI, "Ruminally Degraded Protein Intake, kg/d", description, "", 3, 3, 1, 8, TRUE, FALSE, TRUE, FALSE,
  TRUE, FALSE, FALSE)
    }
    rum.fd.LFAC12.rate <<- ifelse((rum.fd.FA_Adjklip.fracprate + rum.fd.FAC12_kp.fracprate) > 0, anim.fd.FAC12.rate *
  (rum.fd.FA_Adjklip.fracprate/(rum.fd.FA_Adjklip.fracprate + rum.fd.FAC12_kp.fracprate)), 0)
    rum.fd.LFAC14.rate <<- ifelse((rum.fd.FA_Adjklip.fracprate + rum.fd.FAC14_kp.fracprate) > 0, anim.fd.FAC14.rate *
  (rum.fd.FA_Adjklip.fracprate/(rum.fd.FA_Adjklip.fracprate + rum.fd.FAC14_kp.fracprate)), 0)
    rum.fd.LFAC16.rate <<- ifelse((rum.fd.FA_Adjklip.fracprate + rum.fd.FAC16_kp.fracprate) > 0, anim.fd.FAC16.rate *
  (rum.fd.FA_Adjklip.fracprate/(rum.fd.FA_Adjklip.fracprate + rum.fd.FAC16_kp.fracprate)), 0)
    rum.fd.LFAC16_1.rate <<- ifelse((rum.fd.FA_Adjklip.fracprate + rum.fd.FAC16_1_kp.fracprate) > 0, anim.fd.FAC16_1.rate *
  (rum.fd.FA_Adjklip.fracprate/(rum.fd.FA_Adjklip.fracprate + rum.fd.FAC16_1_kp.fracprate)), 0)
    rum.fd.LFAC18.rate <<- ifelse((rum.fd.FA_Adjklip.fracprate + rum.fd.FAC18_kp.fracprate) > 0, anim.fd.FAC18.rate *
  (rum.fd.FA_Adjklip.fracprate/(rum.fd.FA_Adjklip.fracprate + rum.fd.FAC18_kp.fracprate)), 0)
    rum.fd.LFAC18_1c.rate <<- ifelse((rum.fd.FA_Adjklip.fracprate + rum.fd.FAC18_1c_kp.fracprate) > 0, anim.fd.FAC18_1c.rate *
  (rum.fd.FA_Adjklip.fracprate/(rum.fd.FA_Adjklip.fracprate + rum.fd.FAC18_1c_kp.fracprate)), 0)
```

```
    rum.fd.LFAC18_1t.rate <<- ifelse((rum.fd.FA_Adjklip.fracprate + rum.fd.FAC18_1t_kp.fracprate) > 0, anim.fd.FAC18_1t.rate * (rum.fd.FA_Adjklip.fracprate/(rum.fd.FA_Adjklip.fracprate + rum.fd.FAC18_1t_kp.fracprate)), 0)
    rum.fd.LFAC18_2.rate <<- ifelse((rum.fd.FA_Adjklip.fracprate + rum.fd.FAC18_2_kp.fracprate) > 0, anim.fd.FAC18_2.rate * (rum.fd.FA_Adjklip.fracprate/(rum.fd.FA_Adjklip.fracprate + rum.fd.FAC18_2_kp.fracprate)), 0)
    rum.fd.LFAC18_3.rate <<- ifelse((rum.fd.FA_Adjklip.fracprate + rum.fd.FAC18_3_kp.fracprate) > 0, anim.fd.FAC18_3.rate * (rum.fd.FA_Adjklip.fracprate/(rum.fd.FA_Adjklip.fracprate + rum.fd.FAC18_3_kp.fracprate)), 0)
    rum.fd.LFAOther.rate <<- ifelse((rum.fd.FA_Adjklip.fracprate + rum.fd.FAOther_kp.fracprate) > 0, anim.fd.FAOther.rate * (rum.fd.FA_Adjklip.fracprate/(rum.fd.FA_Adjklip.fracprate + rum.fd.FAOther_kp.fracprate)), 0)
    rum.diet.LFAC12.rate <<- sum(rum.fd.LFAC12.rate)
    rum.diet.LFAC14.rate <<- sum(rum.fd.LFAC14.rate)
    rum.diet.LFAC16.rate <<- sum(rum.fd.LFAC16.rate)
    rum.diet.LFAC16_1.rate <<- sum(rum.fd.LFAC16_1.rate)
    rum.diet.LFAC18.rate <<- sum(rum.fd.LFAC18.rate)
    rum.diet.LFAC18_1c.rate <<- sum(rum.fd.LFAC18_1c.rate)
    rum.diet.LFAC18_1t.rate <<- sum(rum.fd.LFAC18_1t.rate)
    rum.diet.LFAC18_2.rate <<- sum(rum.fd.LFAC18_2.rate)
    rum.diet.LFAC18_3.rate <<- sum(rum.fd.LFAC18_3.rate)
    rum.diet.LFAOther.rate <<- sum(rum.fd.LFAOther.rate)
    rum.diet.LFA.rate <<- rum.diet.LFAC12.rate + rum.diet.LFAC14.rate + rum.diet.LFAC16.rate + rum.diet.LFAC16_1.rate + rum.diet.LFAC18.rate + rum.diet.LFAC18_1c.rate + rum.diet.LFAC18_1t.rate + rum.diet.LFAC18_2.rate + rum.diet.LFAC18_3.rate + rum.diet.LFAOther.rate
    if (genRPT)
    {
      rptRLFA_DMI <- fds["FeedName.x"]
      names(rptRLFA_DMI) <- "FeedName"
      rptRLFA_DMI["C12:0"] <- rum.fd.LFAC12.rate
      rptRLFA_DMI["C14:0"] <- rum.fd.LFAC14.rate
      rptRLFA_DMI["C16:0"] <- rum.fd.LFAC16.rate
      rptRLFA_DMI["C16:1"] <- rum.fd.LFAC16_1.rate
      rptRLFA_DMI["C18:0"] <- rum.fd.LFAC18.rate
      rptRLFA_DMI["C18:1c"] <- rum.fd.LFAC18_1c.rate
      rptRLFA_DMI["C18:1t"] <- rum.fd.LFAC18_1t.rate
      rptRLFA_DMI["C18:2"] <- rum.fd.LFAC18_2.rate
      rptRLFA_DMI["C18:3"] <- rum.fd.LFAC18_3.rate
      rptRLFA_DMI["Other FFA"] <- rum.fd.LFAOther.rate
      report(rptRLFA_DMI, "\nRuminally Lipolyzed Fatty Acid Intake, g/d", "", "", 3, 3, 1000, 7, TRUE, FALSE, TRUE, FALSE, TRUE, FALSE, TRUE)
    }
    # ++++++++++++++++++++++++++
    # Bacteria growth submodel
    # ++++++++++++++++++++++++++
    # The Yg1 (FC) adjustment is not computed
    rum.bact.Adj_Yg2 <<- calcBacteriaYg(flag_yg, Parm_rum.bact.Yg2, anim.diet.peNDF.conc)  #NFC bacteria
    rum.bact.imp.factor <<- calcBacteriaYieldImprovement(rum.diet.DPep.rate, rum.diet.DCHOA4.rate, rum.diet.DCHOB1.rate, rum.diet.DCHOB2.rate)
    rum.fd.bact.CHOA1Y <<- calcBacteriaY(Parm_rum.bact.km2, rum.bact.Adj_Yg2, rum.fd.CHOA1_kd.fracprate) * rum.bact.imp.factor
    rum.fd.bact.CHOA2Y <<- calcBacteriaY(Parm_rum.bact.km2, rum.bact.Adj_Yg2, rum.fd.CHOA2_kd.fracprate) * rum.bact.imp.factor
    rum.fd.bact.CHOA3Y <<- calcBacteriaY(Parm_rum.bact.km2, rum.bact.Adj_Yg2, rum.fd.CHOA3_kd.fracprate) * rum.bact.imp.factor
    rum.fd.bact.CHOA4Y <<- calcBacteriaY(Parm_rum.bact.km2, rum.bact.Adj_Yg2, rum.fd.CHOA4_kd.fracprate) * rum.bact.imp.factor
    rum.fd.bact.CHOB1Y <<- calcBacteriaY(Parm_rum.bact.km2, rum.bact.Adj_Yg2, rum.fd.CHOB1_kd.fracprate) * rum.bact.imp.factor
    rum.fd.bact.CHOB2Y <<- calcBacteriaY(Parm_rum.bact.km2, rum.bact.Adj_Yg2, rum.fd.CHOB2_kd.fracprate) * rum.bact.imp.factor
```

```
    rum.fd.bact.CHOB3Y <<- calcBacteriaY(Parm_rum.bact.km1, Parm_rum.bact.Yg1, rum.fd.CHOB3_kd.fracprate)
    if (genRPT)
    {
      FCBacteriaParms["CHOA1 Yld"] <- rum.fd.bact.CHOA1Y
      FCBacteriaParms["CHOA2 Yld"] <- rum.fd.bact.CHOA2Y
      FCBacteriaParms["CHOA3 Yld"] <- rum.fd.bact.CHOA3Y
      FCBacteriaParms["CHOA4 Yld"] <- rum.fd.bact.CHOA4Y
      FCBacteriaParms["CHOB1 Yld"] <- rum.fd.bact.CHOB1Y
      FCBacteriaParms["CHOB2 Yld"] <- rum.fd.bact.CHOB2Y
      FCBacteriaParms["CHOB3 Yld"] <- rum.fd.bact.CHOB3Y
      description <- paste("NFC Bacteria improvement, % : ", formatC((rum.bact.imp.factor - 1) * 100, digits = 5), "\n\n", sep = "")
      if (flag_yg == 0) footnote <- "Algorithm for adjustment of Yg: CNCPS v. 5; Fox et al. (2004)"
      if (flag_yg == 1) footnote <- "Algorithm for adjustment of Yg: CPM Dairy v. 1.08; Boston et al. (2000)"
      report(FCBacteriaParms, "Ruminal Bacterial Parameters", description, footnote, 3, 3, 1, 7, FALSE, FALSE, FALSE, FALSE, FALSE, FALSE, TRUE)
    }
    rum.fd.bact.CHOA1.rate <<- rum.fd.DCHOA1.rate * rum.fd.bact.CHOA1Y
    rum.fd.bact.CHOA2.rate <<- rum.fd.DCHOA2.rate * rum.fd.bact.CHOA2Y
    rum.fd.bact.CHOA3.rate <<- rum.fd.DCHOA3.rate * rum.fd.bact.CHOA3Y
    rum.fd.bact.CHOA4.rate <<- rum.fd.DCHOA4.rate * rum.fd.bact.CHOA4Y
    rum.fd.bact.CHOB1.rate <<- rum.fd.DCHOB1.rate * rum.fd.bact.CHOB1Y
    rum.fd.bact.CHOB2.rate <<- rum.fd.DCHOB2.rate * rum.fd.bact.CHOB2Y
    rum.fd.bact.CHOB3.rate <<- rum.fd.DCHOB3.rate * rum.fd.bact.CHOB3Y
    rum.diet.bact.CHOA1.rate <<- sum(rum.fd.bact.CHOA1.rate)
    rum.diet.bact.CHOA2.rate <<- sum(rum.fd.bact.CHOA2.rate)
    rum.diet.bact.CHOA3.rate <<- sum(rum.fd.bact.CHOA3.rate)
    rum.diet.bact.CHOA4.rate <<- sum(rum.fd.bact.CHOA4.rate)
    rum.diet.bact.CHOB1.rate <<- sum(rum.fd.bact.CHOB1.rate)
    rum.diet.bact.CHOB2.rate <<- sum(rum.fd.bact.CHOB2.rate)
    rum.diet.bact.CHOB3.rate <<- sum(rum.fd.bact.CHOB3.rate)
    rum.fd.bact.NFC.rate <<- rum.fd.bact.CHOA1.rate + rum.fd.bact.CHOA2.rate + rum.fd.bact.CHOA3.rate + rum.fd.bact.CHOA4.rate + rum.fd.bact.CHOB1.rate + rum.fd.bact.CHOB2.rate
    rum.fd.bact.FC.rate <<- rum.fd.bact.CHOB3.rate
    rum.diet.bact.NFC.rate <<- sum(rum.fd.bact.NFC.rate)
    rum.diet.bact.FC.rate <<- sum(rum.fd.bact.FC.rate)
    if (genRPT)
    {
      rptEnergyAllowableBact <- fds["FeedName.x"]
      names(rptEnergyAllowableBact) <- "FeedName"
      rptEnergyAllowableBact["CHO A1"] <- rum.fd.bact.CHOA1.rate
      rptEnergyAllowableBact["CHO A2"] <- rum.fd.bact.CHOA2.rate
      rptEnergyAllowableBact["CHO A3"] <- rum.fd.bact.CHOA3.rate
      rptEnergyAllowableBact["CHO A4"] <- rum.fd.bact.CHOA4.rate
      rptEnergyAllowableBact["CHO B1"] <- rum.fd.bact.CHOB1.rate
      rptEnergyAllowableBact["CHO B2"] <- rum.fd.bact.CHOB2.rate
      rptEnergyAllowableBact["CHO B3"] <- rum.fd.bact.CHOB3.rate
      rptEnergyAllowableBact["NFC"] <- rum.fd.bact.NFC.rate
      rptEnergyAllowableBact["FC"] <- rum.fd.bact.FC.rate
      rptEnergyAllowableBact["NFC+FC"] <- rum.fd.bact.NFC.rate + rum.fd.bact.FC.rate
```

```
    report(rptEnergyAllowableBact, "Energy-Allowable Bacterial Dry Matter, g/d", "", "", 3, 3, 1000, 7, TRUE, FALSE, FALSE, FALSE, FALSE, FALSE, TRUE)
  }
  # ++++++++++++++++++++++++
  # Peptide uptake submodel
  # ++++++++++++++++++++++++
  rum.bact.PepUptake.rate <<- calcPeptideUptake(flag_peptide, Parm_rum.bact.PepUp, rum.kp_forage.fracprate, rum.kp_liquid.fracprate, rum.diet.bact.NFC.rate, rum.diet.DPep.rate, anim.diet.Concentrate.frac)
  # Adjust Ruminally Degraded Protein
  rum.fd.DProtB1_Unadj.rate <<- rum.fd.DProtB1.rate
  rum.fd.DProtB2_Unadj.rate <<- rum.fd.DProtB2.rate
  rum.fd.DProtB3_Unadj.rate <<- rum.fd.DProtB3.rate
  rum.fd.DPep_Unadj.rate <<- rum.fd.DPep.rate
  rum.fd.RDP_Unadj.rate <<- rum.fd.DProt_Unadj.rate <<- rum.fd.RDP.rate
  rum.diet.DProtB1_Unadj.rate <<- sum(rum.fd.DProtB1.rate)
  rum.diet.DProtB2_Unadj.rate <<- sum(rum.fd.DProtB2.rate)
  rum.diet.DProtB3_Unadj.rate <<- sum(rum.fd.DProtB3.rate)
  rum.diet.DPep_Unadj.rate <<- sum(rum.fd.DPep.rate)
  rum.diet.RDP_Unadj.rate <<- rum.diet.DProt_Unadj.rate <<- sum(rum.fd.RDP.rate)
  rum.fd.DProtB1.rate <<- (rum.fd.DProtB1.rate/rum.diet.DPep.rate) * rum.bact.PepUptake.rate
  rum.fd.DProtB2.rate <<- (rum.fd.DProtB2.rate/rum.diet.DPep.rate) * rum.bact.PepUptake.rate
  rum.fd.DProtB3.rate <<- (rum.fd.DProtB3.rate/rum.diet.DPep.rate) * rum.bact.PepUptake.rate
  rum.fd.DPep.rate <<- rum.fd.DProtB1.rate + rum.fd.DProtB2.rate + rum.fd.DProtB3.rate
  rum.fd.RDP.rate <<- rum.fd.DProt.rate <<- rum.fd.DProtA.rate + rum.fd.DPep.rate
  rum.diet.DProtB1.rate <<- sum(rum.fd.DProtB1.rate)
  rum.diet.DProtB2.rate <<- sum(rum.fd.DProtB2.rate)
  rum.diet.DProtB3.rate <<- sum(rum.fd.DProtB3.rate)
  rum.diet.DPep.rate <<- sum(rum.fd.DPep.rate)
  rum.diet.RDP.rate <<- rum.diet.DProt.rate <<- sum(rum.fd.RDP.rate)
  if (genRPT)
  {
    title <- "Peptide Uptake Submodel"
    cat(paste("#Title#", title, "\n", string("=", nchar(title)), "\n\n", sep = ""))
    cat(paste("Unadjusted Ruminally degraded protein (peptide and AA), g/d : ", formatC(rum.diet.DPep_Unadj.rate * 1000, format = "f", digits = 3, width = 7), "\n", sep = ""))
    cat(paste("Peptide uptake rate by NFC bacteria, g/d                    : ", formatC(rum.bact.PepUptake.rate * 1000, format = "f", digits = 3, width = 7), "\n", sep = ""))
    cat(paste("Peptide escape from rumen, g/d                              : ", formatC((rum.diet.DPep_Unadj.rate - rum.bact.PepUptake.rate) * 1000, format = "f", digits = 3, width = 7), "\n", sep = ""))
    cat(paste("Adjusted Ruminally degraded protein (peptide and AA), g/d   : ", formatC(rum.diet.DPep.rate * 1000, format = "f", digits = 3, width = 7), "\n", sep = ""))
    cat(paste("Fractional liquid passage rate, 1/h                         : ", formatC(rum.kp_liquid.fracprate, format = "f", digits = 3, width = 7), "\n", sep = ""))
    cat(paste("Peptide in the rumen, g                                     : ", formatC(isz((rum.diet.DPep_Unadj.rate - rum.bact.PepUptake.rate) * 1000, (rum.kp_liquid.fracprate/100)), format = "f", digits = 3, width = 7), "\n", sep = ""))
    if (flag_peptide == 0) cat("\nAlgorithm for peptide uptake rate: CNCPS v. 5; Fox et al. (2004)")
    if (flag_peptide == 1) cat("\nAlgorithm for peptide uptake rate: RNS v. 1.0")
    cat("\n\n\n")
    rptRDProt_DMI <- fds["FeedName.x"]
    names(rptRDProt_DMI) <- "FeedName"
    rptRDProt_DMI["Prot A"] <- rum.fd.DProtA.rate
```

```
    rptRDProt_DMI["Prot B1"] <- rum.fd.DProtB1.rate
    rptRDProt_DMI["Prot B2"] <- rum.fd.DProtB2.rate
    rptRDProt_DMI["Prot B3"] <- rum.fd.DProtB3.rate
    report(rptRDProt_DMI, "Ruminally Degraded Protein Intake (Revised), g/d", "", "", 3, 3, 1000, 8, TRUE, FALSE, TRUE, FALSE,
TRUE, FALSE, FALSE)
    rptRDProt_DMI <- fds["FeedName.x"]
    names(rptRDProt_DMI) <- "FeedName"
    rptRDProt_DMI["ProtB1 kd"] <- rum.fd.ProtB1_kd.fracprate
    rptRDProt_DMI["Eff. B1 kd"] <- ifelse((rum.fd.DProtB1.rate - anim.fd.ProtB1.rate) != 0, -rum.fd.DProtB1.rate *
rum.fd.ProtB1_kp.fracprate/(rum.fd.DProtB1.rate - anim.fd.ProtB1.rate), rum.fd.ProtB1_kd.fracprate)
    rptRDProt_DMI["ProtB2 kd"] <- rum.fd.ProtB2_kd.fracprate
    rptRDProt_DMI["Eff. B2 kd"] <- ifelse((rum.fd.DProtB2.rate - anim.fd.ProtB2.rate) != 0, -rum.fd.DProtB2.rate *
rum.fd.ProtB2_kp.fracprate/(rum.fd.DProtB2.rate - anim.fd.ProtB2.rate), rum.fd.ProtB2_kd.fracprate)
    rptRDProt_DMI["ProtB3 kd"] <- rum.fd.ProtB3_kd.fracprate
    rptRDProt_DMI["Eff. B3 kd"] <- ifelse((rum.fd.DProtB3.rate - anim.fd.ProtB3.rate) != 0, -rum.fd.DProtB3.rate *
rum.fd.ProtB3_kp.fracprate/(rum.fd.DProtB3.rate - anim.fd.ProtB3.rate), rum.fd.ProtB3_kd.fracprate)
    footnote <- "RDP adjusted for effective peptide uptake"
    report(rptRDProt_DMI, "\nEffective Fractional Rate of Degradation", "", footnote, 3, 3, 1, 8, FALSE, FALSE, FALSE, FALSE,
TRUE, FALSE, TRUE)
  }
  # ++++++++++++++++++++++++++++++++++
  # Rumen nitrogen balance submodel
  # ++++++++++++++++++++++++++++++++++
  # NFC Bacteria
  rum.bact.AminoN_Uptake.rate <<- rum.bact.PepUptake.rate/6.25
  rum.fd.bact.NFC_AminoN.rate <<- rum.fd.bact.NFC.rate * (2/3) * (Parm_rum.bact.CP/100)/6.25
  rum.diet.bact.NFC_AminoN.rate <<- sum(rum.fd.bact.NFC_AminoN.rate)
  rum.fd.bact.NFC_AmmoniaN.rate <<- rum.fd.bact.NFC.rate * (1/3) * (Parm_rum.bact.CP/100)/6.25
  rum.diet.bact.NFC_AmmoniaN.rate <<- sum(rum.fd.bact.NFC_AmmoniaN.rate)
  rum.AminoN_balance.rate <<- rum.bact.AminoN_Uptake.rate - rum.diet.bact.NFC_AminoN.rate
  if (rum.AminoN_balance.rate > 0)
  {
    # NFC Bacteria will convert excess of peptide into ammonia
    # 1 g amino N will yield 1 g of ammonia N
    rum.diet.bact.NFC_SurplusN.rate <<- rum.AminoN_balance.rate
  } else
  {
    rum.diet.bact.NFC_SurplusN.rate <<- 0
  }
  rum.diet.Ammonia.rate <<- rum.diet.DProtA.rate/6.25
  # Recycled N, kg/d
  anim.diet.CP.conc <<- anim.diet.CP.rate * 100/anim.diet.DMI.rate
  # anim.diet.DMI.rate * (1.9472 * anim.diet.CP.conc - 0.19216 * anim.diet.CP.conc^2 + 0.005176 * anim.diet.CP.conc^3), g/d
  if (flag_RecycledN == 0) rum.Recycled_N.rate <<- max(0, ((121.7 - 12.01 * anim.diet.CP.conc + 0.3235 *
anim.diet.CP.conc^2)/100) * (anim.diet.CP.rate/6.25))
  if (flag_RecycledN == 1) rum.Recycled_N.rate <<- max(0, (-0.1113 + 0.966 * exp(-0.0616 * anim.diet.CP.conc)) * (1.192 *
anim.diet.CP.conc * anim.diet.DMI.rate - 11.98)/1000)
  # plot(seq(1,20,1),(121.7-12.01*seq(1,20,1)+0.3235*seq(1,20,1)^2)/100) NRC (1985)
  # FC Bacteria
  rum.AmmoniaN.rate <<- (rum.diet.bact.NFC_SurplusN.rate + rum.diet.Ammonia.rate + rum.Recycled_N.rate) -
rum.diet.bact.NFC_AmmoniaN.rate
```

```
rum.fd.bact.FC_AmmoniaN.rate <<- rum.fd.bact.FC.rate * (Parm_rum.bact.CP/100)/6.25
rum.diet.bact.FC_AmmoniaN.rate <<- sum(rum.fd.bact.FC_AmmoniaN.rate)
rum.N_balance.rate <<- (rum.bact.AminoN_Uptake.rate + rum.diet.Ammonia.rate + rum.Recycled_N.rate) - (rum.diet.bact.NFC_AminoN.rate + rum.diet.bact.NFC_AmmoniaN.rate + rum.diet.bact.FC_AmmoniaN.rate)
if (genRPT)
{
  title <- "Ruminal Bacteria Amino-N and Ammonia-N Balances"
  cat(paste("#Title#", title, "\n", string("=", 47), "\n\n", sep = ""))
  if (rum.AmmoniaN.rate < 0)
  {
    cat("!!Attention: Ruminal ammonia-N available for FC bacteria is negative. Not enough ruminal ammonia-N for FC bacteria growth\n\n")
  }

  cat(paste(string("=", 102), "\n", sep=""))
  cat("Items                        Amino-N, g/d                Ammonia-N, g/d\n")
  cat("                     --------------------------  --------------------------------------------\n")
  cat("                      Supply                                  Supply\n")
  cat("                     --------                   --------------------------\n")
  cat("                        Diet       Reqt.  Balance    Diet    Recycled Ammino-N  Reqt.   Balance   Total\n")
  cat("-------------------- -------- -------- -------- -------- -------- -------- -------- -------- --------\n")
  cat(paste("Nonfiber bacteria    ", " ",
            formatC(rum.bact.AminoN_Uptake.rate * 1000, format = "f", digits = 3, width = 8), " ",
            formatC(rum.diet.bact.NFC_AminoN.rate * 1000, format = "f", digits = 3, width = 8), " ",
            formatC(rum.AminoN_balance.rate * 1000, format = "f", digits = 3, width = 8), " ",
            formatC(rum.diet.Ammonia.rate * 1000, format = "f", digits = 3, width = 8), " ",
            formatC(rum.Recycled_N.rate * 1000, format = "f", digits = 3, width = 8), " ",
            formatC(rum.diet.bact.NFC_SurplusN.rate * 1000, format = "f", digits = 3, width = 8), " ",
            formatC(rum.diet.bact.NFC_AmmoniaN.rate * 1000, format = "f", digits = 3, width = 8), " ",
            formatC(rum.AmmoniaN.rate * 1000, format = "f", digits = 3, width = 8), "\n", sep=""))
  cat(paste("Fiber bacteria       ", " ", string(" ", 27),
            formatC(rum.AmmoniaN.rate * 1000, format = "f", digits = 3, width = 8), " ", string(" ", 18),
            formatC(rum.diet.bact.FC_AmmoniaN.rate * 1000, format = "f", digits = 3, width = 8), " ",
            formatC(rum.N_balance.rate * 1000, format = "f", digits = 3, width = 8), "\n", sep = ""))
  cat(paste(string("=", 102), "\n", sep=""))
  cat(paste("Supply               ", " ",
            formatC(rum.bact.AminoN_Uptake.rate * 1000, format = "f", digits = 3, width = 8), " ", string(" ", 18),
            formatC(rum.diet.Ammonia.rate * 1000, format = "f", digits = 3, width = 8), " ",
            formatC(rum.Recycled_N.rate * 1000, format = "f", digits = 3, width = 8), " ", string(" ", 27),
            formatC((rum.bact.AminoN_Uptake.rate + rum.diet.Ammonia.rate + rum.Recycled_N.rate) * 1000, format = "f", digits = 3, width = 8), "\n", sep = ""))
  cat(paste("Requirement (Reqt.) ", " ", string(" ", 9),
            formatC(rum.diet.bact.NFC_AminoN.rate * 1000, format = "f", digits = 3, width = 8), " ", string(" ", 36),
            formatC((rum.diet.bact.NFC_AmmoniaN.rate + rum.diet.bact.FC_AmmoniaN.rate) * 1000, format = "f", digits = 3, width = 8), " ", string(" ", 9),
            formatC((rum.diet.bact.NFC_AminoN.rate + rum.diet.bact.NFC_AmmoniaN.rate + rum.diet.bact.FC_AmmoniaN.rate) * 1000, format = "f", digits = 3, width = 8), "\n", sep = ""))
  cat(paste("Balance              ", " ", string(" ", 8*9), formatC(rum.N_balance.rate * 1000, format = "f", digits = 3, width = 8), "\n", sep = ""))
  cat(paste(string("=", 102), "\n", sep=""))
  cat("\n")
```

```
    cat(paste("Amino-N Balance, g/d            : ", formatC(rum.AminoN_balance.rate * 1000, format = "f", digits = 3, width =
8), string(" ", 11),
              "Ruminal N Balance (RNB), g/d    : ", formatC(rum.N_balance.rate * 1000, format = "f", digits = 3, width = 8),
"\n", sep = ""))
    cat(paste("   Amino-N, % req               : ", formatC(100 + rum.AminoN_balance.rate * 100/rum.diet.bact.NFC_AminoN.rate,
format = "f", digits = 3, width = 8),  string(" ", 11),
              "   Ruminal N, % req             : ", formatC(100 + rum.N_balance.rate * 100/(rum.diet.bact.NFC_AminoN.rate +
rum.diet.bact.NFC_AmmoniaN.rate + rum.diet.bact.FC_AmmoniaN.rate), format = "f", digits = 3, width = 8), "\n", sep = ""))

    # Ammonia-N Concentration
    Vr <- rum.volume/1000 # m^3
    kl <- rum.kp_liquid.fracprate*24 # %/d
    NH3mM <- rum.N_balance.rate*1000/((kl/100)*Vr*14) # mM
    RNB.ideal <- 3.6 * ((kl/100)*Vr*14) # g/d
    cat("\n")
    cat(paste("Ruminal Ammonia-N (NH3) Concentration", string(" ", 13), "Efficiency of N use, %\n"))
    cat(paste("   Ruminal volume, m^3          : ", formatC(Vr, format = "f", digits = 3, width = 8), string(" ", 11),
              "   Efficiency of amino-N use    : ", formatC(isz(rum.diet.bact.NFC_AminoN.rate * 100, rum.bact.AminoN_Up-
take.rate), format = "f", digits = 3, width = 8), "\n", sep = ""))
    cat(paste("   Liquid passage rate, %/d     : ", formatC(kl, format = "f", digits = 3, width = 8), string(" ", 11),
              "   Efficiency of ammonia-N use : ", formatC(isz((rum.diet.bact.NFC_AmmoniaN.rate + rum.diet.bact.FC_Ammo-
niaN.rate) * 100, (rum.diet.Ammonia.rate + rum.Recycled_N.rate + rum.AminoN_balance.rate)), format = "f", digits = 3, width =
8), "\n", sep = ""))
    cat(paste("   Ruminal ammonia-N, mM        : ", formatC(NH3mM, format = "f", digits = 3, width = 8), string(" ", 11),
              "   Efficiency of N use          : ", formatC(isz(((rum.diet.bact.NFC_AminoN.rate + rum.diet.bact.NFC_Ammo-
niaN.rate + rum.diet.bact.FC_AmmoniaN.rate)) * 100, (rum.bact.AminoN_Uptake.rate + rum.diet.Ammonia.rate + rum.Recy-
cled_N.rate)), format = "f", digits = 3, width = 8), "\n", sep = ""))
    cat(paste("   Ideal RNB, g/d (3.6 mM NH3) : ", formatC(RNB.ideal, format = "f", digits = 3, width = 8), "\n", sep = ""))
    newpage()
  }

  # ++++++++++++++++++++++++++++++++++++++++
  # Ruminal N Balance Allowable Bacteria
  # ++++++++++++++++++++++++++++++++++++++++
  # EAFCB = Energy Allowable FC Bacteria
  # EANFCB = Energy Allowable NFC Bacteria
  # EAB = Energy Allowable Bacteria
  # NAB = Nitrogen Allowable Bacteria
  # NABR = Bacteria Reduction due to Nitrogen Allowable Bacteria
  # NAFCBR = FC Bacteria Reduction due to Nitrogen Allowable Bacteria
  # NANFCBR = NFC Bacteria Reduction due to Nitrogen Allowable Bacteria
  # NAFCB = Nitrogen Allowable FC Bacteria
  # NANFCB = Nitrogen Allowable NFC Bacteria
  # DCHOB3 = Energy Allowable Ruminally Degraded CHO B3
  # NADCHOB3R = Degraded CHO B3 Reduction due to Nitrogen Allowable Bacteria
  # NADCHOB3 = Nitrogen Allowable Ruminally Degraded CHO B3
  rum.fd.EAFCB.rate <<- rum.fd.bact.FC.rate
  rum.fd.EANFCB.rate <<- rum.fd.bact.NFC.rate
  # Protein basis
```

```
rum.diet.NAB.rate <<- ((rum.bact.AminoN_Uptake.rate + rum.diet.Ammonia.rate + rum.Recycled_N.rate)/(Parm_rum.bact.CP/100)) * 6.25
rum.fd.EAB.frac <<- (rum.fd.EAFCB.rate + rum.fd.EANFCB.rate)/(rum.diet.bact.FC.rate + rum.diet.bact.NFC.rate)
rum.fd.NAB.rate <<- rum.fd.EAB.frac * rum.diet.NAB.rate
rum.fd.NABR.rate <<- pmax(0, (rum.fd.EAFCB.rate + rum.fd.EANFCB.rate) - rum.fd.NAB.rate)
rum.fd.EAFCB.frac <<- ifelse((rum.fd.EAFCB.rate + rum.fd.EANFCB.rate) > 0, rum.fd.EAFCB.rate/(rum.fd.EAFCB.rate + rum.fd.EANFCB.rate), 0)
rum.fd.NAFCBR.rate <<- rum.fd.EAFCB.frac * rum.fd.NABR.rate
rum.fd.NANFCBR.rate <<- (1 - rum.fd.EAFCB.frac) * rum.fd.NABR.rate
rum.fd.NANFCB.rate <<- rum.fd.EANFCB.rate - rum.fd.NANFCBR.rate
rum.fd.NAFCB.rate <<- rum.fd.EAFCB.rate - rum.fd.NAFCBR.rate
rum.diet.NANFCB.rate <<- sum(rum.fd.NANFCB.rate)
rum.diet.NAFCB.rate <<- sum(rum.fd.NAFCB.rate)
# CHOB3 Reduction due to reduced FC bacteria growth if ruminal N is limiting
rum.fd.NADCHOB3R.rate <<- ifelse(rum.fd.bact.CHOB3Y > 0, rum.fd.NAFCBR.rate/rum.fd.bact.CHOB3Y, 0)
rum.fd.NADCHOB3.rate <<- pmax(0, rum.fd.DCHOB3.rate - rum.fd.NADCHOB3R.rate)
rum.diet.NADCHOB3.rate <<- sum(rum.fd.NADCHOB3.rate)
# +++++++++++++++++++++++++++++++++++++++++++++++++++++++++++++++
# Ruminal Branched-Chain Amino Acid Balance Allowable Bacteria
# +++++++++++++++++++++++++++++++++++++++++++++++++++++++++++++++
# BCAAAB = BCAA Allowable Bacteria
# BCAABR = Bacteria Reduction due to Ruminal BCAA Deficiency
# BCAAFCBR = FC Bacteria Reduction
# BCAANFCBR = NFC Bacteria Reduction
# BCAAAFCB = BCAA Allowable FC Bacteria
# BCAAANFCB = BCAA Allowable NFC Bacteria
# BCAAADCHOB3 = Ruminally degraded CHO B3 Reduction due to BCAA Deficiency
# Concentration of bacteria BCAA is computed assuming 75% from non-cell wall and 25% from cell wall
rum.bact.Leu.frac <<- (rum.bact.NCW_Leu.conc * (1 - flag_BCAA_CWc) + rum.bact.CW_Leu.conc * flag_BCAA_CWc)/100
rum.bact.Ile.frac <<- (rum.bact.NCW_Ile.conc * (1 - flag_BCAA_CWc) + rum.bact.CW_Ile.conc * flag_BCAA_CWc)/100
rum.bact.Val.frac <<- (rum.bact.NCW_Val.conc * (1 - flag_BCAA_CWc) + rum.bact.CW_Ile.conc * flag_BCAA_CWc)/100
# Bacteria BCAA requirement
NFCB_BCAA_Req <- flag_BCAA_NFC
FCB_BCAA_Req <- flag_BCAA_FC
rum.diet.bact.Leu.rate <<- (NFCB_BCAA_Req * rum.diet.NANFCB.rate + FCB_BCAA_Req * rum.diet.NAFCB.rate) * (Parm_rum.bact.CP/100) * (Parm_rum.bact.TP_CP/100) * rum.bact.Leu.frac
rum.diet.bact.Ile.rate <<- (NFCB_BCAA_Req * rum.diet.NANFCB.rate + FCB_BCAA_Req * rum.diet.NAFCB.rate) * (Parm_rum.bact.CP/100) * (Parm_rum.bact.TP_CP/100) * rum.bact.Ile.frac
rum.diet.bact.Val.rate <<- (NFCB_BCAA_Req * rum.diet.NANFCB.rate + FCB_BCAA_Req * rum.diet.NAFCB.rate) * (Parm_rum.bact.CP/100) * (Parm_rum.bact.TP_CP/100) * rum.bact.Val.frac
# Supply of BCAA from the bacteria predated by the protozoa
rum.bact.BCAAUse.frac <<- flag_BCAA_Eff
ProtozoaPredation <- flag_BCAA_BPP
rum.bact.Recycled.rate <<- (((rum.diet.NANFCB.rate + rum.diet.NAFCB.rate)/(1-ProtozoaPredation)) * ProtozoaPredation) * rum.bact.BCAAUse.frac
rum.diet.protozoa.Leu.rate <<- rum.bact.Recycled.rate * (Parm_rum.bact.CP/100) * (Parm_rum.bact.TP_CP/100) * rum.bact.Leu.frac
rum.diet.protozoa.Ile.rate <<- rum.bact.Recycled.rate * (Parm_rum.bact.CP/100) * (Parm_rum.bact.TP_CP/100) * rum.bact.Ile.frac
rum.diet.protozoa.Val.rate <<- rum.bact.Recycled.rate * (Parm_rum.bact.CP/100) * (Parm_rum.bact.TP_CP/100) * rum.bact.Val.frac
```

```
    # Ration Supply of BCAA
    anim.fd.Leu_CP.frac <<- anim.fd.Leu_CP.conc/100
    anim.fd.Ile_CP.frac <<- anim.fd.Ile_CP.conc/100
    anim.fd.Val_CP.frac <<- anim.fd.Val_CP.conc/100
    if (flag_BCAAProtA == TRUE)
    {
      rum.fd.BCAAUptake.rate <<- (rum.fd.DProtA.rate + rum.fd.DProtB1.rate + rum.fd.DProtB2.rate + rum.fd.DProtB3.rate) * rum.bact.BCAAUse.frac
    } else
    {
      rum.fd.BCAAUptake.rate <<- (rum.fd.DProtB1.rate + rum.fd.DProtB2.rate + rum.fd.DProtB3.rate) * rum.bact.BCAAUse.frac
    }
    rum.fd.DLeu.rate <<- rum.fd.BCAAUptake.rate * anim.fd.Leu_CP.frac
    rum.fd.DIle.rate <<- rum.fd.BCAAUptake.rate * anim.fd.Ile_CP.frac
    rum.fd.DVal.rate <<- rum.fd.BCAAUptake.rate * anim.fd.Val_CP.frac
    rum.diet.DLeu.rate <<- sum(rum.fd.DLeu.rate)
    rum.diet.DIle.rate <<- sum(rum.fd.DIle.rate)
    rum.diet.DVal.rate <<- sum(rum.fd.DVal.rate)
    rum.diet.BCAA_Leu.rate <<- rum.diet.DLeu.rate + rum.diet.protozoa.Leu.rate - rum.diet.bact.Leu.rate
    rum.diet.BCAA_Ile.rate <<- rum.diet.DIle.rate + rum.diet.protozoa.Ile.rate - rum.diet.bact.Ile.rate
    rum.diet.BCAA_Val.rate <<- rum.diet.DVal.rate + rum.diet.protozoa.Val.rate - rum.diet.bact.Val.rate

    # First limiting BCAA as a % of requirement
    rum.BCAA_1stLim <<- which.min(c(rum.diet.BCAA_Leu.rate, rum.diet.BCAA_Ile.rate, rum.diet.BCAA_Val.rate)/c(rum.diet.bact.Leu.rate,rum.diet.bact.Ile.rate,rum.diet.bact.Val.rate))
    # First limiting BCAA as daily amounts
    #rum.BCAA_1stLim <<- which.min(c(rum.diet.BCAA_Leu.rate, rum.diet.BCAA_Ile.rate, rum.diet.BCAA_Val.rate))
    rum.BCAA_balance.rate <<- c(rum.diet.BCAA_Leu.rate, rum.diet.BCAA_Ile.rate, rum.diet.BCAA_Val.rate)[rum.BCAA_1stLim]

    # Because the impact of BCAA deficiency if negligible on NFC bacteria, the adjustment is performed on FC bacteria
    # BCAA Allowable is computed when: rum.diet.bact.Leu.rate=rum.diet.DLeu.rate+rum.diet.protozoa.Leu.rate
    if (rum.BCAA_1stLim == 1)
    {
      # Leucine
      rum.diet.BCAAAFCB.rate <<- (rum.diet.DLeu.rate + rum.diet.protozoa.Leu.rate)/((Parm_rum.bact.CP/100) * (Parm_rum.bact.TP_CP/100) * rum.bact.Leu.frac)
    }
    if (rum.BCAA_1stLim == 2)
    {
      # Isoleucine
      rum.diet.BCAAAFCB.rate <<- (rum.diet.DIle.rate + rum.diet.protozoa.Ile.rate)/((Parm_rum.bact.CP/100) * (Parm_rum.bact.TP_CP/100) * rum.bact.Ile.frac)
    }
    if (rum.BCAA_1stLim == 3)
    {
      # Valine
      rum.diet.BCAAAFCB.rate <<- (rum.diet.DVal.rate + rum.diet.protozoa.Val.rate)/((Parm_rum.bact.CP/100) * (Parm_rum.bact.TP_CP/100) * rum.bact.Val.frac)
    }
    if (flag_NandBCAA == 1 | flag_NandBCAA == 3)
    {
```

```
    # Adjust for N or N and BCAA deficiencies
    rum.diet.BCAAAB.rate <<- min(rum.diet.BCAAAFCB.rate, rum.diet.bact.FC.rate, rum.diet.NAFCB.rate) +
min(rum.diet.bact.NFC.rate, rum.diet.NANFCB.rate)
  } else
  {
    # Adjust for BCAA deficiencies only
    rum.diet.BCAAAB.rate <<- min(rum.diet.BCAAAFCB.rate, rum.diet.bact.FC.rate) + rum.diet.bact.NFC.rate
  }
  rum.fd.BCAAAB.rate <<- rum.fd.EAB.frac * rum.diet.BCAAAB.rate
  if (flag_NandBCAA == 1 | flag_NandBCAA == 3)
  {
    # Adjust for N or N and BCAA deficiencies
    # Firstly, assume the reduction of bacteria occurs on FC bacteria only
    rum.fd.BCAAABR.rate <<- pmax(0, pmin(rum.fd.bact.NFC.rate, rum.fd.NANFCB.rate) + pmin(rum.fd.bact.FC.rate,
rum.fd.NAFCB.rate) - rum.fd.BCAAAB.rate)
    rum.fd.BCAAAFCB.rate <<- pmax(0, pmin(rum.fd.bact.FC.rate, rum.fd.NAFCB.rate) - rum.fd.BCAAABR.rate)
    # Secondly, if the FC reduction does not account for all the bacteria reduction, then NFC is discounted
    rum.fd.BCAAANFCB.rate <<- ifelse((pmin(rum.fd.bact.FC.rate, rum.fd.NAFCB.rate) - rum.fd.BCAAABR.rate) < 0, pmax(0,
pmin(rum.fd.bact.NFC.rate, rum.fd.NANFCB.rate) + (pmin(rum.fd.bact.FC.rate, rum.fd.NAFCB.rate) - rum.fd.BCAAABR.rate)),
pmin(rum.fd.bact.NFC.rate, rum.fd.NANFCB.rate))
    rum.fd.BCAAAFCBR.rate <<- pmax(0, pmin(rum.fd.bact.FC.rate, rum.fd.NAFCB.rate) - rum.fd.BCAAAFCB.rate)
    rum.fd.BCAAANFCBR.rate <<- pmax(0, pmin(rum.fd.bact.NFC.rate, rum.fd.NANFCB.rate) - rum.fd.BCAAANFCB.rate)
  } else
  {
    # Adjust for BCAA deficiencies only
    # Firstly, assume the reduction of bacteria occurs on FC bacteria only
    rum.fd.BCAAABR.rate <<- pmax(0, rum.fd.bact.NFC.rate + rum.fd.bact.FC.rate - rum.fd.BCAAAB.rate)
    rum.fd.BCAAAFCB.rate <<- pmax(0, rum.fd.bact.FC.rate - rum.fd.BCAAABR.rate)
    # Secondly, if the FC reduction does not account for all the bacteria reduction, then NFC is discounted
    rum.fd.BCAAANFCB.rate <<- ifelse((rum.fd.bact.FC.rate - rum.fd.BCAAABR.rate) < 0, pmax(0, rum.fd.bact.NFC.rate +
(rum.fd.bact.FC.rate - rum.fd.BCAAABR.rate)), rum.fd.bact.NFC.rate)
    rum.fd.BCAAAFCBR.rate <<- pmax(0, rum.fd.bact.FC.rate - rum.fd.BCAAAFCB.rate)
    rum.fd.BCAAANFCBR.rate <<- pmax(0, rum.fd.bact.NFC.rate - rum.fd.BCAAANFCB.rate)
  }
  rum.diet.BCAAANFCB.rate <<- sum(rum.fd.BCAAANFCB.rate)
  rum.diet.BCAAAFCB.rate <<- sum(rum.fd.BCAAAFCB.rate)
  # CHOB3 Reduction due to reduced FC bacteria growth of BCAA N is limiting
  # Assume energy spilling for NFC bacteria
  rum.fd.BCAAADCHOB3R.rate <<- ifelse(rum.fd.bact.CHOB3Y > 0, rum.fd.BCAAAFCBR.rate/rum.fd.bact.CHOB3Y, 0)
  if (flag_NandBCAA == 1 | flag_NandBCAA == 3)
  {
    # Use N allowable bacteria for N or N and BCAA adjustments
    rum.fd.BCAAADCHOB3.rate <<- pmax(0, pmin(rum.fd.DCHOB3.rate, rum.fd.NADCHOB3.rate) - rum.fd.BCAAADCHOB3R.rate)
  } else
  {
    rum.fd.BCAAADCHOB3.rate <<- pmax(0, rum.fd.DCHOB3.rate - rum.fd.BCAAADCHOB3R.rate)
  }
  rum.diet.BCAAADCHOB3.rate <<- sum(rum.fd.BCAAADCHOB3.rate)
  if (genRPT)
  {
    rptNandBCAA <- fds["FeedName.x"]
```

```
    names(rptNandBCAA) <- "FeedName"
    rptNandBCAA["EAFCB"] <- rum.fd.EAFCB.rate
    rptNandBCAA["EANFCB"] <- rum.fd.EANFCB.rate
    rptNandBCAA["EAB"] <- rum.fd.EAFCB.rate + rum.fd.EANFCB.rate
    rptNandBCAA["EABRatio"] <- rum.fd.EAB.frac
    rptNandBCAA["EAFCBRatio"] <- rum.fd.EAFCB.frac
    rptNandBCAA["NAB"] <- rum.fd.NAB.rate
    rptNandBCAA["NAFCB"] <- rum.fd.NAFCB.rate
    rptNandBCAA["NANFCB"] <- rum.fd.NANFCB.rate
    rptNandBCAA["NAFCBR"] <- rum.fd.NAFCBR.rate
    rptNandBCAA["NANFCBR"] <- rum.fd.NANFCBR.rate
    rptNandBCAA["NABR"] <- rum.fd.NABR.rate
    rptNandBCAA["BCAAAB"] <- rum.fd.BCAAAB.rate
    rptNandBCAA["BCAAAFCB"] <- rum.fd.BCAAAFCB.rate
    rptNandBCAA["BCAAANFCB"] <- rum.fd.BCAAANFCB.rate
    rptNandBCAA["BCAAAFCBR"] <- rum.fd.BCAAAFCBR.rate
    rptNandBCAA["BCAAANFCBR"] <- rum.fd.BCAAANFCBR.rate
    rptNandBCAA["BCAAABR"] <- rum.fd.BCAAABR.rate
    rptNandBCAA["DCHOB3"] <- rum.fd.DCHOB3.rate
    rptNandBCAA["NADCHOB3R"] <- rum.fd.NADCHOB3R.rate
    rptNandBCAA["NADCHOB3"] <- rum.fd.NADCHOB3.rate
    rptNandBCAA["BCAAADCHOB3R"] <- rum.fd.BCAAADCHOB3R.rate
    rptNandBCAA["BCAAADCHOB3"] <- rum.fd.BCAAADCHOB3.rate
    description <- paste("# BCAAAB = BCAA Allowable Bacteria\n",
                         "# BCAAAFCB = BCAA Allowable FC Bacteria\n",
                         "# BCAAANFCB = BCAA Allowable NFC Bacteria\n",
                         "# BCAAAFCBR = FC Bacteria Reduction due to BCAA Deficiency\n",
                         "# BCAAANFCBR = NFC Bacteria Reduction due to BCAA Deficiency\n",
                         "# BCAAABR = Bacteria Reduction due to ruminal BCAA deficiency\n",
                         "# BCAAADCHOB3R = Reduction of Ruminally degraded CHO B3 due to BCAA Deficiency\n",
                         "# BCAAADCHOB3 = BCAA Allowable Ruminally degraded CHO B3\n",
                         "# DCHOB3 = 'Energy Allowable' Ruminally Degraded CHO B3\n",
                         "# EAFCB = Energy Allowable FC Bacteria\n",
                         "# EANFCB = Energy Allowable NFC Bacteria\n",
                         "# EAB = Energy Allowable Bacteria\n",
                         "# EABRatio = Energy Allowable Bacteria Ratio\n",
                         "# EAFCBRatio = Energy Allowable FC Bacteria Ratio\n",
                         "# NAB = Nitrogen Allowable Bacteria\n",
                         "# NAFCB = Nitrogen Allowable FC Bacteria\n",
                         "# NANFCB = Nitrogen Allowable NFC Bacteria\n",
                         "# NAFCBR = FC Bacteria Reduction due to Nitrogen Deficiency\n",
                         "# NANFCBR = NFC Bacteria Reduction due to Nitrogen Deficiency\n",
                         "# NABR = Bacteria Reduction due to ruminal N deficiency\n",
                         "# NADCHOB3R = Reduction of Ruminally Degraded CHO B3 due to Nitrogen Deficiency\n",
                         "# NADCHOB3 = 'Nitrogen Allowable' Ruminally Degraded CHO B3\n\n", sep = "")
    if (rum.N_balance.rate < 0)
    {
      description <- paste(description,
                           "The ration is deficient in Nitrogen\n",
                           "   Amount deficient, g/d     : ", formatC(rum.N_balance.rate * 1000, format = "f", digits = 3, width = 7), "\n",
```

```
                                    "    FC Bacteria reduction, %   : ", formatC(100 - rum.diet.NAFCB.rate * 100/rum.diet.bact.FC.rate, format = "f", digits = 3, width = 7), "\n",
                                    "    NFC Bacteria reduction, % : ", formatC(100 - rum.diet.NANFCB.rate * 100/rum.diet.bact.NFC.rate, format = "f", digits = 3, width = 7), "\n",
                                    "    RDCHO B3 Reduction, %      : ", formatC(100 - rum.diet.NADCHOB3.rate * 100/rum.diet.DCHOB3.rate, format = "f", digits = 3, width = 7), "\n\n", sep = "")
    } else
    {
      description <- paste(description, "The ration is NOT deficient in Nitrogen\n\n")
    }
    if (rum.BCAA_balance.rate < 0)
    {
      if (rum.BCAA_1stLim == 1) temp <- "Leucine"
      if (rum.BCAA_1stLim == 2) temp <- "Isoleucine"
      if (rum.BCAA_1stLim == 3) temp <- "Valine"
      if (flag_NandBCAA == 1 | flag_NandBCAA == 3)
      {
        description <- paste(description, "The ration is deficient in Branched-Chain Amino Acids\n")
        if (flag_BCAAProtA == TRUE)
        {
          description <- paste(description, "  #The amount of degraded Protein A was added to BCAA uptake\n")
        } else
        {
          description <- paste(description, "  #The amount of degraded Protein A was NOT added to BCAA uptake\n")
        }
        description <- paste(description,
                                    "    Leucine balance, g/d        : ", formatC(rum.diet.BCAA_Leu.rate * 1000, format = "f", digits = 3, width = 7),
                                    " (", formatC(100 + isz(rum.diet.BCAA_Leu.rate * 100, rum.diet.bact.Leu.rate), format = "f", digits = 3, width = 7), "% req)\n",
                                    "    Isoleucine balance, g/d    : ", formatC(rum.diet.BCAA_Ile.rate * 1000, format = "f", digits = 3, width = 7),
                                    " (", formatC(100 + isz(rum.diet.BCAA_Ile.rate * 100, rum.diet.bact.Ile.rate), format = "f", digits = 3, width = 7), "% req)\n",
                                    "    Valine balance, g/d         : ", formatC(rum.diet.BCAA_Val.rate * 1000, format = "f", digits = 3, width = 7),
                                    " (", formatC(100 + isz(rum.diet.BCAA_Val.rate * 100, rum.diet.bact.Val.rate), format = "f", digits = 3, width = 7), "% req)\n\n",
                                    "    The first limiting BCAA     : ", temp, "\n",
                                    "    Amount deficient, g/d       : ", formatC(rum.BCAA_balance.rate * 1000, format = "f", digits = 3, width = 7), "\n",
                                    "    FC Bacteria reduction, %   : ", formatC(100 - rum.diet.BCAAAFCB.rate * 100/min(rum.diet.bact.FC.rate, rum.diet.NAFCB.rate), format = "f", digits = 3, width = 7), "\n",
                                    "    NFC Bacteria reduction, % : ", formatC(100 - rum.diet.BCAAANFCB.rate * 100/min(rum.diet.bact.NFC.rate, rum.diet.NANFCB.rate), format = "f", digits = 3, width = 7), "\n",
                                    "    RDCHO B3 Reduction, %      : ", formatC(100 - rum.diet.BCAAADCHOB3.rate * 100/min(rum.diet.DCHOB3.rate, rum.diet.NADCHOB3.rate), format = "f", digits = 3, width = 7), "\n\n", sep = "")
      } else
      {
        description <- paste(description, "The ration is deficient in Branched-Chain Amino Acids\n")
        if (flag_BCAAProtA == TRUE)
```

```
          {
            description <- paste(description, "  #The amount of degraded Protein A was added to BCAA uptake\n")
          } else
          {
            description <- paste(description, "  #The amount of degraded Protein A was NOT added to BCAA uptake\n")
          }
          description <- paste(description,
                               "    Leucine balance, g/d        : ", formatC(rum.diet.BCAA_Leu.rate * 1000, format = "f", digits = 3, width = 7),
                               " (", formatC(100 + isz(rum.diet.BCAA_Leu.rate * 100, rum.diet.bact.Leu.rate), format = "f", digits = 3, width = 7), "% req)\n",
                               "    Isoleucine balance, g/d     : ", formatC(rum.diet.BCAA_Ile.rate * 1000, format = "f", digits = 3, width = 7),
                               " (", formatC(100 + isz(rum.diet.BCAA_Ile.rate * 100, rum.diet.bact.Ile.rate), format = "f", digits = 3, width = 7), "% req)\n",
                               "    Valine balance, g/d         : ", formatC(rum.diet.BCAA_Val.rate * 1000, format = "f", digits = 3, width = 7),
                               " (", formatC(100 + isz(rum.diet.BCAA_Val.rate * 100, rum.diet.bact.Val.rate), format = "f", digits = 3, width = 7), "% req)\n\n",
                               "    The first limiting BCAA     : ", temp, "\n",
                               "    Amount deficient, g/d       : ", formatC(rum.BCAA_balance.rate * 1000, format = "f", digits = 3, width = 7), "\n",
                               "    FC Bacteria reduction, %    : ", formatC(100 - rum.diet.BCAAAFCB.rate * 100/rum.diet.bact.FC.rate, format = "f", digits = 3, width = 7), "\n",
                               "    NFC Bacteria reduction, %   : ", formatC(100 - rum.diet.BCAAANFCB.rate * 100/rum.diet.bact.NFC.rate, format = "f", digits = 3, width = 7), "\n",
                               "    RDCHO B3 Reduction, %       : ", formatC(100 - rum.diet.BCAAADCHOB3.rate * 100/rum.diet.DCHOB3.rate, format = "f", digits = 3, width = 7), "\n\n", sep = "")
        }
      } else
      {
        description <- paste(description, "The ration is NOT deficient in Branched-Chain Amino Acids\n")
        if (flag_BCAAProtA == TRUE)
        {
          description <- paste(description, "  #The amount of degraded Protein A was added to BCAA uptake\n")
        } else
        {
          description <- paste(description, "  #The amount of degraded Protein A was NOT added to BCAA uptake\n")
        }
      }
      cat(paste("#Title#Ruminal Nitrogen and Branched-Chain Amino Acid (BCAA) Allowable Bacteria Growth, kg/d (Balance)", "\n", string("=", 102), "\n\n", description, "\n", sep = ""))
      newpage()
      description <- ""
      report(rptNandBCAA, "Ruminal Nitrogen and Branched-Chain Amino Acid (BCAA) Allowable Bacteria Growth, kg/d", description, "", 3, 3, 1, 8, TRUE, FALSE, FALSE, FALSE, FALSE, FALSE, TRUE, 3)
      rptBCAA <- fds["FeedName.x"]
      names(rptBCAA) <- "FeedName"
      rptBCAA["Leu, %CP"] <- anim.fd.Leu_CP.conc
      rptBCAA["Ile, %CP"] <- anim.fd.Ile_CP.conc
      rptBCAA["Val, %CP"] <- anim.fd.Val_CP.conc
```

```
    rptBCAA["DLeu,g/d"] <- rum.fd.DLeu.rate
    rptBCAA["DIle,g/d"] <- rum.fd.DIle.rate
    rptBCAA["DVal,g/d"] <- rum.fd.DVal.rate
    rptBCAA_Diet <- data.frame(FeedName = "Ration")
    rptBCAA_Diet["Leu, %CP"] <- ifelse(anim.diet.CP.rate > 0, sum(anim.fd.Leu_CP.conc * anim.fd.CP.rate)/anim.diet.CP.rate, 0)
    rptBCAA_Diet["Ile, %CP"] <- ifelse(anim.diet.CP.rate > 0, sum(anim.fd.Ile_CP.conc * anim.fd.CP.rate)/anim.diet.CP.rate, 0)
    rptBCAA_Diet["Val, %CP"] <- ifelse(anim.diet.CP.rate > 0, sum(anim.fd.Val_CP.conc * anim.fd.CP.rate)/anim.diet.CP.rate, 0)
    rptBCAA_Diet["DLeu,g/d"] <- rum.diet.DLeu.rate
    rptBCAA_Diet["DIle,g/d"] <- rum.diet.DIle.rate
    rptBCAA_Diet["DVal,g/d"] <- rum.diet.DVal.rate
    description <- paste("Efficiency of use of BCAA to BCVFA, %      : ", formatC(flag_BCAA_Eff*100, format = "f", digits = 1, width = 5), " \n",
                         "Bacterial protozoa predation, %            : ", formatC(flag_BCAA_BPP*100, format = "f", digits = 1, width = 5), " \n",
                         "Bacterial cell wall, %                     : ", formatC(flag_BCAA_CWc*100, format = "f", digits = 1, width = 5), " \n",
                         "Bacterial noncell wall, %                  : ", formatC((1 - flag_BCAA_CWc)*100, format = "f", digits = 1, width = 5), " \n",
                         "BCAA synthesis for NFC bacteria, % req     : ", formatC(flag_BCAA_NFC*100, format = "f", digits = 1, width = 5), " \n",
                         "BCAA synthesis for FC bacteria, % req      : ", formatC(flag_BCAA_FC*100, format = "f", digits = 1, width = 5), " \n\n\n",
                         "                                        Leucine   Isoleucine   Valine     Total\n",
                         "                                       ---------- ---------- ---------- ----------\n",
                         "Bacteria BCAA concentration, % DM :    ", formatC(rum.bact.Leu.frac, format = "f", digits = 3, width = 10), " ",
                         formatC(rum.bact.Ile.frac, format = "f", digits = 3, width = 10), " ",
                         formatC(rum.bact.Val.frac, format = "f", digits = 3, width = 10), " \n",
                         "Bacteria BCAA requirement, g/d    :    ", formatC(rum.diet.bact.Leu.rate * 1000, format = "f", digits = 3, width = 10), " ",
                         formatC(rum.diet.bact.Ile.rate * 1000, format = "f", digits = 3, width = 10), " ",
                         formatC(rum.diet.bact.Val.rate * 1000, format = "f", digits = 3, width = 10), " ",
                         formatC((rum.diet.bact.Leu.rate + rum.diet.bact.Ile.rate + rum.diet.bact.Val.rate) * 1000, format = "f", digits = 3, width = 10), " \n",
                         "Protozoa BCAA supply, g/d         :    ", formatC(rum.diet.protozoa.Leu.rate * 1000, format = "f", digits = 3, width = 10), " ",
                         formatC(rum.diet.protozoa.Ile.rate * 1000, format = "f", digits = 3, width = 10), " ",
                         formatC(rum.diet.protozoa.Val.rate * 1000, format = "f", digits = 3, width = 10), " ",
                         formatC((rum.diet.protozoa.Leu.rate + rum.diet.protozoa.Ile.rate + rum.diet.protozoa.Val.rate) * 1000, format = "f", digits = 3, width = 10), " \n",
                         "Diet BCAA supply, g/d             :    ", formatC(rum.diet.DLeu.rate * 1000, format = "f", digits = 3, width = 10), " ",
                         formatC(rum.diet.DIle.rate * 1000, format = "f", digits = 3, width = 10), " ",
                         formatC(rum.diet.DVal.rate * 1000, format = "f", digits = 3, width = 10), " ",
                         formatC((rum.diet.DLeu.rate + rum.diet.DIle.rate + rum.diet.DVal.rate) * 1000, format = "f", digits = 3, width = 10), " \n",
                         "Balance BCAA, g/d                 :    ", formatC(rum.diet.BCAA_Leu.rate * 1000, format = "f", digits = 3, width = 10), " ",
                         formatC(rum.diet.BCAA_Ile.rate * 1000, format = "f", digits = 3, width = 10), " ",
                         formatC(rum.diet.BCAA_Val.rate * 1000, format = "f", digits = 3, width = 10), " ",
```

```
                          formatC((rum.diet.BCAA_Leu.rate + rum.diet.BCAA_Ile.rate + rum.diet.BCAA_Val.rate) * 1000, format = "f", digits = 3, width = 10), " \n",
                          "Balance BCAA, % req                :    ",
                          formatC(100 + isz(rum.diet.BCAA_Leu.rate * 100, rum.diet.bact.Leu.rate), format = "f", digits = 3, width = 10), " ",
                          formatC(100 + isz(rum.diet.BCAA_Ile.rate * 100, rum.diet.bact.Ile.rate), format = "f", digits = 3, width = 10), " ",
                          formatC(100 + isz(rum.diet.BCAA_Val.rate * 100, rum.diet.bact.Val.rate), format = "f", digits = 3, width = 10), " ",
                          formatC(100 + isz((rum.diet.BCAA_Leu.rate + rum.diet.BCAA_Ile.rate + rum.diet.BCAA_Val.rate) * 100, (rum.diet.bact.Leu.rate + rum.diet.bact.Ile.rate + rum.diet.bact.Val.rate)), format = "f", digits = 3, width = 10), " \n", sep = "")
    footnote <- "Concentration of bacteria BCAA is computed assuming the cell wall and noncell wall percentages.\nDLeu, DIle, and DVal are the amounts of BCAA degraded and absorbed by the ruminal bacteria."
    report(rptBCAA, "Branched-Chain Amino Acid (BCAA)", description, footnote, 3, 3, 1, 6, FALSE, FALSE, FALSE, FALSE, FALSE, FALSE, TRUE)
  }
  # Assign the first limiting (Energy, N, BCAA) to FC and NFC bacteria, and ruminally degraded CHO B3
  if (flag_NandBCAA == 1 & rum.N_balance.rate < 0)
  {
    # Use N Deficiency only
    rum.fd.bact.NFC.rate <<- pmin(rum.fd.bact.NFC.rate, rum.fd.NANFCB.rate)
    rum.fd.bact.FC.rate <<- pmin(rum.fd.bact.FC.rate, rum.fd.NAFCB.rate)
    rum.fd.DCHOB3.rate <<- pmin(rum.fd.DCHOB3.rate, rum.fd.NADCHOB3.rate)
  }
  if (flag_NandBCAA == 2 & rum.BCAA_balance.rate < 0)
  {
    # Use BCAA Deficiency only
    rum.fd.bact.NFC.rate <<- pmin(rum.fd.bact.NFC.rate, rum.fd.BCAAANFCB.rate)
    rum.fd.bact.FC.rate <<- pmin(rum.fd.bact.FC.rate, rum.fd.BCAAAFCB.rate)
    rum.fd.DCHOB3.rate <<- pmin(rum.fd.DCHOB3.rate, rum.fd.BCAAADCHOB3.rate)
  }
  if (flag_NandBCAA == 3 & (rum.N_balance.rate < 0 | rum.BCAA_balance.rate < 0))
  {
    # Use N and BCAA Deficiency
    rum.fd.bact.NFC.rate <<- pmin(rum.fd.bact.NFC.rate, rum.fd.NANFCB.rate, rum.fd.BCAAANFCB.rate)
    rum.fd.bact.FC.rate <<- pmin(rum.fd.bact.FC.rate, rum.fd.NAFCB.rate, rum.fd.BCAAAFCB.rate)
    rum.fd.DCHOB3.rate <<- pmin(rum.fd.DCHOB3.rate, rum.fd.NADCHOB3.rate, rum.fd.BCAAADCHOB3.rate)
  }
  rum.fd.DPep.rate <<- rum.fd.DProtB1.rate + rum.fd.DProtB2.rate + rum.fd.DProtB3.rate
  rum.fd.RDP.rate <<- rum.fd.DProt.rate <<- rum.fd.DProtA.rate + rum.fd.DPep.rate
  rum.fd.DCHO.rate <<- rum.fd.DCHOA1.rate + rum.fd.DCHOA2.rate + rum.fd.DCHOA3.rate + rum.fd.DCHOA4.rate + rum.fd.DCHOB1.rate + rum.fd.DCHOB2.rate + rum.fd.DCHOB3.rate + rum.fd.DCHOC.rate
  rum.diet.DPep.rate <<- sum(rum.fd.DPep.rate)
  rum.diet.RDP.rate <<- rum.diet.DProt.rate <<- sum(rum.fd.RDP.rate)
  rum.diet.DCHOB3.rate <<- sum(rum.fd.DCHOB3.rate)
  rum.diet.DCHO.rate <<- sum(rum.fd.DCHO.rate)
  rum.diet.bact.NFC.rate <<- sum(rum.fd.bact.NFC.rate)
  rum.diet.bact.FC.rate <<- sum(rum.fd.bact.FC.rate)
  if (genRPT)
  {
```

```
    if (flag_NandBCAA > 0 & (rum.N_balance.rate < 0 | rum.BCAA_balance.rate < 0))
    {
      rptAllowableBact <- fds["FeedName.x"]
      names(rptAllowableBact) <- "FeedName"
      rptAllowableBact["NFC"] <- rum.fd.bact.NFC.rate
      rptAllowableBact["FC"] <- rum.fd.bact.FC.rate
      rptAllowableBact["NFC+FC"] <- rum.fd.bact.NFC.rate + rum.fd.bact.FC.rate
      rptAllowableBact["RDCHOB3"] <- rum.fd.DCHOB3.rate
      if (flag_NandBCAA == 1) footnote <- "Algorithm for ruminal N and BCAA adjustment: Only for ruminal N deficiency"
      if (flag_NandBCAA == 2) footnote <- "Algorithm for ruminal N and BCAA adjustment: Only for ruminal BCAA deficiency"
      if (flag_NandBCAA == 3) footnote <- "Algorithm for ruminal N and BCAA adjustment: For ruminal N and BCAA deficiencies"
      report(rptAllowableBact, "N- or BCAA-Allowable Bacteria Growth and Ruminally Degraded Carbohydrate B3, g/d", "", footnote, 3, 3, 1000, 8, TRUE, FALSE, FALSE, FALSE, FALSE, FALSE, TRUE)
      rum.bact.PepUptake.rate <- calcPeptideUptake(flag_peptide, Parm_rum.bact.PepUp, rum.kp_forage.fracprate, rum.kp_liquid.fracprate, rum.diet.bact.NFC.rate, rum.diet.DPep.rate, anim.diet.Concentrate.frac)
      title <- "Peptide Uptake Submodel - Revised"
      cat(paste(title, "\n", string("=", nchar(title)), "\n\n", sep = ""))
      cat(paste("Unadjusted Ruminally degraded protein (peptide and AA), g/d : ", formatC(rum.diet.DPep_Unadj.rate * 1000, format = "f", digits = 3, width = 7), "\n", sep = ""))
      cat(paste("Peptide uptake rate by NFC bacteria, g/d                   : ", formatC(rum.bact.PepUptake.rate * 1000, format = "f", digits = 3, width = 7), "\n", sep = ""))
      cat(paste("Peptide escape from rumen, g/d                             : ", formatC((rum.diet.DPep_Unadj.rate - rum.bact.PepUptake.rate) * 1000, format = "f", digits = 3, width = 7), "\n", sep = ""))
      cat(paste("Adjusted Ruminally degraded protein (peptide and AA), g/d   : ", formatC(rum.bact.PepUptake.rate * 1000, format = "f", digits = 3, width = 7), "\n", sep = ""))
      cat(paste("Fractional liquid passage rate, 1/h                        : ", formatC(rum.kp_liquid.fracprate, format = "f", digits = 3, width = 7), "\n", sep = ""))
      cat(paste("Peptide in the rumen, g                                    : ", formatC(isz((rum.diet.DPep.rate - rum.bact.PepUptake.rate) * 1000, (rum.kp_liquid.fracprate/100)), format = "f", digits = 3, width = 7), "\n\n", sep = ""))
      cat("This revised peptide uptake is for information only.\nNo re-adjustment to ruminally degraded protein is performed.\n\n")
    }
  }
  # +++++++++++++++++++++++++++++++++
  # Bacteria CHO and Protein Yield
  # +++++++++++++++++++++++++++++++++
  rum.fd.bact.NFC_CP.rate <<- rum.fd.bact.NFC.rate * (Parm_rum.bact.CP/100)
  rum.fd.bact.FC_CP.rate <<- rum.fd.bact.FC.rate * (Parm_rum.bact.CP/100)
  rum.fd.bact.CP.rate <<- rum.fd.bact.NFC_CP.rate + rum.fd.bact.FC_CP.rate
  rum.fd.bact.NFC_TP.rate <<- rum.fd.bact.NFC_CP.rate * (Parm_rum.bact.TP_CP/100)
  rum.fd.bact.FC_TP.rate <<- rum.fd.bact.FC_CP.rate * (Parm_rum.bact.TP_CP/100)
  rum.fd.bact.TP.rate <<- rum.fd.bact.NFC_TP.rate + rum.fd.bact.FC_TP.rate
  rum.fd.bact.NFC_NA.rate <<- rum.fd.bact.NFC_CP.rate * (Parm_rum.bact.NA_CP/100)
  rum.fd.bact.FC_NA.rate <<- rum.fd.bact.FC_CP.rate * (Parm_rum.bact.NA_CP/100)
  rum.fd.bact.NA.rate <<- rum.fd.bact.NFC_NA.rate + rum.fd.bact.FC_NA.rate
  rum.fd.bact.NFC_CW.rate <<- rum.fd.bact.NFC_CP.rate * (Parm_rum.bact.CW_CP/100)
  rum.fd.bact.FC_CW.rate <<- rum.fd.bact.FC_CP.rate * (Parm_rum.bact.CW_CP/100)
  rum.fd.bact.CW.rate <<- rum.fd.bact.NFC_CW.rate + rum.fd.bact.FC_CW.rate
  rum.diet.bact.NFC_CP.rate <<- sum(rum.fd.bact.NFC_CP.rate)
  rum.diet.bact.FC_CP.rate <<- sum(rum.fd.bact.FC_CP.rate)
  rum.diet.bact.CP.rate <<- sum(rum.fd.bact.CP.rate)
```

```
rum.diet.bact.NFC_TP.rate <<- sum(rum.fd.bact.NFC_TP.rate)
rum.diet.bact.FC_TP.rate <<- sum(rum.fd.bact.FC_TP.rate)
rum.diet.bact.TP.rate <<- sum(rum.fd.bact.TP.rate)
rum.diet.bact.NFC_NA.rate <<- sum(rum.fd.bact.NFC_NA.rate)
rum.diet.bact.FC_NA.rate <<- sum(rum.fd.bact.FC_NA.rate)
rum.diet.bact.NA.rate <<- sum(rum.fd.bact.NA.rate)
rum.diet.bact.NFC_CW.rate <<- sum(rum.fd.bact.NFC_CW.rate)
rum.diet.bact.FC_CW.rate <<- sum(rum.fd.bact.FC_CW.rate)
rum.diet.bact.CW.rate <<- sum(rum.fd.bact.CW.rate)
rum.fd.bact.NFC_CHO.rate <<- rum.fd.bact.NFC.rate * (Parm_rum.bact.CHO/100)
rum.fd.bact.FC_CHO.rate <<- rum.fd.bact.FC.rate * (Parm_rum.bact.CHO/100)
rum.fd.bact.CHO.rate <<- rum.fd.bact.NFC_CHO.rate + rum.fd.bact.FC_CHO.rate
rum.fd.bact.NFC_CHOA.rate <<- rum.fd.bact.NFC_CHO.rate * (Parm_rum.bact.CHOA/100)
rum.fd.bact.FC_CHOA.rate <<- rum.fd.bact.FC_CHO.rate * (Parm_rum.bact.CHOA/100)
rum.fd.bact.CHOA.rate <<- rum.fd.bact.NFC_CHOA.rate + rum.fd.bact.FC_CHOA.rate
rum.fd.bact.NFC_CHOB1.rate <<- rum.fd.bact.NFC_CHO.rate * (Parm_rum.bact.CHOB1/100)
rum.fd.bact.FC_CHOB1.rate <<- rum.fd.bact.FC_CHO.rate * (Parm_rum.bact.CHOB1/100)
rum.fd.bact.CHOB1.rate <<- rum.fd.bact.NFC_CHOB1.rate + rum.fd.bact.FC_CHOB1.rate
rum.diet.bact.NFC_CHO.rate <<- sum(rum.fd.bact.NFC_CHO.rate)
rum.diet.bact.FC_CHO.rate <<- sum(rum.fd.bact.FC_CHO.rate)
rum.diet.bact.CHO.rate <<- sum(rum.fd.bact.CHO.rate)
rum.diet.bact.NFC_CHOA.rate <<- sum(rum.fd.bact.NFC_CHOA.rate)
rum.diet.bact.FC_CHOA.rate <<- sum(rum.fd.bact.FC_CHOA.rate)
rum.diet.bact.CHOA.rate <<- sum(rum.fd.bact.CHOA.rate)
rum.diet.bact.NFC_CHOB1.rate <<- sum(rum.fd.bact.NFC_CHOB1.rate)
rum.diet.bact.FC_CHOB1.rate <<- sum(rum.fd.bact.FC_CHOB1.rate)
rum.diet.bact.CHOB1.rate <<- sum(rum.fd.bact.CHOB1.rate)
rum.fd.bact.NFC_Fat.rate <<- rum.fd.bact.NFC.rate * (Parm_rum.bact.Fat/100)
rum.fd.bact.FC_Fat.rate <<- rum.fd.bact.FC.rate * (Parm_rum.bact.Fat/100)
rum.fd.bact.fat.rate <<- rum.fd.bact.NFC_Fat.rate + rum.fd.bact.FC_Fat.rate
rum.diet.bact.NFC_Fat.rate <<- sum(rum.fd.bact.NFC_Fat.rate)
rum.diet.bact.FC_Fat.rate <<- sum(rum.fd.bact.FC_Fat.rate)
rum.diet.bact.fat.rate <<- sum(rum.fd.bact.fat.rate)
rum.fd.bact.NFC_Ash.rate <<- rum.fd.bact.NFC.rate * (Parm_rum.bact.Ash/100)
rum.fd.bact.FC_Ash.rate <<- rum.fd.bact.FC.rate * (Parm_rum.bact.Ash/100)
rum.fd.bact.ash.rate <<- rum.fd.bact.NFC_Ash.rate + rum.fd.bact.FC_Ash.rate
rum.diet.bactNFC_Ash.rate <<- sum(rum.fd.bact.NFC_Ash.rate)
rum.diet.bact.FC_Ash.rate <<- sum(rum.fd.bact.FC_Ash.rate)
rum.diet.bact.ash.rate <<- sum(rum.fd.bact.ash.rate)
if (genRPT)
{
  rptREBactComp_DMI <- fds["FeedName.x"]
  names(rptREBactComp_DMI) <- "FeedName"
  rptREBactComp_DMI["NFC CP"] <- rum.fd.bact.NFC_CP.rate
  rptREBactComp_DMI["FC CP"] <- rum.fd.bact.FC_CP.rate
  rptREBactComp_DMI["NFC TP"] <- rum.fd.bact.NFC_TP.rate
  rptREBactComp_DMI["FC TP"] <- rum.fd.bact.FC_TP.rate
  rptREBactComp_DMI["NFC NA"] <- rum.fd.bact.NFC_NA.rate
  rptREBactComp_DMI["FC NA"] <- rum.fd.bact.FC_NA.rate
  rptREBactComp_DMI["NFC CW"] <- rum.fd.bact.NFC_CW.rate
  rptREBactComp_DMI["FC CW"] <- rum.fd.bact.FC_CW.rate
```

```
    rptREBactComp_DMI["NFC CHO"] <- rum.fd.bact.NFC_CHO.rate
    rptREBactComp_DMI["FC CHO"] <- rum.fd.bact.FC_CHO.rate
    rptREBactComp_DMI["NFC CHOA"] <- rum.fd.bact.NFC_CHOA.rate
    rptREBactComp_DMI["FC CHOA"] <- rum.fd.bact.FC_CHOA.rate
    rptREBactComp_DMI["NFC CHOB1"] <- rum.fd.bact.NFC_CHOB1.rate
    rptREBactComp_DMI["FC CHOB1"] <- rum.fd.bact.FC_CHOB1.rate
    rptREBactComp_DMI["NFC Fat"] <- rum.fd.bact.NFC_Fat.rate
    rptREBactComp_DMI["FC Fat"] <- rum.fd.bact.FC_Fat.rate
    rptREBactComp_DMI["NFC Ash"] <- rum.fd.bact.NFC_Ash.rate
    rptREBactComp_DMI["FC Ash"] <- rum.fd.bact.FC_Ash.rate
    description <- paste("Bacterial Growth Efficiency\n",
                         "   g Bacteria DM/kg ruminally degraded CHO              : ", formatC((rum.diet.bact.NFC.rate +
rum.diet.bact.FC.rate) * 1000/(rum.diet.DCHO.rate), format = "f", digits = 3, width = 7), "\n",
                         "      g NFC Bacteria DM/kg ruminally degraded NFC CHO     : ", formatC((rum.diet.bact.NFC.rate) *
1000/(rum.diet.DCHOA1.rate + rum.diet.DCHOA2.rate + rum.diet.DCHOA3.rate + rum.diet.DCHOA4.rate + rum.diet.DCHOB1.rate +
rum.diet.DCHOB2.rate), format = "f", digits = 3, width = 7), "\n",
                         "      g FC Bacteria DM/kg ruminally degraded FC CHO       : ", formatC((rum.diet.bact.FC.rate) *
1000/(rum.diet.DCHOB3.rate), format = "f", digits = 3, width = 7), "\n\n",
                         "   g Bacteria N/kg ruminally degraded CHO               : ", formatC((rum.diet.bact.NFC.rate +
rum.diet.bact.FC.rate) * (Parm_rum.bact.CP/100/6.25) * 1000/(rum.diet.DCHO.rate), format = "f", digits = 3, width = 7), "\n",
                         "      g NFC Bacteria N/kg ruminally degraded NFC CHO      : ", formatC((rum.diet.bact.NFC.rate) *
(Parm_rum.bact.CP/100/6.25) * 1000/(rum.diet.DCHOA1.rate + rum.diet.DCHOA2.rate + rum.diet.DCHOA3.rate + rum.diet.DCHOA4.rate
+ rum.diet.DCHOB1.rate + rum.diet.DCHOB2.rate), format = "f", digits = 3, width = 7), "\n",
                         "      g FC Bacteria N/kg ruminally degraded FC CHO        : ", formatC((rum.diet.bact.FC.rate) *
(Parm_rum.bact.CP/100/6.25) * 1000/(rum.diet.DCHOB3.rate), format = "f", digits = 3, width = 7), "\n\n",
                         "   g Bacteria DM/kg Ruminally degraded CHO & CP          : ", formatC((rum.diet.bact.NFC.rate +
rum.diet.bact.FC.rate) * 1000/(rum.diet.DCHO.rate + rum.diet.DProt.rate), format = "f", digits = 3, width = 7), "\n",
                         "   g Bacteria DM/kg Ruminally degraded Organic Matter    : ", formatC((rum.diet.bact.NFC.rate +
rum.diet.bact.FC.rate) * 1000/(rum.diet.DCHO.rate + rum.diet.DPep.rate), format = "f", digits = 3, width = 7), "\n",
                         "   g Bacteria N/kg Ruminally degraded CHO & CP           : ", formatC((rum.diet.bact.NFC.rate +
rum.diet.bact.FC.rate) *(Parm_rum.bact.CP/100/6.25) * 1000/(rum.diet.DCHO.rate + rum.diet.DProt.rate), format = "f", digits =
3, width = 7), "\n",
                         "   g Bacteria N/kg Ruminally degraded Organic Matter     : ", formatC((rum.diet.bact.NFC.rate +
rum.diet.bact.FC.rate) * (Parm_rum.bact.CP/100/6.25) * 1000/(rum.diet.DCHO.rate + rum.diet.DPep.rate), format = "f", digits =
3, width = 7), "\n\n", sep = "")
    report(rptREBactComp_DMI, "Ruminal Bacteria Contents, g/d", description, "", 2, 2, 1000, 9, TRUE, FALSE, FALSE, FALSE,
TRUE, FALSE, TRUE)
  }
  # ++++++++++++++++++++++++++++++++++++++
  # Ruminal Fatty Acids Biohydrogenation
  # ++++++++++++++++++++++++++++++++++++++
  # E = Escaped
  # L = Lipolyzed = Non-Esterified
  # B = Biohydrogenized
  # Moate et al. (2004; Anim. Feed Sci. Technol. 112:79-105)
  rum.diet.LFA.rate_g <<- rum.diet.LFA.rate * 1000
  # C18:3
  rum.fd.FAC18_3_kb.fracprate <<- 500 * (exp(-0.0187884381 * rum.diet.LFA.rate_g/anim.diet.DMI.rate))
  rum.fd.LEFAC18_3.rate <<- ifelse((rum.fd.FAC18_3_kb.fracprate + rum.fd.FAC18_3_kp.fracprate) > 0, rum.fd.LFAC18_3.rate *
(rum.fd.FAC18_3_kp.fracprate/(rum.fd.FAC18_3_kb.fracprate + rum.fd.FAC18_3_kp.fracprate)), 0)
  rum.fd.LBFAC18_3.rate <<- rum.fd.LFAC18_3.rate - rum.fd.LEFAC18_3.rate
```

```
  # C18:2
  rum.fd.FAC18_2_kb.fracprate <<- 87.56241579
  rum.fd.LEFAC18_2.rate <<- ifelse((rum.fd.FAC18_2_kb.fracprate + rum.fd.FAC18_2_kp.fracprate) > 0, (rum.fd.LFAC18_2.rate + rum.fd.LBFAC18_3.rate) * (rum.fd.FAC18_2_kp.fracprate/(rum.fd.FAC18_2_kb.fracprate + rum.fd.FAC18_2_kp.fracprate)), 0)
  rum.fd.LBFAC18_2.rate <<- ifelse((rum.fd.FAC18_2_kb.fracprate + rum.fd.FAC18_2_kp.fracprate) > 0, (rum.fd.LFAC18_2.rate + rum.fd.LBFAC18_3.rate) * (rum.fd.FAC18_2_kb.fracprate/(rum.fd.FAC18_2_kb.fracprate + rum.fd.FAC18_2_kp.fracprate)), 0)
  # C18:1t
  rum.fd.FAC18_1t_kb.fracprate <<- 54.4618963 * (exp(-0.022844773 * rum.diet.LFA.rate_g/anim.diet.DMI.rate))
  rum.fd.LEFAC18_1t.rate <<- ifelse((rum.fd.FAC18_1t_kb.fracprate + rum.fd.FAC18_1t_kp.fracprate) > 0, (rum.fd.LFAC18_1t.rate + rum.fd.LBFAC18_2.rate) * (rum.fd.FAC18_1t_kp.fracprate/(rum.fd.FAC18_1t_kb.fracprate + rum.fd.FAC18_1t_kp.fracprate)), 0)
  rum.fd.LBFAC18_1t.rate <<- ifelse((rum.fd.FAC18_1t_kb.fracprate + rum.fd.FAC18_1t_kp.fracprate) > 0, (rum.fd.LFAC18_1t.rate + rum.fd.LBFAC18_2.rate) * (rum.fd.FAC18_1t_kb.fracprate/(rum.fd.FAC18_1t_kb.fracprate + rum.fd.FAC18_1t_kp.fracprate)), 0)
  # C18:1c
  rum.fd.FAC18_1c_kb.fracprate <<- 27.34532619
  rum.fd.LEFAC18_1c.rate <<- ifelse((rum.fd.FAC18_1c_kb.fracprate + rum.fd.FAC18_1c_kp.fracprate) > 0, rum.fd.LFAC18_1c.rate * (rum.fd.FAC18_1c_kp.fracprate/(rum.fd.FAC18_1c_kb.fracprate + rum.fd.FAC18_1c_kp.fracprate)), 0)
  rum.fd.LBFAC18_1c.rate <<- rum.fd.LFAC18_1c.rate - rum.fd.LEFAC18_1c.rate
  # C18:0
  rum.fd.LEFAC18.rate <<- rum.fd.LFAC18.rate + rum.fd.LBFAC18_1t.rate + rum.fd.LBFAC18_1c.rate
  # C16:1
  rum.fd.FAC16_1_kb.fracprate <<- 300 * (exp(-0.030486193 * rum.diet.LFA.rate_g/anim.diet.DMI.rate))
  rum.fd.LEFAC16_1.rate <<- ifelse((rum.fd.FAC16_1_kb.fracprate + rum.fd.FAC16_1_kp.fracprate) > 0, rum.fd.LFAC16_1.rate * (rum.fd.FAC16_1_kp.fracprate/(rum.fd.FAC16_1_kb.fracprate + rum.fd.FAC16_1_kp.fracprate)), 0)
  rum.fd.LBFAC16_1.rate <<- rum.fd.LFAC16_1.rate - rum.fd.LEFAC16_1.rate
  # C16:0
  rum.fd.LEFAC16.rate <<- rum.fd.LFAC16.rate + rum.fd.LBFAC16_1.rate
  # C14:0
  rum.fd.LEFAC14.rate <<- rum.fd.LFAC14.rate
  # C12:0
  rum.fd.LEFAC12.rate <<- rum.fd.LFAC12.rate
  # Other Lipids
  rum.fd.LEFAOther.rate <<- rum.fd.LFAOther.rate
  rum.diet.LEFAC18_1c.rate <<- sum(rum.fd.LEFAC18_1c.rate)
  rum.diet.LEFAC18_3.rate <<- sum(rum.fd.LEFAC18_3.rate)
  rum.diet.LEFAC18_2.rate <<- sum(rum.fd.LEFAC18_2.rate)
  rum.diet.LEFAC18_1t.rate <<- sum(rum.fd.LEFAC18_1t.rate)
  rum.diet.LEFAC18.rate <<- sum(rum.fd.LEFAC18.rate)
  rum.diet.LEFAC16_1.rate <<- sum(rum.fd.LEFAC16_1.rate)
  rum.diet.LEFAC16.rate <<- sum(rum.fd.LEFAC16.rate)
  rum.diet.LEFAC14.rate <<- sum(rum.fd.LEFAC14.rate)
  rum.diet.LEFAC12.rate <<- sum(rum.fd.LEFAC12.rate)
  rum.diet.LEFAOther.rate <<- sum(rum.fd.LEFAOther.rate)
  rum.diet.LBFAC18_1c.rate <<- sum(rum.fd.LBFAC18_1c.rate)
  rum.diet.LBFAC18_3.rate <<- sum(rum.fd.LBFAC18_3.rate)
  rum.diet.LBFAC18_2.rate <<- sum(rum.fd.LBFAC18_2.rate)
  rum.diet.LBFAC18_1t.rate <<- sum(rum.fd.LBFAC18_1t.rate)
  rum.diet.LBFAC16_1.rate <<- sum(rum.fd.LBFAC16_1.rate)
  if (genRPT)
  {
    rptRumFA_DMI <- fds["FeedName.x"]
    names(rptRumFA_DMI) <- "FeedName"
```

```
    rptRumFA_DMI["C12:0"] <- rum.fd.LEFAC12.rate
    rptRumFA_DMI["C14:0"] <- rum.fd.LEFAC14.rate
    rptRumFA_DMI["C16:0"] <- rum.fd.LEFAC16.rate
    rptRumFA_DMI["C16:1"] <- rum.fd.LEFAC16_1.rate
    rptRumFA_DMI["C18:0"] <- rum.fd.LEFAC18.rate
    rptRumFA_DMI["C18:1c"] <- rum.fd.LEFAC18_1c.rate
    rptRumFA_DMI["C18:1t"] <- rum.fd.LEFAC18_1t.rate
    rptRumFA_DMI["C18:2"] <- rum.fd.LEFAC18_2.rate
    rptRumFA_DMI["C18:3"] <- rum.fd.LEFAC18_3.rate
    rptRumFA_DMI["Other"] <- rum.fd.LEFAOther.rate
    report(rptRumFA_DMI, "Ruminally Escaped Lipolyzed Fatty Acids, g/d", "", "", 2, 2, 1000, 8, TRUE, FALSE, TRUE, FALSE, TRUE, FALSE, FALSE)
    rptRumFA_DMI <- fds["FeedName.x"]
    names(rptRumFA_DMI) <- "FeedName"
    rptRumFA_DMI["C16:1"] <- rum.fd.LBFAC16_1.rate
    rptRumFA_DMI["C18:1c"] <- rum.fd.LBFAC18_1c.rate
    rptRumFA_DMI["C18:1t"] <- rum.fd.LBFAC18_1t.rate
    rptRumFA_DMI["C18:2"] <- rum.fd.LBFAC18_2.rate
    rptRumFA_DMI["C18:3"] <- rum.fd.LBFAC18_3.rate
    footnote <- "Note that C18:3, C18:2, C18:1c, C18:1t, and C16:1 values are double accounted due to biohydrogenation.\nThey are also included in the Ruminally Escaped Lipolyzed Fatty Acids report."
    report(rptRumFA_DMI, "\nRuminally Biohydrogenized Fatty Acids, g/d", "", footnote, 2, 2, 1000, 7, TRUE, FALSE, TRUE, FALSE, TRUE, FALSE, TRUE)
  }
  # Non-Esterified Fatty Acids
  rum.diet.NEFAC16.rate <<- rum.diet.LEFAC16.rate
  rum.diet.NEFAC16_1.rate <<- rum.diet.LEFAC16_1.rate
  rum.diet.NEFAC18.rate <<- rum.diet.LEFAC18.rate
  rum.diet.NEFAOther.rate <<- rum.diet.LEFAOther.rate
  # De novo synthesis, g/d
  rum.fd.DNFAC16.rate <<- ifelse(anim.diet.DMI.rate > 0, 5.76 * rum.fd.DCHO.rate * exp(-0.269 * rum.diet.NEFAC16.rate * 1000/anim.diet.DMI.rate)/1000, 0)
  rum.fd.DNFAC16_1.rate <<- ifelse(anim.diet.DMI.rate > 0, 0.6241 * rum.fd.DCHO.rate * exp(-1.23 * rum.diet.NEFAC16_1.rate * 1000/anim.diet.DMI.rate)/1000, 0)
  rum.fd.DNFAC18.rate <<- ifelse(anim.diet.DMI.rate > 0, 27.3 * rum.fd.DCHO.rate * exp(-0.117 * rum.diet.NEFAC18.rate * 1000/anim.diet.DMI.rate)/1000, 0)
  rum.fd.DNFAOther.rate <<- ifelse(anim.diet.DMI.rate > 0, 5.02 * rum.fd.DCHO.rate * exp(-0.332 * rum.diet.NEFAOther.rate * 1000/anim.diet.DMI.rate)/1000, 0)
  # CPM Dairy 3.0.8 equations
  #rum.fd.DNFAC16.rate<<-if(anim.diet.DMI.rate>0) {10.32130161*rum.fd.DCHO.rate*exp(-0.401822896*rum.diet.NEFAC16.rate*1000/anim.diet.DMI.rate)/1000} else 0
  #rum.fd.DNFAC16_1.rate<<-if(anim.diet.DMI.rate>0) {0.45513344*rum.fd.DCHO.rate*exp(-4.891359211*rum.diet.NEFAC16_1.rate*1000/anim.diet.DMI.rate)/1000} else 0
  #rum.fd.DNFAC18.rate<<-if(anim.diet.DMI.rate>0) {27.26414196*rum.fd.DCHO.rate*exp(-0.116927153*rum.diet.NEFAC18.rate*1000/anim.diet.DMI.rate)/1000} else 0
  #rum.fd.DNFAOther.rate<<-if(anim.diet.DMI.rate>0) {5.02406278*rum.fd.DCHO.rate*exp(-0.332150761*rum.diet.NEFAOther.rate*1000/anim.diet.DMI.rate)/1000} else 0
  rum.diet.DNFAC16.rate <<- sum(rum.fd.DNFAC16.rate)
  rum.diet.DNFAC16_1.rate <<- sum(rum.fd.DNFAC16_1.rate)
  rum.diet.DNFAC18.rate <<- sum(rum.fd.DNFAC18.rate)
  rum.diet.DNFAOther.rate <<- sum(rum.fd.DNFAOther.rate)
```

```
  if (genRPT)
  {
    rptRumDNFA_DMI <- fds["FeedName.x"]
    names(rptRumDNFA_DMI) <- "FeedName"
    rptRumDNFA_DMI["C16:0"] <- rum.fd.DNFAC16.rate
    rptRumDNFA_DMI["C16:1"] <- rum.fd.DNFAC16_1.rate
    rptRumDNFA_DMI["C18:0"] <- rum.fd.DNFAC18.rate
    rptRumDNFA_DMI["Other FA"] <- rum.fd.DNFAOther.rate
    footnote <- "De novo synthesis of fatty acids (C16:0, C16:1, C18:0, and other fatty acids) by ruminal bacteria."
    report(rptRumDNFA_DMI, "Ruminally Synthesized 'de novo' Fatty Acids, g/d", "", "", 2, 2, 1000, 8, TRUE, FALSE, TRUE, FALSE, TRUE, FALSE, FALSE)
  }
  # Fat & Fatty Acids - Feed
  rum.fd.EFat.rate <<- anim.fd.EE.rate
  rum.fd.EFAC12.rate <<- anim.fd.FAC12.rate - rum.fd.LFAC12.rate
  rum.fd.EFAC14.rate <<- anim.fd.FAC14.rate - rum.fd.LFAC14.rate
  rum.fd.EFAC16.rate <<- anim.fd.FAC16.rate - rum.fd.LFAC16.rate
  rum.fd.EFAC16_1.rate <<- anim.fd.FAC16_1.rate - rum.fd.LFAC16_1.rate
  rum.fd.EFAC18.rate <<- anim.fd.FAC18.rate - rum.fd.LFAC18.rate
  rum.fd.EFAC18_1c.rate <<- anim.fd.FAC18_1c.rate - rum.fd.LFAC18_1c.rate
  rum.fd.EFAC18_1t.rate <<- anim.fd.FAC18_1t.rate - rum.fd.LFAC18_1t.rate
  rum.fd.EFAC18_2.rate <<- anim.fd.FAC18_2.rate - rum.fd.LFAC18_2.rate
  rum.fd.EFAC18_3.rate <<- anim.fd.FAC18_3.rate - rum.fd.LFAC18_3.rate
  rum.fd.EFAOther.rate <<- anim.fd.FAOther.rate - rum.fd.LFAOther.rate
  rum.fd.EGlycerol.rate <<- anim.fd.Glycerol.rate - rum.fd.LGlycerol.rate
  rum.fd.EPigment.rate <<- anim.fd.Pigment.rate
  rum.diet.EFat.rate <<- sum(rum.fd.EFat.rate)
  rum.diet.EFAC12.rate <<- sum(rum.fd.EFAC12.rate)
  rum.diet.EFAC14.rate <<- sum(rum.fd.EFAC14.rate)
  rum.diet.EFAC16.rate <<- sum(rum.fd.EFAC16.rate)
  rum.diet.EFAC16_1.rate <<- sum(rum.fd.EFAC16_1.rate)
  rum.diet.EFAC18.rate <<- sum(rum.fd.EFAC18.rate)
  rum.diet.EFAC18_1c.rate <<- sum(rum.fd.EFAC18_1c.rate)
  rum.diet.EFAC18_1t.rate <<- sum(rum.fd.EFAC18_1t.rate)
  rum.diet.EFAC18_2.rate <<- sum(rum.fd.EFAC18_2.rate)
  rum.diet.EFAC18_3.rate <<- sum(rum.fd.EFAC18_3.rate)
  rum.diet.EFAOther.rate <<- sum(rum.fd.EFAOther.rate)
  rum.diet.EGlycerol.rate <<- sum(rum.fd.EGlycerol.rate)
  rum.diet.EPigment.rate <<- sum(rum.fd.EPigment.rate)
  if (genRPT)
  {
    rptREFA_DMI <- feeds3["FeedName.x"]
    names(rptREFA_DMI) <- "FeedName"
    rptREFA_DMI["C12:0"] <- rum.fd.EFAC12.rate
    rptREFA_DMI["C14:0"] <- rum.fd.EFAC14.rate
    rptREFA_DMI["C16:0"] <- rum.fd.EFAC16.rate
    rptREFA_DMI["C16:1"] <- rum.fd.EFAC16_1.rate
    rptREFA_DMI["C18:0"] <- rum.fd.EFAC18.rate
    rptREFA_DMI["C18:1c"] <- rum.fd.EFAC18_1c.rate
    rptREFA_DMI["C18:2"] <- rum.fd.EFAC18_2.rate
    rptREFA_DMI["C18:3"] <- rum.fd.EFAC18_3.rate
```

```
    rptREFA_DMI["Other FFA"] <- rum.fd.EFAOther.rate
    description <- paste("Escaped glycerol, g/d : ", formatC(rum.diet.EGlycerol.rate * 1000, format = "f", digits = 3, width = 7), "\n",
                         "Escaped pigments, g/d : ", formatC(rum.diet.EPigment.rate * 1000, format = "f", digits = 3, width = 7), "\n\n", sep = "")
    report(rptREFA_DMI, "\nRuminally Escaped Esterified Fatty Acids, g/d", description, "", 3, 3, 1000, 7, TRUE, FALSE, TRUE, FALSE, TRUE, FALSE, TRUE)
  }
}
```

4.3.9 Ruminal volatile fatty acids

```
calcVFA <- function(fds = feeds3, pH = NA, CECNDF = 500, genRPT = TRUE)
{
  # Substrates
  # ++++++++++
  # CHOA1 = C2 + C3 + C4
  # CHOA2 = Lactate
  # CHOA3 = Other organic acids
  # CHOA4 = Sugars
  # CHOB1 = Starch
  # CHOB2 = Soluble fiber (e.g., pectin)
  # CHOB3 = Available NDF

  # Acid product
  # ++++++++++++
  # CHOA4, CHOB1, CHOB2
  fracA4 <- isz(rum.fd.bact.CHOA4.rate, (rum.fd.bact.CHOA1.rate + rum.fd.bact.CHOA2.rate + rum.fd.bact.CHOA3.rate + rum.fd.bact.CHOA4.rate + rum.fd.bact.CHOB1.rate + rum.fd.bact.CHOB2.rate))
  fracB1 <- isz(rum.fd.bact.CHOB1.rate, (rum.fd.bact.CHOA1.rate + rum.fd.bact.CHOA2.rate + rum.fd.bact.CHOA3.rate + rum.fd.bact.CHOA4.rate + rum.fd.bact.CHOB1.rate + rum.fd.bact.CHOB2.rate))
  fracB2 <- isz(rum.fd.bact.CHOB2.rate, (rum.fd.bact.CHOA1.rate + rum.fd.bact.CHOA2.rate + rum.fd.bact.CHOA3.rate + rum.fd.bact.CHOA4.rate + rum.fd.bact.CHOB1.rate + rum.fd.bact.CHOB2.rate))
  rum.fd.CHOA4.acid.rate <<- pmax(0, (1 - 0.344) * rum.fd.DCHOA4.rate - (1 - (Parm_rum.bact.Ash/100)) * rum.fd.bact.CHOA4.rate + (rum.fd.bact.NFC_AmmoniaN.rate + 6.25 * rum.fd.bact.NFC_AminoN.rate) * fracA4)
  rum.fd.CHOB1.acid.rate <<- pmax(0, (1 - 0.344) * rum.fd.DCHOB1.rate - (1 - (Parm_rum.bact.Ash/100)) * rum.fd.bact.CHOB1.rate + (rum.fd.bact.NFC_AmmoniaN.rate + 6.25 * rum.fd.bact.NFC_AminoN.rate) * fracB1)
  rum.fd.CHOB2.acid.rate <<- pmax(0, (1 - 0.344) * rum.fd.DCHOB2.rate - (1 - (Parm_rum.bact.Ash/100)) * rum.fd.bact.CHOB2.rate + (rum.fd.bact.NFC_AmmoniaN.rate + 6.25 * rum.fd.bact.NFC_AminoN.rate) * fracB2)
  # CHOB3
  rum.fd.CHOB3.acid.rate <<- pmax(0, (1 - 0.54) * rum.fd.DCHOB3.rate - (rum.fd.bact.CHOB3.rate - rum.fd.bact.FC_Ash.rate - rum.fd.bact.FC_AmmoniaN.rate))
  # VFA (acetate, propionate, butyrate) and lactate production
  # ++++++++++++++++++++++++++++++++++++++++++++++++++++++++++
  if (is.na(pH) == TRUE)
  {
    if (exists("rum.pH")) pH <- rum.pH
    if (exists("rum.pH_peNDF")) pH <- rum.pH_peNDF
  }
  ratio.CHOA4.Lact <<- max(0, 2.4444 - 0.3075 * pH)
  ratio.CHOB1.Lact <<- max(0, 3.2989 - 0.4744 * pH)
  ratio.CHOB2.Lact <<- 0
  ratio.CHOB3.Lact <<- max(0, 2.4278 - 0.3532 * pH)
  ratio.CHOA4.But <<- max(0, 0.5733 - 0.0585 * pH)
  ratio.CHOB1.But <<- max(0, 0.7359 - 0.0921 * pH)
  ratio.CHOB2.But <<- max(0, 0.3621 - 0.0504 * pH)
  ratio.CHOB3.But <<- max(0, 0.5015 - 0.0631 * pH)
  ratio.CHOA4.C2C3 <<- max(0, -1.3209 + 0.468 * pH)
  ratio.CHOB1.C2C3 <<- max(0, 5.6265 - 0.627 * pH)
  ratio.CHOB2.C2C3 <<- max(0, 2.5186 + 0.5643 * pH)
```

```
ratio.CHOB3.C2C3 <<- max(0, -0.2662 + 0.3267 * pH)
rum.fd.CHOA4.lactate.rate <<- ratio.CHOA4.Lact * rum.fd.CHOA4.acid.rate
rum.fd.CHOB1.lactate.rate <<- ratio.CHOB1.Lact * rum.fd.CHOB1.acid.rate
rum.fd.CHOB2.lactate.rate <<- ratio.CHOB2.Lact * rum.fd.CHOB2.acid.rate
rum.fd.CHOB3.lactate.rate <<- ratio.CHOB3.Lact * rum.fd.CHOB3.acid.rate
rum.fd.CHOA4.VFA.rate <<- rum.fd.CHOA4.acid.rate - rum.fd.CHOA4.lactate.rate
rum.fd.CHOB1.VFA.rate <<- rum.fd.CHOB1.acid.rate - rum.fd.CHOB1.lactate.rate
rum.fd.CHOB2.VFA.rate <<- rum.fd.CHOB2.acid.rate - rum.fd.CHOB2.lactate.rate
rum.fd.CHOB3.VFA.rate <<- rum.fd.CHOB3.acid.rate - rum.fd.CHOB3.lactate.rate
rum.fd.CHOA4.butyrate.rate <<- ratio.CHOA4.But * rum.fd.CHOA4.VFA.rate
rum.fd.CHOB1.butyrate.rate <<- ratio.CHOB1.But * rum.fd.CHOB1.VFA.rate
rum.fd.CHOB2.butyrate.rate <<- ratio.CHOB2.But * rum.fd.CHOB2.VFA.rate
rum.fd.CHOB3.butyrate.rate <<- ratio.CHOB3.But * rum.fd.CHOB3.VFA.rate
rum.fd.CHOA4.propionate.rate <<- (1 - ratio.CHOA4.But) * rum.fd.CHOA4.VFA.rate/(1 + ratio.CHOA4.C2C3)
rum.fd.CHOB1.propionate.rate <<- (1 - ratio.CHOB1.But) * rum.fd.CHOB1.VFA.rate/(1 + ratio.CHOB1.C2C3)
rum.fd.CHOB2.propionate.rate <<- (1 - ratio.CHOB2.But) * rum.fd.CHOB2.VFA.rate/(1 + ratio.CHOB2.C2C3)
rum.fd.CHOB3.propionate.rate <<- (1 - ratio.CHOB3.But) * rum.fd.CHOB3.VFA.rate/(1 + ratio.CHOB3.C2C3)
rum.fd.CHOA4.acetate.rate <<- ratio.CHOA4.C2C3 * rum.fd.CHOA4.propionate.rate
rum.fd.CHOB1.acetate.rate <<- ratio.CHOB1.C2C3 * rum.fd.CHOB1.propionate.rate
rum.fd.CHOB2.acetate.rate <<- ratio.CHOB2.C2C3 * rum.fd.CHOB2.propionate.rate
rum.fd.CHOB3.acetate.rate <<- ratio.CHOB3.C2C3 * rum.fd.CHOB3.propionate.rate
rum.fd.acetate.rate <<- rum.fd.CHOA4.acetate.rate + rum.fd.CHOB1.acetate.rate + rum.fd.CHOB2.acetate.rate + rum.fd.CHOB3.acetate.rate
rum.fd.propionate.rate <<- rum.fd.LGlycerol.propionate.rate + rum.fd.CHOA4.propionate.rate + rum.fd.CHOB1.propionate.rate + rum.fd.CHOB2.propionate.rate + rum.fd.CHOB3.propionate.rate
rum.fd.butyrate.rate <<- rum.fd.CHOA4.butyrate.rate + rum.fd.CHOB1.butyrate.rate + rum.fd.CHOB2.butyrate.rate + rum.fd.CHOB3.butyrate.rate
rum.fd.lactate.rate <<- rum.fd.CHOA4.lactate.rate + rum.fd.CHOB1.lactate.rate + rum.fd.CHOB2.lactate.rate + rum.fd.CHOB3.lactate.rate
rum.diet.CHOA4.acetate.rate <<- sum(rum.fd.CHOA4.acetate.rate)
rum.diet.CHOA4.propionate.rate <<- sum(rum.fd.CHOA4.propionate.rate)
rum.diet.CHOA4.butyrate.rate <<- sum(rum.fd.CHOA4.butyrate.rate)
rum.diet.CHOA4.lactate.rate <<- sum(rum.fd.CHOA4.lactate.rate)
rum.diet.CHOB1.acetate.rate <<- sum(rum.fd.CHOB1.acetate.rate)
rum.diet.CHOB1.propionate.rate <<- sum(rum.fd.CHOB1.propionate.rate)
rum.diet.CHOB1.butyrate.rate <<- sum(rum.fd.CHOB1.butyrate.rate)
rum.diet.CHOB1.lactate.rate <<- sum(rum.fd.CHOB1.lactate.rate)
rum.diet.CHOB2.acetate.rate <<- sum(rum.fd.CHOB2.acetate.rate)
rum.diet.CHOB2.propionate.rate <<- sum(rum.fd.CHOB2.propionate.rate)
rum.diet.CHOB2.butyrate.rate <<- sum(rum.fd.CHOB2.butyrate.rate)
rum.diet.CHOB2.lactate.rate <<- sum(rum.fd.CHOB2.lactate.rate)
rum.diet.CHOB3.acetate.rate <<- sum(rum.fd.CHOB3.acetate.rate)
rum.diet.CHOB3.propionate.rate <<- sum(rum.fd.CHOB3.propionate.rate)
rum.diet.CHOB3.butyrate.rate <<- sum(rum.fd.CHOB3.butyrate.rate)
rum.diet.CHOB3.lactate.rate <<- sum(rum.fd.CHOB3.lactate.rate)
# Methane production
# +++++++++++++++++++
fracP.CHOA4 <- ifelse(rum.diet.CHOA4.acetate.rate + rum.diet.CHOA4.propionate.rate + rum.diet.CHOA4.butyrate.rate > 0, (rum.diet.CHOA4.propionate.rate/74)/(rum.diet.CHOA4.acetate.rate/60 + rum.diet.CHOA4.propionate.rate/74 + rum.diet.CHOA4.butyrate.rate/88), 0)
rum.CHOA4.methane.Y.frac <- ifelse(fracP.CHOA4 != 0, max(0, (1/(2 * fracP.CHOA4) - 3/4) * 16/74), 0)
```

```
rum.fd.CHOA4.methane.rate <<- rum.fd.CHOA4.propionate.rate * rum.CHOA4.methane.Y.frac
fracP.CHOB1 <- ifelse(rum.diet.CHOB1.acetate.rate + rum.diet.CHOB1.propionate.rate + rum.diet.CHOB1.butyrate.rate > 0, (rum.diet.CHOB1.propionate.rate/74)/(rum.diet.CHOB1.acetate.rate/60 + rum.diet.CHOB1.propionate.rate/74 + rum.diet.CHOB1.butyrate.rate/88), 0)
rum.CHOB1.methane.Y.frac <- ifelse(fracP.CHOB1 != 0, max(0, (1/(2 * fracP.CHOB1) - 3/4) * 16/74), 0)
rum.fd.CHOB1.methane.rate <<- rum.fd.CHOB1.propionate.rate * rum.CHOB1.methane.Y.frac
fracP.CHOB2 <- ifelse(rum.diet.CHOB2.acetate.rate + rum.diet.CHOB2.propionate.rate + rum.diet.CHOB2.butyrate.rate > 0, (rum.diet.CHOB2.propionate.rate/74)/(rum.diet.CHOB2.acetate.rate/60 + rum.diet.CHOB2.propionate.rate/74 + rum.diet.CHOB2.butyrate.rate/88), 0)
rum.CHOB2.methane.Y.frac <- ifelse(fracP.CHOB2 != 0, max(0, (1/(2 * fracP.CHOB2) - 3/4) * 16/74), 0)
rum.fd.CHOB2.methane.rate <<- rum.fd.CHOB2.propionate.rate * rum.CHOB2.methane.Y.frac
fracP.CHOB3 <- ifelse(rum.diet.CHOB3.acetate.rate + rum.diet.CHOB3.propionate.rate + rum.diet.CHOB3.butyrate.rate > 0, (rum.diet.CHOB3.propionate.rate/74)/(rum.diet.CHOB3.acetate.rate/60 + rum.diet.CHOB3.propionate.rate/74 + rum.diet.CHOB3.butyrate.rate/88), 0)
rum.CHOB3.methane.Y.frac <- ifelse(fracP.CHOB3 != 0, max(0, (1/(2 * fracP.CHOB3) - 3/4) * 16/74), 0)
rum.fd.CHOB3.methane.rate <<- rum.fd.CHOB3.propionate.rate * rum.CHOB3.methane.Y.frac
rum.fd.methane.rate <<- rum.fd.CHOA4.methane.rate + rum.fd.CHOB1.methane.rate + rum.fd.CHOB2.methane.rate + rum.fd.CHOB3.methane.rate
rum.diet.methane.rate <<- sum(rum.fd.methane.rate)
# Lactate fermentation
# +++++++++++++++++++++
# Megasphaera elsdenii growth
rum.bact.elsdenii.Yg <<- ifelse(pH < 5.07, 0, -1.176 + 0.232 * pH)
rum.bact.elsdenii.m <<- -2.779 + 0.664 * pH
rum.bact.elsdenii.u <<- ifelse(pH < 4.18 | pH > 7.33, 0, ifelse(pH >= 4.18 & pH <= 6.07, -3.631 + 1.255 * pH - 0.0925 * pH^2, -6.906 + 2.636 * pH - 0.2311 * pH^2))
rum.bact.elsdenii.Y <<- 1/(rum.bact.elsdenii.m/rum.bact.elsdenii.u + 1/rum.bact.elsdenii.Yg)
# lactate fractional degradation rate, %/d
kdL <- rum.diet.lactate_kd.fracprate <<- (rum.bact.elsdenii.u + rum.bact.elsdenii.m * rum.bact.elsdenii.Yg) * 24 * 100
# lactate fractional absorption rate, %/d
Ar <- rum.area <<- calcRumenArea(anim.diet.NDF.rate * 100/anim.diet.DMI.rate)
Vr <- rum.volume/1000
fLu <- (1 + 10^(pH - 3.86))^-1
kaL <- rum.diet.lactate_ka.fracprate <<- (Ar/Vr) * (0.00405 * fLu + 0.00139 * (1 - fLu)) * 100 # %/d
# lactate fractional passage rate, %/d
kl <- rum.kp_liquid.fracprate * 24
# lactate degradation and VFA formation
rum.fd.lactate.rate <- rum.fd.CHOA4.lactate.rate + rum.fd.CHOB1.lactate.rate + rum.fd.CHOB2.lactate.rate + rum.fd.CHOB3.lactate.rate + anim.fd.lactate.rate
rum.fd.RDL.rate <<- rum.fd.lactate.rate * kdL/(kdL + kl + kaL)
rum.fd.bact.elsdenii.rate <<- rum.fd.RDL.rate * rum.bact.elsdenii.Y
ratio.lactate.C2 <<- ifelse(pH < 4 | pH > 8, 0, ifelse(pH >= 4 & pH <= 5.65, 1.035 - 0.154 * pH, -1.089 + 0.222 * pH))
ratio.lactate.C3 <<- ifelse(pH < 4 | pH > 8, 0, ifelse(pH >= 4 & pH <= 6, 1.568 - 0.206 * pH, -1.408 + 0.29 * pH))
ratio.lactate.C4 <<- ifelse(pH < 4.4 | pH > 7, 0, ifelse(pH >= 4.4 & pH <= 5.5, -1.181 + 0.27 * pH, 1.316 - 0.184 * pH))
rum.fd.lactate.VFA.rate <<- rum.fd.RDL.rate * (1 - 0.856 * rum.bact.elsdenii.Y)/(1 + ratio.lactate.C2 * 44/60)
rum.fd.lactate.acetate.rate <<- rum.fd.lactate.VFA.rate * ratio.lactate.C2
rum.fd.lactate.propionate.rate <<- rum.fd.lactate.VFA.rate * ratio.lactate.C3
rum.fd.lactate.butyrate.rate <<- rum.fd.lactate.VFA.rate * ratio.lactate.C4
rum.diet.bact.elsdenii.rate <<- sum(rum.fd.bact.elsdenii.rate)
rum.diet.lactate.VFA.rate <<- sum(rum.fd.lactate.rate)
rum.diet.lactate.acetate.rate <<- sum(rum.fd.lactate.acetate.rate)
```

```
  rum.diet.lactate.propionate.rate <<- sum(rum.fd.lactate.propionate.rate)
  rum.diet.lactate.butyrate.rate <<- sum(rum.fd.lactate.butyrate.rate)
  # Ruminal concentration of VFA and lactate
  fAu <- (1 + 10^(pH - 4.76))^-1
  fPu <- (1 + 10^(pH - 4.87))^-1
  fBu <- (1 + 10^(pH - 4.81))^-1
  kaA <- rum.diet.acetate_ka.fracprate <<- (Ar/Vr) * (0.48 * fAu + 0.12 * (1 - fAu)) * 100  # %/d
  kaP <- rum.diet.propionate_ka.fracprate <<- (Ar/Vr) * (0.67 * fPu + 0.21 * (1 - fPu)) * 100  # %/d
  kaB <- rum.diet.butyrate_ka.fracprate <<- (Ar/Vr) * (1.43 * fBu + 0.15 * (1 - fBu)) * 100  # %/d
  rum.fd.acetate.rate <<- rum.fd.CHOA4.acetate.rate + rum.fd.CHOB1.acetate.rate + rum.fd.CHOB2.acetate.rate + rum.fd.CHOB3.acetate.rate + rum.fd.lactate.acetate.rate + anim.fd.acetate.rate
  rum.fd.propionate.rate <<- rum.fd.LGlycerol.propionate.rate + rum.fd.CHOA4.propionate.rate + rum.fd.CHOB1.propionate.rate + rum.fd.CHOB2.propionate.rate + rum.fd.CHOB3.propionate.rate + rum.fd.lactate.propionate.rate + anim.fd.propionate.rate
  rum.fd.butyrate.rate <<- rum.fd.CHOA4.butyrate.rate + rum.fd.CHOB1.butyrate.rate + rum.fd.CHOB2.butyrate.rate + rum.fd.CHOB3.butyrate.rate + rum.fd.lactate.butyrate.rate + anim.fd.butyrate.rate
  rum.diet.lactate.rate <<- sum(rum.fd.lactate.rate)
  rum.diet.RDL.rate <<- sum(rum.fd.RDL.rate)
  rum.diet.acetate.rate <<- sum(rum.fd.acetate.rate)
  rum.diet.propionate.rate <<- sum(rum.fd.propionate.rate)
  rum.diet.butyrate.rate <<- sum(rum.fd.butyrate.rate)
  rum.lactate.conc <<- rum.diet.lactate.rate * 1000/((kdL/100 + kl/100 + kaL/100) * Vr * 90)
  rum.acetate.conc <<- rum.diet.acetate.rate * 1000/((kl/100 + kaA/100) * Vr * 60)
  rum.propionate.conc <<- rum.diet.propionate.rate * 1000/((kl/100 + kaP/100) * Vr * 74)
  rum.butyrate.conc <<- rum.diet.butyrate.rate * 1000/((kl/100 + kaB/100) * Vr * 88)
  # Rumen buffering capacity
  # ++++++++++++++++++++++++++
  # Saliva
  # Pitt et al. (1996; JAS 74(1):226-244)
  Ds <- max(100, -177.2 + 0.01638 * (anim.diet.DMI.rate * 1000) + 4.766 * anim.diet.peNDF.conc) # L/d
  # Argyle and Baldwin (1988; JDS 71(5):1178-1188)
  EatSa <- (3.2 * anim.diet.DMI.rate) # Eating saliva, L/d
  Cwcf <- 0.5085 * anim.diet.NDF.rate/anim.diet.DMI.rate + 0.174 # Cell wall factor
  RumSa <- 255 * Cwcf # Rumination saliva, L/d
  RestSa <- 6 * anim.diet.DMI.rate * (1 - Cwcf) # Resting saliva, L/d
  SaIn <- EatSa + RumSa + RestSa
  anim.saliva.rate <<- max(Ds, SaIn)
  anim.saliva.conc <<- anim.saliva.rate/(1000 * Vr * kl/100) # L/L
  anim.saliva.buffer <<- -33.3 + 165.8/(1 + 10^(pH - 6.4)) # mEq/L
  # Fiber
  rum.NDF.conc <<- sum(ifelse(rum.fd.CHOB3_kd.fracprate <=0, 0, rum.fd.DCHOB3.rate * 1000/(rum.fd.CHOB3_kd.fracprate*24/100)))/(1000 * Vr) # g/L
  rum.NDF.pHc <<- 2.388 + 0.00078 * CECNDF # mmol/kg NDF
  rum.NDF.buffer <<- -0.004 + 0.3 * exp(-(pH - rum.NDF.pHc)) # mEq/g NDF
  rum.buffer <<- anim.saliva.conc * anim.saliva.buffer + rum.NDF.conc * rum.NDF.buffer # mEq/L
  rum.acidity <<- rum.acetate.conc * (1 - fAu) + rum.propionate.conc * (1 - fPu) + rum.butyrate.conc * (1 - fBu) + rum.lactate.conc * (1 - fLu) # mEq/L
  rum.pH_ArgyleBaldwin <<- 7.2 - 0.01 * (rum.acetate.conc + rum.propionate.conc + rum.butyrate.conc) + 0.0015 * (rum.lactate.conc)
  if (genRPT == TRUE)
  {
    rptMethane <- fds["FeedName.x"]
```

```
    names(rptMethane) <- "FeedName"
    rptMethane["Acid A4"] <- rum.fd.CHOA4.acid.rate * 1000
    rptMethane["Acid B1"] <- rum.fd.CHOB1.acid.rate * 1000
    rptMethane["Acid B2"] <- rum.fd.CHOB2.acid.rate * 1000
    rptMethane["Acid B3"] <- rum.fd.CHOB3.acid.rate * 1000
    rptMethane["Ac A4"] <- rum.fd.CHOA4.acetate.rate * 1000
    rptMethane["Ac B1"] <- rum.fd.CHOB1.acetate.rate * 1000
    rptMethane["Ac B2"] <- rum.fd.CHOB2.acetate.rate * 1000
    rptMethane["Ac B3"] <- rum.fd.CHOB3.acetate.rate * 1000
    rptMethane["Acetate"] <- rum.fd.acetate.rate * 1000
    rptMethane["Prop A4"] <- rum.fd.CHOA4.propionate.rate * 1000
    rptMethane["Prop B1"] <- rum.fd.CHOB1.propionate.rate * 1000
    rptMethane["Prop B2"] <- rum.fd.CHOB2.propionate.rate * 1000
    rptMethane["Prop B3"] <- rum.fd.CHOB3.propionate.rate * 1000
    rptMethane["Propionate"] <- rum.fd.propionate.rate * 1000
    rptMethane["But A4"] <- rum.fd.CHOA4.butyrate.rate * 1000
    rptMethane["But B1"] <- rum.fd.CHOB1.butyrate.rate * 1000
    rptMethane["But B2"] <- rum.fd.CHOB2.butyrate.rate * 1000
    rptMethane["But B3"] <- rum.fd.CHOB3.butyrate.rate * 1000
    rptMethane["Butyrate"] <- rum.fd.butyrate.rate * 1000
    rptMethane["Lact A4"] <- rum.fd.CHOA4.lactate.rate * 1000
    rptMethane["Lact B1"] <- rum.fd.CHOB1.lactate.rate * 1000
    rptMethane["Lact B2"] <- rum.fd.CHOB2.lactate.rate * 1000
    rptMethane["Lact B3"] <- rum.fd.CHOB3.lactate.rate * 1000
    rptMethane["Lactate"] <- rum.fd.lactate.rate * 1000
    rptMethane["CH4 A4"] <- rum.fd.CHOA4.methane.rate * 1000
    rptMethane["CH4 B1"] <- rum.fd.CHOB1.methane.rate * 1000
    rptMethane["CH4 B2"] <- rum.fd.CHOB2.methane.rate * 1000
    rptMethane["CH4 B3"] <- rum.fd.CHOB3.methane.rate * 1000
    rptMethane["CH4"] <- rum.fd.methane.rate * 1000
    # Methane conversions
    # 13.3 Mcal/kg and 16 g/mol
    # 0.6556 g/L (kg/m^3) at 25 oC and 1 atm
    # 0.716 g/L (kg/m^3) at 0 oC and 1 atm
    CH4_VFA_g <- sum(rum.fd.methane.rate * 1000)
    CH4_VFA_L <- CH4_VFA_g/0.6556
    CH4_VFA_Mcal <- (CH4_VFA_g/1000)*13.3
    CH4_VFA_FOM <- CH4_VFA_g/anim.diet.FOMI.rate
    CH4_VFA_DM <- CH4_VFA_g/anim.diet.DMI.rate
    CH4_VFAL_g <- CH4_VFA_g + (rum.diet.RDL.rate*1000)*0.08*(16/90)
    CH4_VFAL_L <- CH4_VFAL_g/0.6556
    CH4_VFAL_Mcal <- (CH4_VFAL_g/1000)*13.3
    CH4_VFAL_FOM <- CH4_VFAL_g/anim.diet.FOMI.rate
    CH4_VFAL_DM <- CH4_VFAL_g/anim.diet.DMI.rate
    description <- paste("Ruminal pH                    Methane production\n",
                     "   Current pH              : ", formatC(pH, format="f", digits=3, width=5),
" Source                     g/d       L/d   Mcal/d  g/kg OM  g/kg DM\n",
                     "   peNDF pH                : ", formatC(ifelse(existsnonNA("rum.pH_peNDF"), rum.pH_peNDF, 0), for-
mat="f", digits=3, width=5),   "     VFA             : ", formatC(CH4_VFA_g, format="f", digits=2, width=7), "  ",
formatC(CH4_VFA_L, format="f", digits=3, width=7), "  ", formatC(CH4_VFA_Mcal, format="f", digits=3, width=7), "  ",
formatC(CH4_VFA_FOM, format="f", digits=3, width=7), "  ", formatC(CH4_VFA_DM, format="f", digits=3, width=7), "\n",
```

```
"   VFA pH (optimized)         : ", ifelse(existsnonNA("rum.pH_VFA"), formatC(rum.pH_VFA, format="f", digits=3, width=5), "   NA"), "       VFA + lactate : ", formatC(CH4_VFAL_g, format="f", digits=2, width=7), "  ", formatC(CH4_VFAL_L, format="f", digits=3, width=7), "  ", formatC(CH4_VFAL_Mcal, format="f", digits=3, width=7), "  ", formatC(CH4_VFAL_FOM, format="f", digits=3, width=7), "  ", formatC(CH4_VFAL_DM, format="f", digits=3, width=7), "\n",
"      Equivalent peNDF        : ", ifelse(existsnonNA("rum.pH_VFA"), formatC(optimize(function(x) abs(calcRumenpH_peNDF(flag_ph, x) - rum.pH_VFA),interval=c(1, 40),maximum=F)$minimum, format="f", digits=3, width=7), "   NA"), "\n",
"   Argyle and Baldwin (1988): ", formatC(rum.pH_ArgyleBaldwin, format="f", digits=3, width=5), "\n",
"      Equivalent peNDF        : ", formatC(optimize(function(x) abs(calcRumenpH_peNDF(flag_ph, x) - rum.pH_ArgyleBaldwin),interval=c(1, 40),maximum=F)$minimum, format="f", digits=3, width=7), "\n",
"Mass fractions                      Mass fractions\n",
"   CHOA4 -> lactate           : ", formatC(ratio.CHOA4.Lact, format="f", digits=3, width=5), "     CHOB1 -> lactate          : ", formatC(ratio.CHOB1.Lact, format="f", digits=3, width=5), "\n",
"   CHOB2 -> lactate           : ", formatC(ratio.CHOB2.Lact, format="f", digits=3, width=5), "     CHOB3 -> lactate          : ", formatC(ratio.CHOB3.Lact, format="f", digits=3, width=5), "\n",
"   CHOA4 -> butyrate          : ", formatC(ratio.CHOA4.But, format="f", digits=3, width=5), "     CHOB1 -> butyrate         : ", formatC(ratio.CHOB1.But, format="f", digits=3, width=5), "\n",
"   CHOB2 -> butyrate          : ", formatC(ratio.CHOB2.But, format="f", digits=3, width=5), "     CHOB3 -> butyrate         : ", formatC(ratio.CHOB3.But, format="f", digits=3, width=5), "\n",
"   CHOA4 -> C2:C3             : ", formatC(ratio.CHOA4.C2C3, format="f", digits=3, width=5), "     CHOB1 -> C2:C3            : ", formatC(ratio.CHOB1.C2C3, format="f", digits=3, width=5), "\n",
"   CHOB2 -> C2:C3             : ", formatC(ratio.CHOB2.C2C3, format="f", digits=3, width=5), "     CHOB3 -> C2:C3            : ", formatC(ratio.CHOB3.C2C3, format="f", digits=3, width=5), "\n",
"Proportion of C3/(C2 + C3 + C4)       Methane yield, g/g\n",
"   CHO A4 (sugars)            : ", formatC(fracP.CHOA4, format="f", digits=3, width=5), "      CHO A4 (sugars)          : ", formatC(rum.CHOA4.methane.Y.frac, format="f", digits=3, width=5), "\n",
"   CHO B1 (starch)            : ", formatC(fracP.CHOB1, format="f", digits=3, width=5), "      CHO B1 (starch)          : ", formatC(rum.CHOB1.methane.Y.frac, format="f", digits=3, width=5), "\n",
"   CHO B2 (Soluble fiber)     : ", formatC(fracP.CHOB2, format="f", digits=3, width=5), "      CHO B2 (Soluble fiber)   : ", formatC(rum.CHOB2.methane.Y.frac, format="f", digits=3, width=5), "\n",
"   CHO B3 (Available fiber) : ", formatC(fracP.CHOB3, format="f", digits=3, width=5), "      CHO B3 (Available fiber) : ", formatC(rum.CHOB3.methane.Y.frac, format="f", digits=3, width=5), "\n\n", sep="")
    footnote <- "Methane production from VFA + lactate assumes an yield of 0.01422 mol methane/mol degraded lactate."
    if (existsnonNA("pH.optimum") == TRUE)
    {
      if (pH == pH.optimum)
      {
        report(rptMethane, "Volatile Fatty Acids, Lactate, and Methane Productions, g/d (* using VFA ruminal pH *)", description, footnote, 2, 2, 1, 8, TRUE, FALSE, FALSE, FALSE, FALSE, FALSE, TRUE, 2)
      } else
      {
        if (pH == rum.pH_peNDF)
        {
          report(rptMethane, "Volatile Fatty Acids, Lactate, and Methane Productions, g/d (* using peNDF ruminal pH *)", description, footnote, 2, 2, 1, 8, TRUE, FALSE, FALSE, FALSE, FALSE, FALSE, TRUE, 2)
        } else
        {
          report(rptMethane, "Volatile Fatty Acids, Lactate, and Methane Productions, g/d (* using VFA ruminal pH *)", description, footnote, 2, 2, 1, 8, TRUE, FALSE, FALSE, FALSE, FALSE, FALSE, TRUE, 2)
        }
      }
```

```
    } else
    {
      if (pH == rum.pH_peNDF)
      {
        report(rptMethane, "Volatile Fatty Acids, Lactate, and Methane Productions, g/d (* using peNDF ruminal pH *)", description, footnote, 2, 2, 1, 8, TRUE, FALSE, FALSE, FALSE, FALSE, FALSE, TRUE, 2)
      } else
      {
        report(rptMethane, "Volatile Fatty Acids, Lactate, and Methane Productions, g/d (* using VFA ruminal pH *)", description, footnote, 2, 2, 1, 8, TRUE, FALSE, FALSE, FALSE, FALSE, FALSE, TRUE, 2)
      }
    }

    # Lactate
    rptLactate <- fds["FeedName.x"]
    names(rptLactate) <- "FeedName"
    rptLactate["A4->Lact"] <- rum.fd.CHOA4.lactate.rate * 1000
    rptLactate["B1->Lact"] <- rum.fd.CHOB1.lactate.rate * 1000
    rptLactate["B2->Lact"] <- rum.fd.CHOB2.lactate.rate * 1000
    rptLactate["B3->Lact"] <- rum.fd.CHOB3.lactate.rate * 1000
    rptLactate["Diet Lact"] <- anim.fd.lactate.rate * 1000
    rptLactate["Total Lact"] <- rum.fd.lactate.rate * 1000
    rptLactate["RDL"] <- rum.fd.RDL.rate * 1000
    rptLactate["M.e."] <- rum.fd.bact.elsdenii.rate * 1000
    rptLactate["Lactate"] <- rum.fd.lactate.rate * 1000 - rum.fd.RDL.rate * 1000
    rptLactate["RDL->VFA"] <- rum.fd.lactate.VFA.rate * 1000
    rptLactate["Lact->Ac"] <- rum.fd.lactate.acetate.rate * 1000
    rptLactate["Lact->Prop"] <- rum.fd.lactate.propionate.rate * 1000
    rptLactate["Lact->But"] <- rum.fd.lactate.butyrate.rate * 1000
    rptLactate["Ac"] <- rum.fd.acetate.rate * 1000
    rptLactate["Prop"] <- rum.fd.propionate.rate * 1000
    rptLactate["But"] <- rum.fd.butyrate.rate * 1000
    description <- paste("Megasphaera elsdenii (M.e.)                              Lactate (Lact) fractional rates, %/d\n",
                        "   Maximum yield (Yg), g/g                    : ", formatC(rum.bact.elsdenii.Yg, format="f", digits=3, width=8), "      Degradation (kd)                    : ", formatC(kdL, format="f", digits=3, width=8), "\n",
                        "   Maintenance coefficient (m), g/(g.d)  : ", formatC(rum.bact.elsdenii.m, format="f", digits=3, width=8), "      Liquid passage (kp)                   : ", formatC(kl, format="f", digits=3, width=8), "\n",
                        "   Net growth rate on lactate, 1/h           : ", formatC(rum.bact.elsdenii.u, format="f", digits=3, width=8), "      Absorption (ka)                       : ", formatC(kaL, format="f", digits=3, width=8), "\n",
                        "   Yield (Y), g/g                             : ", formatC(rum.bact.elsdenii.Y, format="f", digits=3, width=8), "\n",
                        "   Mass, g/d                                  : ", formatC(rum.diet.bact.elsdenii.rate, format="f", digits=3, width=8), "\n",
                        "Rumen dimensions                                          Mass fractions\n",
                        "   Volume, L                                  : ", formatC(rum.volume, format="f", digits=3, width=8), "      Lactate -> acetate                 : ", formatC(ratio.lactate.C2, format="f", digits=3, width=8), "\n",
                        "   Volume, m^3                                : ", formatC(Vr, format="f", digits=3, width=8),                "      Lactate -> propionate              : ", formatC(ratio.lactate.C3, format="f", digits=3, width=8), "\n",
                        "   Surface (epithelial) area, m^2             : ", formatC(Ar, format="f", digits=3, width=8),                "      Lactate -> butyrate                : ", formatC(ratio.lactate.C4, format="f", digits=3, width=8), "\n",
                        "Absorption rates, %/d                                     Rumen acid concentration, mM (mol/m^3)\n",
```

```
                  "   Acetate (Ac)                          : ", formatC(kaA, format="f", digits=3, width=8), "
Lactate (Lact)                  : ", formatC(rum.lactate.conc, format="f", digits=3, width=8), "\n",
                  "   Propionate (Prop)                     : ", formatC(kaP, format="f", digits=3, width=8), "      Ac-
etate (Ac)                  : ", formatC(rum.acetate.conc, format="f", digits=3, width=8), "\n",
                  "   Butyrate (But)                        : ", formatC(kaB, format="f", digits=3, width=8), "
Propionate (Prop)               : ", formatC(rum.propionate.conc, format="f", digits=3, width=8), "\n",
                  "Rumen buffering capacity                                  Butyrate (But)                  : ",
formatC(rum.butyrate.conc, format="f", digits=3, width=8), "\n",
                  "   Saliva rate, L/d                      : ", formatC(anim.saliva.rate, format="f", digits=3,
width=8), "\n",
                  "   Saliva concentration, L/L             : ", formatC(anim.saliva.conc, format="f", digits=3,
width=8), "\n",
                  "   Saliva buffering capacity, mEq/L      : ", formatC(anim.saliva.buffer, format="f", digits=3,
width=8), "\n",
                  "   NDF concentration, g/L                : ", formatC(rum.NDF.conc, format="f", digits=3, width=8),
"\n",
                  "   NDF buffering capacity, mEq/L         : ", formatC(rum.NDF.buffer, format="f", digits=3, width=8),
"\n",
                  "   Rumen buffering capacity, mEq/L       : ", formatC(rum.buffer, format="f", digits=3, width=8),
"\n",
                  "   Rumen acidity, mEq/L                  : ", formatC(rum.acidity, format="f", digits=3, width=8),
"\n\n", sep="")
    footnote <- paste("RDL is Ruminally degraded lactate, M.e. is Megasphaera elsdenii\n", "Saliva rate lower than 100 L/d
might be incorrect.\nEstimates were ", formatC(Ds, format="f", digits=1, width=5), " L/d for Pitt et al. (1996) and ",
formatC(SaIn, format="f", digits=1, width=5), " L/d for Argyle and Baldwin (1988).", sep="")
    if (pH == rum.pH_peNDF)
    {
      report(rptLactate, "Lactate Fermentation, g/d (* using peNDF ruminal pH *)", description, footnote, 2, 2, 1, 8, TRUE,
FALSE, FALSE, FALSE, FALSE, FALSE, TRUE, 3)
    } else
    {
      report(rptLactate, "Lactate Fermentation, g/d (* using VFA ruminal pH *)", description, footnote, 2, 2, 1, 8, TRUE,
FALSE, FALSE, FALSE, FALSE, FALSE, TRUE, 3)
    }
  }
  diff <- (rum.acidity-rum.buffer)^2
  return(invisible(diff))
}
```

4.3.10 Duodenum submodel

```
calcDuodenum <- function(fds = feeds3, genRPT = TRUE)
{
  # +++++++++++++++++++
  # Duodenal Submodel
  # +++++++++++++++++++
  # E = Escaped
  # U = Undegraded
  # Carbohydrate - Feed
  duo.fd.CHOA1.rate <<- rum.fd.ECHOA1.rate <<- anim.fd.CHOA1.rate + rum.fd.LGlycerol.propionate.rate - rum.fd.DCHOA1.rate
  duo.fd.CHOA2.rate <<- rum.fd.ECHOA2.rate <<- anim.fd.CHOA2.rate - rum.fd.DCHOA2.rate
  duo.fd.CHOA3.rate <<- rum.fd.ECHOA3.rate <<- anim.fd.CHOA3.rate - rum.fd.DCHOA3.rate
  duo.fd.CHOA4.rate <<- rum.fd.ECHOA4.rate <<- anim.fd.CHOA4.rate - rum.fd.DCHOA4.rate
  duo.fd.CHOB1.rate <<- rum.fd.ECHOB1.rate <<- anim.fd.CHOB1.rate - rum.fd.DCHOB1.rate
  duo.fd.CHOB2.rate <<- rum.fd.ECHOB2.rate <<- anim.fd.CHOB2.rate - rum.fd.DCHOB2.rate
  duo.fd.CHOB3.rate <<- rum.fd.ECHOB3.rate <<- anim.fd.CHOB3.rate - rum.fd.DCHOB3.rate
  duo.fd.CHOC.rate <<- rum.fd.ECHOC.rate <<- anim.fd.CHOC.rate - rum.fd.DCHOC.rate
  duo.fd.CHO.rate <<- duo.fd.CHOA1.rate + duo.fd.CHOA2.rate + duo.fd.CHOA3.rate + duo.fd.CHOA4.rate + duo.fd.CHOB1.rate +
duo.fd.CHOB2.rate + duo.fd.CHOB3.rate + duo.fd.CHOC.rate
  duo.diet.CHOA1.rate <<- rum.diet.ECHOA1.rate <<- sum(rum.fd.ECHOA1.rate)
  duo.diet.CHOA2.rate <<- rum.diet.ECHOA2.rate <<- sum(rum.fd.ECHOA2.rate)
  duo.diet.CHOA3.rate <<- rum.diet.ECHOA3.rate <<- sum(rum.fd.ECHOA3.rate)
  duo.diet.CHOA4.rate <<- rum.diet.ECHOA4.rate <<- sum(rum.fd.ECHOA4.rate)
  duo.diet.CHOB1.rate <<- rum.diet.ECHOB1.rate <<- sum(rum.fd.ECHOB1.rate)
  duo.diet.CHOB2.rate <<- rum.diet.ECHOB2.rate <<- sum(rum.fd.ECHOB2.rate)
  duo.diet.CHOB3.rate <<- rum.diet.ECHOB3.rate <<- sum(rum.fd.ECHOB3.rate)
  duo.diet.CHOC.rate <<- rum.diet.ECHOC.rate <<- sum(rum.fd.ECHOC.rate)
  if (genRPT)
  {
    rptDuoCHO_DMI <- fds["FeedName.x"]
    names(rptDuoCHO_DMI) <- "FeedName"
    rptDuoCHO_DMI["CHO A1"] <- duo.fd.CHOA1.rate
    rptDuoCHO_DMI["CHO A2"] <- duo.fd.CHOA2.rate
    rptDuoCHO_DMI["CHO A3"] <- duo.fd.CHOA3.rate
    rptDuoCHO_DMI["CHO A4"] <- duo.fd.CHOA4.rate
    rptDuoCHO_DMI["CHO B1"] <- duo.fd.CHOB1.rate
    rptDuoCHO_DMI["CHO B2"] <- duo.fd.CHOB2.rate
    rptDuoCHO_DMI["CHO B3"] <- duo.fd.CHOB3.rate
    report(rptDuoCHO_DMI, "Duodenal Dietary Carbohydrate (Ruminally Escaped Carbohydrate), g/d", "", "", 3, 3, 1000, 8, TRUE,
FALSE, TRUE, FALSE, TRUE, FALSE, FALSE)
  }
  # Carbohydrate - Bacteria
  duo.fd.bact.NFC_CHO.rate <<- rum.fd.bact.NFC_CHO.rate
  duo.fd.bact.FC_CHO.rate <<- rum.fd.bact.FC_CHO.rate
  duo.fd.bact.CHO.rate <<- rum.fd.bact.CHO.rate
  duo.fd.bact.NFC_CHOA.rate <<- rum.fd.bact.NFC_CHOA.rate
  duo.fd.bact.FC_CHOA.rate <<- rum.fd.bact.FC_CHOA.rate
  duo.fd.bact.CHOA.rate <<- rum.fd.bact.CHOA.rate
  duo.fd.bact.NFC_CHOB1.rate <<- rum.fd.bact.NFC_CHOB1.rate
```

```
  duo.fd.bact.FC_CHOB1.rate <<- rum.fd.bact.FC_CHOB1.rate
  duo.fd.bact.CHOB1.rate <<- rum.fd.bact.CHOB1.rate
  duo.diet.bact.NFC_CHO.rate <<- rum.diet.bact.NFC_CHO.rate
  duo.diet.bact.FC_CHO.rate <<- rum.diet.bact.FC_CHO.rate
  duo.diet.bact.CHO.rate <<- rum.diet.bact.CHO.rate
  duo.diet.bact.NFC_CHOA.rate <<- rum.diet.bact.NFC_CHOA.rate
  duo.diet.bact.FC_CHOA.rate <<- rum.diet.bact.FC_CHOA.rate
  duo.diet.bact.CHOA.rate <<- rum.diet.bact.CHOA.rate
  duo.diet.bact.NFC_CHOB1.rate <<- rum.diet.bact.NFC_CHOB1.rate
  duo.diet.bact.FC_CHOB1.rate <<- rum.diet.bact.FC_CHOB1.rate
  duo.diet.bact.CHOB1.rate <<- rum.diet.bact.CHOB1.rate
  if (genRPT)
  {
    rptDuoCHO_DMI <- fds["FeedName.x"]
    names(rptDuoCHO_DMI) <- "FeedName"
    rptDuoCHO_DMI["CHOA"] <- duo.fd.bact.CHOA.rate
    rptDuoCHO_DMI["CHO B1"] <- duo.fd.bact.CHOB1.rate
    report(rptDuoCHO_DMI, "\nDuodenal Bacterial Carbohydrate, g/d", "", "", 3, 3, 1000, 8, TRUE, FALSE, TRUE, FALSE, TRUE,
FALSE, TRUE)
  }
  # Protein - Feed
  duo.fd.ProtA.rate <<- rum.fd.EProtA.rate <<- anim.fd.ProtA.rate - rum.fd.DProtA.rate
  duo.fd.ProtB1.rate <<- rum.fd.EProtB1.rate <<- anim.fd.ProtB1.rate - rum.fd.DProtB1.rate
  duo.fd.ProtB2.rate <<- rum.fd.EProtB2.rate <<- anim.fd.ProtB2.rate - rum.fd.DProtB2.rate
  duo.fd.ProtB3.rate <<- rum.fd.EProtB3.rate <<- anim.fd.ProtB3.rate - rum.fd.DProtB3.rate
  duo.fd.ProtC.rate <<- rum.fd.EProtC.rate <<- anim.fd.ProtC.rate - rum.fd.DProtC.rate
  duo.fd.RUTP.rate <<- rum.fd.RUTP.rate <<- rum.fd.EProtB1.rate + rum.fd.EProtB2.rate + rum.fd.EProtB3.rate
  duo.fd.RUCP.rate <<- rum.fd.RUCP.rate <<- rum.fd.EProtA.rate + rum.fd.RUTP.rate + rum.fd.EProtC.rate
  duo.diet.ProtA.rate <<- rum.diet.EProtA.rate <<- sum(rum.fd.EProtA.rate)
  duo.diet.ProtB1.rate <<- rum.diet.EProtB1.rate <<- sum(rum.fd.EProtB1.rate)
  duo.diet.ProtB2.rate <<- rum.diet.EProtB2.rate <<- sum(rum.fd.EProtB2.rate)
  duo.diet.ProtB3.rate <<- rum.diet.EProtB3.rate <<- sum(rum.fd.EProtB3.rate)
  duo.diet.ProtC.rate <<- rum.diet.EProtC.rate <<- sum(rum.fd.EProtC.rate)
  duo.diet.RUTP.rate <<- rum.diet.RUTP.rate <<- sum(rum.fd.RUTP.rate)
  duo.diet.RUCP.rate <<- rum.diet.RUCP.rate <<- sum(rum.fd.RUCP.rate)
  if (genRPT)
  {
    rptDuoProt_DMI <- fds["FeedName.x"]
    names(rptDuoProt_DMI) <- "FeedName"
    rptDuoProt_DMI["Prot A"] <- duo.fd.ProtA.rate
    rptDuoProt_DMI["Prot B1"] <- duo.fd.ProtB1.rate
    rptDuoProt_DMI["Prot B2"] <- duo.fd.ProtB2.rate
    rptDuoProt_DMI["Prot B3"] <- duo.fd.ProtB3.rate
    rptDuoProt_DMI["Prot C"] <- duo.fd.ProtC.rate
    report(rptDuoProt_DMI, "Duodenal Dietary Protein (Ruminally Escaped Protein), g/d", "", "", 3, 3, 1000, 8, TRUE, FALSE,
TRUE, FALSE, TRUE, FALSE, FALSE)
  }
  # Protein - Bacteria
  duo.fd.bact.NFC_CP.rate <<- rum.fd.bact.NFC_CP.rate
  duo.fd.bact.FC_CP.rate <<- rum.fd.bact.FC_CP.rate
  duo.fd.bact.CP.rate <<- rum.fd.bact.CP.rate
```

```
    duo.fd.bact.NFC_TP.rate <<- rum.fd.bact.NFC_TP.rate
    duo.fd.bact.FC_TP.rate <<- rum.fd.bact.FC_TP.rate
    duo.fd.bact.TP.rate <<- rum.fd.bact.TP.rate
    duo.fd.bact.NFC_NA.rate <<- rum.fd.bact.NFC_NA.rate
    duo.fd.bact.FC_NA.rate <<- rum.fd.bact.FC_NA.rate
    duo.fd.bact.NA.rate <<- rum.fd.bact.NA.rate
    duo.fd.bact.NFC_CW.rate <<- rum.fd.bact.NFC_CW.rate
    duo.fd.bact.FC_CW.rate <<- rum.fd.bact.FC_CW.rate
    duo.fd.bact.CW.rate <<- rum.fd.bact.CW.rate
    duo.diet.bact.NFC_CP.rate <<- rum.diet.bact.NFC_CP.rate
    duo.diet.bact.FC_CP.rate <<- rum.diet.bact.FC_CP.rate
    duo.diet.bact.CP.rate <<- rum.diet.bact.CP.rate
    duo.diet.bact.NFC_TP.rate <<- rum.diet.bact.NFC_TP.rate
    duo.diet.bact.FC_TP.rate <<- rum.diet.bact.FC_TP.rate
    duo.diet.bact.TP.rate <<- rum.diet.bact.TP.rate
    duo.diet.bact.NFC_NA.rate <<- rum.diet.bact.NFC_NA.rate
    duo.diet.bact.FC_NA.rate <<- rum.diet.bact.FC_NA.rate
    duo.diet.bact.NA.rate <<- rum.diet.bact.NA.rate
    duo.diet.bact.NFC_CW.rate <<- rum.diet.bact.NFC_CW.rate
    duo.diet.bact.FC_CW.rate <<- rum.diet.bact.FC_CW.rate
    duo.diet.bact.CW.rate <<- rum.diet.bact.CW.rate
    if (genRPT)
    {
      rptDuoProt_DMI <- fds["FeedName.x"]
      names(rptDuoProt_DMI) <- "FeedName"
      rptDuoProt_DMI["Bact CP"] <- duo.fd.bact.CP.rate
      rptDuoProt_DMI["Bact TP"] <- duo.fd.bact.TP.rate
      rptDuoProt_DMI["Bact CW"] <- duo.fd.bact.CW.rate
      report(rptDuoProt_DMI, "\nDuodenal Bacterial Protein, g/d", "", "", 3, 3, 1000, 8, TRUE, FALSE, TRUE, FALSE, TRUE, FALSE, TRUE)
    }
    # Amino Acids - Feed
    duo.fd.RUCP.rate <<- rum.fd.RUCP.rate
    duo.fd.RUTP.rate <<- rum.fd.RUTP.rate
    duo.fd.Met.rate <<- (fds[, "Met_RUP"]/100) * duo.fd.RUTP.rate
    duo.fd.Lys.rate <<- (fds[, "Lys_RUP"]/100) * duo.fd.RUTP.rate
    duo.fd.Arg.rate <<- (fds[, "Arg_RUP"]/100) * duo.fd.RUTP.rate
    duo.fd.Thr.rate <<- (fds[, "Thr_RUP"]/100) * duo.fd.RUTP.rate
    duo.fd.Leu.rate <<- (fds[, "Leu_RUP"]/100) * duo.fd.RUTP.rate
    duo.fd.Ile.rate <<- (fds[, "Ile_RUP"]/100) * duo.fd.RUTP.rate
    duo.fd.Val.rate <<- (fds[, "Val_RUP"]/100) * duo.fd.RUTP.rate
    duo.fd.His.rate <<- (fds[, "His_RUP"]/100) * duo.fd.RUTP.rate
    duo.fd.Phe.rate <<- (fds[, "Phe_RUP"]/100) * duo.fd.RUTP.rate
    duo.fd.Trp.rate <<- (fds[, "Trp_RUP"]/100) * duo.fd.RUTP.rate
    duo.diet.RUCP.rate <<- sum(duo.fd.RUCP.rate)
    duo.diet.RUTP.rate <<- sum(duo.fd.RUTP.rate)
    duo.diet.Met.rate <<- sum(duo.fd.Met.rate)
    duo.diet.Lys.rate <<- sum(duo.fd.Lys.rate)
    duo.diet.Arg.rate <<- sum(duo.fd.Arg.rate)
    duo.diet.Thr.rate <<- sum(duo.fd.Thr.rate)
    duo.diet.Leu.rate <<- sum(duo.fd.Leu.rate)
```

```
duo.diet.Ile.rate <<- sum(duo.fd.Ile.rate)
duo.diet.Val.rate <<- sum(duo.fd.Val.rate)
duo.diet.His.rate <<- sum(duo.fd.His.rate)
duo.diet.Phe.rate <<- sum(duo.fd.Phe.rate)
duo.diet.Trp.rate <<- sum(duo.fd.Trp.rate)
if (genRPT)
{
  rptDuoAA_DMI <- fds["FeedName.x"]
  names(rptDuoAA_DMI) <- "FeedName"
  rptDuoAA_DMI["Met"] <- duo.fd.Met.rate
  rptDuoAA_DMI["Lys"] <- duo.fd.Lys.rate
  rptDuoAA_DMI["Arg"] <- duo.fd.Arg.rate
  rptDuoAA_DMI["Thr"] <- duo.fd.Thr.rate
  rptDuoAA_DMI["Leu"] <- duo.fd.Leu.rate
  rptDuoAA_DMI["Ile"] <- duo.fd.Ile.rate
  rptDuoAA_DMI["His"] <- duo.fd.His.rate
  rptDuoAA_DMI["Phe"] <- duo.fd.Phe.rate
  rptDuoAA_DMI["Trp"] <- duo.fd.Trp.rate
  report(rptDuoAA_DMI, "Duodenal Dietary Amino Acids, g/d", "", "", 3, 3, 1000, 8, TRUE, FALSE, TRUE, FALSE, TRUE, FALSE, TRUE)
}
# Amino Acids - Bacteria
duo.fd.bact.Met.rate <<- rum.fd.bact.TP.rate * rum.bact.NCW_Met.frac + rum.fd.bact.CW.rate * rum.bact.CW_Met.frac
duo.fd.bact.Lys.rate <<- rum.fd.bact.TP.rate * rum.bact.NCW_Lys.frac + rum.fd.bact.CW.rate * rum.bact.CW_Lys.frac
duo.fd.bact.Arg.rate <<- rum.fd.bact.TP.rate * rum.bact.NCW_Arg.frac + rum.fd.bact.CW.rate * rum.bact.CW_Arg.frac
duo.fd.bact.Thr.rate <<- rum.fd.bact.TP.rate * rum.bact.NCW_Thr.frac + rum.fd.bact.CW.rate * rum.bact.CW_Thr.frac
duo.fd.bact.Leu.rate <<- rum.fd.bact.TP.rate * rum.bact.NCW_Leu.frac + rum.fd.bact.CW.rate * rum.bact.CW_Leu.frac
duo.fd.bact.Ile.rate <<- rum.fd.bact.TP.rate * rum.bact.NCW_Ile.frac + rum.fd.bact.CW.rate * rum.bact.CW_Ile.frac
duo.fd.bact.Val.rate <<- rum.fd.bact.TP.rate * rum.bact.NCW_Val.frac + rum.fd.bact.CW.rate * rum.bact.CW_Val.frac
duo.fd.bact.His.rate <<- rum.fd.bact.TP.rate * rum.bact.NCW_His.frac + rum.fd.bact.CW.rate * rum.bact.CW_His.frac
duo.fd.bact.Phe.rate <<- rum.fd.bact.TP.rate * rum.bact.NCW_Phe.frac + rum.fd.bact.CW.rate * rum.bact.CW_Phe.frac
duo.fd.bact.Trp.rate <<- rum.fd.bact.TP.rate * rum.bact.NCW_Trp.frac + rum.fd.bact.CW.rate * rum.bact.CW_Trp.frac
duo.diet.bact.Met.rate <<- sum(duo.fd.bact.Met.rate)
duo.diet.bact.Lys.rate <<- sum(duo.fd.bact.Lys.rate)
duo.diet.bact.Arg.rate <<- sum(duo.fd.bact.Arg.rate)
duo.diet.bact.Thr.rate <<- sum(duo.fd.bact.Thr.rate)
duo.diet.bact.Leu.rate <<- sum(duo.fd.bact.Leu.rate)
duo.diet.bact.Ile.rate <<- sum(duo.fd.bact.Ile.rate)
duo.diet.bact.Val.rate <<- sum(duo.fd.bact.Val.rate)
duo.diet.bact.His.rate <<- sum(duo.fd.bact.His.rate)
duo.diet.bact.Phe.rate <<- sum(duo.fd.bact.Phe.rate)
duo.diet.bact.Trp.rate <<- sum(duo.fd.bact.Trp.rate)
if (genRPT)
{
  rptDuoBactAA_DMI <- fds["FeedName.x"]
  names(rptDuoBactAA_DMI) <- "FeedName"
  rptDuoBactAA_DMI["Met"] <- duo.fd.bact.Met.rate
  rptDuoBactAA_DMI["Lys"] <- duo.fd.bact.Lys.rate
  rptDuoBactAA_DMI["Arg"] <- duo.fd.bact.Arg.rate
  rptDuoBactAA_DMI["Thr"] <- duo.fd.bact.Thr.rate
  rptDuoBactAA_DMI["Leu"] <- duo.fd.bact.Leu.rate
```

```
    rptDuoBactAA_DMI["Ile"] <- duo.fd.bact.Ile.rate
    rptDuoBactAA_DMI["Val"] <- duo.fd.bact.Val.rate
    rptDuoBactAA_DMI["His"] <- duo.fd.bact.His.rate
    rptDuoBactAA_DMI["Phe"] <- duo.fd.bact.Phe.rate
    rptDuoBactAA_DMI["Trp"] <- duo.fd.bact.Trp.rate
    report(rptDuoBactAA_DMI, "Duodenal Bacterial Amino Acids, g/d", "", "", 3, 3, 1000, 8, TRUE, FALSE, TRUE, FALSE, TRUE,
FALSE, TRUE)
    rptDuoAA_DMI <- fds["FeedName.x"]
    names(rptDuoAA_DMI) <- "FeedName"
    rptDuoAA_DMI["Met"] <- duo.fd.Met.rate + duo.fd.bact.Met.rate
    rptDuoAA_DMI["Lys"] <- duo.fd.Lys.rate + duo.fd.bact.Lys.rate
    rptDuoAA_DMI["Arg"] <- duo.fd.Arg.rate + duo.fd.bact.Arg.rate
    rptDuoAA_DMI["Thr"] <- duo.fd.Thr.rate + duo.fd.bact.Thr.rate
    rptDuoAA_DMI["Leu"] <- duo.fd.Leu.rate + duo.fd.bact.Leu.rate
    rptDuoAA_DMI["Ile"] <- duo.fd.Ile.rate + duo.fd.bact.Ile.rate
    rptDuoAA_DMI["Val"] <- duo.fd.Val.rate + duo.fd.bact.Val.rate
    rptDuoAA_DMI["His"] <- duo.fd.His.rate + duo.fd.bact.His.rate
    rptDuoAA_DMI["Phe"] <- duo.fd.Phe.rate + duo.fd.bact.Phe.rate
    rptDuoAA_DMI["Trp"] <- duo.fd.Trp.rate + duo.fd.bact.Trp.rate
    report(rptDuoAA_DMI, "Duodenal Amino Acids (Feed + Bacteria), g/d", "", "", 3, 3, 1000, 8, TRUE, FALSE, TRUE, FALSE, TRUE,
FALSE, TRUE)
  }
  duo.fd.EE.rate <<- rum.fd.EFat.rate
  duo.diet.EE.rate <<- sum(duo.fd.EE.rate)
  duo.fd.FAC12.rate <<- rum.fd.EFAC12.rate + rum.fd.LEFAC12.rate
  duo.fd.FAC14.rate <<- rum.fd.EFAC14.rate + rum.fd.LEFAC14.rate
  duo.fd.FAC16.rate <<- rum.fd.EFAC16.rate + rum.fd.LEFAC16.rate + rum.fd.DNFAC16.rate
  duo.fd.FAC16_1.rate <<- rum.fd.EFAC16_1.rate + rum.fd.LEFAC16_1.rate + rum.fd.DNFAC16_1.rate
  duo.fd.FAC18.rate <<- rum.fd.EFAC18.rate + rum.fd.LEFAC18.rate + rum.fd.DNFAC18.rate
  duo.fd.FAC18_1c.rate <<- rum.fd.EFAC18_1c.rate + rum.fd.LEFAC18_1c.rate
  duo.fd.FAC18_1t.rate <<- rum.fd.EFAC18_1t.rate + rum.fd.LEFAC18_1t.rate
  duo.fd.FAC18_2.rate <<- rum.fd.EFAC18_2.rate + rum.fd.LEFAC18_2.rate
  duo.fd.FAC18_3.rate <<- rum.fd.EFAC18_3.rate + rum.fd.LEFAC18_3.rate
  duo.fd.FAOther.rate <<- rum.fd.EFAOther.rate + rum.fd.LEFAOther.rate + rum.fd.DNFAOther.rate
  duo.fd.Glycerol.rate <<- rum.fd.EGlycerol.rate
  duo.fd.Pigment.rate <<- rum.fd.EPigment.rate
  duo.diet.FAC12.rate <<- sum(duo.fd.FAC12.rate)
  duo.diet.FAC14.rate <<- sum(duo.fd.FAC14.rate)
  duo.diet.FAC16.rate <<- sum(duo.fd.FAC16.rate)
  duo.diet.FAC16_1.rate <<- sum(duo.fd.FAC16_1.rate)
  duo.diet.FAC18.rate <<- sum(duo.fd.FAC18.rate)
  duo.diet.FAC18_1c.rate <<- sum(duo.fd.FAC18_1c.rate)
  duo.diet.FAC18_1t.rate <<- sum(duo.fd.FAC18_1t.rate)
  duo.diet.FAC18_2.rate <<- sum(duo.fd.FAC18_2.rate)
  duo.diet.FAC18_3.rate <<- sum(duo.fd.FAC18_3.rate)
  duo.diet.FAOther.rate <<- sum(duo.fd.FAOther.rate)
  duo.diet.Glycerol.rate <<- sum(duo.fd.Glycerol.rate)
  duo.diet.Pigment.rate <<- sum(duo.fd.Pigment.rate)
  if (genRPT)
  {
    rptDuoFA_DMI <- fds["FeedName.x"]
```

```
      names(rptDuoFA_DMI) <- "FeedName"
      rptDuoFA_DMI["C12:0"] <- duo.fd.FAC12.rate
      rptDuoFA_DMI["C14:0"] <- duo.fd.FAC14.rate
      rptDuoFA_DMI["C16:0"] <- duo.fd.FAC16.rate
      rptDuoFA_DMI["C16:1"] <- duo.fd.FAC16_1.rate
      rptDuoFA_DMI["C18:0"] <- duo.fd.FAC18.rate
      rptDuoFA_DMI["C18:1c"] <- duo.fd.FAC18_1c.rate
      rptDuoFA_DMI["C18:1t"] <- duo.fd.FAC18_1t.rate
      rptDuoFA_DMI["C18:2"] <- duo.fd.FAC18_2.rate
      rptDuoFA_DMI["C18:3"] <- duo.fd.FAC18_3.rate
      rptDuoFA_DMI["Other FFA"] <- duo.fd.FAOther.rate
      description <- paste("Duodenal glycerol, g/d : ", formatC(duo.diet.Glycerol.rate * 1000, format = "f", digits = 3, width = 7), "\n",
                           "Duodenal pigments, g/d : ", formatC(duo.diet.Pigment.rate * 1000, format = "f", digits = 3, width = 7), "\n\n", sep = "")
      report(rptDuoFA_DMI, "Duodenal Dietary Fatty Acids, g/d", description, "", 3, 3, 1000, 8, TRUE, FALSE, TRUE, FALSE, TRUE, FALSE, TRUE)
    }
    # Fat - Bacteria
    duo.fd.bact.NFC_Fat.rate <<- rum.fd.bact.NFC_Fat.rate
    duo.fd.bact.FC_Fat.rate <<- rum.fd.bact.FC_Fat.rate
    duo.fd.bact.fat.rate <<- rum.fd.bact.fat.rate
    duo.fd.bact.FAC12.rate <<- duo.fd.bact.fat.rate * mean(c(0.4,1.2,4.6))/100
    duo.fd.bact.FAC14.rate <<- duo.fd.bact.fat.rate * mean(c(2.3,3.7,3.9))/100
    duo.fd.bact.FAC16.rate <<- duo.fd.bact.fat.rate * mean(c(25.4,31,35.2))/100
    duo.fd.bact.FAC16_1.rate <<- duo.fd.bact.fat.rate * mean(c(4))/100
    duo.fd.bact.FAC18.rate <<- duo.fd.bact.fat.rate * mean(c(15,20.8,32))/100
    duo.fd.bact.FAC18_1.rate <<- duo.fd.bact.fat.rate * mean(c(3.9,6,19.7))/100
    duo.fd.bact.FAC18_2.rate <<- duo.fd.bact.fat.rate * mean(c(2.7,3.5,5.6))/100
    duo.fd.bact.FAC18_3.rate <<- duo.fd.bact.fat.rate * mean(c(1))/100
    duo.fd.bact.FAOther.rate <<- duo.fd.bact.fat.rate * mean(c(8.8,20.2))/100
    duo.diet.bact.NFC_Fat.rate <<- rum.diet.bact.NFC_Fat.rate
    duo.diet.bact.FC_Fat.rate <<- rum.diet.bact.FC_Fat.rate
    duo.diet.bact.fat.rate <<- rum.diet.bact.fat.rate
    duo.diet.bact.FAC12.rate <<- sum(duo.fd.bact.FAC12.rate)
    duo.diet.bact.FAC14.rate <<- sum(duo.fd.bact.FAC14.rate)
    duo.diet.bact.FAC16.rate <<- sum(duo.fd.bact.FAC16.rate)
    duo.diet.bact.FAC16_1.rate <<- sum(duo.fd.bact.FAC16_1.rate)
    duo.diet.bact.FAC18.rate <<- sum(duo.fd.bact.FAC18.rate)
    duo.diet.bact.FAC18_1.rate <<- sum(duo.fd.bact.FAC18_1.rate)
    duo.diet.bact.FAC18_2.rate <<- sum(duo.fd.bact.FAC18_2.rate)
    duo.diet.bact.FAC18_3.rate <<- sum(duo.fd.bact.FAC18_3.rate)
    duo.diet.bact.FAOther.rate <<- sum(duo.fd.bact.FAOther.rate)
    if (genRPT)
    {
      rptDuoFA_DMI <- fds["FeedName.x"]
      names(rptDuoFA_DMI) <- "FeedName"
      rptDuoFA_DMI["C12:0"] <- duo.fd.bact.FAC12.rate
      rptDuoFA_DMI["C14:0"] <- duo.fd.bact.FAC14.rate
      rptDuoFA_DMI["C16:0"] <- duo.fd.bact.FAC16.rate
      rptDuoFA_DMI["C16:1"] <- duo.fd.bact.FAC16_1.rate
```

```
      rptDuoFA_DMI["C18:0"] <- duo.fd.bact.FAC18.rate
      rptDuoFA_DMI["C18:1"] <- duo.fd.bact.FAC18_1.rate
      rptDuoFA_DMI["C18:2"] <- duo.fd.bact.FAC18_2.rate
      rptDuoFA_DMI["C18:3"] <- duo.fd.bact.FAC18_3.rate
      rptDuoFA_DMI["Other FFA"] <- duo.fd.bact.FAOther.rate
      footnote <- "There is no Bacterial FA C18:1t."
      report(rptDuoFA_DMI, "Duodenal Bacteria Fatty Acids, g/d", "", footnote, 3, 3, 1000, 8, TRUE, FALSE, TRUE, FALSE, TRUE, FALSE, TRUE)
    }
    # Ash - Bacteria
    duo.fd.bact.NFC_Ash.rate <<- rum.fd.bact.NFC_Ash.rate
    duo.fd.bact.FC_Ash.rate <<- rum.fd.bact.FC_Ash.rate
    duo.fd.bact.ash.rate <<- rum.fd.bact.ash.rate
    duo.diet.bactNFC_Ash.rate <<- rum.diet.bactNFC_Ash.rate
    duo.diet.bact.FC_Ash.rate <<- rum.diet.bact.FC_Ash.rate
    duo.diet.bact.ash.rate <<- rum.diet.bact.ash.rate
  }
```

4.3.11 Small and large intestine submodels

```
calcSI <- function(fds = feeds3, genRPT = TRUE)
{
  # +++++++++++++++++++++++++++
  # Small Intestine Submodel
  # +++++++++++++++++++++++++++
  # G = Digested
  # Digested Carbohydrate - Feeds
  si.fd.CHOA1_ID.frac <<- as.numeric(fds[, "CHO_A1_ID"])/100
  si.fd.CHOA2_ID.frac <<- as.numeric(fds[, "CHO_A2_ID"])/100
  si.fd.CHOA3_ID.frac <<- as.numeric(fds[, "CHO_A3_ID"])/100
  si.fd.CHOA4_ID.frac <<- as.numeric(fds[, "CHO_A4_ID"])/100
  si.fd.CHOB1_ID.frac <<- as.numeric(fds[, "CHO_B1_ID"])/100
  si.fd.CHOB2_ID.frac <<- as.numeric(fds[, "CHO_B2_ID"])/100
  si.fd.CHOB3_ID.frac <<- as.numeric(fds[, "CHO_B3_ID"])/100
  si.fd.CHOC_ID.frac <<- 0
  si.fd.GCHOA1.rate <<- duo.fd.CHOA1.rate * si.fd.CHOA1_ID.frac
  si.fd.GCHOA2.rate <<- duo.fd.CHOA2.rate * si.fd.CHOA2_ID.frac
  si.fd.GCHOA3.rate <<- duo.fd.CHOA3.rate * si.fd.CHOA3_ID.frac
  si.fd.GCHOA4.rate <<- duo.fd.CHOA4.rate * si.fd.CHOA4_ID.frac
  si.fd.GCHOB1.rate <<- duo.fd.CHOB1.rate * si.fd.CHOB1_ID.frac
  si.fd.GCHOB2.rate <<- duo.fd.CHOB2.rate * si.fd.CHOB2_ID.frac
  si.fd.GCHOB3.rate <<- duo.fd.CHOB3.rate * si.fd.CHOB3_ID.frac
  si.fd.GCHOC.rate <<- duo.fd.CHOC.rate * si.fd.CHOC_ID.frac
  si.fd.GCHO.rate <<- si.fd.GCHOA1.rate + si.fd.GCHOA2.rate + si.fd.GCHOA3.rate + si.fd.GCHOA4.rate + si.fd.GCHOB1.rate +
si.fd.GCHOB2.rate + si.fd.GCHOB3.rate + si.fd.GCHOC.rate
  si.diet.GCHOA1.rate <<- sum(si.fd.GCHOA1.rate)
  si.diet.GCHOA2.rate <<- sum(si.fd.GCHOA2.rate)
  si.diet.GCHOA3.rate <<- sum(si.fd.GCHOA3.rate)
  si.diet.GCHOA4.rate <<- sum(si.fd.GCHOA4.rate)
  si.diet.GCHOB1.rate <<- sum(si.fd.GCHOB1.rate)
  si.diet.GCHOB2.rate <<- sum(si.fd.GCHOB2.rate)
  si.diet.GCHOB3.rate <<- sum(si.fd.GCHOB3.rate)
  si.diet.GCHOC.rate <<- sum(si.fd.GCHOC.rate)
  si.diet.GCHO.rate <<- sum(si.fd.GCHO.rate)
  if (genRPT)
  {
    rptIDCHO_DMI <- fds["FeedName.x"]
    names(rptIDCHO_DMI) <- "FeedName"
    rptIDCHO_DMI["CHO A1"] <- si.fd.GCHOA1.rate
    rptIDCHO_DMI["CHO A2"] <- si.fd.GCHOA2.rate
    rptIDCHO_DMI["CHO A3"] <- si.fd.GCHOA3.rate
    rptIDCHO_DMI["CHO A4"] <- si.fd.GCHOA4.rate
    rptIDCHO_DMI["CHO B1"] <- si.fd.GCHOB1.rate
    rptIDCHO_DMI["CHO B2"] <- si.fd.GCHOB2.rate
    rptIDCHO_DMI["CHO B3"] <- si.fd.GCHOB3.rate
    rptIDCHO_DMI["CHO C"] <- si.fd.GCHOC.rate
    report(rptIDCHO_DMI, "Small Intestinally Digested Feed Carbohydrate, g/d", "", "", 3, 3, 1000, 9, TRUE, FALSE, TRUE,
FALSE, TRUE, FALSE, FALSE)
```

```
    }
    # Digested Carbohydrate - Bacteria
    si.fd.bact.GCHOA.rate <<- (Parm_rum.bact.IDCHOA/100) * duo.fd.bact.NFC_CHOA.rate + (Parm_rum.bact.IDCHOA/100) * duo.fd.bact.FC_CHOA.rate
    si.fd.bact.GCHOB1.rate <<- (Parm_rum.bact.IDCHOB1/100) * duo.fd.bact.NFC_CHOB1.rate + (Parm_rum.bact.IDCHOB1/100) * duo.fd.bact.FC_CHOB1.rate
    si.fd.bact.GCHO.rate <<- si.fd.bact.GCHOA.rate + si.fd.bact.GCHOB1.rate
    si.diet.bact.GCHOA.rate <<- sum(si.fd.bact.GCHOA.rate)
    si.diet.bact.GCHOB1.rate <<- sum(si.fd.bact.GCHOB1.rate)
    si.diet.bact.GCHO.rate <<- sum(si.fd.bact.GCHO.rate)
    si.GCHO.rate <<- si.fd.GCHO.rate + si.fd.bact.GCHO.rate
    if (genRPT)
    {
      rptIDProt_DMI <- fds["FeedName.x"]
      names(rptIDProt_DMI) <- "FeedName"
      rptIDProt_DMI["Bact CHOA"] <- si.fd.bact.GCHOA.rate
      rptIDProt_DMI["Bact CHOB1"] <- si.fd.bact.GCHOB1.rate
      description <- paste("Small Intestinally Digested Carbohydrate, g/d\n",
                           "   Ration    : ", formatC(si.diet.GCHO.rate * 1000, format = "f", digits = 3, width = 8), "\n",
                           "   Bacteria : ", formatC(si.diet.bact.GCHO.rate * 1000, format = "f", digits = 3, width = 8), "\n",
                           "   Total     : ", formatC(sum(si.GCHO.rate) * 1000, format = "f", digits = 3, width = 8), "\n", sep = "")
      report(rptIDProt_DMI, "\nSmall Intestinally Digested Bacterial Carbohydrate, g/d", description, "", 3, 3, 1000, 8, TRUE, FALSE, TRUE, FALSE, TRUE, FALSE, TRUE)
    }
    # Digested Protein - Feeds
    si.fd.ProtA_ID.frac <<- as.numeric(fds[, "Prot_A_ID"])/100
    si.fd.ProtB1_ID.frac <<- as.numeric(fds[, "Prot_B1_ID"])/100
    si.fd.ProtB2_ID.frac <<- as.numeric(fds[, "Prot_B2_ID"])/100
    si.fd.ProtB3_ID.frac <<- as.numeric(fds[, "Prot_B3_ID"])/100
    si.fd.ProtC_ID.frac <<- 0
    si.fd.GProtA.rate <<- duo.fd.ProtA.rate * si.fd.ProtA_ID.frac
    si.fd.GProtB1.rate <<- duo.fd.ProtB1.rate * si.fd.ProtB1_ID.frac
    si.fd.GProtB2.rate <<- duo.fd.ProtB2.rate * si.fd.ProtB2_ID.frac
    si.fd.GProtB3.rate <<- duo.fd.ProtB3.rate * si.fd.ProtB3_ID.frac
    si.fd.GProtC.rate <<- duo.fd.ProtC.rate * si.fd.ProtC_ID.frac
    si.fd.GProt.rate <<- si.fd.GProtA.rate + si.fd.GProtB1.rate + si.fd.GProtB2.rate + si.fd.GProtB3.rate
    si.diet.GProtA.rate <<- sum(si.fd.GProtA.rate)
    si.diet.GProtB1.rate <<- sum(si.fd.GProtB1.rate)
    si.diet.GProtB2.rate <<- sum(si.fd.GProtB2.rate)
    si.diet.GProtB3.rate <<- sum(si.fd.GProtB3.rate)
    si.diet.GProtC.rate <<- sum(si.fd.GProtC.rate)
    si.diet.GProt.rate <<- sum(si.fd.GProt.rate)
    if (genRPT)
    {
      rptIDProt_DMI <- fds["FeedName.x"]
      names(rptIDProt_DMI) <- "FeedName"
      rptIDProt_DMI["Prot A"] <- si.fd.GProtA.rate
      rptIDProt_DMI["Prot B1"] <- si.fd.GProtB1.rate
      rptIDProt_DMI["Prot B2"] <- si.fd.GProtB2.rate
      rptIDProt_DMI["Prot B3"] <- si.fd.GProtB3.rate
```

```
        rptIDProt_DMI["Prot C"] <- si.fd.GProtC.rate
        rptIDProt_DMI["Digested"] <- si.fd.GProt.rate
        rptIDProt_DMI["RUTPD"] <- isz(si.fd.GProt.rate/10, duo.fd.RUTP.rate)  # Converting g to %
        rptIDProt_DMI["RUCPD"] <- isz(si.fd.GProt.rate/10, duo.fd.RUCP.rate)  # Converting g to %
        rptIDProt_DMI2 <- data.frame(FeedName = "Ration")
        rptIDProt_DMI2["Prot A"] <- si.diet.GProtA.rate
        rptIDProt_DMI2["Prot B1"] <- si.diet.GProtB1.rate
        rptIDProt_DMI2["Prot B2"] <- si.diet.GProtB2.rate
        rptIDProt_DMI2["Prot B3"] <- si.diet.GProtB3.rate
        rptIDProt_DMI2["Prot C"] <- si.diet.GProtC.rate
        rptIDProt_DMI2["Digested"] <- si.diet.GProt.rate
        rptIDProt_DMI2["RUTPD"] <- isz(si.diet.GProt.rate/10, duo.diet.RUTP.rate)  # Converting g to %
        rptIDProt_DMI2["RUCPD"] <- isz(si.diet.GProt.rate/10, duo.diet.RUCP.rate)  # Converting g to %
        rptIDProt_DMI <- rbind(rptIDProt_DMI, rptIDProt_DMI2)
        description <- paste("# RUTPD = Ruminally Undegraded True Protein Digestibility (PB1 + PB2 + PB3), %\n",
                             "# RUCPD = Ruminally Undegraded Crude Protein Digestibility (PA + RUTP + PC), %\n",
                             "Ration RUTP digestibility : ", formatC(isz(si.diet.GProt.rate * 100, rum.diet.RUTP.rate), format = "f", digits = 3, width = 7), "\n",
                             "Ration RUCP digestibility : ", formatC(isz(si.diet.GProt.rate * 100, rum.diet.RUCP.rate), format = "f", digits = 3, width = 7), "\n\n", sep = "")
        report(rptIDProt_DMI, "Small Intestinally Digested Feed Protein, g/d", description, "", 3, 3, 1000, 8, FALSE, FALSE, FALSE, FALSE, FALSE, FALSE, FALSE)
      }
      # Digested Protein - Bacteria
      si.fd.bact.GTP.rate <<- (Parm_rum.bact.IDTP/100) * duo.fd.bact.NFC_TP.rate + (Parm_rum.bact.IDTP/100) * duo.fd.bact.FC_TP.rate
      si.fd.bact.GNA.rate <<- (Parm_rum.bact.IDNA/100) * duo.fd.bact.NFC_NA.rate + (Parm_rum.bact.IDNA/100) * duo.fd.bact.FC_NA.rate
      si.fd.bact.GCW.rate <<- (Parm_rum.bact.IDCW/100) * duo.fd.bact.NFC_CW.rate + (Parm_rum.bact.IDCW/100) * duo.fd.bact.FC_CW.rate
      si.fd.bact.GProt.rate <<- si.fd.bact.GTP.rate + si.fd.bact.GNA.rate + si.fd.bact.GCW.rate
      si.diet.bact.GTP.rate <<- sum(si.fd.bact.GTP.rate)
      si.diet.bact.GNA.rate <<- sum(si.fd.bact.GNA.rate)
      si.diet.bact.GCW.rate <<- sum(si.fd.bact.GCW.rate)
      si.diet.bact.GProt.rate <<- sum(si.fd.bact.GProt.rate)
      si.GProt.rate <<- si.fd.GProt.rate + si.fd.bact.GProt.rate
      if (genRPT)
      {
        rptIDProt_DMI <- fds["FeedName.x"]
        names(rptIDProt_DMI) <- "FeedName"
        rptIDProt_DMI["Bact TP"] <- si.fd.bact.GTP.rate
        rptIDProt_DMI["Bact NA"] <- si.fd.bact.GNA.rate
        rptIDProt_DMI["Bact CW"] <- si.fd.bact.GCW.rate
        description <- paste("Small Intestinally Digested Protein, g/d\n",
                             "  Ration   : ", formatC(si.diet.GProt.rate * 1000, format = "f", digits = 3, width = 8), "\n",
                             "  Bacteria : ", formatC(si.diet.bact.GProt.rate * 1000, format = "f", digits = 3, width = 8), "\n",
                             "  Total    : ", formatC(sum(si.GProt.rate) * 1000, format = "f", digits = 3, width = 8), "\n", sep = "")
        report(rptIDProt_DMI, "\nSmall Intestinally Digested Bacterial Protein, g/d", description, "", 3, 3, 1000, 8, TRUE, FALSE, TRUE, FALSE, TRUE, FALSE, TRUE)
      }
```

```
    # Digested Amino Acids - Feeds
    si.fd.GMet.rate <<- (fds[, "Met_RUP"]/100) * (si.fd.GProtB1.rate + si.fd.GProtB2.rate + si.fd.GProtB3.rate)
    si.fd.GLys.rate <<- (fds[, "Lys_RUP"]/100) * (si.fd.GProtB1.rate + si.fd.GProtB2.rate + si.fd.GProtB3.rate)
    si.fd.GArg.rate <<- (fds[, "Arg_RUP"]/100) * (si.fd.GProtB1.rate + si.fd.GProtB2.rate + si.fd.GProtB3.rate)
    si.fd.GThr.rate <<- (fds[, "Thr_RUP"]/100) * (si.fd.GProtB1.rate + si.fd.GProtB2.rate + si.fd.GProtB3.rate)
    si.fd.GLeu.rate <<- (fds[, "Leu_RUP"]/100) * (si.fd.GProtB1.rate + si.fd.GProtB2.rate + si.fd.GProtB3.rate)
    si.fd.GIle.rate <<- (fds[, "Ile_RUP"]/100) * (si.fd.GProtB1.rate + si.fd.GProtB2.rate + si.fd.GProtB3.rate)
    si.fd.GVal.rate <<- (fds[, "Val_RUP"]/100) * (si.fd.GProtB1.rate + si.fd.GProtB2.rate + si.fd.GProtB3.rate)
    si.fd.GHis.rate <<- (fds[, "His_RUP"]/100) * (si.fd.GProtB1.rate + si.fd.GProtB2.rate + si.fd.GProtB3.rate)
    si.fd.GPhe.rate <<- (fds[, "Phe_RUP"]/100) * (si.fd.GProtB1.rate + si.fd.GProtB2.rate + si.fd.GProtB3.rate)
    si.fd.GTrp.rate <<- (fds[, "Trp_RUP"]/100) * (si.fd.GProtB1.rate + si.fd.GProtB2.rate + si.fd.GProtB3.rate)
    si.diet.GMet.rate <<- sum(si.fd.GMet.rate)
    si.diet.GLys.rate <<- sum(si.fd.GLys.rate)
    si.diet.GArg.rate <<- sum(si.fd.GArg.rate)
    si.diet.GThr.rate <<- sum(si.fd.GThr.rate)
    si.diet.GLeu.rate <<- sum(si.fd.GLeu.rate)
    si.diet.GIle.rate <<- sum(si.fd.GIle.rate)
    si.diet.GVal.rate <<- sum(si.fd.GVal.rate)
    si.diet.GHis.rate <<- sum(si.fd.GHis.rate)
    si.diet.GPhe.rate <<- sum(si.fd.GPhe.rate)
    si.diet.GTrp.rate <<- sum(si.fd.GTrp.rate)
    if (genRPT)
    {
      rptIDAA_DMI <- fds["FeedName.x"]
      names(rptIDAA_DMI) <- "FeedName"
      rptIDAA_DMI["Met"] <- si.fd.GMet.rate
      rptIDAA_DMI["Lys"] <- si.fd.GLys.rate
      rptIDAA_DMI["Arg"] <- si.fd.GArg.rate
      rptIDAA_DMI["Thr"] <- si.fd.GThr.rate
      rptIDAA_DMI["Leu"] <- si.fd.GLeu.rate
      rptIDAA_DMI["Ile"] <- si.fd.GIle.rate
      rptIDAA_DMI["Val"] <- si.fd.GVal.rate
      rptIDAA_DMI["His"] <- si.fd.GHis.rate
      rptIDAA_DMI["Phe"] <- si.fd.GPhe.rate
      rptIDAA_DMI["Trp"] <- si.fd.GTrp.rate
      footnote <- "The Digested AA is also the Metabolizable AA."
      report(rptIDAA_DMI, "Small Intestinally Digested Feed Amino Acids, g/d", "", footnote, 3, 3, 1000, 7, TRUE, FALSE, TRUE,
  FALSE, TRUE, FALSE, FALSE)
    }
    # Digested Amino Acids - Bacteria
    si.fd.bact.GMet.rate <<- si.fd.bact.GTP.rate * rum.bact.NCW_Met.frac + si.fd.bact.GCW.rate * rum.bact.CW_Met.frac
    si.fd.bact.GLys.rate <<- si.fd.bact.GTP.rate * rum.bact.NCW_Lys.frac + si.fd.bact.GCW.rate * rum.bact.CW_Lys.frac
    si.fd.bact.GArg.rate <<- si.fd.bact.GTP.rate * rum.bact.NCW_Arg.frac + si.fd.bact.GCW.rate * rum.bact.CW_Arg.frac
    si.fd.bact.GThr.rate <<- si.fd.bact.GTP.rate * rum.bact.NCW_Thr.frac + si.fd.bact.GCW.rate * rum.bact.CW_Thr.frac
    si.fd.bact.GLeu.rate <<- si.fd.bact.GTP.rate * rum.bact.NCW_Leu.frac + si.fd.bact.GCW.rate * rum.bact.CW_Leu.frac
    si.fd.bact.GIle.rate <<- si.fd.bact.GTP.rate * rum.bact.NCW_Ile.frac + si.fd.bact.GCW.rate * rum.bact.CW_Ile.frac
    si.fd.bact.GVal.rate <<- si.fd.bact.GTP.rate * rum.bact.NCW_Val.frac + si.fd.bact.GCW.rate * rum.bact.CW_Val.frac
    si.fd.bact.GHis.rate <<- si.fd.bact.GTP.rate * rum.bact.NCW_His.frac + si.fd.bact.GCW.rate * rum.bact.CW_His.frac
    si.fd.bact.GPhe.rate <<- si.fd.bact.GTP.rate * rum.bact.NCW_Phe.frac + si.fd.bact.GCW.rate * rum.bact.CW_Phe.frac
    si.fd.bact.GTrp.rate <<- si.fd.bact.GTP.rate * rum.bact.NCW_Trp.frac + si.fd.bact.GCW.rate * rum.bact.CW_Trp.frac
    si.diet.bact.Met.rate <<- sum(si.fd.bact.GMet.rate)
```

```
  si.diet.bact.Lys.rate <<- sum(si.fd.bact.GLys.rate)
  si.diet.bact.Arg.rate <<- sum(si.fd.bact.GArg.rate)
  si.diet.bact.Thr.rate <<- sum(si.fd.bact.GThr.rate)
  si.diet.bact.Leu.rate <<- sum(si.fd.bact.GLeu.rate)
  si.diet.bact.Ile.rate <<- sum(si.fd.bact.GIle.rate)
  si.diet.bact.Val.rate <<- sum(si.fd.bact.GVal.rate)
  si.diet.bact.His.rate <<- sum(si.fd.bact.GHis.rate)
  si.diet.bact.Phe.rate <<- sum(si.fd.bact.GPhe.rate)
  si.diet.bact.Trp.rate <<- sum(si.fd.bact.GTrp.rate)
  if (genRPT)
  {
    rptIDBactAA_DMI <- fds["FeedName.x"]
    names(rptIDBactAA_DMI) <- "FeedName"
    rptIDBactAA_DMI["Met"] <- si.fd.bact.GMet.rate
    rptIDBactAA_DMI["Lys"] <- si.fd.bact.GLys.rate
    rptIDBactAA_DMI["Arg"] <- si.fd.bact.GArg.rate
    rptIDBactAA_DMI["Thr"] <- si.fd.bact.GThr.rate
    rptIDBactAA_DMI["Leu"] <- si.fd.bact.GLeu.rate
    rptIDBactAA_DMI["Ile"] <- si.fd.bact.GIle.rate
    rptIDBactAA_DMI["Val"] <- si.fd.bact.GVal.rate
    rptIDBactAA_DMI["His"] <- si.fd.bact.GHis.rate
    rptIDBactAA_DMI["Phe"] <- si.fd.bact.GPhe.rate
    rptIDBactAA_DMI["Trp"] <- si.fd.bact.GTrp.rate
    footnote <- "The Digested AA is also the Metabolizable AA."
    report(rptIDBactAA_DMI, "\nSmall Intestinally Digested Bacterial Amino Acids, g/d", "", footnote, 3, 3, 1000, 7, TRUE, FALSE, TRUE, FALSE, TRUE, FALSE, TRUE)
  }
  si.GMet.rate <<- si.fd.GMet.rate + si.fd.bact.GMet.rate
  si.GLys.rate <<- si.fd.GLys.rate + si.fd.bact.GLys.rate
  si.GArg.rate <<- si.fd.GArg.rate + si.fd.bact.GArg.rate
  si.GThr.rate <<- si.fd.GThr.rate + si.fd.bact.GThr.rate
  si.GLeu.rate <<- si.fd.GLeu.rate + si.fd.bact.GLeu.rate
  si.GIle.rate <<- si.fd.GIle.rate + si.fd.bact.GIle.rate
  si.GVal.rate <<- si.fd.GVal.rate + si.fd.bact.GVal.rate
  si.GHis.rate <<- si.fd.GHis.rate + si.fd.bact.GHis.rate
  si.GPhe.rate <<- si.fd.GPhe.rate + si.fd.bact.GPhe.rate
  si.GTrp.rate <<- si.fd.GTrp.rate + si.fd.bact.GTrp.rate
  si.diet.GMet.rate <<- sum(si.GMet.rate)
  si.diet.GLys.rate <<- sum(si.GLys.rate)
  si.diet.GArg.rate <<- sum(si.GArg.rate)
  si.diet.GThr.rate <<- sum(si.GThr.rate)
  si.diet.GLeu.rate <<- sum(si.GLeu.rate)
  si.diet.GIle.rate <<- sum(si.GIle.rate)
  si.diet.GVal.rate <<- sum(si.GVal.rate)
  si.diet.GHis.rate <<- sum(si.GHis.rate)
  si.diet.GPhe.rate <<- sum(si.GPhe.rate)
  si.diet.GTrp.rate <<- sum(si.GTrp.rate)
  if (genRPT)
  {
    rptIDAA_DMI <- fds["FeedName.x"]
    names(rptIDAA_DMI) <- "FeedName"
```

```
      rptIDAA_DMI["Met"] <- si.GMet.rate
      rptIDAA_DMI["Lys"] <- si.GLys.rate
      rptIDAA_DMI["Arg"] <- si.GArg.rate
      rptIDAA_DMI["Thr"] <- si.GThr.rate
      rptIDAA_DMI["Leu"] <- si.GLeu.rate
      rptIDAA_DMI["Ile"] <- si.GIle.rate
      rptIDAA_DMI["Val"] <- si.GVal.rate
      rptIDAA_DMI["His"] <- si.GHis.rate
      rptIDAA_DMI["Phe"] <- si.GPhe.rate
      rptIDAA_DMI["Trp"] <- si.GTrp.rate
      footnote <- "The Digested AA is also the Metabolizable AA."
      report(rptIDAA_DMI, "Small Intestinally Digested Amino Acids (Feed + Bacteria), g/d", "", footnote, 3, 3, 1000, 7, TRUE,
    FALSE, TRUE, FALSE, TRUE, FALSE, TRUE)
    }
    # Digested Fat - Feed
    si.fd.EE_ID.frac <<- as.numeric(fds[, "EE_ID"])/100
    si.fd.GEE.rate <<- duo.fd.EE.rate * si.fd.EE_ID.frac
    si.diet.GEE.rate <<- sum(si.fd.GEE.rate)
    si.fd.FAC12_ID.frac <<- as.numeric(fds[, "C12_0_ID"])/100
    si.fd.FAC14_ID.frac <<- as.numeric(fds[, "C14_0_ID"])/100
    si.fd.FAC16_ID.frac <<- as.numeric(fds[, "C16_0_ID"])/100
    si.fd.FAC16_1_ID.frac <<- as.numeric(fds[, "C16_1_ID"])/100
    si.fd.FAC18_ID.frac <<- as.numeric(fds[, "C18_0_ID"])/100
    si.fd.FAC18_1c_ID.frac <<- as.numeric(fds[, "C18_1c_ID"])/100
    si.fd.FAC18_1t_ID.frac <<- as.numeric(fds[, "C18_1t_ID"])/100
    si.fd.FAC18_2_ID.frac <<- as.numeric(fds[, "C18_2_ID"])/100
    si.fd.FAC18_3_ID.frac <<- as.numeric(fds[, "C18_3_ID"])/100
    si.fd.FAOther_ID.frac <<- as.numeric(fds[, "OtherLipids_ID"])/100
    si.fd.FAC12NL_ID.frac <<- as.numeric(fds[, "C12_0NL_ID"])/100
    si.fd.FAC14NL_ID.frac <<- as.numeric(fds[, "C14_0NL_ID"])/100
    si.fd.FAC16NL_ID.frac <<- as.numeric(fds[, "C16_0NL_ID"])/100
    si.fd.FAC16_1NL_ID.frac <<- as.numeric(fds[, "C16_1NL_ID"])/100
    si.fd.FAC18NL_ID.frac <<- as.numeric(fds[, "C18_0NL_ID"])/100
    si.fd.FAC18_1cNL_ID.frac <<- as.numeric(fds[, "C18_1cNL_ID"])/100
    si.fd.FAC18_1tNL_ID.frac <<- as.numeric(fds[, "C18_1tNL_ID"])/100
    si.fd.FAC18_2NL_ID.frac <<- as.numeric(fds[, "C18_2NL_ID"])/100
    si.fd.FAC18_3NL_ID.frac <<- as.numeric(fds[, "C18_3NL_ID"])/100
    si.fd.FAOtherNL_ID.frac <<- as.numeric(fds[, "OtherLipidsNL_ID"])/100
    si.fd.GFAC12.rate <<- rum.fd.LEFAC12.rate * si.fd.FAC12_ID.frac + rum.fd.EFAC12.rate * si.fd.FAC12NL_ID.frac
    si.fd.GFAC14.rate <<- rum.fd.LEFAC14.rate * si.fd.FAC14_ID.frac + rum.fd.EFAC14.rate * si.fd.FAC14NL_ID.frac
    si.fd.GFAC16.rate <<- (rum.fd.LEFAC16.rate + rum.fd.DNFAC16.rate) * si.fd.FAC16_ID.frac + rum.fd.EFAC16.rate *
  si.fd.FAC16NL_ID.frac
    si.fd.GFAC16_1.rate <<- (rum.fd.LEFAC16_1.rate + rum.fd.DNFAC16_1.rate) * si.fd.FAC16_1_ID.frac + rum.fd.EFAC16_1.rate *
  si.fd.FAC16_1NL_ID.frac
    si.fd.GFAC18.rate <<- (rum.fd.LEFAC18.rate + rum.fd.DNFAC18.rate) * si.fd.FAC18_ID.frac + rum.fd.EFAC18.rate *
  si.fd.FAC18NL_ID.frac
    si.fd.GFAC18_1c.rate <<- rum.fd.LEFAC18_1c.rate * si.fd.FAC18_1c_ID.frac + rum.fd.EFAC18_1c.rate * si.fd.FAC18_1cNL_ID.frac
    si.fd.GFAC18_1t.rate <<- rum.fd.LEFAC18_1t.rate * si.fd.FAC18_1t_ID.frac + rum.fd.EFAC18_1t.rate * si.fd.FAC18_1tNL_ID.frac
    si.fd.GFAC18_2.rate <<- rum.fd.LEFAC18_2.rate * si.fd.FAC18_2_ID.frac + rum.fd.EFAC18_2.rate * si.fd.FAC18_2NL_ID.frac
    si.fd.GFAC18_3.rate <<- rum.fd.LEFAC18_3.rate * si.fd.FAC18_3_ID.frac + rum.fd.EFAC18_3.rate * si.fd.FAC18_3NL_ID.frac
```

```
    si.fd.GFAOther.rate <<- (rum.fd.LEFAOther.rate + rum.fd.DNFAOther.rate) * si.fd.FAOther_ID.frac + rum.fd.EFAOther.rate * si.fd.FAOtherNL_ID.frac
    si.fd.GFA.rate <<- si.fd.GFAC12.rate + si.fd.GFAC14.rate + si.fd.GFAC16.rate + si.fd.GFAC16_1.rate + si.fd.GFAC18.rate + si.fd.GFAC18_1c.rate + si.fd.GFAC18_1t.rate + si.fd.GFAC18_2.rate + si.fd.GFAC18_3.rate + si.fd.GFAOther.rate
    si.fd.GGlycerol.rate <<- rum.fd.EGlycerol.rate * si.fd.CHOA1_ID.frac
    si.fd.GPigment.rate <<- rum.fd.EPigment.rate * 0  # Assume pigments and waxes have zero intestinal digestibility
    si.diet.GFAC12.rate <<- sum(si.fd.GFAC12.rate)
    si.diet.GFAC14.rate <<- sum(si.fd.GFAC14.rate)
    si.diet.GFAC16.rate <<- sum(si.fd.GFAC16.rate)
    si.diet.GFAC16_1.rate <<- sum(si.fd.GFAC16_1.rate)
    si.diet.GFAC18.rate <<- sum(si.fd.GFAC18.rate)
    si.diet.GFAC18_1c.rate <<- sum(si.fd.GFAC18_1c.rate)
    si.diet.GFAC18_1t.rate <<- sum(si.fd.GFAC18_1t.rate)
    si.diet.GFAC18_2.rate <<- sum(si.fd.GFAC18_2.rate)
    si.diet.GFAC18_3.rate <<- sum(si.fd.GFAC18_3.rate)
    si.diet.GFAOther.rate <<- sum(si.fd.GFAOther.rate)
    si.diet.GFA.rate <<- sum(si.fd.GFA.rate)
    si.diet.GGlycerol.rate <<- sum(si.fd.GGlycerol.rate)
    si.diet.GPigment.rate <<- sum(si.fd.GPigment.rate)
    if (genRPT)
    {
      rptIDFA_DMI <- fds["FeedName.x"]
      names(rptIDFA_DMI) <- "FeedName"
      rptIDFA_DMI["C12:0"] <- si.fd.GFAC12.rate
      rptIDFA_DMI["C14:0"] <- si.fd.GFAC14.rate
      rptIDFA_DMI["C16:0"] <- si.fd.GFAC16.rate
      rptIDFA_DMI["C16:1"] <- si.fd.GFAC16_1.rate
      rptIDFA_DMI["C18:0"] <- si.fd.GFAC18.rate
      rptIDFA_DMI["C18:1c"] <- si.fd.GFAC18_1c.rate
      rptIDFA_DMI["C18:1t"] <- si.fd.GFAC18_1t.rate
      rptIDFA_DMI["C18:2"] <- si.fd.GFAC18_2.rate
      rptIDFA_DMI["C18:3"] <- si.fd.GFAC18_3.rate
      rptIDFA_DMI["Other FFA"] <- si.fd.GFAOther.rate
      description <- paste("Digested glycerol, g/d       : ", formatC(si.diet.GGlycerol.rate * 1000, format = "f", digits = 3, width = 7), "\n",
                           "Digested pigments, g/d       : ", formatC(si.diet.GPigment.rate * 1000, format = "f", digits = 3, width = 7), "\n", sep = "")
      report(rptIDFA_DMI, "#Title#Small Intestinally Digested Fatty Acids, g/d", description, "", 3, 3, 1000, 7, TRUE, FALSE, TRUE, FALSE, TRUE, FALSE, TRUE)
    }
    # Fatty Acid Digestibility
    if (genRPT)
    {
      rptGFA_DMI <- fds["FeedName.x"]
      names(rptGFA_DMI) <- "FeedName"
      rptGFA_DMI["C12:0"] <- isz(si.fd.GFAC12.rate * 100, rum.fd.LEFAC12.rate + rum.fd.EFAC12.rate)
      rptGFA_DMI["C14:0"] <- isz(si.fd.GFAC14.rate * 100, rum.fd.LEFAC14.rate + rum.fd.EFAC14.rate)
      rptGFA_DMI["C16:0"] <- isz(si.fd.GFAC16.rate * 100, (rum.fd.LEFAC16.rate + rum.fd.DNFAC16.rate) + rum.fd.EFAC16.rate)
      rptGFA_DMI["C16:1"] <- isz(si.fd.GFAC16_1.rate * 100, (rum.fd.LEFAC16_1.rate + rum.fd.DNFAC16_1.rate) + rum.fd.EFAC16_1.rate)
      rptGFA_DMI["C18:0"] <- isz(si.fd.GFAC18.rate * 100, (rum.fd.LEFAC18.rate + rum.fd.DNFAC18.rate) + rum.fd.EFAC18.rate)
```

```
    rptGFA_DMI["C18:1c"] <- isz(si.fd.GFAC18_1c.rate * 100, rum.fd.LEFAC18_1c.rate + rum.fd.EFAC18_1c.rate)
    rptGFA_DMI["C18:1t"] <- isz(si.fd.GFAC18_1t.rate * 100, rum.fd.LEFAC18_1t.rate + rum.fd.EFAC18_1t.rate)
    rptGFA_DMI["C18:2"] <- isz(si.fd.GFAC18_2.rate * 100, rum.fd.LEFAC18_2.rate + rum.fd.EFAC18_2.rate)
    rptGFA_DMI["C18:3"] <- isz(si.fd.GFAC18_3.rate * 100, rum.fd.LEFAC18_3.rate + rum.fd.EFAC18_3.rate)
    rptGFA_DMI["Other FFA"] <- isz(si.fd.GFAOther.rate * 100, (rum.fd.LEFAOther.rate + rum.fd.DNFAOther.rate) + rum.fd.EFAOther.rate)
    rptGFA_DMI2 <- data.frame(FeedName = "Ration")
    rptGFA_DMI2["C12:0"] <- isz(si.diet.GFAC12.rate * 100, rum.diet.LEFAC12.rate + rum.diet.EFAC12.rate)
    rptGFA_DMI2["C14:0"] <- isz(si.diet.GFAC14.rate * 100, rum.diet.LEFAC14.rate + rum.diet.EFAC14.rate)
    rptGFA_DMI2["C16:0"] <- isz(si.diet.GFAC16.rate * 100, (rum.diet.LEFAC16.rate + rum.diet.DNFAC16.rate) + rum.diet.EFAC16.rate)
    rptGFA_DMI2["C16:1"] <- isz(si.diet.GFAC16_1.rate * 100, (rum.diet.LEFAC16_1.rate + rum.diet.DNFAC16_1.rate) + rum.diet.EFAC16_1.rate)
    rptGFA_DMI2["C18:0"] <- isz(si.diet.GFAC18.rate * 100, (rum.diet.LEFAC18.rate + rum.diet.DNFAC18.rate) + rum.diet.EFAC18.rate)
    rptGFA_DMI2["C18:1c"] <- isz(si.diet.GFAC18_1c.rate * 100, rum.diet.LEFAC18_1c.rate + rum.diet.EFAC18_1c.rate)
    rptGFA_DMI2["C18:1t"] <- isz(si.diet.GFAC18_1t.rate * 100, rum.diet.LEFAC18_1t.rate + rum.diet.EFAC18_1t.rate)
    rptGFA_DMI2["C18:2"] <- isz(si.diet.GFAC18_2.rate * 100, rum.diet.LEFAC18_2.rate + rum.diet.EFAC18_2.rate)
    rptGFA_DMI2["C18:3"] <- isz(si.diet.GFAC18_3.rate * 100, rum.diet.LEFAC18_3.rate + rum.diet.EFAC18_3.rate)
    rptGFA_DMI2["Other FFA"] <- isz(si.diet.GFAOther.rate * 100, (rum.diet.LEFAOther.rate + rum.diet.DNFAOther.rate) + rum.diet.EFAOther.rate)
    rptGFA_DMI <- rbind(rptGFA_DMI, rptGFA_DMI2)
    footnote <- "Digested FA/(Escaped Esterified FA + Escaped Non-Esterified FA + De novo FA)"
    report(rptGFA_DMI, "Small Intestinal Digestibility of Fatty Acids, %", "", footnote, 1, 1, 1, 10, FALSE, FALSE, FALSE, FALSE, FALSE, FALSE, FALSE)
  }
  # Digested Fat - Bacteria
  si.fd.bact.GFat.rate <<- (Parm_rum.bact.IDFat/100) * duo.fd.bact.NFC_Fat.rate + (Parm_rum.bact.IDFat/100) * duo.fd.bact.FC_Fat.rate
  si.diet.bact.GFat.rate <<- sum(si.fd.bact.GFat.rate)
  si.GEE.rate <<- si.fd.GEE.rate + si.fd.bact.GFat.rate
  si.fd.bact.GFAC12.rate <<- si.fd.bact.GFat.rate * mean(c(0.4,1.2,4.6))/100
  si.fd.bact.GFAC14.rate <<- si.fd.bact.GFat.rate * mean(c(2.3,3.7,3.9))/100
  si.fd.bact.GFAC16.rate <<- si.fd.bact.GFat.rate * mean(c(25.4,31,35.2))/100
  si.fd.bact.GFAC16_1.rate <<- si.fd.bact.GFat.rate * mean(c(4))/100
  si.fd.bact.GFAC18.rate <<- si.fd.bact.GFat.rate * mean(c(15,20.8,32))/100
  si.fd.bact.GFAC18_1.rate <<- si.fd.bact.GFat.rate * mean(c(3.9,6,19.7))/100
  si.fd.bact.GFAC18_2.rate <<- si.fd.bact.GFat.rate * mean(c(2.7,3.5,5.6))/100
  si.fd.bact.GFAC18_3.rate <<- si.fd.bact.GFat.rate * mean(c(1))/100
  si.fd.bact.GFAOther.rate <<- si.fd.bact.GFat.rate * mean(c(8.8,20.2))/100
  si.diet.bact.GFAC12.rate <<- sum(si.fd.bact.GFAC12.rate)
  si.diet.bact.GFAC14.rate <<- sum(si.fd.bact.GFAC14.rate)
  si.diet.bact.GFAC16.rate <<- sum(si.fd.bact.GFAC16.rate)
  si.diet.bact.GFAC16_1.rate <<- sum(si.fd.bact.GFAC16_1.rate)
  si.diet.bact.GFAC18.rate <<- sum(si.fd.bact.GFAC18.rate)
  si.diet.bact.GFAC18_1.rate <<- sum(si.fd.bact.GFAC18_1.rate)
  si.diet.bact.GFAC18_2.rate <<- sum(si.fd.bact.GFAC18_2.rate)
  si.diet.bact.GFAC18_3.rate <<- sum(si.fd.bact.GFAC18_3.rate)
  si.diet.bact.GFAOther.rate <<- sum(si.fd.bact.GFAOther.rate)
  if (genRPT)
  {
```

```
      rptIDBactFA_DMI <- fds["FeedName.x"]
      names(rptIDBactFA_DMI) <- "FeedName"
      rptIDBactFA_DMI["C12:0"] <- si.fd.bact.GFAC12.rate
      rptIDBactFA_DMI["C14:0"] <- si.fd.bact.GFAC14.rate
      rptIDBactFA_DMI["C16:0"] <- si.fd.bact.GFAC16.rate
      rptIDBactFA_DMI["C16:1"] <- si.fd.bact.GFAC16_1.rate
      rptIDBactFA_DMI["C18:0"] <- si.fd.bact.GFAC18.rate
      rptIDBactFA_DMI["C18:1"] <- si.fd.bact.GFAC18_1.rate
      rptIDBactFA_DMI["C18:2"] <- si.fd.bact.GFAC18_2.rate
      rptIDBactFA_DMI["C18:3"] <- si.fd.bact.GFAC18_3.rate
      rptIDBactFA_DMI["Other FA"] <- si.fd.bact.GFAOther.rate
      footnote <- "There is no Bacterial FA C18:1t."
      description <- paste("Digested bacterial fat, g/d : ", formatC(si.diet.bact.GFat.rate * 1000, format = "f", digits = 3, width = 7), "\n", sep = "")
      report(rptIDBactFA_DMI, "\nSmall Intestinally Digested Bacterial Fatty Acids, g/d", description, footnote, 3, 3, 1000, 7, TRUE, FALSE, TRUE, FALSE, TRUE, FALSE, TRUE)
    }
    si.GFAC12.rate <<- si.fd.GFAC12.rate + si.fd.bact.GFAC12.rate
    si.GFAC14.rate <<- si.fd.GFAC14.rate + si.fd.bact.GFAC14.rate
    si.GFAC16.rate <<- si.fd.GFAC16.rate + si.fd.bact.GFAC16.rate
    si.GFAC16_1.rate <<- si.fd.GFAC16_1.rate + si.fd.bact.GFAC16_1.rate
    si.GFAC18.rate <<- si.fd.GFAC18.rate + si.fd.bact.GFAC18.rate
    si.GFAC18_1c.rate <<- si.fd.GFAC18_1c.rate + si.fd.bact.GFAC18_1.rate
    si.GFAC18_1t.rate <<- si.fd.GFAC18_1t.rate + 0 # Assume zero for bacterial FA C18:1t
    si.GFAC18_2.rate <<- si.fd.GFAC18_2.rate + si.fd.bact.GFAC18_2.rate
    si.GFAC18_3.rate <<- si.fd.GFAC18_3.rate + si.fd.bact.GFAC18_3.rate
    si.GFAOther.rate <<- si.fd.GFAOther.rate + si.fd.bact.GFAOther.rate
    si.GFA.rate <<- si.GFAC12.rate + si.GFAC14.rate + si.GFAC16.rate + si.GFAC16_1.rate + si.GFAC18.rate + si.GFAC18_1c.rate + si.GFAC18_1t.rate + si.GFAC18_2.rate + si.GFAC18_3.rate + si.GFAOther.rate
    if (genRPT)
    {
      rptIDFA_DMI <- fds["FeedName.x"]
      names(rptIDFA_DMI) <- "FeedName"
      rptIDFA_DMI["C12:0"] <- si.GFAC12.rate
      rptIDFA_DMI["C14:0"] <- si.GFAC14.rate
      rptIDFA_DMI["C16:0"] <- si.GFAC16.rate
      rptIDFA_DMI["C16:1"] <- si.GFAC16_1.rate
      rptIDFA_DMI["C18:0"] <- si.GFAC18.rate
      rptIDFA_DMI["C18:1c"] <- si.GFAC18_1c.rate
      rptIDFA_DMI["C18:1t"] <- si.GFAC18_1t.rate
      rptIDFA_DMI["C18:2"] <- si.GFAC18_2.rate
      rptIDFA_DMI["C18:3"] <- si.GFAC18_3.rate
      rptIDFA_DMI["Other FFA"] <- si.GFAOther.rate
      report(rptIDFA_DMI, "Small Intestinally Digested Fatty Acids (Feed + Bacteria), g/d", "", "", 3, 3, 1000, 7, TRUE, FALSE, TRUE, FALSE, TRUE, FALSE, TRUE)
    }
    # Digested Ash - Feed
    si.fd.Ash_ID.frac <<- as.numeric(fds[, "Ash_ID"])/100
    si.fd.GAsh.rate <<- anim.fd.ash.rate * si.fd.Ash_ID.frac
    si.diet.GAsh.rate <<- sum(si.fd.GAsh.rate)
    # Digested Ash - Bacteria
```

```
  si.fd.bact.GAsh.rate <<- (Parm_rum.bact.IDAsh/100) * duo.fd.bact.NFC_Ash.rate + (Parm_rum.bact.IDAsh/100) *
duo.fd.bact.FC_Ash.rate
  si.diet.bact.GAsh.rate <<- sum(si.fd.bact.GAsh.rate)
  si.GAsh.rate <<- si.fd.GAsh.rate + si.fd.bact.GAsh.rate
  if (genRPT)
  {
    rptIDAsh_DMI <- fds["FeedName.x"]
    names(rptIDAsh_DMI) <- "FeedName"
    rptIDAsh_DMI["Feed Ash"] <- si.fd.GAsh.rate
    rptIDAsh_DMI["Bact Ash"] <- si.fd.bact.GAsh.rate
    report(rptIDAsh_DMI, "Small Intestinally Digested Ash (Feed + Bacteria), g/d", "", "", 3, 3, 1000, 8, TRUE, FALSE, TRUE,
FALSE, TRUE, FALSE, TRUE)
  }
}
```

4.3.12 Fecal submodel

```
calcFecal <- function(fds = feeds3, genRPT = TRUE)
{
  # ++++++++++++++++
  # Fecal Submodel
  # ++++++++++++++++
  # Feeds
  fc.fd.CP.rate <<- anim.fd.CP.rate - (rum.fd.DProt.rate + si.fd.GProt.rate)
  fc.fd.CHO.rate <<- (anim.fd.CHO.rate + rum.fd.LGlycerol.propionate.rate) - (rum.fd.DCHO.rate + si.fd.GCHO.rate)  # Includes lipolyzed glycerol
  fc.fd.EE.rate <<- anim.fd.EE.rate - si.fd.GEE.rate
  fc.fd.ash.rate <<- anim.fd.ash.rate - si.fd.GAsh.rate
  if (genRPT)
  {
    rptFecalFeed_DMI <- fds["FeedName.x"]
    names(rptFecalFeed_DMI) <- "FeedName"
    rptFecalFeed_DMI["CP"] <- fc.fd.CP.rate
    rptFecalFeed_DMI["CHO"] <- fc.fd.CHO.rate
    rptFecalFeed_DMI["EE"] <- fc.fd.EE.rate
    rptFecalFeed_DMI["Ash"] <- fc.fd.ash.rate
    footnote <- "CHO includes lipolyzed glycerol"
    report(rptFecalFeed_DMI, "Fecal Feed Matter, g/d", "", footnote, 3, 3, 1000, 8, TRUE, FALSE, TRUE, FALSE, TRUE, FALSE, FALSE)
  }
  fc.fd.Glycerol.rate <<- (anim.fd.Glycerol.rate - rum.fd.LGlycerol.propionate.rate) - si.fd.GGlycerol.rate  # Excludes lipolyzed glycerol
  fc.fd.Pigment.rate <<- anim.fd.Pigment.rate - si.fd.GPigment.rate
  fc.fd.FAC12.rate <<- duo.fd.FAC12.rate - si.fd.GFAC12.rate
  fc.fd.FAC14.rate <<- duo.fd.FAC14.rate - si.fd.GFAC14.rate
  fc.fd.FAC16.rate <<- duo.fd.FAC16.rate - si.fd.GFAC16.rate
  fc.fd.FAC16_1.rate <<- duo.fd.FAC16_1.rate - si.fd.GFAC16_1.rate
  fc.fd.FAC18.rate <<- duo.fd.FAC18.rate - si.fd.GFAC18.rate
  fc.fd.FAC18_1c.rate <<- duo.fd.FAC18_1c.rate - si.fd.GFAC18_1c.rate
  fc.fd.FAC18_1t.rate <<- duo.fd.FAC18_1t.rate - si.fd.GFAC18_1t.rate
  fc.fd.FAC18_2.rate <<- duo.fd.FAC18_2.rate - si.fd.GFAC18_2.rate
  fc.fd.FAC18_3.rate <<- duo.fd.FAC18_3.rate - si.fd.GFAC18_3.rate
  fc.fd.FAOther.rate <<- duo.fd.FAOther.rate - si.fd.GFAOther.rate
  fc.fd.TFA.rate <<- fc.fd.FAC12.rate + fc.fd.FAC14.rate + fc.fd.FAC16.rate + fc.fd.FAC16_1.rate + fc.fd.FAC18.rate + fc.fd.FAC18_1c.rate + fc.fd.FAC18_1t.rate + fc.fd.FAC18_2.rate + fc.fd.FAC18_3.rate + fc.fd.FAOther.rate
  fc.fd.bact.FAC12.rate <<- duo.fd.bact.FAC12.rate - si.fd.bact.GFAC12.rate
  fc.fd.bact.FAC14.rate <<- duo.fd.bact.FAC14.rate - si.fd.bact.GFAC14.rate
  fc.fd.bact.FAC16.rate <<- duo.fd.bact.FAC16.rate  - si.fd.bact.GFAC16.rate
  fc.fd.bact.FAC16_1.rate <<- duo.fd.bact.FAC16_1.rate - si.fd.bact.GFAC16_1.rate
  fc.fd.bact.FAC18.rate <<- duo.fd.bact.FAC18.rate - si.fd.bact.GFAC18.rate
  fc.fd.bact.FAC18_1.rate <<- duo.fd.bact.FAC18_1.rate - si.fd.bact.GFAC18_1.rate
  fc.fd.bact.FAC18_2.rate <<- duo.fd.bact.FAC18_2.rate - si.fd.bact.GFAC18_2.rate
  fc.fd.bact.FAC18_3.rate <<- duo.fd.bact.FAC18_3.rate - si.fd.bact.GFAC18_3.rate
  fc.fd.bact.FAOther.rate <<- duo.fd.bact.FAOther.rate - si.fd.bact.GFAOther.rate
  if (genRPT)
```

```
  {
    rptFecalFA_DMI <- fds["FeedName.x"]
    names(rptFecalFA_DMI) <- "FeedName"
    rptFecalFA_DMI["C12:0"] <- fc.fd.FAC12.rate
    rptFecalFA_DMI["C14:0"] <- fc.fd.FAC14.rate
    rptFecalFA_DMI["C16:0"] <- fc.fd.FAC16.rate
    rptFecalFA_DMI["C16:1"] <- fc.fd.FAC16_1.rate
    rptFecalFA_DMI["C18:0"] <- fc.fd.FAC18.rate
    rptFecalFA_DMI["C18:1c"] <- fc.fd.FAC18_1c.rate
    rptFecalFA_DMI["C18:1t"] <- fc.fd.FAC18_1t.rate
    rptFecalFA_DMI["C18:2"] <- fc.fd.FAC18_2.rate
    rptFecalFA_DMI["C18:3"] <- fc.fd.FAC18_3.rate
    rptFecalFA_DMI["Other FA"] <- fc.fd.FAOther.rate
    footnote <- "Note that glycerol excludes lipolyzed glycerol"
    description <- paste("Fecal glycerol, g/d      : ", formatC(sum(fc.fd.Glycerol.rate) * 1000, format = "f", digits = 3, width = 7), "\n",
                         "Fecal pigments, g/d      : ", formatC(sum(fc.fd.Pigment.rate) * 1000, format = "f", digits = 3, width = 7), "\n", sep = "")
    report(rptFecalFA_DMI, "\nFecal Feed Fatty Acid Matter, g/d", description, footnote, 3, 3, 1000, 7, TRUE, FALSE, TRUE, FALSE, TRUE, FALSE, TRUE)
    # Bacteria FA
    rptFecalFA_DMI <- fds["FeedName.x"]
    names(rptFecalFA_DMI) <- "FeedName"
    rptFecalFA_DMI["C12:0"] <- fc.fd.bact.FAC12.rate
    rptFecalFA_DMI["C14:0"] <- fc.fd.bact.FAC14.rate
    rptFecalFA_DMI["C16:0"] <- fc.fd.bact.FAC16.rate
    rptFecalFA_DMI["C16:1"] <- fc.fd.bact.FAC16_1.rate
    rptFecalFA_DMI["C18:0"] <- fc.fd.bact.FAC18.rate
    rptFecalFA_DMI["C18:1"] <- fc.fd.bact.FAC18_1.rate
    rptFecalFA_DMI["C18:2"] <- fc.fd.bact.FAC18_2.rate
    rptFecalFA_DMI["C18:3"] <- fc.fd.bact.FAC18_3.rate
    rptFecalFA_DMI["Other FA"] <- fc.fd.bact.FAOther.rate
    footnote <- "There is no Bacterial FA C18:1t."
    report(rptFecalFA_DMI, "Fecal Bacteria Fatty Acid Matter, g/d", "", footnote, 3, 3, 1000, 7, TRUE, FALSE, TRUE, FALSE, TRUE, FALSE, TRUE)
  }
  if (flag_fecal == 0)
  {
    # Fox et al., (2004; Anim. Feed Sci. Technol. 112:29-78) Endogenous
    fc.fd.Endogenous.fat.rate <<- (1.19/100) * anim.fd.DMI.rate
    fc.fd.Endogenous.ash.rate <<- (1.7/100) * anim.fd.DMI.rate
    # Bacteria
    fc.fd.bact.CHO.rate <<- (duo.fd.bact.CHOA.rate + duo.fd.bact.CHOB1.rate) - (si.fd.bact.GCHOA.rate + si.fd.bact.GCHOB1.rate)
    fc.fd.bact.CP.rate <<- duo.fd.bact.CP.rate - si.fd.bact.GProt.rate
    fc.fd.bact.EE.rate <<- duo.fd.bact.fat.rate - si.fd.bact.GFat.rate
    fc.fd.bact.ash.rate <<- duo.fd.bact.ash.rate - si.fd.bact.GAsh.rate
    fc.fd.bact.rate <<- fc.fd.bact.CP.rate + fc.fd.bact.CHO.rate + fc.fd.bact.EE.rate + fc.fd.bact.ash.rate
    fc.CHO.rate <<- fc.fd.CHO.rate + fc.fd.bact.CHO.rate
    fc.CP.rate <<- fc.fd.CP.rate + fc.fd.bact.CP.rate
    fc.EE.rate <<- fc.fd.EE.rate + fc.fd.bact.EE.rate + fc.fd.Endogenous.fat.rate
```

```
        fc.ash.rate <<- fc.fd.ash.rate + fc.fd.bact.ash.rate + fc.fd.Endogenous.ash.rate
        fc.fd.IDM.rate <<- (fc.CP.rate + fc.CHO.rate + fc.EE.rate + fc.ash.rate)/0.91
        fc.fd.IOM.rate <<- fc.fd.IDM.rate - fc.ash.rate
        fc.fd.Endogenous.CP.rate <<- fc.fd.IDM.rate * 0.09
        fc.CP.rate <<- fc.fd.CP.rate + fc.fd.bact.CP.rate + fc.fd.Endogenous.CP.rate  # Add the endogenous contribution
    }
    if (flag_fecal == 1)
    {
        # Cannas et al. (2004; J. Anim. Sci. 82:149-169) Endogenous and bacterial CP, EE, and Ash contributions are computed together
        fc.fd.Endogenous.CP.rate <<- 0
        fc.fd.Endogenous.fat.rate <<- 0
        fc.fd.Endogenous.ash.rate <<- 0
        # Bacteria + Endogenous
        fc.fd.bact.CHO.rate <<- (duo.fd.bact.CHOA.rate + duo.fd.bact.CHOB1.rate) - (si.fd.bact.GCHOA.rate + si.fd.bact.GCHOB1.rate)
        fc.fd.bact.CP.rate <<- (30/1000) * anim.fd.DMI.rate
        fc.fd.bact.EE.rate <<- (11.9/1000) * anim.fd.DMI.rate
        fc.fd.bact.ash.rate <<- (17/1000) * anim.fd.DMI.rate
        fc.fd.bact.rate <<- fc.fd.bact.CP.rate + fc.fd.bact.CHO.rate + fc.fd.bact.EE.rate + fc.fd.bact.ash.rate
        fc.CHO.rate <<- fc.fd.CHO.rate + fc.fd.bact.CHO.rate
        fc.CP.rate <<- fc.fd.CP.rate + fc.fd.bact.CP.rate + fc.fd.Endogenous.CP.rate
        fc.EE.rate <<- fc.fd.EE.rate + fc.fd.bact.EE.rate + fc.fd.Endogenous.fat.rate
        fc.ash.rate <<- fc.fd.ash.rate + fc.fd.bact.ash.rate + fc.fd.Endogenous.ash.rate
        fc.fd.IDM.rate <<- fc.CP.rate + fc.CHO.rate + fc.EE.rate + fc.ash.rate
        fc.fd.IOM.rate <<- fc.CP.rate + fc.CHO.rate + fc.EE.rate
    }
    if (flag_fecal == 2)
    {
        # Tedeschi et al. (2010; Small Ruminant Res. 89:174-184) Endogenous: assumes that only 15% was from endogenous origin
        fc.fd.Endogenous.CP.rate <<- 0.15 * (30/1000) * anim.fd.DMI.rate
        fc.fd.Endogenous.fat.rate <<- (11.9/1000) * anim.fd.DMI.rate
        fc.fd.Endogenous.ash.rate <<- (17/1000) * anim.fd.DMI.rate
        # Bacteria
        fc.fd.bact.CHO.rate <<- (duo.fd.bact.CHOA.rate + duo.fd.bact.CHOB1.rate) - (si.fd.bact.GCHOA.rate + si.fd.bact.GCHOB1.rate)
        fc.fd.bact.CP.rate <<- duo.fd.bact.CP.rate - si.fd.bact.GProt.rate
        fc.fd.bact.EE.rate <<- duo.fd.bact.fat.rate - si.fd.bact.GFat.rate
        fc.fd.bact.ash.rate <<- duo.fd.bact.ash.rate - si.fd.bact.GAsh.rate
        fc.fd.bact.rate <<- fc.fd.bact.CP.rate + fc.fd.bact.CHO.rate + fc.fd.bact.EE.rate + fc.fd.bact.ash.rate
        fc.CHO.rate <<- fc.fd.CHO.rate + fc.fd.bact.CHO.rate
        fc.CP.rate <<- fc.fd.CP.rate + fc.fd.bact.CP.rate + fc.fd.Endogenous.CP.rate
        fc.EE.rate <<- fc.fd.EE.rate + fc.fd.bact.EE.rate + fc.fd.Endogenous.fat.rate
        fc.ash.rate <<- fc.fd.ash.rate + fc.fd.bact.ash.rate + fc.fd.Endogenous.ash.rate
        fc.fd.IDM.rate <<- fc.CP.rate + fc.CHO.rate + fc.EE.rate + fc.ash.rate
        fc.fd.IOM.rate <<- fc.CP.rate + fc.CHO.rate + fc.EE.rate
    }
    fc.fd.Mi_CP.rate <<- fc.fd.Endogenous.CP.rate + fc.fd.bact.CP.rate
    fc.fd.Mi_CHO.rate <<- fc.fd.bact.CHO.rate
    fc.fd.Mi_Fat.rate <<- fc.fd.Endogenous.fat.rate + fc.fd.bact.EE.rate
    fc.fd.Mi_Ash.rate <<- fc.fd.Endogenous.ash.rate + fc.fd.bact.ash.rate
```

```
    fc.fd.Mi.rate <<- fc.fd.Mi_CP.rate + fc.fd.Mi_CHO.rate + fc.fd.Mi_Fat.rate + fc.fd.Mi_Ash.rate
    fc.diet.Mi.rate <<- sum(fc.fd.Mi.rate)
    fc.diet.IDM.rate <<- sum(fc.fd.IDM.rate)
    fc.diet.fd_IOM.rate <<- sum(fc.fd.IOM.rate)
    fc.diet.bact.CP.rate <<- sum(fc.fd.bact.CP.rate)
    fc.diet.bact.CHO.rate <<- sum(fc.fd.bact.CHO.rate)
    fc.diet.bact.EE.rate <<- sum(fc.fd.bact.EE.rate)
    fc.diet.bact.ash.rate <<- sum(fc.fd.bact.ash.rate)
    fc.diet.Endogenous.CP.rate <<- sum(fc.fd.Endogenous.CP.rate)
    fc.diet.Endogenous.fat.rate <<- sum(fc.fd.Endogenous.fat.rate)
    fc.diet.Endogenous.ash.rate <<- sum(fc.fd.Endogenous.ash.rate)
    fc.diet.CP.rate <<- sum(fc.CP.rate)
    fc.diet.CHO.rate <<- sum(fc.CHO.rate)
    fc.diet.EE.rate <<- sum(fc.EE.rate)
    fc.diet.ash.rate <<- sum(fc.ash.rate)
    if (genRPT)
    {
      rptFecalBact_DMI <- fds["FeedName.x"]
      names(rptFecalBact_DMI) <- "FeedName"
      rptFecalBact_DMI["Bact CP"] <- fc.fd.bact.CP.rate
      rptFecalBact_DMI["Bact CHO"] <- fc.fd.bact.CHO.rate
      rptFecalBact_DMI["Bact Fat"] <- fc.fd.bact.EE.rate
      rptFecalBact_DMI["Bact Ash"] <- fc.fd.bact.ash.rate
      rptFecalBact_DMI["Endo CP"] <- fc.fd.Endogenous.CP.rate
      rptFecalBact_DMI["Endo Fat"] <- fc.fd.Endogenous.fat.rate
      rptFecalBact_DMI["Endo Ash"] <- fc.fd.Endogenous.ash.rate
      description <- "Endo = endogenous source\n"
      if (flag_fecal == 0) footnote <- "Algorithm for fecal endogenous matter: CNCPS 5 & CPM 3.0.8 (Fox et al., 2004; Boston et al., 2000)"
      if (flag_fecal == 1) footnote <- "Algorithm for fecal endogenous matter: SRNS v. 1.8.11; Cannas et al. (2004)\nBacterial and endogenous protein, fat, and ash are computed together"
      if (flag_fecal == 2) footnote <- "Algorithm for fecal endogenous matter: RNS v. 1; Tedeschi and Fox (2016)"
      report(rptFecalBact_DMI, "Fecal Bacterial and Endogenous Matter, g/d", description, footnote, 3, 3, 1000, 8, TRUE, FALSE, TRUE, FALSE, TRUE, FALSE, FALSE)
      rptFecalTotal_DMI <- fds["FeedName.x"]
      names(rptFecalTotal_DMI) <- "FeedName"
      rptFecalTotal_DMI["CP"] <- fc.CP.rate
      rptFecalTotal_DMI["CHO"] <- fc.CHO.rate
      rptFecalTotal_DMI["Fat"] <- fc.EE.rate
      rptFecalTotal_DMI["Ash"] <- fc.ash.rate
      rptFecalTotal_DMI["IDM"] <- fc.fd.IDM.rate
      rptFecalTotal_DMI["IDM, %DMI"] <- isz(fc.fd.IDM.rate/10, anim.fd.DMI.rate)  # g to %
      rptFecalTotal_DMI["IOM"] <- fc.fd.IOM.rate
      rptFecalTotal_DMI["IOM, %DMI"] <- isz(fc.fd.IOM.rate/10, anim.fd.DMI.rate)  # g to %
      rptFecalTotal_DMI["IOM, %IDM"] <- isz(fc.fd.IOM.rate/10, fc.fd.IDM.rate)  # g to %
      rptFecalTotal_DMI2 <- data.frame(FeedName = "Ration")
      rptFecalTotal_DMI2["CP"] <- fc.diet.CP.rate
      rptFecalTotal_DMI2["CHO"] <- fc.diet.CHO.rate
      rptFecalTotal_DMI2["Fat"] <- fc.diet.EE.rate
      rptFecalTotal_DMI2["Ash"] <- fc.diet.ash.rate
      rptFecalTotal_DMI2["IDM"] <- fc.diet.IDM.rate
```

```
        rptFecalTotal_DMI2["IDM, %DMI"] <- isz(fc.diet.IDM.rate/10, anim.diet.DMI.rate)  # g to %
        rptFecalTotal_DMI2["IOM"] <- fc.diet.fd_IOM.rate
        rptFecalTotal_DMI2["IOM, %DMI"] <- isz(fc.diet.fd_IOM.rate/10, anim.diet.DMI.rate)  # g to %
        rptFecalTotal_DMI2["IOM, %IDM"] <- isz(fc.diet.fd_IOM.rate/10, fc.diet.IDM.rate)  # g to %
        rptFecalTotal_DMI <- rbind(rptFecalTotal_DMI, rptFecalTotal_DMI2)
        description <- "DMI = dry matter intake\nIDM = indigestible dry matter\nIOM = indigestible organic matter\n"
        if (flag_fecal == 0) footnote <- "Algorithm for fecal endogenous matter: CNCPS 5 & CPM 3.0.8 (Fox et al., 2004; Boston et al., 2000)"
        if (flag_fecal == 1) footnote <- "Algorithm for fecal endogenous matter: SRNS v. 1.8.11; Cannas et al. (2004)"
        if (flag_fecal == 2) footnote <- "Algorithm for fecal endogenous matter: RNS v. 1; Tedeschi and Fox (2016)"
        report(rptFecalTotal_DMI, "\nFecal Feed, Bacterial, and Endogenous Matter, g/d", description, footnote, 3, 3, 1000, 5, FALSE, FALSE, FALSE, FALSE, FALSE, FALSE, TRUE)
    }
}
```

4.3.13 Digestibility

```
calcDIG <- function(fds = feeds3, genRPT = TRUE)
{
  # ++++++++++++++++++++++++++++
  # Digestibility Calculations
  # ++++++++++++++++++++++++++++
  if (SolutionLevel == 2)
  {
    # aDDM = apparent digestible dry matter
    # aDMD = apparent dry matter digestibility
    anim.fd.aDDM.rate <<- (anim.fd.DMI.rate - fc.fd.IDM.rate)
    anim.fd.aDMD.conc <<- isz(anim.fd.aDDM.rate * 100, anim.fd.DMI.rate)
    anim.diet.aDDM.rate <<- sum(anim.fd.aDDM.rate)
    anim.diet.aDMD.conc <<- isz(anim.diet.aDDM.rate * 100, anim.diet.DMI.rate)
    # tDDM = true digestible dry matter
    # tDMD = true dry matter digestibility
    # Rf - Mi = Ra (Van Soest, 1994)
    anim.fd.tDDM.rate <<- (anim.fd.DMI.rate - fc.fd.IDM.rate + fc.fd.Mi.rate)
    anim.fd.tDMD.conc <<- isz(anim.fd.tDDM.rate * 100, anim.fd.DMI.rate)
    anim.diet.tDDM.rate <<- sum(anim.fd.tDDM.rate)
    anim.diet.tDMD.conc <<- isz(anim.diet.tDDM.rate * 100, anim.diet.DMI.rate)
    # aDOM = apparent digestible organic matter
    # aOMD = apparent organic matter digestibility
    anim.fd.aDOM.rate <<- (anim.fd.OMI.rate - fc.fd.IOM.rate)
    anim.fd.aOMD.conc <<- isz(anim.fd.aDOM.rate * 100, anim.fd.OMI.rate)
    anim.diet.aDOM.rate <<- sum(anim.fd.aDOM.rate)
    anim.diet.aOMD.conc <<- isz(anim.diet.aDOM.rate * 100, anim.diet.OMI.rate)
    # tDOM = true digestible organic matter
    # tOMD = true organic matter digestibility
    # Rf - Mi = Ra (Van Soest, 1994)
    anim.fd.tDOM.rate <<- (anim.fd.OMI.rate - fc.fd.IOM.rate + (fc.fd.Mi.rate - fc.fd.Mi_Ash.rate))
    anim.fd.tOMD.conc <<- isz(anim.fd.tDOM.rate * 100, anim.fd.OMI.rate)
    anim.diet.tDOM.rate <<- sum(anim.fd.tDOM.rate)
    anim.diet.tOMD.conc <<- isz(anim.diet.tDOM.rate * 100, anim.diet.OMI.rate)
    if (genRPT)
    {
      rptBioValues <- fds["FeedName.x"]
      names(rptBioValues) <- "FeedName"
      rptBioValues["tDDM, kg/d"] <- anim.fd.tDDM.rate
      rptBioValues["tDMD, % DM"] <- anim.fd.tDMD.conc
      rptBioValues["aDDM, kg/d"] <- anim.fd.aDDM.rate
      rptBioValues["aDMD, % DM"] <- anim.fd.aDMD.conc
      rptBioValues["tDOM, kg/d"] <- anim.fd.tDOM.rate
      rptBioValues["tOMD, % DM"] <- anim.fd.tOMD.conc
      rptBioValues["aDOM, kg/d"] <- anim.fd.aDOM.rate
      rptBioValues["aOMD, % DM"] <- anim.fd.aOMD.conc
      rptBioValues2 <- data.frame(FeedName = "Ration")
      rptBioValues2["tDDM, kg/d"] <- anim.diet.tDDM.rate
      rptBioValues2["tDMD, % DM"] <- anim.diet.tDMD.conc
```

```
            rptBioValues2["aDDM, kg/d"] <- anim.diet.aDDM.rate
            rptBioValues2["aDMD, % DM"] <- anim.diet.aDMD.conc
            rptBioValues2["tDOM, kg/d"] <- anim.diet.tDOM.rate
            rptBioValues2["tOMD, % DM"] <- anim.diet.tOMD.conc
            rptBioValues2["aDOM, kg/d"] <- anim.diet.aDOM.rate
            rptBioValues2["aOMD, % DM"] <- anim.diet.aOMD.conc
            rptBioValues <- rbind(rptBioValues, rptBioValues2)
            description <- paste("# a    = apparent\n", "# t    = true\n",
                                 "# DDM = digestible dry matter\n",
                                 "# DOM = digestible organic matter\n",
                                 "# DMD = dry matter digestibility\n",
                                 "# OMD = organic matter digestibility\n", sep = "")
            report(rptBioValues, "Dry Matter and Organic Matter Digestibility", description, "", 3, 3, 1, 4, FALSE, FALSE, FALSE,
    FALSE, FALSE, FALSE, TRUE)
        }
      } else
      {
        # aDDM = apparent digestible dry matter
        # aDMD = apparent dry matter digestibility
        anim.fd.aDDM.rate <<- rep(0, length(anim.fd.DMI.rate))
        anim.fd.aDMD.conc <<- rep(0, length(anim.fd.DMI.rate))
        anim.diet.aDDM.rate <<- 0
        anim.diet.aDMD.conc <<- 0
        # tDDM = true digestible dry matter
        # tDMD = true dry matter digestibility
        anim.fd.tDDM.rate <<- rep(0, length(anim.fd.DMI.rate))
        anim.fd.tDMD.conc <<- rep(0, length(anim.fd.DMI.rate))
        anim.diet.tDDM.rate <<- 0
        anim.diet.tDMD.conc <<- 0
        # aDOM = apparent digestible organic matter
        # aOMD = apparent organic matter digestibility
        anim.fd.aDOM.rate <<- rep(0, length(anim.fd.DMI.rate))
        anim.fd.aOMD.conc <<- rep(0, length(anim.fd.DMI.rate))
        anim.diet.aDOM.rate <<- 0
        anim.diet.aOMD.conc <<- 0
        # tDOM = true digestible organic matter
        # tOMD = true organic matter digestibility
        anim.fd.tDOM.rate <<- rep(0, length(anim.fd.DMI.rate))
        anim.fd.tOMD.conc <<- rep(0, length(anim.fd.DMI.rate))
        anim.diet.tDOM.rate <<- 0
        anim.diet.tOMD.conc <<- 0
      }
    }
```

4.3.14 Total digestible nutrients, and gross, digestible, metabolizable, and net energies

```
calcTDN <- function(fds = feeds3, genRPT = TRUE)
{
  # ++++++++++++++
  # Gross Energy
  # ++++++++++++++
  # Atwater factors
  anim.fd.GE.rate <<- anim.fd.EE.rate * 9.4 + anim.fd.CP.rate * 5.65 + (anim.fd.NFC.rate + anim.fd.FC.rate) * 4.1
  anim.fd.GE.frac <<- isz(anim.fd.GE.rate, anim.fd.DMI.rate)
  anim.diet.GE.rate <<- sum(anim.fd.GE.rate)
  anim.diet.GE.frac <<- isz(anim.diet.GE.rate, anim.diet.DMI.rate)
  # ++++++++++++++++++++++++++++
  # Total Digestible Nutrients
  # ++++++++++++++++++++++++++++
  # Apparent TDN
  anim.fd.aTDProt.rate <<- anim.fd.CP.rate - fc.CP.rate
  if (flag_TDN_EE == 0)
  {
    anim.fd.aTDEE.rate <<- 2.25 * (anim.fd.EE.rate - fc.EE.rate)
    anim.fd.aTDCHO.rate <<- anim.fd.CHO.rate - fc.CHO.rate
  }
  if (flag_TDN_EE == 1)
  {
    # Note that si.fd.GFA.rate =
(anim.fd.TFA.rate+rum.fd.DNFAC16.rate+rum.fd.DNFAC16_1.rate+rum.fd.DNFAC18.rate+rum.fd.DNFAOther.rate-fc.fd.TFA.rate)
    # Note that si.GFA.rate = si.fd.GFA.rate + si.fd.bact.GFAC12.rate + si.fd.bact.GFAC14.rate + si.fd.bact.GFAC16.rate +
    #                         si.fd.bact.GFAC16_1.rate + si.fd.bact.GFAC18.rate + si.fd.bact.GFAC18_1.rate +
si.fd.bact.GFAC18_2.rate +
    #                         si.fd.bact.GFAC18_3.rate + si.fd.bact.GFAOther.rate
    if (flag_TDN_BactFA == FALSE) anim.fd.aTDEE.rate <<- 2.25 * si.fd.GFA.rate
    if (flag_TDN_BactFA == TRUE) anim.fd.aTDEE.rate <<- 2.25 * si.GFA.rate
    anim.fd.aTDCHO.rate <<- (anim.fd.CHO.rate + anim.fd.Glycerol.rate) - fc.CHO.rate - 2.25 * (rum.fd.DNFAC16.rate +
rum.fd.DNFAC16_1.rate + rum.fd.DNFAC18.rate + rum.fd.DNFAOther.rate)
  }
  if (flag_TDN_EE == 2)
  {
    # Note that si.fd.GFA.rate =
(anim.fd.TFA.rate+rum.fd.DNFAC16.rate+rum.fd.DNFAC16_1.rate+rum.fd.DNFAC18.rate+rum.fd.DNFAOther.rate-fc.fd.TFA.rate)
    # Note that si.GFA.rate = si.fd.GFA.rate + si.fd.bact.GFAC12.rate + si.fd.bact.GFAC14.rate + si.fd.bact.GFAC16.rate +
    #                         si.fd.bact.GFAC16_1.rate + si.fd.bact.GFAC18.rate + si.fd.bact.GFAC18_1.rate +
si.fd.bact.GFAC18_2.rate +
    #                         si.fd.bact.GFAC18_3.rate + si.fd.bact.GFAOther.rate
    # Assuming that bacterial and endogenous fat (Mi_Fat) are 100% fatty acids
    if (flag_TDN_BactFA == FALSE) anim.fd.aTDEE.rate <<- 2.25 * (si.fd.GFA.rate - fc.fd.Mi_Fat.rate)
    if (flag_TDN_BactFA == TRUE) anim.fd.aTDEE.rate <<- 2.25 * (si.GFA.rate - fc.fd.Mi_Fat.rate)
    anim.fd.aTDCHO.rate <<- (anim.fd.CHO.rate + anim.fd.Glycerol.rate) - fc.CHO.rate - 2.25 * (rum.fd.DNFAC16.rate +
rum.fd.DNFAC16_1.rate + rum.fd.DNFAC18.rate + rum.fd.DNFAOther.rate)
  }
  anim.fd.aTDN.rate <<- pmax(0, anim.fd.aTDProt.rate + anim.fd.aTDCHO.rate + anim.fd.aTDEE.rate)
```

```
anim.fd.aTDN.conc <<- isz(anim.fd.aTDN.rate * 100, anim.fd.DMI.rate)
anim.diet.aTDProt.rate <<- sum(anim.fd.aTDProt.rate)
anim.diet.aTDCHO.rate <<- sum(anim.fd.aTDCHO.rate)
anim.diet.aTDEE.rate <<- sum(anim.fd.aTDEE.rate)
anim.diet.aTDN.rate <<- sum(anim.fd.aTDN.rate)
anim.diet.aTDN.conc <<- isz(anim.diet.aTDN.rate * 100, anim.diet.DMI.rate)
# True TDN
anim.fd.tTDProt.rate <<- anim.fd.CP.rate - fc.CP.rate + fc.fd.Mi_CP.rate
if (flag_TDN_EE == 0)
{
  anim.fd.tTDEE.rate <<- 2.25 * (anim.fd.EE.rate - fc.EE.rate + fc.fd.Mi_Fat.rate)
  anim.fd.tTDCHO.rate <<- anim.fd.CHO.rate - fc.CHO.rate + fc.fd.Mi_CHO.rate
} else
{
  # Note that si.fd.GFA.rate =
(anim.fd.TFA.rate+rum.fd.DNFAC16.rate+rum.fd.DNFAC16_1.rate+rum.fd.DNFAC18.rate+rum.fd.DNFAOther.rate-fc.fd.TFA.rate)
  # Note that si.GFA.rate = si.fd.GFA.rate + si.fd.bact.GFAC12.rate + si.fd.bact.GFAC14.rate + si.fd.bact.GFAC16.rate +
  #                         si.fd.bact.GFAC16_1.rate + si.fd.bact.GFAC18.rate + si.fd.bact.GFAC18_1.rate +
si.fd.bact.GFAC18_2.rate +
  #                         si.fd.bact.GFAC18_3.rate + si.fd.bact.GFAOther.rate
  if (flag_TDN_BactFA == FALSE) anim.fd.tTDEE.rate <<- 2.25 * si.fd.GFA.rate
  if (flag_TDN_BactFA == TRUE) anim.fd.tTDEE.rate <<- 2.25 * si.GFA.rate
  anim.fd.tTDCHO.rate <<- (anim.fd.CHO.rate + anim.fd.Glycerol.rate) - fc.CHO.rate + fc.fd.Mi_CHO.rate - 2.25 *
(rum.fd.DNFAC16.rate + rum.fd.DNFAC16_1.rate + rum.fd.DNFAC18.rate + rum.fd.DNFAOther.rate)
}
anim.fd.tTDN.rate <<- pmax(0, anim.fd.tTDProt.rate + anim.fd.tTDCHO.rate + anim.fd.tTDEE.rate)
anim.fd.tTDN.conc <<- isz(anim.fd.tTDN.rate * 100, anim.fd.DMI.rate)
anim.diet.tTDProt.rate <<- sum(anim.fd.tTDProt.rate)
anim.diet.tTDCHO.rate <<- sum(anim.fd.tTDCHO.rate)
anim.diet.tTDEE.rate <<- sum(anim.fd.tTDEE.rate)
anim.diet.tTDN.rate <<- sum(anim.fd.tTDN.rate)
anim.diet.tTDN.conc <<- isz(anim.diet.tTDN.rate * 100, anim.diet.DMI.rate)
# ++++++++++++++++++++
# Digestible Energy
# ++++++++++++++++++++
# Mcal/d
anim.fd.DEProt.rate <<- 4.409 * pmax(0, anim.fd.aTDProt.rate)
anim.fd.DECHO.rate <<- 4.409 * pmax(0, anim.fd.aTDCHO.rate)
anim.fd.DEEE.rate <<- 4.409 * pmax(0, anim.fd.aTDEE.rate)
anim.fd.DE.rate <<- anim.fd.DEProt.rate + anim.fd.DECHO.rate + anim.fd.DEEE.rate
anim.diet.DEProt.rate <<- 4.409 * pmax(0, anim.diet.aTDProt.rate)
anim.diet.DECHO.rate <<- 4.409 * pmax(0, anim.diet.aTDCHO.rate)
anim.diet.DEEE.rate <<- 4.409 * pmax(0, anim.diet.aTDEE.rate)
anim.diet.DE.rate <<- anim.diet.DEProt.rate + anim.diet.DECHO.rate + anim.diet.DEEE.rate
# Mcal/kg
anim.fd.DEProt.frac <<- isz(anim.fd.DEProt.rate, anim.fd.DMI.rate)
anim.fd.DECHO.frac <<- isz(anim.fd.DECHO.rate, anim.fd.DMI.rate)
anim.fd.DEEE.frac <<- isz(anim.fd.DEEE.rate, anim.fd.DMI.rate)
anim.fd.DE.frac <<- isz(anim.fd.DE.rate, anim.fd.DMI.rate)
anim.diet.DEProt.frac <<- isz(anim.diet.DEProt.rate, anim.diet.DMI.rate)
anim.diet.DECHO.frac <<- isz(anim.diet.DECHO.rate, anim.diet.DMI.rate)
```

```
    anim.diet.DEEE.frac <<- isz(anim.diet.DEEE.rate, anim.diet.DMI.rate)
    anim.diet.DE.frac <<- isz(anim.diet.DE.rate, anim.diet.DMI.rate)
    # ++++++++++++++++++++++
    # Metabolizable Energy
    # ++++++++++++++++++++++
    if (anim.type == "Milk" & (anim.stage_type == "Lactating" | anim.stage_type == "Dry"))
    {
      # Dairy Remove negative values and adjust for high fat feeds
      anim.fd.ME.frac <<- pmax(0, ifelse(anim.fd.EE.conc <= 3, 1.01 * anim.fd.DE.frac - 0.45, 1.01 * anim.fd.DE.frac - 0.45 + 0.0046 * (anim.fd.EE.conc - 3)))
    } else
    {
      # Remove negative values and adjust for high fat feeds
      anim.fd.ME.frac <<- pmax(0, 0.82 * anim.fd.DE.frac)
    }
    if (anim.diet.ionophore == TRUE & flag_Ionophore == 1) anim.fd.ME.frac <<- 1.023 * anim.fd.ME.frac
    anim.fd.ME.rate <<- anim.fd.ME.frac * anim.fd.DMI.rate
    anim.diet.ME.rate <<- sum(anim.fd.ME.rate)
    anim.diet.ME.frac <<- isz(anim.diet.ME.rate, anim.diet.DMI.rate)
    # ++++++++++++
    # Net Energy
    # ++++++++++++
    # Feeds
    anim.fd.NEm.frac <<- ifelse(anim.fd.ME.frac > 0, 1.37 * anim.fd.ME.frac - 0.138 * anim.fd.ME.frac^2 + 0.0105 * anim.fd.ME.frac^3 - 1.12, 0)
    anim.fd.NEg.frac <<- ifelse(anim.fd.ME.frac > 0, 1.42 * anim.fd.ME.frac - 0.174 * anim.fd.ME.frac^2 + 0.0122 * anim.fd.ME.frac^3 - 1.65, 0)
    anim.fd.NEl.frac <<- ifelse(anim.fd.ME.frac > 0, 0.644 * anim.fd.ME.frac, 0)
    if (anim.type == "Milk" & anim.stage_type == "Lactating") anim.fd.NEm.frac <<- anim.fd.NEl.frac
    if (anim.diet.ionophore == TRUE & flag_Ionophore == 0) anim.fd.NEm.frac <<- 1.12 * anim.fd.NEm.frac
    anim.fd.NEm.rate <<- anim.fd.NEm.frac * anim.fd.DMI.rate
    anim.fd.NEg.rate <<- anim.fd.NEg.frac * anim.fd.DMI.rate
    anim.fd.NEl.rate <<- anim.fd.NEl.frac * anim.fd.DMI.rate
    # Ration
    anim.diet.NEm.frac <<- ifelse(anim.diet.ME.frac > 0, 1.37 * anim.diet.ME.frac - 0.138 * anim.diet.ME.frac^2 + 0.0105 * anim.diet.ME.frac^3 - 1.12, 0)
    anim.diet.NEg.frac <<- ifelse(anim.diet.ME.frac > 0, 1.42 * anim.diet.ME.frac - 0.174 * anim.diet.ME.frac^2 + 0.0122 * anim.diet.ME.frac^3 - 1.65, 0)
    anim.diet.NEl.frac <<- ifelse(anim.diet.ME.frac > 0, 0.644 * anim.diet.ME.frac, 0)
    if (anim.type == "Milk" & anim.stage_type == "Lactating") anim.diet.NEm.frac <<- anim.diet.NEl.frac
    if (anim.diet.ionophore == TRUE & flag_Ionophore == 0) anim.diet.NEm.frac <<- 1.12 * anim.diet.NEm.frac
    anim.diet.NEm.rate <<- anim.diet.NEm.frac * anim.diet.DMI.rate
    anim.diet.NEg.rate <<- anim.diet.NEg.frac * anim.diet.DMI.rate
    anim.diet.NEl.rate <<- anim.diet.NEl.frac * anim.diet.DMI.rate
    if (genRPT)
    {
      rptBioValues <- feeds3["FeedName.x"]
      names(rptBioValues) <- "FeedName"
      rptBioValues["GE, Mcal/d"] <- anim.fd.GE.rate
      rptBioValues["GE, Mcal/kg"] <- anim.fd.GE.frac
      rptBioValues["tTDN, kg/d"] <- anim.fd.tTDN.rate
```

```
        rptBioValues["aTDN, kg/d"] <- anim.fd.aTDN.rate
        rptBioValues["tTDN, % DM"] <- anim.fd.tTDN.conc
        rptBioValues["aTDN, % DM"] <- anim.fd.aTDN.conc
        rptBioValues["DE, Mcal/d"] <- anim.fd.DE.rate
        rptBioValues["DE, Mcal/kg"] <- anim.fd.DE.frac
        rptBioValues["ME, Mcal/d"] <- anim.fd.ME.rate
        rptBioValues["ME, Mcal/kg"] <- anim.fd.ME.frac
        rptBioValues["NEm, Mcal/d"] <- anim.fd.NEm.rate
        rptBioValues["NEm, Mcal/kg"] <- anim.fd.NEm.frac
        rptBioValues["NEg, Mcal/d"] <- anim.fd.NEg.rate
        rptBioValues["NEg, Mcal/kg"] <- anim.fd.NEg.frac
        rptBioValues["NEl, Mcal/d"] <- anim.fd.NEl.rate
        rptBioValues["NEl, Mcal/kg"] <- anim.fd.NEl.frac
        rptBioValues2 <- data.frame(FeedName = "Ration")
        rptBioValues2["GE, Mcal/d"] <- anim.diet.GE.rate
        rptBioValues2["GE, Mcal/kg"] <- anim.diet.GE.frac
        rptBioValues2["tTDN, kg/d"] <- anim.diet.tTDN.rate
        rptBioValues2["aTDN, kg/d"] <- anim.diet.aTDN.rate
        rptBioValues2["tTDN, % DM"] <- anim.diet.tTDN.conc
        rptBioValues2["aTDN, % DM"] <- anim.diet.aTDN.conc
        rptBioValues2["DE, Mcal/d"] <- anim.diet.DE.rate
        rptBioValues2["DE, Mcal/kg"] <- anim.diet.DE.frac
        rptBioValues2["ME, Mcal/d"] <- anim.diet.ME.rate
        rptBioValues2["ME, Mcal/kg"] <- anim.diet.ME.frac
        rptBioValues2["NEm, Mcal/d"] <- anim.diet.NEm.rate
        rptBioValues2["NEm, Mcal/kg"] <- anim.diet.NEm.frac
        rptBioValues2["NEg, Mcal/d"] <- anim.diet.NEg.rate
        rptBioValues2["NEg, Mcal/kg"] <- anim.diet.NEg.frac
        rptBioValues2["NEl, Mcal/d"] <- anim.diet.NEl.rate
        rptBioValues2["NEl, Mcal/kg"] <- anim.diet.NEl.frac
        rptBioValues <- rbind(rptBioValues, rptBioValues2)
        description <- paste("# a    = apparent\n", "# t    = true\n",
                             "# TDN = total digestible nutrients\n",
                             "# GE  = gross energy\n",
                             "# DE  = digestible energy\n",
                             "# ME  = metabolizable energy\n",
                             "# NEm = net energy for maintenance\n",
                             "# NEg = net energy for growth\n",
                             "# NEl = net energy for lactation\n", sep = "")
        report(rptBioValues, "Gross Energy, Total Digestible Nutrients, Digestible Energy, Metabolizable Energy, and Net Energy",
    description, "", 3, 3, 1, 6, FALSE, FALSE, FALSE, FALSE, FALSE, FALSE, TRUE)
      }
    }
```

4.3.15 Metabolizable protein

```
calcMP <- function(fds = feeds3, genRPT = TRUE)
{
  # +++++++++++++++++++++++
  # Metabolizable Protein
  # +++++++++++++++++++++++
  anim.fd.bact.MP.rate <<- si.fd.bact.GProt.rate - si.fd.bact.GNA.rate
  anim.fd.fd.MP.rate <<- si.fd.GProt.rate
  anim.fd.MP.rate <<- anim.fd.bact.MP.rate + anim.fd.fd.MP.rate
  anim.diet.bact.MP.rate <<- sum(anim.fd.bact.MP.rate)
  anim.diet.fd.MP.rate <<- sum(anim.fd.fd.MP.rate)
  anim.diet.MP.rate <<- sum(anim.fd.MP.rate)
  if (genRPT)
  {
    rptBioValues <- fds["FeedName.x"]
    names(rptBioValues) <- "FeedName"
    rptBioValues["RDP, g/d"] <- (anim.fd.CP.rate - rum.fd.RUCP.rate) * 1000
    rptBioValues["RDP, %CP"] <- isz((anim.fd.CP.rate - rum.fd.RUCP.rate) * 100, anim.fd.CP.rate)
    rptBioValues["RUP, g/d"] <- rum.fd.RUCP.rate * 1000
    rptBioValues["RUP, %CP"] <- isz(rum.fd.RUCP.rate * 100, anim.fd.CP.rate)
    rptBioValues["MP Bact, g/d"] <- anim.fd.bact.MP.rate * 1000
    rptBioValues["MP Fd, g/d"] <- anim.fd.fd.MP.rate * 1000
    rptBioValues["MP, g/d"] <- anim.fd.MP.rate * 1000
    rptBioValues2 <- data.frame(FeedName = "Ration")
    rptBioValues2["RDP, g/d"] <- (anim.diet.CP.rate - rum.diet.RUCP.rate) * 1000
    rptBioValues2["RDP, %CP"] <- isz((anim.diet.CP.rate - rum.diet.RUCP.rate) * 100, anim.diet.CP.rate)
    rptBioValues2["RUP, g/d"] <- rum.diet.RUCP.rate * 1000
    rptBioValues2["RUP, %CP"] <- isz(rum.diet.RUCP.rate * 100, anim.diet.CP.rate)
    rptBioValues2["MP Bact, g/d"] <- anim.diet.bact.MP.rate * 1000
    rptBioValues2["MP Fd, g/d"] <- anim.diet.fd.MP.rate * 1000
    rptBioValues2["MP, g/d"] <- anim.diet.MP.rate * 1000
    rptBioValues <- rbind(rptBioValues, rptBioValues2)
    description <- paste("# MP  = metabolizable protein\n",
                         "# RDP = ruminally degraded protein (i.e., DIP: digestible intake protein)\n",
                         "# RUP = ruminally undegradable protein (i.e., UIP: undegradable intake protein)\n", sep = "")
    report(rptBioValues, "Metabolizable Protein, Ruminally Degraded Protein, and Ruminally Undegradable Protein", description,
"", 3, 3, 1, 7, FALSE, FALSE, FALSE, FALSE, FALSE, FALSE, TRUE)
  }
}
```

Part II. Calculations of Energy and Nutrient Requirements

"*Dans les champs de l'observation le hasard ne favorise que les esprits prepares* (in the fields of observation chance favors the prepared mind)."
Louis Pasteur (Lecture at the University of Lille, 1854)

(This page intentionally left blank)

5 Energy and Nutrient Requirements

5.1 Flowchart of the calculation logic

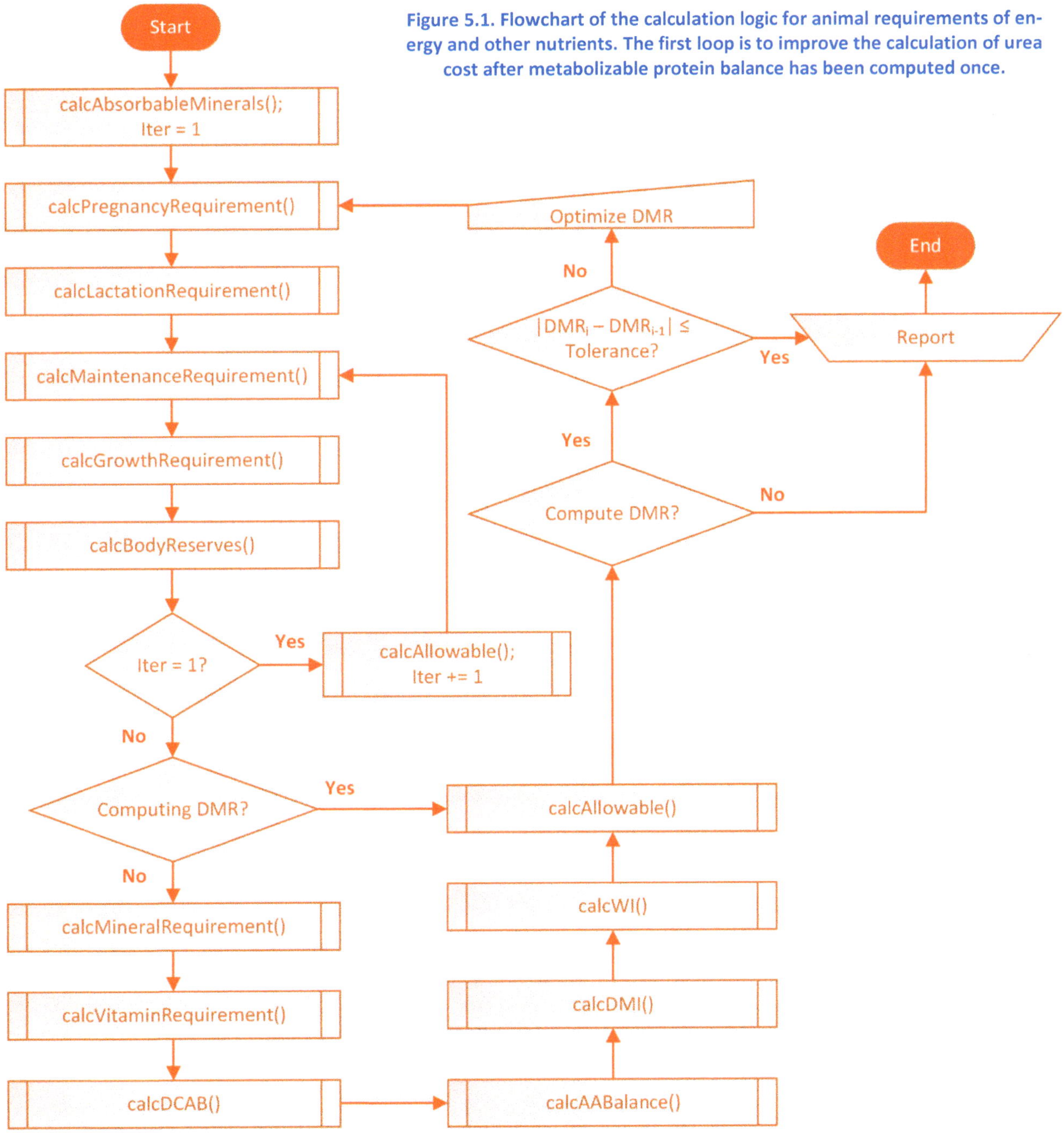

Figure 5.1. Flowchart of the calculation logic for animal requirements of energy and other nutrients. The first loop is to improve the calculation of urea cost after metabolizable protein balance has been computed once.

5.2 Equations

5.2.1 Basic calculations: calcBW(), calcBCS(), and calcDMINursingCalves()

#	Variable[1]	Description	Equation[2]
1:	*SBW*		$0.96 * FBW$
2:	*EBW*		$0.891 * SBW$
3:	$BCS_{[0\text{-}5]}$		$\left(\frac{5}{4}\right) * (BCS_{[1-5]} - 1)$
4:	$BCS_{[0\text{-}5]}$		$\left(\frac{5}{8}\right) * (BCS_{[1-9]} - 1)$
5:	$BCS_{[1\text{-}5]}$		$\left(\frac{1}{5}\right) * (5 + 4 * BCS_{[0-5]})$
6:	$BCS_{[1\text{-}5]}$		$\frac{BCS_{[1-9]} + 1}{2}$
7:	$BCS_{[1\text{-}9]}$		$\left(\frac{8}{5}\right) * BCS_{[0-5]} + 1$
8:	$BCS_{[1\text{-}9]}$		$2 * BCS_{[1-5]} + 1$
9:	$BCS_{[1\text{-}8]}$		$\left(\frac{1}{5}\right) * (5 + 7 * BCS_{[0-5]})$
10:	$BCS_{[1\text{-}8]}$		$\left(\frac{1}{4}\right) * (7 * BCS_{[1-5]} - 3)$
11:	$BCS_{[1\text{-}8]}$		$\left(\frac{1}{8}\right) * (1 + 7 * BCS_{[1-9]})$
12:	$BCS_{[1\text{-}10]}$		$\left(\frac{1}{5}\right) * (9 * BCS_{[0-5]} + 5)$
13:	$BCS_{[1\text{-}10]}$		$\left(\frac{1}{4}\right) * (9 * BCS_{[1-5]} - 5)$
14:	$BCS_{[1\text{-}10]}$		$\left(\frac{1}{8}\right) * (9 * BCS_{[1-9]} - 1)$
15:	*ForageDMI*		$Max\left[0, \left(\frac{1}{ForageDE^2}\right) * \left(\left(CalfBW^{-0.3895-0.0197*PML^2}\right) * \text{Exp}(CalfBW * (-0.00244 - 0.00337 * PML) - 1.3594 * PML) * \left(\left(CalfBW^{0.4477*PML}\right) * (-32.5704 + (27.9016 - 7.66732 * ForageDE) * ForageDE) * \text{Exp}((0.0588 + 0.00018 * CalfBW) * (PML^2)) + \left(CalfBW^{1.3895+0.0197*PML^2}\right) * \text{Exp}(CalfBW * (0.00244 + 0.00337 * PML) + 1.3594 * PML) * (0.4738 + ForageDE * (-0.4059 + ForageDE * (0.11154 - 0.003273 * PML) + 0.01191 * PML) - 0.0139046 * PML) + \left(CalfBW^{0.3895+0.0197*PML^2}\right) * \text{Exp}(CalfBW * (0.00244 + 0.00337 * PML) + 1.3594 * PML) * (-10.3049 + ForageDE * (8.82778 + ForageDE * (-2.42586 + 0.362681 * PML) - 1.31981 * PML) + 1.54065 * PML)\right)\right)\right]$

(1) ***BCS*** is body condition score, dimensionless; ***CalfBW*** is calf body weight, kg; ***EBW*** is empty body weight, kg; ***ForageDE*** is forage digestible energy, Mcal/kg; ***ForageDMI*** is forage dry matter intake, kg/d; ***PML*** is peak milk level, kg/d; and ***SBW*** is shrunk body weight, kg.

(2) Figure 5.2 depicts the pattern of forage dry matter intake of nursing calves given calf body weight, peak milk level, and forage digestible energy content.

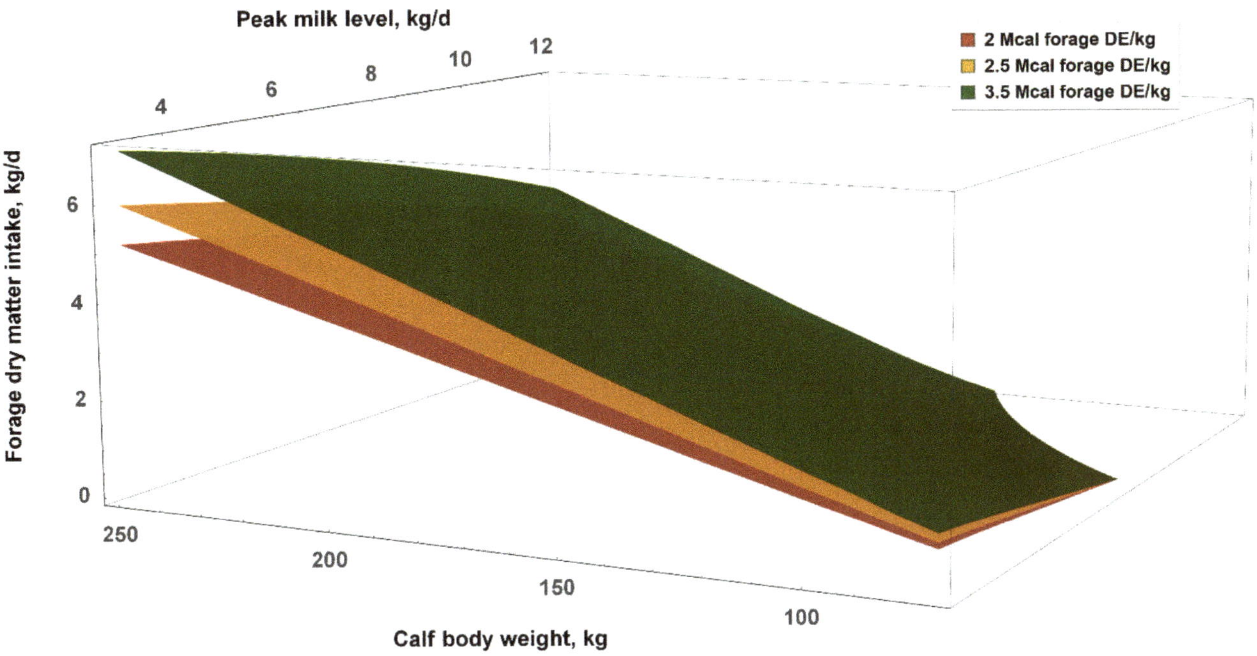

Figure 5.2. Predicted forage dry matter intake of nursing calves of different body weights and levels of cow's peak milk, assuming three forage digestible energy contents.

5.2.2 Maintenance requirements: calcMaintenanceRequirement()

#	Variable[1]	Description	Equation[2]
1:	*COMP*	growing/finishing or replacement heifer	$0.8 + 0.05 * (BCS_{[1-9]} - 1)$
2:		otherwise	1
3:	*PETI*	Tp>20	$27.88 - 0.456 * Tp + 0.010754 * Tp^2 - 0.4905 * RHp + 0.00088 * RHp + 1.1507 * \left(\frac{1000}{3600}\right) * WS - 0.126447 * \left(\frac{1000}{3600}\right) * WS^2 + 0.019876 * Tp * RHp - 0.046313 * Tp * \left(\frac{1000}{3600}\right) * WS + 0.4167 * HRS$
4:		otherwise	Tp
5:	*a2*		$\frac{88.426 - 0.785 * PETI + 0.0116 * PETI^2 - 77}{1000}$
6:	*L*	lactating beef or dual-purpose cows	1.2
7:		otherwise	1
8:	*sex*	intact males	1.15
9:		otherwise	1
10:	$NEmr_{Basal}$		$(a1 * L * COMP * sex + a2) * (SBW - GUW)^{0.75}$
11:	$NEmr_{Act}$		$\left(0.1 * Standing + 0.062 * Position + 0.621 * \frac{Distance_{horizontal}}{1000} + 6.69 * \frac{Distance_{vertical}}{1000}\right) * FBW * 0.001$
12:	*HE*		$[ME] * DMI - (NEmr_{Basal} + NEgr + NEpr + NElr)$
13:	*SA*		$0.09 * FBW^{0.67}$
14:	*mud*	hair coat = 0	1
15:		hair coat = 1	0.8
16:		hair coat = 2	0.5
17:		hair coat = 3	0.3
18:	*hide*	thin	0.8
19:		medium	1
20:		thick	1.2

#	Variable[(1)]	Description	Equation[(2)]
21:	*EI*		$(6.1816 - 0.5575 * WS + 0.0152 * WS^2 + 5.298 * HD - 0.5297 * HD^2 - 0.1029 * WS * HD) * mud * hide$
22:	*TI*	age<30 days	2.5
23:		30<age<183 days	6.5
24:		184<age<363 days	$5.1875 + 0.3125 * BCS_{[1-9]}$
25:		age>363 days	$5.25 + 0.75 * BCS_{[1-9]}$
26:	*IN*		$EI + TI$
27:	*LCT*		$39 - 0.85 * IN * \frac{HE}{SA}$
28:	*MEmr_{CS}*	LCT>Tc	$SA * (LCT - Tc)/IN$
29:		otherwise	0
30:	$NEmr_{CS}$		$MEmr_{CS} * k_m$
31:	*CETI*		$27.88 - 0.456 * Tc + 0.010754 * Tc^2 - 0.4905 * RHc + 0.00088 * RHc + 1.1507 * \left(\frac{1000}{3600}\right) * WS - 0.126447 * \left(\frac{1000}{3600}\right) * WS^2 + 0.019876 * Tc * RHc - 0.046313 * Tc * \left(\frac{1000}{3600}\right) * WS + 0.4167 * HRS$
32:	*HSF*	*Bos indicus* & panting score=0	1
33:		*Bos indicus* & panting score=1	1.07
34:		*Bos indicus* & panting score=2	1.18
35:		*Bos taurus* & CETI≥20	$1.09857 - 0.1343 * CETI + 0.000457 * CETI^2$
36:		*Bos taurus* & CETI<20	1
37:	$NEmr_{HS}$		$NEmr_{Basal} * HSF$
38:	*MPB*		$\sum_{f=1}^{nf} MP_f - (MPmr + MPpr + MPlr + MPgr + MPrr)$
39:	$NEmr_{Urea}$		$(\Delta RuminalN - RecycledN + MPB) * 0.0073 * k_m$
40:	*NEmr*		$NEmr_{Basal} + NEmr_{Act} + NEmr_{CS} + NEmr_{HS} + NEmr_{Urea}$
41:	*UPA*	SolutionLevel=2	$2.75 * \frac{SBW^{0.5}}{0.67}$
42:	*SPA*	SolutionLevel=2	$0.2 * \frac{SBW^{0.6}}{0.67}$
43:	*FPN*	SolutionLevel=2	$0.09 * IDM$
44:	*MPmr*	SolutionLevel=2	$UPA + SPA + FPN$
45:		otherwise	$3.8 * SBW^{0.75}$
46:	*NPmr*	SolutionLevel=2	$FPN * 0.5 + (UPA + SPA) * 0.67$
47:		otherwise	$MPmr * 0.5$
48:	*a2*		$1 + 0.0091 * (20 - PETI)$
49:	$NEmr_{Basal}$		$a1 * a2 * \left(Exp\left(-0.03 * \left(\frac{age}{30.4}\right)\right)\right) * (SBW - GUW)^{0.75}$
50:	$NEmr_{Act}$	sheep	$\left(0.62 * \frac{Distance_{horizontal}}{1000} + 6.69 * \frac{Distance_{vertizal}}{1000}\right) * FBW * 0.001$
51:		goats	$\left(0.836 * \frac{Distance_{horizontal}}{1000} + 6.69 * \frac{Distance_{vertizal}}{1000}\right) * FBW * 0.001$
52:	*E*		$\frac{1.3}{4.184}$
53:	*z*	sheep	0.141
54:		goats	0.11
55:	*r*	age<365	50
56:		otherwise	120
57:	*TI*		$1.3 * 4.184$
58:	*EI*		$4.184 * \left(\left(\left(\frac{r}{(0.481 + 0.326 * \sqrt{WS}) * (r + WD)}\right) + r * Log\left(\frac{r + WD}{r}\right)\right) * \left(z - 0.017 * \sqrt{WS}\right)\right)$
59:	*IN*		$TI + \left(1 - 0.3 * \left(1 - Exp\left(-1.5 * \frac{RF}{WD}\right)\right)\right) * EI$

#	Variable[(1)]	Description	Equation[(2)]
60:	*LCT*		$39 + E * EI - IN * \frac{HE}{SA}$
61:	$MEmr_{CS}$	LCT>Tc	$SA * (LCT - Tc)/IN$
62:		otherwise	0
63:	$NEmr_{CS}$		$MEmr_{CS} * k_m$
64:	$NEmr_{HS}$		0
65:	*NEmr*		$NEmr_{Basal} + NEmr_{Act} + NEmr_{CS} + NEmr_{HS} + NEmr_{Urea}$
66:	*UPA*		$\frac{0.147 * (SBW - GUW) + 3.375}{0.67}$
67:	*SPA*	*sheep*	$\frac{CW}{0.6 * 365}$
68:		*goats*	$0.1125 * FBW^{0.75}$
69:	*FPN*		$15.2 * \frac{DMI}{0.67}$
70:	*MPmr*		$UPA + SPA + FPN$
71:	*NPmr*		$MPmr * 0.67$
72:	$MAAmr_j$		$\frac{NPmr * \frac{TiAA_j}{100}}{k_{TiAA_j}}$
73:	*FFM*		$NEmr/[NEm]$
74:	L_{DMI}		DMI/FFM

(1) ***[ME]*** is the dietary content of metabolizable energy, Mcal/kg (dry matter basis); ***a1*** is the basal metabolism coefficient that is breed-specific, Mcal/kg$^{0.75}$/d; ***a2*** is the adjustment for previous temperature (acclimatization), Mcal/kg$^{0.75}$/d; ***age*** is the animal age, days; ***BCS*** is body condition score (1 to 9 scale), dimensionless; ***CETI*** is the current effective temperature index, °C; ***COMP*** is the adjustment for compensatory growth (i.e., previous plane of nutrition), dimensionless; ***CW*** is clean wool, g/yr; ***$Distance_{horizontal}$*** is the distance traveled daily, km; ***$Distance_{vertical}$*** is the distance traveled daily as any vertical movement, km; ***DMI*** is dry matter intake, kg/d; ***EI*** is external insulation, °C·m^2·d/Mcal; ***FBW*** is the full (unshrunk) body weight, kg; ***FFM*** is feed required for maintenance, kg/d; ***FPN*** is the fecal protein nitrogen, g/d; ***GUW*** is the gravid uterus weight for pregnant animals, kg; ***HD*** is the hair depth, cm; ***HE*** is the heat production, Mcal/d; ***hide*** is the hide thickness adjustment factor, dimensionless; ***HRS*** is the hours under the sunlight, h; ***HSF*** is heat stress factor, dimensionless; ***IDM*** is the indigestible dry matter, g/d; ***IN*** is the total insulation (tissue and external), °C·m^2·d/Mcal; ***j*** is the jth amino acid; ***k_m*** is the partial efficiency of utilization of metabolizable energy for net energy for maintenance, dimensionless; ***$K_{TiAA,j}$*** is the jth tissue amino acid efficiency (Arg: 0.85, His: 0.85, Ile: 0.66, Leu: 0.66, Lys: 0.85, Met: 0.85, Phe: 0.85, Thr: 0.85, Trp: 0.85, and Val: 0.66), dimensionless; ***L*** is the adjustment factor for lactating beef or dual-purpose cows to account for increased organ size during lactation, dimensionless; ***LCT*** is the lower critical temperature, °C; ***L_{DMI}*** is the level of intake as multiples of feed required for maintenance, dimensionless; ***$MAAmr_j$*** is the metabolizable jth amino acid required for maintenance, g/d; ***MP*** is the dietary metabolizable energy, g/d; ***MPB*** is the metabolizable protein balance, g/d; ***MPgr*** is the metabolizable protein required for growth, g/d; ***MPlr*** is the metabolizable protein required for lactation, g/d; ***MPmr*** is the metabolizable protein required for maintenance, g/d; ***MPpr*** is the metabolizable protein required for pregnancy, g/d; ***MPrr*** is the metabolizable protein required for body reserves, g/d; ***mud*** is the mud adjustment factor for clean and dry (hair coat = 0), some mud on lower body (hair coat = 1), wet and matted (hair coat = 2), and covered with wet snow or mud (hair coat = 3), dimensionless; ***NEgr*** is the net energy required for growth, Mcal/d; ***NElr*** is the net energy required for lactation, Mcal/d; ***[NEm]*** is dietary content of net energy for maintenance, Mcal/kg; ***NEmr*** is the net energy required for maintenance, Mcal/d; ***$NEmr_{Act}$*** is the net energy required for physical activity, Mcal/d; ***$NEmr_{Basal}$*** is the net energy required for basal metabolism, Mcal/d; ***$NEmr_{CS}$*** is the net energy required for maintenance for cold stress, Mcal/d; ***$NEmr_{HS}$*** is the net energy required for maintenance for heat stress, Mcal/d; ***$NEmr_{Urea}$*** is the net energy required for maintenance for excess of nitrogen (i.e., plasma urea), Mcal/d; ***NEpr*** is the net energy required for pregnancy, Mcal/d; ***NPmr*** is the net protein required for maintenance, g/d; ***PETI*** is the previous effective temperature index, °C; ***Position*** is the number of daily standing and lying changes; ***RecycledN*** is the amount of nitrogen recycled back to the rumen, g/d; ***RF*** is rainfall, mm/d; ***RHc*** is the current relative humidity, %; ***RHp*** is the previous relative humidity, %; ***SA*** is the body surface area, m^2; ***SBW*** is the shrunk body weight, kg; ***sex*** is the adjustment factor for sex, dimensionless; ***SPA*** is the scurf protein, g/d; ***Standing*** is the hours standing, h; ***Tc*** is the current temperature, °C; ***TI*** is tissue insulation, °C·m^2·d/Mcal; ***TiAA*** is the jth tissue amino acid content (Arg: 6.6, His: 2.47, Ile: 2.84, Leu: 6.7, Lys: 6.37, Met: 1.97, Phe: 3.53, Thr: 3.9, Trp: 1.18, and Val: 4.03), %; ***Tp*** is the previous temperature, °C; ***UPA*** is urinary protein, g/d; ***WD*** is wool depth, mm; ***WS*** is the wind speed, km/h; and ***ΔRuminalN*** is the ruminal nitrogen balance (a negative balance indicates there is not enough ammonia-N in the rumen to support the energy-allowable growth of fiber carbohydrate-degrading bacteria), g/d.

(2) Equations 1 to 47 are for cattle, and Equations 48 to 71 have replacement equations for sheep and goats. Note that PETI and CETI use the same wind speed (WS) and hours of sunlight (HRS) when it would be ideal to have used the corresponding values for previous and current situations. Figure 5.3 shows the simulation of the $MEmr_{CS}$, given different combinations of SBW, BCS, WS, and HD.

Figure 5.3 depicts the additional metabolizable energy required due to cold stress given the combined effects of current temperature (-20°C or -10°C), hair depth, and wind speed for animals with 350 or 550

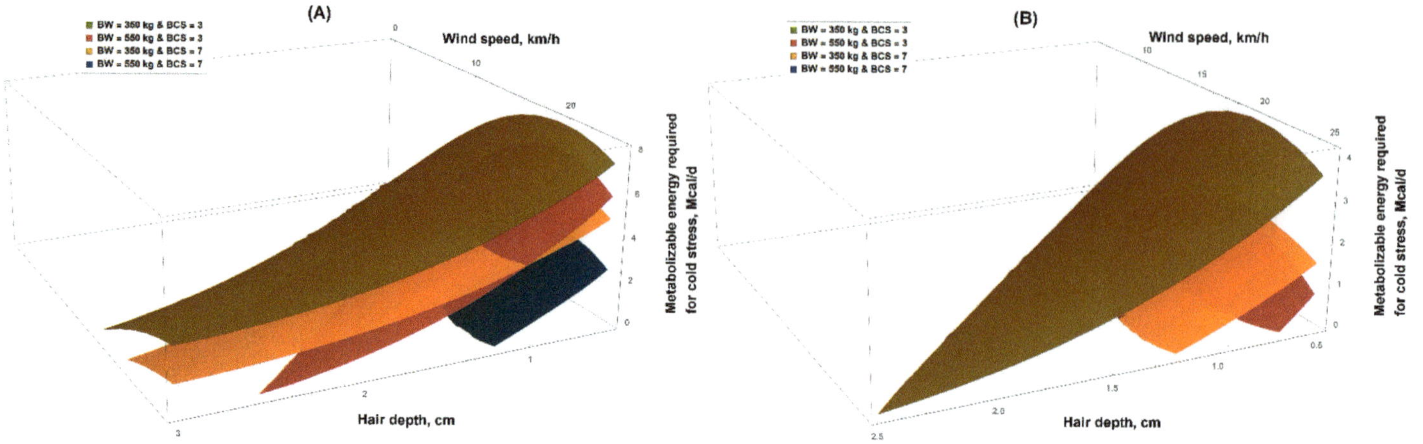

Figure 5.3. Metabolizable energy required for cold stress at different wind speeds and hair depths, assuming current temperature of (A) - 20°C and (B) -10°C, and combinations of body weight (BW: 350 and 550 kg) and body condition score (BCS: 3 and 7).

kg and body condition score of 3 or 7. The calculations were performed assuming a fixed dry matter intake of 2.3% of body weight and dietary metabolizable energy of 2.9 Mcal/kg. The external insulation equation developed by the NASEM (2016) used the data from Table 5 of Fox et al. (1988), who reported wind speeds varying from 1.6 to 25.6 km/h and hair depth ranging from 0.5 to 3 cm. Therefore, the external insulation equations should be used within these limits to avoid extrapolating beyond the limits of the dataset. Figure 5.3A indicates that under a cold environment (current temperature of -20°C), a 350-kg animal having short hair depth and BCS of 3 would require up to 8 Mcal /d of metabolizable energy for windy conditions. This extra energy requirement corresponds to approximately an additional daily intake of 2.7 kg of dry matter to survive the cold stress (assuming dietary metabolizable energy of 2.9 Mcal/kg) compared to a similar animal at the thermoneutral condition. Figure 5.3B indicates that the same animal in a warmer environment (current temperature of -10°C) would require an additional daily intake of about 1.4 kg of dry matter. The ability of animals to consume these additional ration amounts will depend on the quality of the ration and the level of production of the animal, i.e., additional energy needed to support animal performance (growth, pregnancy, and lactation) above that required for basal metabolism.

5.2.3 Lactation requirements: calcLactationRequirement()

#	Variable[(1)]	Description	Equation[(2)]
1:	T	beef cattle	8.5
2:		beef cattle & age ≤ 2 years	$0.74 * \frac{DIM * (0.125 * RelMY + 0.375) * PKYD * Exp(1)}{7 * T * Exp\left(\frac{DIM}{7 * T}\right)}$
3:		beef cattle & 2 < age ≤ 3 years	$0.88 * \frac{DIM * (0.125 * RelMY + 0.375) * PKYD * Exp(1)}{7 * T * Exp\left(\frac{DIM}{7 * T}\right)}$
4:	PMY	beef cattle & age > 3 years	$\frac{DIM * (0.125 * RelMY + 0.375) * PKYD * Exp(1)}{7 * T * Exp\left(\frac{DIM}{7 * T}\right)}$
5:		dairy cattle & lactation = 1	$27.34059 * DIM^{0.08} * Exp(-0.002 * DIM) * Exp(-0.001 * DG)$
6:		dairy cattle & lactation = 2	$35.92915 * DIM^{0.12} * Exp(-0.004 * DIM) * Exp(-0.002 * DG)$
7:		dairy cattle & lactation	$35.92915 * DIM^{0.16} * Exp(-0.005 * DIM) * Exp(-0.002 * DG)$

#	Variable[(1)]	Description	Equation[(2)]
		≥ 3	
8:	*PMkFat*	cattle	$\frac{\left(MkFat * \left(\left(\frac{DIM+1}{7}\right)^{-0.13}\right) * Exp\left(0.02 * \frac{DIM+1}{7}\right)\right)}{0.9922}$
9:	*PMkProt*	cattle	$\frac{\left(MkTP * \left(\left(\frac{DIM+1}{7}\right)^{-0.12}\right) * Exp\left(0.01 * \frac{DIM+1}{7}\right)\right)}{0.875}$
10:	*NElr*	beef cattle	$PMY * \left(0.0929 * MkFat + 0.0547 * \frac{MkTP}{0.93} + 0.0395 * MkL\right)$
11:		dairy cattle	$MY * \left(0.0929 * MkFat + 0.0547 * \frac{MkTP}{0.93} + 0.0395 * MkL\right)$
12:	*MElr*		$\frac{NElr}{0.644}$
13:	*NPlr*	beef cattle	$PMY * \left(\frac{MkTP}{100}\right) * 1000$
14:		dairy cattle	$MY * \left(\frac{MkTP}{100}\right) * 1000$
15:	*MPlr*	cattle	$\frac{NPlr}{0.67}$
16:	*MAAlr$_j$*	cattle	$\frac{NPlr * \frac{MkAA_j}{100}}{k_{MkAA_j}}$
17:	*NElr*	sheep	$MY * \left(0.25173 + 0.08964 * MkFat + 0.03785 * \frac{MkTP}{0.93}\right)$
18:	*MElr*	sheep	$\frac{NElr}{0.644}$
19:	*NPlr*	sheep	$MY * \left(\frac{MkTP}{100}\right) * 1000$
20:	*MPlr*	sheep	$\frac{NPlr}{0.58}$
21:	*NElr*	goats	$MY * \left(0.28972 + 0.07193 * MkFat + 0.04828 * \frac{MkTP}{0.92}\right)$
22:	*MElr*	goats	$\frac{NElr}{0.644}$
23:	*NPlr*	goats	$MY * \left(\frac{MkTP}{100}\right) * 1000$
24:	*MPlr*	goats	$\frac{NPlr}{0.64}$
25:	*FFL*		$NElr/[NEl]$

(1) ***DG*** is days of gestation (i.e., days pregnant); ***DIM*** is the days in milk; ***FFL*** is feed required for lactation, kg/d; ***j*** is the jth amino acid; $K_{MkAA,j}$ is the jth milk amino acid efficiency (Arg: 0.35, His: 0.96, Ile: 0.66, Leu: 0.72, Lys: 0.82, Met: 1.0, Phe: 0.98, Thr: 0.78, Trp: 0.85, and Val: 0.62), dimensionless; ***MAAlr$_j$*** is the metabolizable jth amino acid required for lactation, g/d; ***MElr*** is the metabolizable energy required for lactation, Mcal/d; ***MkAA*** is the jth milk amino acid content (Arg: 3.4, His: 2.74, Ile: 5.79, Leu: 9.18, Lys: 7.62, Met: 2.71, Phe: 4.75, Thr: 3.72, Trp: 1.51, and Val: 5.89), %; ***MkFat*** is milk fat content, %; ***MkL*** is milk lactose content (default is 4.85), %; ***MkTP*** is milk true protein content (for cattle it is 92% of milk crude protein and for sheep and goats it is 93% of milk crude protein), %; ***MPlr*** is the metabolizable protein required for lactation, g/d; ***MY*** is milk yield, kg/d; ***[NEl]*** is dietary content of net energy for lactation, Mcal/kg; ***NElr*** is the net energy required for lactation, Mcal/d; ***NPlr*** is the net protein required for lactation, g/d; ***PKYD*** is peak milk yield, kg/d; ***PMkFat*** is predicted milk fat content adjusted for days in milk, %; ***PMkTP*** is predicted milk true protein content adjusted for days in milk, %; ***PMY*** is predicted milk yield, kg/d; ***RelMY*** is relative milk yield factor (1 to 9 scale: 1 = low, 5 = average, and 9 = high); and ***T*** is the average week of peak milk yield for beef cows.

(2) Equations 1 to 16 are for cattle and Equations 17 to 24 have replacement equations for sheep and goats. Figure 5.4 shows the prediction of the daily and accumulated metabolizable energy and metabolizable protein required for beef cattle.

Figure 5.4 has the predicted daily and accumulated metabolizable energy and metabolizable protein required for a lactating beef cow for 210 days in milk, assuming peak milk of 8 kg/d and milk contents of fat, true protein, and lactose of 4%, 3.8%, and 4.85%, respectively. The shape of metabolizable energy and metabolizable protein are identical, but they do not overlap in Figure 5.4 because the y-axes scaling was

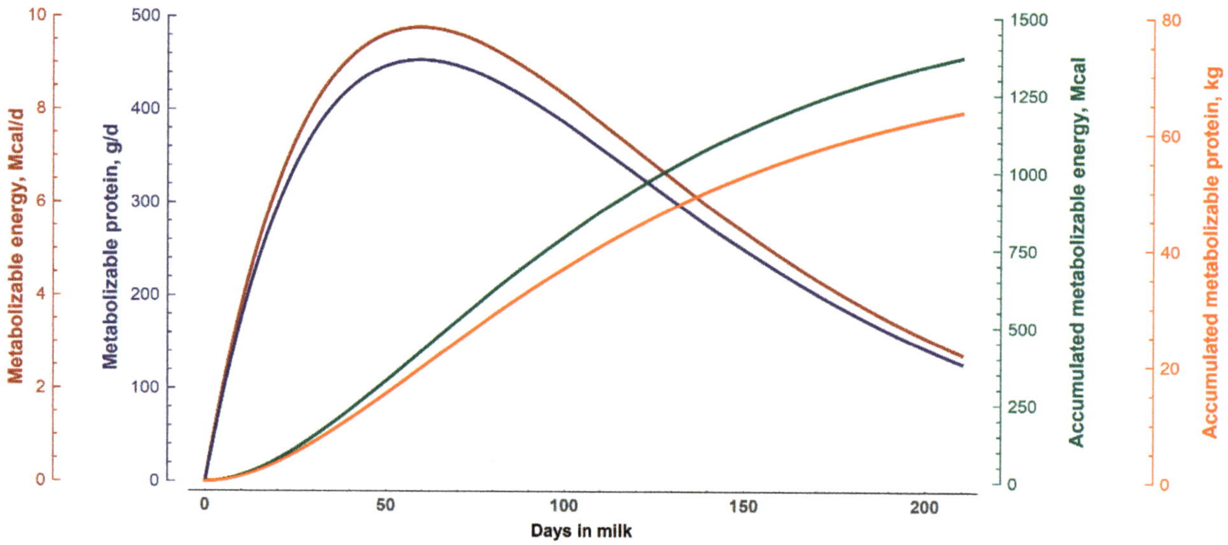

Figure 5.4. Predicted daily and accumulated metabolizable energy and protein required for lactation of beef cattle, assuming peak milk yield of 8 kg/d, and milk fat, true protein, and lactose contents of 4%, 3.8%, and 4.85%, respectively.

set to prevent the overlapping. The equations in the RNS model predicted 9.6% more metabolizable energy and 3.1% less metabolizable protein when compared to the equations adopted by the NASEM (2016). This discrepancy is likely due to a combination of different equations and milk components to compute milk energy content and the efficiency of the utilization of metabolizable energy and metabolizable protein. The daily and accumulated milk yield are identical between the NASEM (2016) and the RNS models. The accumulated milk yield was computed by integrating the RNS model's predict milk yield equation, as follows: $2.3785 * Exp\left(-\frac{DIM}{7*T}\right) * PKYD * (3 + 1 * RelMY) * \left(-0.142857 * DIM + \left(Exp\left(\frac{DIM}{7*T}\right) - 1\right) * T\right)$.

5.2.4 Pregnancy requirements: calcPregnancyRequirement()

#	Variable[1]	Description	Equation
1:	*GUW*	dairy cattle	$\left(\frac{CBW}{47}\right) * 0.1436 * Exp(0.03729 * DG - 0.00005164 * DG^2)$
2:	*ADG_{GU}*	dairy cattle	$\left(\frac{CBW}{47}\right) * 0.1436 * (0.03729 - 0.00010328 * DG) * Exp(0.03729 * DG - 0.00005164 * DG^2)$
3:	*NEpr*	dairy cattle & DG>0	$\left(\frac{CBW}{47}\right) * (0.00318 * DG - 0.0352)$
4:	*MEpr*	dairy cattle & DG>0	$\frac{NEpr}{0.14}$
5:	*NPpr*	dairy cattle & DG>0	$\left(\frac{CBW}{47}\right) * (0.69 * DG - 69.2)$
6:	*MPpr*	dairy cattle & DG>0	$\frac{NPpr}{0.13}$
7:	*GUW*	beef cattle	$\left(\frac{CBW}{41}\right) * 0.7439 * Exp(0.02 * DG - 0.0000143 * DG^2)$
8:	*ADG_{GU}*	beef cattle	$\left(\frac{CBW}{41}\right) * 0.7439 * (0.02 - 0.0000286 * DG) * Exp(0.02 * DG - 0.0000143 * DG^2)$

#	Variable(1)	Description	Equation
9:	*NEpr*	beef cattle	$\left(\frac{CBW}{41}\right) * 69.73 * (0.0323 - 0.000055 * DG) * \frac{Exp(0.0323 * DG - 0.0000275 * DG^2)}{1000}$
10:	*MEpr*	beef cattle	$\frac{NEpr}{0.13}$
11:	*NPpr*	beef cattle	$\left(\frac{CBW}{41}\right) * 2.312 * (0.0278 - 0.0000352 * DG) * \frac{Exp(0.0278 * DG - 0.0000176 * DG^2)}{0.16}$
12:	*MPpr*	beef cattle	$\frac{NPpr}{0.5}$
13:	*MAApr*		$\frac{NPpr * \frac{TiAA_j}{100}}{k_{GUAA_j}}$
14:	*GUW*	sheep or goats	$\left(\frac{LBW}{4}\right) * 175.915 * Exp(-8.38 * Exp(-0.00608 * DG))$
15:	*ADG_{GU}*	sheep or goats	$\left(\frac{LBW}{4}\right) * 8.96293 * Exp(-8.38 * Exp(-0.00608 * DG) - 0.00608 * DG)$
16:	*NEpr*	sheep or goats	$\left(\frac{LBW}{4}\right) * 36.628 * Exp(-11.465 * Exp(-0.00643 * DG) - 0.00643 * DG)$
17:	*MEpr*	sheep or goats	$\frac{NEpr}{0.13}$
18:	*NPpr*	sheep or goats	$\left(\frac{LBW}{4}\right) * 5712.24 * Exp(-11.22 * Exp(-0.00601 * DG) - 0.00601 * DG)$
19:	*MPpr*	sheep	$\frac{NPpr}{0.7}$
20:	*MPpr*	goats	$\frac{NPpr}{0.33}$
21:	*FFP*		$MEpr/[ME]$

(1) ***[ME]*** is the dietary content of metabolizable energy, Mcal/kg; ***ADG_{GU}*** is the gravid uterus average dairy gain, kg/d; ***CBW*** is the calf birth weight, kg; ***DG*** is days of gestation (i.e., days pregnant); ***FFP*** is the feed required for pregnancy, kg/d; ***GUW*** is the gravid uterus weight, kg; ***$K_{GUAA,j}$*** is the jth gravid uterus amino acid efficiency (Arg: 0.38, His: 0.32, Ile: 0.32, Leu: 0.42, Lys: 0.53, Met: 0.35, Phe: 0.48, Thr: 0.57, Trp: 0.85, and Val: 0.32), dimensionless; ***LBW*** is lamb(s) or kid(s) total body weight, kg/d; ***$MAApr_j$*** is the metabolizable jth amino acid required for pregnancy, g/d; ***MEpr*** is the metabolizable energy required for pregnancy, Mcal/d; ***MPpr*** is the metabolizable protein required for pregnancy, g/d; ***NEpr*** is the net energy required for pregnancy, Mcal/d; ***NPpr*** is the net protein required for pregnancy, g/d; and ***TiAA*** is the jth tissue amino acid content (Arg: 6.6, His: 2.47, Ile: 2.84, Leu: 6.7, Lys: 6.37, Met: 1.97, Phe: 3.53, Thr: 3.9, Trp: 1.18, and Val: 4.03), %.

5.2.5 Growth requirements: calcGrowthRequirement()

5.2.5.1 Target weights and daily gains for cattle replacement heifers, and dry and lactating cows

#	Variable(1)	Description	Equation(2)
1:	*TPW1*	dual-purpose or dairy breeds	$MSBW * 0.55$
2:		*Bos taurus* breeds	$MSBW * 0.60$
3:		*Bos indicus* breeds	$MSBW * 0.65$
4:	*TPA1*		$TCA - 280$
5:	*ADG_{BP}*		$\frac{TPW1 - WW}{TPA1 - WA}$
6:	*TCW1*	dairy breeds	$MSBW * 0.85$
7:		otherwise	$MSBW * 0.8$
8:	*ADG_{AP}*		$\frac{TCW1 - TPW1}{280 - DG}$
9:	*TCW2*		$MSBW * 0.92$
10:	*ADG_{AC1}*		$\frac{TCW2 - TCW1}{CvI}$
11:	*TCW3*		$MSBW * 0.96$

#	Variable[1]	Description	Equation[2]
12:	ADG_{AC2}		$\frac{TCW3 - TCW2}{CvI}$
13:	$TCW4$		$MSBW$
14:	ADG_{AC3}		$\frac{TCW4 - TCW3}{CvI}$
15:	CA		$TCA + parity * CvI$
16:	$EqSBW$		$(SBW - GUW) * \frac{SRW}{MSBW}$
17:	$EqEBW$		$EqSBW * 0.891$
18:		age<TPA1	$\frac{TPW1 - SBW}{TPA1 - age}$
19:		otherwise	$\frac{TCW1 - SBW}{280 - DG}$
20:	SWG	parity=1	$\frac{TCW2 - SBW}{CA - age}$
21:		parity=2	$\frac{TCW3 - SBW}{CA - age}$
22:		Parity≥3	$\frac{TCW4 - SBW}{CA - age}$
23:	EWG	SWG is known	$SWG * 0.956$
24:	$NEgr$	SWG is known	$0.0625 * EqEBW^{0.75} * EWG^{1.097}$
25:	$NEgr$	SWG is unknown	$(DMI - (FFM + FFL + FFP)) * NEga$
26:	$MEgr$		$\frac{NEgr}{k_g}$
27:	SWG	SWG is unknown	$13.91 * EqEBW^{-0.6837} * NEgr^{0.9116}$
28:	EWG	SWG is unknown	$12.341 * EqSBW^{-0.6837} * NEgr^{0.9116}$
29:	PIG		$\left(268 - 29.4 * \frac{NEgr}{SWG}\right) * 0.1$
30:	$NPgr$		$SWG * (PIG * 0.01) * 1000$
31:	FIG		$100 * \frac{\frac{NEgr - NPgr * 0.0057}{9.4}}{SWG}$
32:		option 1	$If[EqSBW \leq 300, 0.834 - EqSBW * 0.00114, 0.492]$
33:	Eff_{MPtoNP}	option 2	$If[EqSBW \leq 478, 0.834 - EqSBW * 0.00114, 0.289]$
34:		option 3	$0.492 + 104.93 * Exp(-0.0486 * SBW)$
35:		option 4	$0.112 + 2.271 * Exp(-0.01887 * EqSBW)$
36:	$MPgr$		$\frac{NPgr}{Eff_{MPtoNP}}$
37:	$MEmm$	DG>259 & replacement heifer or dry cow	$\frac{1}{k_g}$
38:	$MPmm$		$\frac{80}{Eff_{MPtoNP}}$
39:	$MAAgr$		$\frac{NPgr * \frac{TiAA_j}{100}}{Eff_{MPtoNP}}$
40:	FFG		$\frac{MEgr}{[ME]}$

[1] ***[ME]*** is the dietary content of metabolizable energy, Mcal/kg; ***ADG_{AC1}*** is the target average daily gain after first calving, kg/d; ***ADG_{AC2}*** is the target average daily gain after second calving, kg/d; ***ADG_{AC3}*** is the target average daily gain after third calving, kg/d; ***ADG_{AP}*** is the average daily gain after first conception, assuming gestion length of 280 days, kg/d; ***ADG_{BP}*** is the average daily gain before first conception, kg/d; ***age*** is the animal age, d; ***CA*** is the calving age, d; ***CvI*** is the calving interval, d; ***DG*** is days of gestation (i.e., days pregnant); ***DMI*** is the dry matter intake, kg/d; ***Eff_{MPtoNP}*** is the efficiency of conversion of metabolizable protein to net protein, dimensionless; ***EqEBW*** is the equivalent empty body weight, kg; ***EqSBW*** is the equivalent shrunk body weight, kg; ***EWG*** is the empty weight gain, kg/d; ***FFG*** is the feed required for growth, kg/d; ***FFL*** is the feed required for lactation, kg/d; ***FFM*** is the feed required for maintenance, kg/d; ***FFP*** is the feed required for pregnancy, kg/d; ***FIG*** is the fat in the gain, %; ***GUW*** is the gravid uterus weight, kg; ***k_g*** is the partial efficiency of utilization of metabolizable energy for net energy for growth, dimensionless; ***MEgr*** is the metabolizable energy required for growth, Mcal/d; ***MEmm*** is the metabolizable energy required for mammogenesis, Mcal/d; ***MPgr*** is the metabolizable protein required for growth, g/d; ***MPmm*** is the metabolizable protein required for mammogenesis, g/d; ***MSBW*** is the mature shrunk body weight at the same chemical fat composition as the standard reference weight, kg; ***NEga*** is the dietary content of net energy available for growth (also known as ***[NEg]***), Mcal/kg; ***NEgr*** is the net energy required for growth, Mcal/d; ***NPgr*** is the net protein required for growth, g/d; ***parity*** is the parity number of the animal, dimensionless; ***PIG*** is the protein in the gain, %; ***SBW*** is the shrunk body weight, kg; ***SRW*** is the standard reference weight (default is 478 kg for replacement heifers), kg; ***SWG*** is the shrunk weight gain, kg/d; ***TCA*** is target first

calving age, d; ***TCW1*** is the target first calving weight, kg; ***TCW2*** is the target second post-calving weight, kg; ***TCW3*** is the target third post-calving weight, kg; ***TCW4*** is the target fourth post-calving weight, kg; ***TiAA*** is the jth tissue amino acid content (Arg: 6.6, His: 2.47, Ile: 2.84, Leu: 6.7, Lys: 6.37, Met: 1.97, Phe: 3.53, Thr: 3.9, Trp: 1.18, and Val: 4.03), %; ***TPA1*** is the target age at first pregnancy, assuming gestion length of 280 days, d; ***TPW1*** is the target first pregnant weight, kg; ***WA*** is the weaning age, d; and ***WW*** is the weaning weight, kg.

(2) There are four options to compute the efficiency of conversion of metabolizable protein to net protein (***Eff_{MPtoNP}***): option 1 is based on the NRC (1996, 2000), option 2 is based on Fox et al. (2004), option 3 is based on the NASEM (2016), and option 4 is based on the RNS model (Tedeschi and Fox, 2020). Figure 5.5 depicts the graphical representation of consecutive reproductive stages (Tedeschi and Fox, 2020).

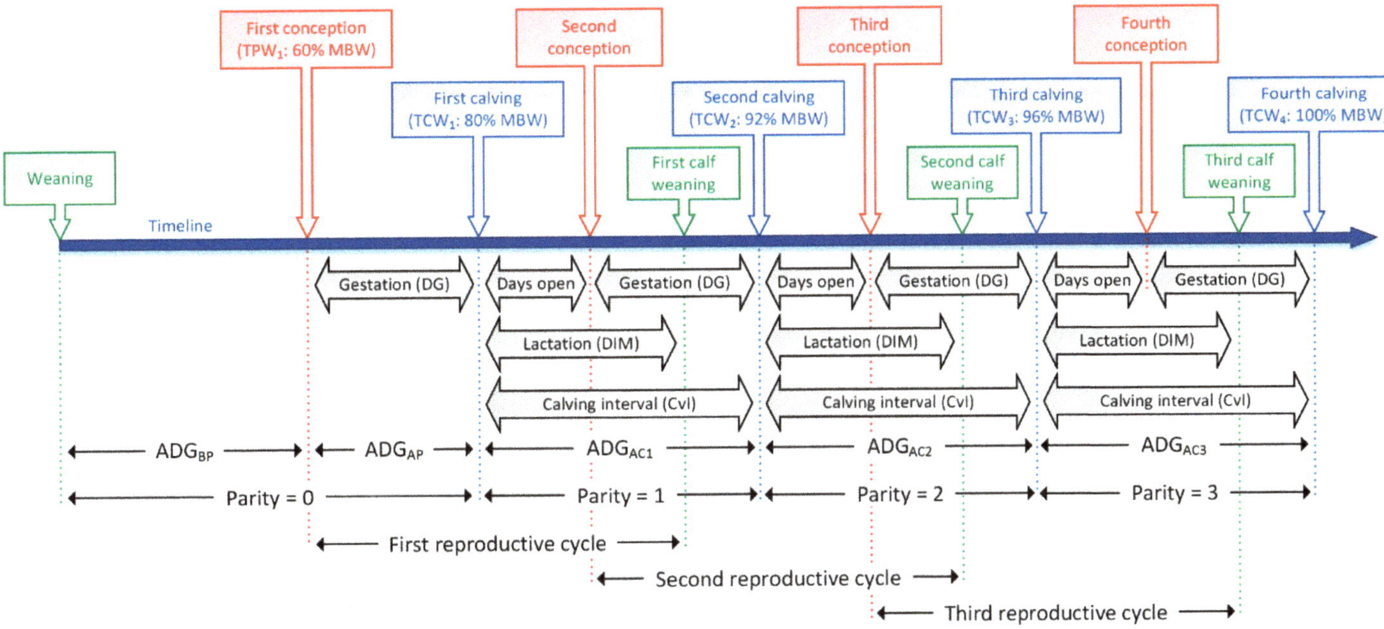

Figure 5.5. Schematic representation of target body weight (BW) and average daily gain (ADG) calculations for three reproductive cycles of beef and dairy cows. CvI is calving interval, DIM is days in milk, DG is days in gestation (i.e., days pregnant), MBW is mature BW, TCW is target calving weight, and TPW is target first pregnancy weight. Reprinted with permission from Tedeschi and Fox (2020).

5.2.5.2 Daily gains for growing or finishing cattle, sheep, and goats

#	Variable[1]	Description	Equation[2]
1:	*EqSBW*	cattle	$SBW * \frac{SRW}{AFSBW}$
2:	*EqEBW*	cattle	$EqSBW * 0.891$
3:	*NEgr*	cattle	$(DMI - FFM) * NEga$
4:	*MEgr*	cattle	$\frac{NEgr}{k_g}$
5:	*SWG*	cattle	$13.91 * EqEBW^{-0.6837} * NEgr^{0.9116}$
6:	*EWG*	cattle	$12.341 * EqSBW^{-0.6837} * NEgr^{0.9116}$
7:	*PIG*	cattle	$\left(268 - 29.4 * \frac{NEgr}{SWG}\right) * 0.1$
8:	*NPgr*	cattle	$SWG * (PIG * 0.01) * 1000$
9:	*FIG*	cattle	$100 * \frac{\frac{NEgr - NPgr * 0.0057}{9.4}}{SWG}$
10:	Eff_{MPtoNP}	cattle: option 1	$If[EqSBW \leq 300, 0.834 - EqSBW * 0.00114, 0.492]$
11:		cattle: option 2	$If[EqSBW \leq 478, 0.834 - EqSBW * 0.00114, 0.289]$
12:		cattle: option 3	$0.492 + 104.93 * Exp(-0.0486 * SBW)$
13:		cattle: option 4	$0.112 + 2.271 * Exp(-0.01887 * EqSBW)$

#	Variable[(1)]	Description	Equation[(2)]
14:	*MEgr*	sheep and goats	$DMI * [ME] - MEmr$
15:	*P*	sheep and goats	$\frac{FBW}{MFBW}$
16:	*R*	sheep and goats	$2 * (L - 1)$
17:	*PIG*	sheep and goats	$\frac{\left(212 - 4 * R - \frac{120 - 4 * R}{1 + Exp(-6 * (P - 0.4))}\right)}{10}$
18:	*FIG*	sheep and goats	$\frac{\left(43 + 28 * R + \frac{(490 - 28 * R)}{1 + Exp(-6 * (P - 0.4))}\right)}{10}$
19:	*RE$_P$*		$\frac{PIG * 5.7}{PIG * 5.7 + FIG * 9.4}$
20:	*k$_g$*	sheep and goats	$\frac{18.36}{27 + 41 * RE_P}$
21:	*NEgr*	sheep and goats	$MEgr * k_g$
22:	*EVG*	sheep and goats	$\frac{6.7 + R + \left(\frac{(16.5 - R)}{1 + Exp(-6 * (P - 0.4))}\right)}{4.184}$
23:	*SWG*	sheep and goats	$\frac{NEgr}{0.92 * EVG}$
24:	*EWG*	sheep and goats	$0.92 * SWG$
25:	*NPgr*	sheep and goats	$1000 * EWG * \left(\frac{PIG}{100}\right)$
26:	*Eff$_{MPtoNP}$*	sheep and goats	0.7
27:	*MPgr*		$\frac{NPgr}{Eff_{MPtoNP}}$
28:	*MAAgr*		$\frac{NPgr * \frac{TiAA_j}{100}}{Eff_{MPtoNP}}$
29:	*FFG*		$\frac{MEgr}{[ME]}$

[(1)] ***[ME]*** is the dietary content of metabolizable energy, Mcal/kg; ***AFFBW*** is the adjusted final full body weight, which is the FBW at the same chemical fat composition as the standard reference weight (also known as the mature full body weight, ***MFBW***), kg; ***AFSBW*** is the adjusted final shrunk body weight, which is the SBW at the same chemical fat composition as the standard reference weight (also known as the mature shrunk body weight, ***MSBW***), kg; ***DMI*** is the dry matter intake, kg/d; ***Eff$_{MPtoNP}$*** is the efficiency of conversion of metabolizable protein to net protein, dimensionless; ***EqEBW*** is the equivalent empty body weight, kg; ***EqSBW*** is the equivalent shrunk body weight, kg; ***EVG*** is the energy content of gain, Mcal/kg; ***EWG*** is the empty weight gain, kg/d; ***FBW*** is the full body weight, kg; ***FFG*** is the feed required for growth, kg/d; ***FFM*** is the feed required for maintenance, kg/d; ***FIG*** is the fat in the gain, %; ***k$_g$*** is the partial efficiency of utilization of metabolizable energy for net energy for growth, dimensionless; ***L$_{DMI}$*** is the level of intake as multiples of feed required for maintenance, dimensionless; ***MEgr*** is the metabolizable energy required for growth, Mcal/d; ***MFBW*** is the mature full body weight (also known as the adjusted final full body weight, ***AFFBW***), kg; ***MPgr*** is the metabolizable protein required for growth, g/d; ***MSBW*** is the mature shrunk body weight (also known as the adjusted final shrunk body weight, ***AFSBW***), kg; ***NEga*** is the dietary content of net energy available for growth (also known as ***[NEg]***), Mcal/kg; ***NEgr*** is the net energy required for growth, Mcal/d; ***NPgr*** is the net protein required for growth, g/d; ***PIG*** is the protein in the gain, %; ***R*** a growth parameter, dimensionless; ***RE$_p$*** is the proportion of protein retained, dimensionless; ***SBW*** is the shrunk body weight, kg; ***SRW*** is the standard reference weight (default is 478 kg for replacement heifers), kg; ***SWG*** is the shrunk weight gain, kg/d; and ***TiAA*** is the jth tissue amino acid content (Arg: 6.6, His: 2.47, Ile: 2.84, Leu: 6.7, Lys: 6.37, Met: 1.97, Phe: 3.53, Thr: 3.9, Trp: 1.18, and Val: 4.03), %.

[(2)] For cattle, there are four options to compute the efficiency of conversion of metabolizable protein to net protein (***Eff$_{MPtoNP}$***): option 1 is based on the NRC (1996, 2000), option 2 is based on Fox et al. (2004), option 3 is based on the NASEM (2016), and option 4 is based on the RNS model (Tedeschi and Fox, 2020). These equations are also used for replacement females for sheep or goats.

5.2.6 Body reserves: calcBodyReserves()

#	Variable[(1)]	Description	Equation
1:	*MEB*		$(DMI - FFM - FFG - FFP - FFL) * [ME]$
2:	*EBW1*		$0.851 * (SBW - GUW)$
3:	*Fat1*		$-0.040604 + 0.046814 * BCS1$
4:	*Prot1*		$0.218778 - 0.008893 * BCS1$

#	Variable[1]	Description	Equation
5:	*Ash1*		$0.068589 - 0.0035539 * BCS1$
6:	*Water1*		$1 - (Fat1 + Prot1 + Ash1)$
7:	*BF1*		$Fat1 * EBW1$
8:	*BP1*		$Prot1 * EBW1$
9:	*BA1*		$Ash1 * EBW1$
10:	*BW1*		$Water1 * EBW1$
11:	*BE1*		$9.4 * BF1 + 5.7 * BP1$
12:	*BCS2*	MEB<0 & BCS1>1	$BCS1 - 1$
13:		MEB>0 & BCS1<9	$BCS1 + 1$
14:	*WAF1*		$1 - \Delta SBW/\Delta BCS * (5 - BCS1)$
15:	*WAF2*		$1 - \Delta SBW/\Delta BCS * (5 - BCS2)$
16:	*EBW2*		$\frac{EBW1}{WAF1} * WAF2$
17:	*Fat2*		$-0.040604 + 0.046814 * BCS2$
18:	*Prot2*		$0.218778 - 0.008893 * BCS2$
19:	*Ash2*		$0.068589 - 0.0035539 * BCS2$
20:	*Water2*		$1 - (Fat2 + Prot2 + Ash2)$
21:	*BF2*		$Fat2 * EBW2$
22:	*BP2*		$Prot2 * EBW2$
23:	*BA2*		$Ash2 * EBW2$
24:	*BW2*		$Water2 * EBW2$
25:	*BE2*		$9.4 * BF2 + 5.7 * BP2$
26:	*ΔBE*		$BE2 - BE1$
27:	*ΔBP*		$BP2 - BP1$
28:	*NEB*	MEB>0 & lactating dairy	$MEB * 0.75$
29:		MEB>0 & not lactating dairy	$MEB * 0.6$
30:		MEB<0 & lactating dairy	$MEB * \left(\frac{0.644}{0.82}\right)$
31:		MEB<0 & not lactating dairy	$MEB * \left(\frac{0.6}{0.8}\right)$
32:	*Days$_{\Delta BCS}$*		$\frac{\Delta BE}{NEB}$
33:	*EWG$_{\Delta BCS}$*		$\frac{EBW2 - EBW1}{Days_{\Delta BCS}}$
34:	*FBW25*	BCS1=2.5	$FBW - GUW$
35:		otherwise	$FBW * \frac{2.796 * BCS1 - 5.311}{0.692 + 0.11 * BCS1}$
36:	*EBW1*	BCS1=2.5	$0.8513 * 0.96 * FBW25$
37:		otherwise	$0.8513 * \left(0.96 * \left(FBW25 * (0.692 + 0.111 * BCS1) + (2.795 * BCS1 - 5.311)\right)\right)$
38:	*Fat1*	sheep	$0.0269 + 0.0868 * BCS1$
39:		goats	$0.0289 + 0.0708 * BCS1$
40:	*Prot1*		$0.1449 + 0.0279 * BCS1 - 0.0039 * BCS1^2$
41:	*BF1*		$Fat1 * EBW1$
42:	*BP1*		$Prot1 * EBW1$
43:	*BE1*		$9.4 * BF1 + 5.7 * BP1$
44:	*BCS2*	MEB<0 & BCS1>0	$BCS1 - 0.5$
45:		MEB>0 & BCS1<5	$BCS1 + 0.5$
46:	*EBW2*	BCS2=2.5	$0.8513 * 0.96 * FBW25$
47:		otherwise	$0.8513 * \left(0.96 * \left(FBW25 * (0.692 + 0.111 * BCS2) + (2.795 * BCS2 - 5.311)\right)\right)$
48:	*Fat2*	sheep	$0.0269 + 0.0868 * BCS2$
49:		goats	$0.0289 + 0.0708 * BCS2$
50:	*Prot2*		$0.1449 + 0.0279 * BCS2 - 0.0039 * BCS2^2$
51:	*BF2*		$Fat2 * EBW2$
52:	*BP2*		$Prot2 * EBW2$
53:	*BE2*		$9.4 * BF2 + 5.7 * BP2$
54:	*ΔBE*		$BE2 - BE1$
55:	*ΔBP*		$BP2 - BP1$
56:	*NEB*	MEB>0	$MEB * 0.6$

#	Variable[1]	Description	Equation
57:		MEB<0	$MEB * \left(\frac{0.6}{0.8}\right)$
58:	$Days_{\Delta BCS}$		$\frac{\Delta BE}{NEB}$
59:	$EWG_{\Delta BCS}$		$\frac{EBW2 - EBW1}{Days_{\Delta BCS}}$

[1] ***[ME]*** is the dietary content of metabolizable energy, Mcal/kg; ***ASh1*** is the proportion of body ash at BCS1, dimensionless; ***BA1*** is the amount of body ash at BCS1, kg; ***BCS1*** is the animal's current body condition score (1 to 9 scale for cattle or 0 to 5 for sheep and goats), dimensionless; ***BCS2*** is the animal's next body condition score (1 to 9 scale for cattle or 0 to 5 for sheep and goats), dimensionless; ***BE1*** is the body energy at BCS1, Mcal; ***BF1*** is the amount of body fat at BCS1, kg; ***BP1*** is the amount of body protein at BCS1, kg; ***BW1*** is the amount of body water at BCS1, kg; ***$Days_{\Delta BCS}$*** is the days to change body condition score, d; ***EBW1*** is the empty body weight at BCS1, kg; ***EBW2*** is the empty body weight at BCS2, kg; ***$EWG_{\Delta BCS}$*** is the empty weight gain due to the change in body condition score, kg/d; ***Fat1*** is the proportion of body fat at BCS1, dimensionless; ***FBW25*** is the full body weight at BCS 2.5, kg; ***GUW*** is the gravid uterus weight, kg; ***MEB*** is the metabolizable energy balance, Mcal/d; ***NEB*** is the net energy balance, Mcal/d; ***Prot1*** is the proportion of body protein at BCS1, dimensionless; ***SBW*** is the shrunk body weight, kg; ***WAF1*** is the weight adjustment factor at BCS1, dimensionless; ***WAF2*** is the weight adjustment factor at BCS2, dimensionless; ***Water1*** is the proportion of body water at BCS1, dimensionless; ***ΔBE*** is the change in body energy from BCS1 to BCS2, Mcal; ***ΔBP*** is the change in body protein from BCS1 to BCS2, kg; and ***ΔSBWΔBCS*** is the change in shrunk body weight per change in the body condition score (default is 0.0743), dimensionless.

[2] Equations 1 to 33 are for cattle body reserves that use 1 to 9 scale for body condition score, and Equations 34 to 59 are for sheep and goats body reserves that use 0 to 5 scale for body condition score. Figure 5.6 applies the body reserves model for cattle.

Figure 5.6 shows the body energy (i.e., net energy) required (gain) or provided (loss) for changing one body condition score of cattle for four body reserves models. As discussed by Tedeschi and Fox (2020), the body reserves developed by the NRC (1996, 2000) assumed that the amount of empty body ash was constant as animals changed body condition score, leading to a constant 5.83 Mcal/kg of shrunk body

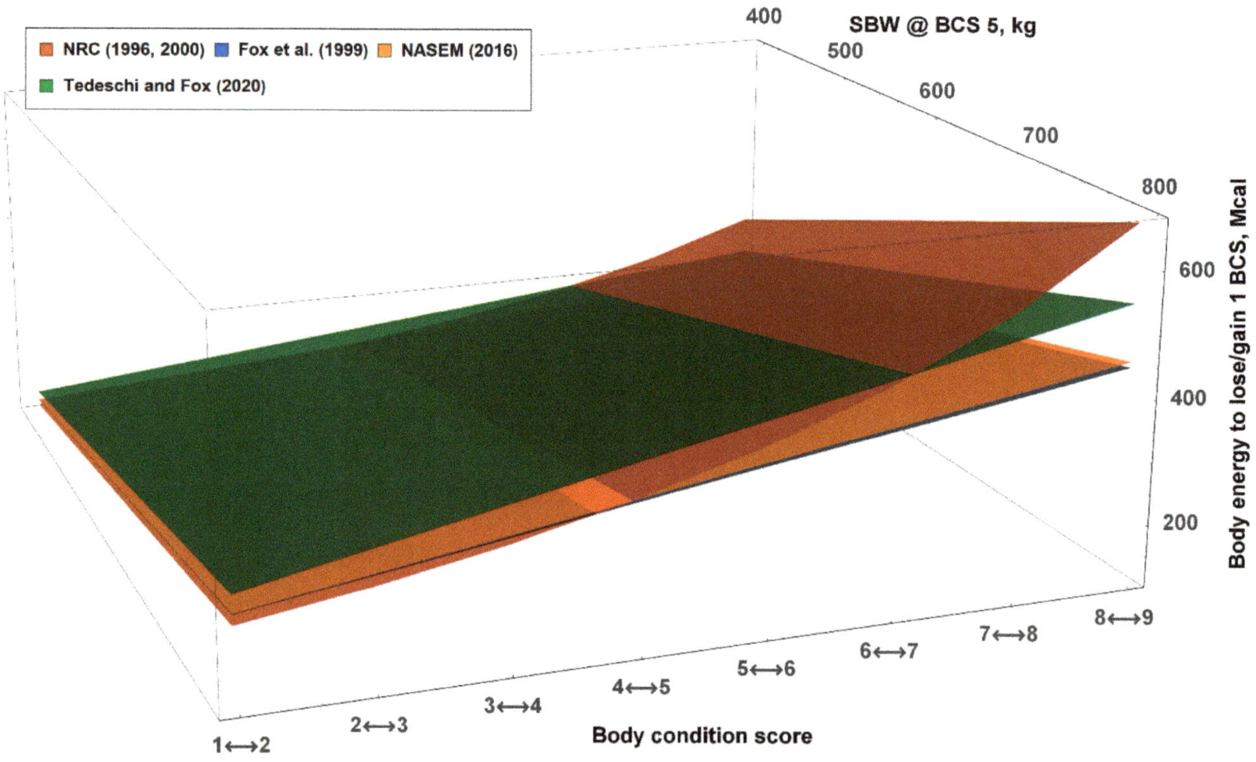

Figure 5.6. Body energy (net energy) required or provided for changing one body condition score (BCS) of mature cows at different shrunk body weight (SBW) at BCS 5.

weight change. As shown in Figure 5.6, the NRC (1996, 2000) body reserves model indicated that the change in the body energy tended to increase exponentially as body weight and condition score increased. The change in the body energy was linear with changes in body weight and condition score for Fox et al. (1999), NASEM (2016), and Tedeschi and Fox (2020) because their body reserves models assumed a fixed change in shrunk body weight per change in body condition score (ΔSBW/ΔBCS) as 6.85%, 7.105%, and 7.43% of the mean shrunk body weight, respectively. As expected, given the closeness of the estimates proposed by Fox et al. (1999) and NASEM (2016), their body reserves models predicted nearly identical body energy fluxes (Figure 5.6).

5.2.7 Mineral requirements: calcMineralRequirement()

5.2.7.1 Dairy cattle

#	Variable[(1)]	Description	Equation
1:	*FCM*		$0.4 * MY + 0.15 * MkFat * MY$
2:	Ca_M	lactating	$0.031 * FBW + 0.0008 * FBW$
3:		nonlactating	$0.0154 * FBW + 0.0008 * FBW$
4:	Ca_P	DG≥190	$0.02456 * Exp((0.05581 - 0.00007 * DG) * DG) - 0.02456 * Exp\left((0.05581 - 0.00007 * (DG-1)) * (DG-1)\right)$
5:	Ca_L	Holstein	$1.22 * FCM$
6:		Jersey	$1.45 * FCM$
7:		otherwise	$1.37 * FCM$
8:	Ca_G		$9.83 * \frac{MFBW^{0.22}}{FBW} * \frac{ADG}{0.96}$
9:	P_M	lactating or dry	$1 * DMI + 0.002 * FBW$
10:		otherwise	$0.8 * DMI + 0.002 * FBW$
11:	P_P	DG≥190	$0.02743 * Exp((0.05527 - 0.000075 * DG) * DG) - 0.02743 * Exp\left((0.05527 - 0.000075 * (DG-1)) * (DG-1)\right)$
12:	P_L		$0.9 * FCM$
13:	P_G		$1.2 + 4.635 * \left(\frac{MFBW}{FBW}\right)^{0.22} * \frac{ADG}{0.96}$
14:	Mg_M		$0.003 * FBW$
15:	Mg_P	DG≥190	0.33
16:	Mg_L		$0.15 * FCM$
17:	Mg_G		$0.45 * \frac{ADG}{0.96}$
18:	S_M		$2 * DMI$
19:	Cl_M		$0.0225 * FBW$
20:	Cl_P	DG≥190	1
21:	Cl_L		$1.15 * FCM$
22:	Cl_G		$1 * \frac{ADG}{0.96}$
23:		lactating & Tc≤25°C	$6.1 * DMI + 0.038 * FBW$
24:		lactating & 25 °C <Tc<30 °C	$6.1 * DMI + 0.038 * FBW + 0.0004 * FBW$
25:		lactating & Tc≥30 °C	$6.1 * DMI + 0.038 * FBW + 0.004 * FBW$
26:	K_M	nonlactating & Tc≤25°C	$2.6 * DMI + 0.038 * FBW$
27:		nonlactating & 25 °C <Tc<30 °C	$2.6 * DMI + 0.038 * FBW + 0.0004 * FBW$
28:		nonlactating & Tc≥30 °C	$2.6 * DMI + 0.038 * FBW + 0.004 * FBW$
29:	K_P	DG≥190	1.027

#	Variable[1]	Description	Equation
30:	K_L		$1.5 * FCM$
31:	K_G		$1.6 * \frac{ADG}{0.96}$
32:		lactating & Tc≤25°C	$0.038 * FBW$
33:		lactating & 25 °C <Tc<30 °C	$0.038 * FBW + 0.001 * FBW$
34:		lactating & Tc≥30 °C	$0.038 * FBW + 0.005 * FBW$
35:	Na_M	nonlactating & Tc≤25°C	$0.015 * FBW$
36:		nonlactating & 25 °C <Tc<30 °C	$0.015 * FBW + 0.001 * FBW$
37:		nonlactating & Tc≥30 °C	$0.015 * FBW + 0.005 * FBW$
38:	Na_P	DG≥190	1.39
39:	Na_L		$0.63 * FCM$
40:	Na_G		$1.4 * \frac{ADG}{0.96}$
41:	Cu_M		$0.0071 * FBW$
42:		0<DG<100	0.5
43:	Cu_P	100≤DG≤225	1.5
44:		DG>225	2
45:	Cu_L		$0.15 * FCM$
46:	Cu_G		$1.15 * \frac{ADG}{0.96}$
47:	I_M	lactating	$0.015 * FBW$
48:		nonlactating	$0.006 * FBW$
49:	Fe_P	DG≥190	18
50:	Fe_L		$1 * FCM$
51:	Fe_G		$34 * \frac{ADG}{0.96}$
52:	Mn_M		$0.002 * FBW$
53:	Mn_P	DG≥190	0.3
54:	Mn_L		$0.03 * FCM$
55:	Mn_G		$0.7 * \frac{ADG}{0.96}$
56:	Zn_M		$0.033 * FBW + 0.012 * FBW$
57:	Zn_P	DG≥190	12
58:	Zn_L		$4 * FCM$
59:	Zn_G		$24 * \frac{ADG}{0.96}$
60:	Co_M		$0.11 * DMI$
61:	Se_M		$0.3 * DMI$
62:	Cr_M	lactating	7.75
63:	Cr_M	nonlactating	0.6

[1] ***ADG*** is the average daily gain, kg/d; ***DG*** is days of gestation (i.e., days pregnant); ***DMI*** is the dry matter intake, kg/d; ***FBW*** is the full body weight, kg; ***FCM*** is the fat-corrected milk, kg/d; ***MFBW*** is the mature full body weight, kg; ***MkFat*** is milk fat content, %; ***MY*** is milk yield, kg/d; ***Tc*** is the current temperature, °C; and X_M, X_P, X_L, ***and*** X_G are the mineral X requirement for maintenance, pregnancy, lactation, and growth, respectively. Ca, P, Mg, S, Cl, K, and Na are expressed as g/d and Cu, I, Fe, Mn, Zn, Co, Se, and Cr are expressed as mg/d.

5.2.7.2 Beef cattle

#	Variable[1]	Description	Equation
1:	Ca_M		$0.0154 * SBW$
2:	Ca_P	DG>90	$CBW * \frac{13.7}{90}$
3:	Ca_L		$1.23 * MY$

#	Variable[1]	Description	Equation
4:	Ca_G		$0.071 * PIG$
5:	P_M		$0.016 * SBW$
6:	P_P	DG>90	$CBW * \frac{7.6}{90}$
7:	P_L		$0.95 * MY$
8:	P_G		$0.039 * PIG$
9:		lactating	$\left(\frac{0.2}{100}\right) * DMI * 1000$
10:	Mg_M	nonlactating & DG>0	$\left(\frac{0.12}{100}\right) * DMI * 1000$
11:		otherwise	$\left(\frac{0.1}{100}\right) * DMI * 1000$
12:	K_M	lactating	$\left(\frac{0.7}{100}\right) * DMI * 1000$
13:		otherwise	$\left(\frac{0.6}{100}\right) * DMI * 1000$
14:	Na_M	lactating	$\left(\frac{0.1}{100}\right) * DMI * 1000$
15:		otherwise	$\left(\frac{0.07}{100}\right) * DMI * 1000$
16:	S_M		$\left(\frac{0.15}{100}\right) * DMI * 1000$
17:	Co_M		$0.15 * DMI$
18:	Cu_M		$10 * DMI$
19:	I_M		$0.5 * DMI$
20:	Fe_M		$50 * DMI$
21:	Mn_M	lactating or DG>0	$40 * DMI$
22:		otherwise	$20 * DMI$
23:	Se_M		$0.1 * DMI$
24:	Zn_M		$30 * DMI$
25:	Cr_M	lactating	7.75
26:	Cr_M	nonlactating	0.6

(1) ***CBW*** is the calf birth weight, kg; ***DG*** is days of gestation (i.e., days pregnant); ***MY*** is milk yield, kg/d; ***PIG*** is the net protein in the gain, g/d; ***SBW*** is the shrunk body weight, kg; and X_M, X_P, X_L, **and** X_G are the mineral X requirement for maintenance, pregnancy, lactation, and growth, respectively. Ca, P, Mg, S, Cl, K, and Na are expressed as g/d and Cu, I, Fe, Mn, Zn, Co, Se, and Cr are expressed as mg/d.

5.2.7.3 Sheep

#	Variable[1]	Description	Equation
1:	FCM		$0.3688 * MY + 0.0971 * MkFat * MY$
2:	Ca_M	age<3 months	$0.3 * FBW^{0.75}$
3:		otherwise	$0.18 * FBW^{0.75}$
4:	Ca_P	DG>117 days	$0.6 * LBW$
5:		otherwise	$1.1 * LBW$
6:	Ca_L	lactating	$6 * FCM$
7:	Ca_G		$0.018 * ADG$
8:	P_M	age<3 months	$0.175 * FBW^{0.75}$
9:		otherwise	$0.12 * FBW^{0.75}$
10:	P_P	DG>117 days	$0.25 * LBW$
11:		otherwise	$0.5 * LBW$
12:	P_L	lactating	$2.5 * FCM$
13:	P_G		$0.008 * ADG$
14:	Na_M		$\frac{0.0108}{0.91} * SBW$
15:	Na_P	105≤DG<133 days	$\frac{0.021}{0.91} * LBW$

#	Variable[1]	Description	Equation
16:		DG>133 days	$\frac{0.013}{0.91} * LBW$
17:	Na_L	lactating	$\frac{0.4}{0.91} * MY$
18:	Na_G		$\frac{1.1}{0.91} * ADG$
19:	Cl_M		$\frac{0.0079}{0.85} * SBW$
20:	Cl_P	105≤DG<133 days	$\frac{0.015}{0.85} * LBW$
21:	Cl_P	DG>133 days	$\frac{0.009}{0.85} * LBW$
22:	Cl_L	lactating	$\frac{1.1}{0.85} * MY$
23:	Cl_G		$\frac{0.8}{0.85} * ADG$
24:	K_M		$\frac{0.038}{0.9} * SBW + \frac{2.6}{0.9} * DMI$
25:	K_P	105≤DG<133 days	$\frac{0.029}{0.9} * LBW$
26:	K_P	DG>133 days	$\frac{0.023}{0.9} * LBW$
27:	K_L	lactating	$\frac{1.4}{0.9} * MY$
28:	K_G		$\frac{1.8}{0.9} * ADG$
29:	Mg_M		$\frac{0.003}{0.17} * SBW$
30:	Mg_P	105≤DG<133 days	$\frac{0.009}{0.17} * LBW$
31:	Mg_P	DG>133 days	$\frac{0.013}{0.17} * LBW$
32:	Mg_L	lactating	$\frac{0.17}{0.17} * MY$
33:	Mg_G		$\frac{0.41}{0.17} * ADG$
34:	S_M		$\frac{0.18}{100} * DMI * 1000$
35:	Co_M		$0.2 * DMI$
36:	Cu_{AC}	growing/finishing & age<3 months & SBW≤5 kg	0.9
37:	Cu_{AC}	growing/finishing & age<3 months & 5<SBW≤10 kg	0.53
38:	Cu_{AC}	growing/finishing & age<3 months & SBW>5 kg	0.2
39:	Cu_{AC}	growing/finishing & age≥3 months & conc>50%	0.06
40:	Cu_{AC}	growing/finishing & age≥3 months & conc≤50%	0.045
41:	Cu_{AC}	lactating	0.045
42:	Cu_{AC}	otherwise	0.06
43:	Cu_M		$\frac{0.004}{Cu_{AC}} * SBW$
44:	Cu_P		$\frac{0.05}{Cu_{AC}} * LBW$
45:	Cu_L	lactating	$\frac{0.2}{Cu_{AC}} * MY$
46:	Cu_G		$\frac{1.06}{Cu_{AC}} * ADG + \frac{0.0137}{Cu_{AC}} * CFW$

#	Variable[(1)]	Description	Equation
47:	I_L	lactating	$0.8 * DMI$
48:	I_M	nonlactating	$0.5 * DMI$
49:	Fe_M		$\left(\frac{0.014}{0.1}\right) * SBW$
50:	Fe_P	DG≥105 days	$\frac{0.5}{0.1} * LBW$
51:	Fe_L	lactating	$\frac{0.9}{0.1} * MY$
52:	Fe_G	age<3 months	$\left(\frac{55}{0.5}\right) * ADG + \left(\frac{30}{365 * 0.1}\right) * CFW$
53:		otherwise	$\left(\frac{55}{0.19}\right) * ADG + \left(\frac{30}{365 * 0.1}\right) * CFW$
54:	Mn_M		$\left(\frac{0.002}{0.0075}\right) * SBW$
55:	Mn_P	DG≥105 days	$\frac{0.02}{0.0075} * LBW$
56:	Mn_L	lactating	$\frac{0.055}{0.0075} * MY$
57:	Mn_G		$\left(\frac{0.47}{0.0075}\right) * ADG + \left(\frac{2.5}{365 * 0.0075}\right) * CFW$
58:	Mo_M		$0.5 * DMI$
59:	Se_{AC}	conc>50%	0.6
60:		conc≤50%	0.31
61:	Se_M		$\left(\frac{0.00025}{Se_{AC}}\right) * SBW$
62:	Se_P	DG≥105 days	$\frac{0.0025}{Se_{AC}} * LBW$
63:	Se_L	lactating	$\frac{0.14}{Se_{AC}} * MY$
64:	Se_G		$\left(\frac{0.5}{Se_{AC}}\right) * ADG + \left(\frac{0.38}{Se_{AC}}\right) * CFW$
65:	Zn_{AC}	growing/finishing & SBW<10 kg	0.55
66:		growing/finishing & 10≤SBW<40 kg	0.3
67:		growing/finishing & SBW≥40 kg	0.2
68:		otherwise	0.15
69:	Zn_M		$0.076 * SBW$
70:	Zn_P	DG≥105 days	$\frac{0.375}{Zn_{AC}} * LBW$
71:	Zn_L		$\frac{7.4}{Zn_{AC}} * MY$
72:	Zn_G		$\frac{24}{Zn_{AC}} * ADG + \frac{115}{365 * Zn_{AC}} * CFW$

(1) ***AC*** is the absorption coefficient, dimensionless; ***ADG*** is the average daily gain, kg/d; ***age*** is the animal age, month; ***CFW*** is the clean fleece weight, kg/yr; ***conc*** is the dietary percentage of concentrates, %; ***DG*** is days of gestation (i.e., days pregnant); ***DMI*** is the dry matter intake, kg/d; ***FBW*** is the full body weight, kg; ***FCM*** is the fat-corrected milk, kg/d; ***LBW*** is lamb(s) or kid(s) total body weight, kg/d; ***MkFat*** is milk fat content, %; ***MY*** is milk yield, kg/d; ***SBW*** is the shrunk body weight, kg; and X_M, X_P, X_L, ***and*** X_G are the mineral X requirement for maintenance, pregnancy, lactation, and growth, respectively. Ca, P, Mg, S, Cl, K, and Na are expressed as g/d and Cu, I, Fe, Mn, Zn, Co, Se, Mo, and Cr are expressed as mg/d.

5.2.7.4 Goats

#	Variable[(1)]	Description	Equation
1:	FCM		$0.3688 * MY + 0.0971 * MkFat * MY$
2:	Ca_M	age<3 months	$0.3 * FBW^{0.75}$
3:		otherwise	$0.18 * FBW^{0.75}$

#	Variable[1]	Description	Equation
4:	Ca_P	DG>117 days	$0.6 * LBW$
5:		otherwise	$1.1 * LBW$
6:	Ca_L	lactating	$6 * FCM$
7:	Ca_G		$0.018 * ADG$
8:	P_M	age<3 months	$0.175 * FBW^{0.75}$
9:		otherwise	$0.12 * FBW^{0.75}$
10:	P_P	DG>117 days	$0.25 * LBW$
11:		otherwise	$0.5 * LBW$
12:	P_L	lactating	$2.5 * FCM$
13:	P_G		$0.008 * ADG$
14:	Na_M		$\frac{0.015}{0.8} * SBW$
15:	Na_P	DG>105 days	$\frac{0.034}{0.8} * LBW$
16:	Na_L	lactating	$\frac{0.4}{0.8} * MY$
17:	Na_G		$\frac{1.6}{0.8} * ADG$
18:	Cl_M		$\frac{0.022}{0.8} * SBW$
19:	Cl_P	DG≥105 days	$\frac{0.024}{0.8} * LBW$
20:	Cl_L	lactating	$\frac{1.1}{0.8} * MY$
21:	Cl_G		$\frac{1}{0.8} * ADG$
22:	K_M		$\frac{0.05}{0.9} * SBW + \frac{2.6}{0.9} * DMI$
23:	K_P	DG≥105 days	$\frac{0.042}{0.9} * LBW$
24:	K_L	lactating	$\frac{2}{0.9} * MY$
25:	K_G		$\frac{2.4}{0.9} * ADG$
26:	Mg_M		$\frac{0.0035}{0.2} * SBW$
27:	Mg_P	DG≥105 days	$\frac{0.006}{0.2} * LBW$
28:	Mg_L	lactating	$\frac{0.14}{0.2} * MY$
29:	Mg_G		$\frac{0.4}{0.2} * ADG$
30:	S_M	nonlactating	$\frac{0.22}{100} * DMI * 1000$
31:	S_L	lactating	$\frac{0.26}{100} * DMI * 1000$
32:	Co_M		$0.11 * DMI$
33:	Cu_M	growing/finishing	$25 * DMI$
34:		nonlactating	$20 * DMI$
35:	Cu_L	lactating	$15 * DMI$
36:	I_L	lactating	$0.8 * DMI$
37:	I_M	nonlactating	$0.5 * DMI$
38:	Fe_M	growing/finishing	$95 * DMI$
39:	Fe_M	otherwise	$35 * DMI$
40:	Mn_M		$\left(\frac{0.002}{0.0075}\right) * SBW$
41:	Mn_P	DG≥105 days	$\frac{0.025}{0.0075} * LBW$
42:	Mn_L	lactating	$\frac{0.03}{0.0075} * MY$
43:	Mn_G		$\left(\frac{0.7}{0.0075}\right) * ADG + \left(\frac{2.5}{365 * 0.0075}\right) * CFW$
44:	Mo_M		$1 * DMI$
45:	Se_{AC}	conc>50%	0.6

#	Variable[1]	Description	Equation
46:		conc≤50%	0.31
47:	Se_M		$\left(\frac{0.083}{Se_{AC}}\right) * SBW + 0.015 * DMI$
48:	Se_P	DG≥105 days	$\frac{0.0021}{Se_{AC}} * LBW$
49:	Se_L	lactating	$\frac{0.1}{Se_{AC}} * MY$
50:	Se_G		$\left(\frac{0.5}{Se_{AC}}\right) * ADG + \left(\frac{0.38}{Se_{AC}}\right) * CFW$
51:		growing/finishing & age<3 months	0.5
52:	Zn_{AC}	growing/finishing & age≥3 months	0.3
53:		otherwise	0.15
54:	Zn_M		$\frac{0.045}{Zn_{AC}} * SBW$
55:	Zn_P	DG≥105 days	$\frac{0.5}{Zn_{AC}} * LBW$
56:	Zn_L		$\frac{5.5}{Zn_{AC}} * MY$
57:	Zn_G		$\frac{24}{Zn_{AC}} * ADG + \frac{115}{365 * Zn_{AC}} * CFW$

[1] ***AC*** is the absorption coefficient, dimensionless; ***ADG*** is the average daily gain, kg/d; ***age*** is the animal age, month; ***CFW*** is the clean fleece weight, kg/yr; ***conc*** is the dietary percentage of concentrates, %; ***DG*** is days of gestation (i.e., days pregnant); ***DMI*** is the dry matter intake, kg/d; ***FBW*** is the full body weight, kg; ***FCM*** is the fat-corrected milk, kg/d; ***LBW*** is lamb(s) or kid(s) total body weight, kg/d; ***MkFat*** is milk fat content, %; ***MY*** is milk yield, kg/d; ***SBW*** is the shrunk body weight, kg; and ***X_M, X_P, X_L, and X_G*** are the mineral X requirement for maintenance, pregnancy, lactation, and growth, respectively. Ca, P, Mg, S, Cl, K, and Na are expressed as g/d and Cu, I, Fe, Mn, Zn, Co, Se, Mo, and Cr are expressed as mg/d.

5.2.8 Vitamin requirements: calcVitaminRequirement()

#	Variable[1]	Description	Equation
1:		dairy: lactating	$110 * FBW$
2:	VitA	dairy: dry	$110 * FBW$
3:		dairy: otherwise	$80 * FBW$
4:	VitD	dairy	$30 * FBW$
5:		dairy: lactating	$0.8 * FBW$
6:	VitE	dairy: dry	$1.6 * FBW$
7:		dairy: otherwise	$0.8 * FBW$
8:		beef: lactating or bulls	$3900 * DMI$
9:	VitA	beef: dry or replacement	$2800 * DMI$
10:		beef: otherwise	$2200 * DMI$
11:	VitD	beef	$275 * DMI$
12:	VitE	beef	$35 * DMI$
13:		sheep or goats: lactating	$178 * FBW$
14:		sheep or goats: female and DG<101	$105 * FBW$
15:	VitA	sheep or goats: female and DG≥101	$152 * FBW$
16:		sheep or goats: otherwise	$333 * FBW$
17:		sheep or goats: lactating	$5.6 * FBW + 716$
18:	VitD	sheep or goats: female	$5.6 * FBW$

#	Variable[1]	Description	Equation
		and DG<101	
19:		sheep or goats: female and DG≥101	$5.6 * FBW + 213$
20:		sheep or goats: otherwise	$If(age < 4,1.1,1) * (5.6 * FBW + 1.08 * ADG * 1000)$
21:	*VitE*	sheep or goats: lactating	$5.6 * FBW$
22:		sheep or goats: female and DG<101	$5.3 * FBW$
23:		sheep or goats: female and DG≥101	$5.6 * FBW$
24:		sheep or goats: otherwise	$10 * FBW$

[1] ***ADG*** is the average daily gain, kg/d; ***age*** is the animal age, month; ***DG*** is the days of gestation (i.e., days pregnant); ***DMI*** is the dry matter intake, kg/d; ***VitA*** is the required vitamin A, IU/d; ***VitD*** is the required vitamin D, IU/d; and ***VitE*** is the required vitamin E, IU/d.

5.3 Code

5.3.1 Basic calculations

```
calcBW <- function(FBWtoSBW = 0.96, SBWtoEBW = 0.891)
{
  anim.iFBW <<- 0
  anim.fFBW <<- 0
  anim.FBW <<- 0
  anim.iSBW <<- 0
  anim.fSBW <<- 0
  anim.SBW <<- 0
  anim.iEBW <<- 0
  anim.fEBW <<- 0
  anim.EBW <<- 0
  anim.FMtBW <<- 0
  anim.MSBW <<- 0
  anim.MEBW <<- 0
  if (tolower(anim.body.weight_type) == "full")
  {
    if (tolower(anim.stage_option) == "mean")
    {
      anim.FBW <<- anim.body.weight_mean
      anim.SBW <<- anim.FBW * FBWtoSBW
      anim.EBW <<- anim.SBW * SBWtoEBW
    } else
    {
      anim.iFBW <<- anim.body.weight_initial
      anim.fFBW <<- anim.body.weight_final
      anim.FBW <<- (anim.iFBW + anim.fFBW)/2
      anim.iSBW <<- anim.iFBW * FBWtoSBW
      anim.fSBW <<- anim.fFBW * FBWtoSBW
      anim.SBW <<- anim.FBW * FBWtoSBW
      anim.iEBW <<- anim.iSBW * SBWtoEBW
      anim.fEBW <<- anim.fSBW * SBWtoEBW
      anim.EBW <<- anim.SBW * SBWtoEBW
    }
    anim.MFBW <<- anim.body.weight_mature
    anim.MSBW <<- anim.MFBW * FBWtoSBW
    anim.MEBW <<- anim.MSBW * SBWtoEBW
  }
  if (tolower(anim.body.weight_type) == "shrunk")
  {
    if (tolower(anim.stage_option) == "mean")
    {
      anim.SBW <<- anim.body.weight_mean
      anim.FBW <<- anim.SBW/FBWtoSBW
```

```
        anim.EBW <<- anim.SBW * SBWtoEBW
      } else
      {
        anim.iSBW <<- anim.body.weight_initial
        anim.fSBW <<- anim.body.weight_final
        anim.SBW <<- (anim.iSBW + anim.fSBW)/2
        anim.iFBW <<- anim.iSBW/FBWtoSBW
        anim.fFBW <<- anim.fSBW/FBWtoSBW
        anim.FBW <<- anim.SBW/FBWtoSBW
        anim.iEBW <<- anim.iSBW * SBWtoEBW
        anim.fEBW <<- anim.fSBW * SBWtoEBW
        anim.EBW <<- anim.SBW * SBWtoEBW
      }
      anim.MSBW <<- anim.body.weight_mature
      anim.MFBW <<- anim.MSBW/FBWtoSBW
      anim.MEBW <<- anim.MSBW * SBWtoEBW
    }
    if (tolower(anim.body.weight_type) == "empty")
    {
      if (tolower(anim.stage_option) == "mean")
      {
        anim.EBW <<- anim.body.weight_mean
        anim.SBW <<- anim.EBW/SBWtoEBW
        anim.FBW <<- anim.SBW/FBWtoSBW
      } else
      {
        anim.iEBW <<- anim.body.weight_initial
        anim.fEBW <<- anim.body.weight_final
        anim.EBW <<- (anim.iEBW + anim.fEBW)/2
        anim.iSBW <<- anim.iEBW/SBWtoEBW
        anim.fSBW <<- anim.fEBW/SBWtoEBW
        anim.SBW <<- anim.EBW/SBWtoEBW
        anim.iFBW <<- anim.iSBW/FBWtoSBW
        anim.fFBW <<- anim.fSBW/FBWtoSBW
        anim.FBW <<- anim.SBW/FBWtoSBW
      }
      anim.MEBW <<- anim.body.weight_mature
      anim.MSBW <<- anim.MEBW/SBWtoEBW
      anim.MFBW <<- anim.MSBW/FBWtoSBW
    }
    if (exists("anim.pregnancy.uterus.weight"))
    {
      # Note that GUW is fixed, GU does not change weight when animal is shrunk or empty
      GUW <- anim.pregnancy.uterus.weight
      anim.FBW_GU <<- anim.FBW - GUW
      anim.SBW_GU <<- anim.SBW - GUW
      anim.EBW_GU <<- anim.EBW - GUW
    } else
    {
      anim.FBW_GU <<- anim.FBW
      anim.SBW_GU <<- anim.SBW
```

```
      anim.EBW_GU <<- anim.EBW
    }
    anim.u.frac <<- ifelse(anim.MFBW > 0, anim.FBW/anim.MFBW, 1)
    return(invisible(TRUE))
  }

  calcBCS <- function(bcs = NA, scale = "1-9")
  {
    tmp <- 5
    if (is.na(bcs) == FALSE)
    {
      if (anim.body.condition_type == "0_5")
      {
        if (scale == "0-5") tmp <- bcs
        if (scale == "1-5") tmp <- (1/5) * (5 + 4 * bcs)
        if (scale == "1-9") tmp <- (8/5) * bcs + 1
        if (scale == "1-8") tmp <- (1/5) * (5 + 7 * bcs)
        if (scale == "1-10") tmp <- (1/5) * (9 * bcs + 5)
      }
      if (anim.body.condition_type == "1_5")
      {
        if (scale == "0-5") tmp <- (5/4) * (bcs - 1)
        if (scale == "1-5") tmp <- bcs
        if (scale == "1-9") tmp <- 2 * bcs - 1
        if (scale == "1-8") tmp <- (1/4) * (7 * bcs - 3)
        if (scale == "1-10") tmp <- (1/4) * (9 * bcs - 5)
      }
      if (anim.body.condition_type == "1_9")
      {
        if (scale == "0-5") tmp <- (5/8) * (bcs - 1)
        if (scale == "1-5") tmp <- (bcs + 1)/2
        if (scale == "1-9") tmp <- bcs
        if (scale == "1-8") tmp <- (1/8) * (1 + 7 * bcs)
        if (scale == "1-10") tmp <- (1/8) * (9 * bcs - 1)
      }
    }
    return(tmp)
  }

  calcDMINursingCalves <- function(PML, ForageDE, CalfBW)
  {
    ForageDMI <- max((1/(ForageDE^2)) *
               ((CalfBW^(-0.3895 - 0.0197 * (PML^2))) * exp(CalfBW * (-0.00244 - 0.00337 * PML) - 1.3594 * PML) *
               ((CalfBW^(0.4477 * PML)) * (-32.5704 + (27.9016 - 7.66732 * ForageDE) * ForageDE) *
               exp((0.0588 + 0.00018 * CalfBW) * (PML^2)) + (CalfBW^(1.3895 + 0.0197 * (PML^2))) *
               exp(CalfBW * (0.00244 + 0.00337 * PML) + 1.3594 * PML) *
               (0.4738 + ForageDE * (-0.4059 + ForageDE * (0.11154 - 0.003273 * PML) + 0.01191 * PML) - 0.0139046 * PML) +
               (CalfBW^(0.3895 + 0.0197 *  (PML^2))) * exp(CalfBW * (0.00244 + 0.00337 * PML) + 1.3594 * PML) *
               (-10.3049 + ForageDE * (8.82778 + ForageDE * (-2.42586 + 0.362681 * PML) - 1.31981 * PML) + 1.54065 * PML))), 0)
    return(ForageDMI)
  }
```

5.3.2 Maintenance requirements

```
calcMaintenanceRequirement <- function(blnReturnNEmr = FALSE, DMI = NA, ME = NA, NEma = NA, NEga = NA, NEla = NA)
{
  if (is.na(anim.species) | (is.na(DMI) == TRUE & anim.diet.DMI.rate <= 0))
  {
    ratio.NEmr.MEmr <<- 0
    anim.comp <<- 0
    env.PETI <<- 0
    anim.a2 <<- 0
    anim.sex_factor <<- 0
    anim.NEmrBasa.rate <<- 0
    anim.NEmrAct.rate <<- 0
    anim.HE.rate <<- 0
    anim.body.SA <<- 0
    env.mud.factor <<- 0
    anim.hide.factor <<- 0
    anim.body.EI <<- 0
    anim.bodyTI <<- 0
    anim.body.IN <<- 0
    anim.body.LCT <<- 0
    anim.MEmrCS.rate <<- 0
    anim.NEmrCS.rate <<- 0
    anim.panting.factor <<- 0
    anim.NEmrHS.rate <<- 0
    env.CETI <<- 0
    anim.NEmrUrea.rate <<- 0
    anim.NEmr.rate <<- 0
    anim.MEmr.rate <<- 0
    anim.UPA.rate <<- 0
    anim.SPA.rate <<- 0
    anim.FPN.rate <<- 0
    anim.MPmr.rate <<- 0
    ratio.NPmr.MPmr <<- 0
    anim.NPmr.rate <<- 0
    anim.MAAmr.rate <<- rep(0, 10)
    anim.body.E_factor <<- 0
    anim.body.z_factor <<- 0
    anim.body.r_factor <<- 0
    anim.FFM.rate <<- 0
    anim.DMI.L.frac <<- 0
    return(invisible(NULL))
  }
  # Returns anim.NEmr.rate, Mcal/d
  if (is.na(DMI) == TRUE) DMI <- anim.diet.DMI.rate
  if (is.na(ME) == TRUE) ME <- anim.diet.ME.frac
  if (is.na(NEma) == TRUE) NEma <- anim.diet.NEm.frac
  if (is.na(NEga) == TRUE) NEga <- anim.diet.NEg.frac
  if (is.na(NEla) == TRUE) NEla <- anim.diet.NEl.frac
  km <- ratio.NEmr.MEmr <<- NEma/ME
```

```
    WS <- env.wind.rate
    Tp <- env.temp_prev
    Tc <- env.temp_curr
    Tn <- env.temp_night
    RHp <- env.hum_prev
    RHc <- env.hum_curr
    HRS <- env.sunlight
    bcs <- ifelse(tolower(anim.stage_option) == "mean",
                  calcBCS(anim.body.condition_mean,"1-9"),
                  (calcBCS(anim.body.condition_initial,"1-9")+calcBCS(anim.body.condition_final,"1-9"))/2)
    panting <- anim.panting
    if (anim.species == "Cattle")
    {
      # +++++++++++++++++++++++++++++++++
      # Basal metabolic rate (NEmrBasal)
      # +++++++++++++++++++++++++++++++++
      # Adjustment for previous plane of nutrition for growing cattle
      if (anim.stage_type == "Growing/Finishing" | anim.stage_type == "Replacement")
        anim.comp <<- 0.8 + (bcs - 1) * 0.05 else anim.comp <<- 1
        # Adjustment for previous temperature
        if (Tp > 20)
        {
          env.PETI <<- 27.88 - 0.456 * Tp + 0.010754 * Tp^2 - 0.4905 * RHp + 0.00088 * RHp + 1.1507 * (1000/3600) * WS -
0.126447 * (1000/3600) * WS^2 + 0.019876 * Tp * RHp - 0.046313 * Tp * (1000/3600) * WS + 0.4167 * HRS
        } else
        {
          env.PETI <<- Tp
        }
        anim.a2 <<- (88.426 - 0.785 * env.PETI + 0.0116 * env.PETI^2 - 77)/1000
        # Adjustment for lactation (beef and dual-purpose cows)
        if (anim.type != "Milk" & anim.stage_type == "Lactating") L <- anim.L.factor else L <- anim.L.factor <<- 1
        # Adjustment for sex
        if (anim.sex == "Male") sex <- anim.sex_factor <<- 1.15 else sex <- anim.sex_factor <<- 1
        anim.NEmrBasal.rate <<- (anim.a1 * L * anim.comp * sex + anim.a2) * anim.SBW_GU^0.75
        # +++++++++++++++++++++++++++++++++++++
        # NEmr for physical activity (NEmrAct)
        # +++++++++++++++++++++++++++++++++++++
        anim.NEmrAct.rate <<- (0.1 * anim.standing + 0.062 * anim.poschanges + 0.621 * (anim.walk.horiz.rate/1000) + 6.69 *
(anim.walk.vert.rate/1000)) * anim.FBW/1000
        # ++++++++++++++++++++++++++++++
        # NEmr for cold stress (NEmrCS)
        # ++++++++++++++++++++++++++++++
        if (exists("anim.NEpr.rate") == FALSE) anim.NEpr.rate <<- 0
        if (exists("anim.NElr.rate") == FALSE) anim.NElr.rate <<- 0
        if (exists("anim.NEgr.rate") == FALSE) anim.NEgr.rate <<- 0
        anim.HE.rate <<- ME * DMI - (anim.NEmrBasal.rate + anim.NEgr.rate + anim.NEpr.rate + anim.NElr.rate)
        anim.body.SA <<- 0.09 * anim.FBW^0.67
        if (anim.body.haircoat == 0) env.mud.factor <<- 1
        if (anim.body.haircoat == 1) env.mud.factor <<- 0.8
        if (anim.body.haircoat == 2) env.mud.factor <<- 0.5
        if (anim.body.haircoat == 3) env.mud.factor <<- 0.3
```

```
    if (anim.hide == "Thin") anim.hide.factor <<- 0.8
    if (anim.hide == "Medium") anim.hide.factor <<- 1
    if (anim.hide == "Thick") anim.hide.factor <<- 1.2
    anim.body.EI <<- max(0, (6.1816 - 0.5575 * WS + 0.0152 * WS^2 + 5.298 * anim.hair.depth - 0.5297 * anim.hair.depth^2 - 
0.1029 * WS * anim.hair.depth) * env.mud.factor * anim.hide.factor)
    if (anim.age * 30.4 <= 30) anim.body.TI <<- 2.5
    if (anim.age * 30.4 > 30 & anim.age * 30.4 <= 183) anim.body.TI <<- 6.5
    if (anim.age * 30.4 > 183 & anim.age * 30.4 <= 363) anim.body.TI <<- 5.1875 + 0.3125 * bcs
    if (anim.age * 30.4 > 363) anim.body.TI <<- 5.25 + 0.75 * bcs
    anim.body.IN <<- anim.body.EI + anim.body.TI
    anim.body.LCT <<- 39 - 0.85 * anim.body.IN * (anim.HE.rate/anim.body.SA)
    if (anim.body.LCT > Tc)
    {
      anim.MEmrCS.rate <<- anim.body.SA * (anim.body.LCT - Tc)/anim.body.IN
    } else anim.MEmrCS.rate <<- 0
    anim.NEmrCS.rate <<- anim.MEmrCS.rate * km
    # ++++++++++++++++++++++++++++++
    # NEmr for heat stress (NEmrHS)
    # ++++++++++++++++++++++++++++++
    env.CETI <<- 27.88 - 0.456 * Tc + 0.010754 * Tc^2 - 0.4905 * RHc + 0.00088 * RHc + 1.1507 * (1000/3600) * WS - 0.126447 
* (1000/3600) * WS^2 + 0.019876 * Tc * RHc - 0.046313 * Tc * (1000/3600) * WS + 0.4167 * HRS
    breeds_bosindicus <- c("Braford", "Brahman", "Brangus", "Canchin", "Gir", "Guzerat", "Nellore", "Sahiwal", "Salers", 
"Santa Gertudis")
    anim.panting.factor <<- 1
    if ((anim.breeding == "Straightbred" & length(which(breeds_bosindicus == anim.breed)) > 0) |
        (anim.breeding == "2-way" & length(which(breeds_bosindicus == anim.breed.dam)) > 0) |
        (anim.breeding == "2-way" & length(which(breeds_bosindicus == anim.breed.sire)) > 0))
    {
      if (panting == 0) anim.panting.factor <<- 1  # no panting
      if (panting == 1) anim.panting.factor <<- 1.07  # rapid shallow panting
      if (panting == 2) anim.panting.factor <<- 1.18  # open mouth panting
      anim.NEmrHS.rate <<- anim.NEmrBasal.rate * (anim.panting.factor - 1)
    } else
    {
      if (env.CETI > 20)
      {
        anim.NEmrHS.rate <<- anim.NEmrBasal.rate * ((1.09857 - 0.01343 * env.CETI + 0.000457 * env.CETI^2) - 1)
      } else anim.NEmrHS.rate <<- 0
    }
    # ++++++++++++++++++++++++++
    # NEmr for urea (NEmrUrea)
    # ++++++++++++++++++++++++++
    if (exists("rum.N_balance.rate") == T) RNB <- TOkg(rum.N_balance.rate) else RNB <- 0
    if (exists("rum.Recycled_N.rate") == T) RRN <- TOkg(rum.Recycled_N.rate) else RRN <- 0
    if (exists("anim.MPe_balance.rate") == T) MPB <- TOkg(anim.MPe_balance.rate/1000)/6.25 else MPB <- 0
    anim.NEmrUrea.rate <<- max(0, (RNB - RRN + MPB)) * 1000 * 0.0073 * km
    anim.NEmr.rate <<- anim.NEmrBasal.rate + anim.NEmrAct.rate + anim.NEmrCS.rate + anim.NEmrHS.rate + anim.NEmrUrea.rate
    anim.MEmr.rate <<- anim.NEmr.rate/ratio.NEmr.MEmr
    # ++++++++++++++++++++++++++++++++
    # Metabolizable protein (MPmr)
    # ++++++++++++++++++++++++++++++++
```

```
      if (SolutionLevel == 0 | SolutionLevel == 1 | flag_ForceEmpiricalMPm == TRUE)
      {
        anim.UPA.rate <<- 0
        anim.SPA.rate <<- 0
        anim.FPN.rate <<- 0
        anim.MPmr.rate <<- 3.8 * anim.SBW^0.75
        ratio.NPmr.MPmr <<- 0.5
      } else
      {
        anim.UPA.rate <<- (2.75 * anim.SBW^0.5)/0.67
        anim.SPA.rate <<- (0.2 * anim.SBW^0.6)/0.67
        if (exists("fc.diet.IDM.rate") == T) IDM <- fc.diet.IDM.rate * 1000 else IDM <- 0
        anim.FPN.rate <<- 0.09 * IDM
        anim.MPmr.rate <<- anim.UPA.rate + anim.SPA.rate + anim.FPN.rate
        ratio.NPmr.MPmr <<- (anim.FPN.rate * 0.5 + (anim.UPA.rate + anim.SPA.rate) * 0.67)/anim.MPmr.rate
      }
      anim.NPmr.rate <<- anim.MPmr.rate * ratio.NPmr.MPmr
      # +++++++++++++++++++++++++++++++++++
      # Metabolizable amino acids (MAA)
      # +++++++++++++++++++++++++++++++++++
      # AA are Met, Lys, His, Phe, Trp, Thr, Leu, Ile, Val, Arg
      anim.MAAmr.rate <<- anim.NPmr.rate * (anim.tissue.AA.conc/100)/anim.tissue.AA_Eff.frac  # g metabolizable AA/d
  } else
  {
    CW <- anim.wool.rate * 1000  # g/yr
    WD <- anim.wool.depth * 10  # mm
    RF <- env.rain.rate  # mm/d
    # ++++++++++++++++++++++++++++++++++++
    # Basal metabolic rate (NEmrBasal)
    # ++++++++++++++++++++++++++++++++++++
    env.CETI <<- 27.88 - 0.456 * Tc + 0.010754 * Tc^2 - 0.4905 * RHc + 0.00088 * RHc + 1.1507 * (1000/3600) * WS - 0.126447 *
(1000/3600) * WS^2 + 0.019876 * Tc * RHc - 0.046313 * Tc * (1000/3600) * WS + 0.4167 * HRS
    # Adjustment for previous temperature
    if (Tp > 20)
    {
      env.PETI <<- 27.88 - 0.456 * Tp + 0.010754 * Tp^2 - 0.4905 * RHp + 0.00088 * RHp + 1.1507 * (1000/3600) * WS - 0.126447
* (1000/3600) * WS^2 + 0.019876 * Tp * RHp - 0.046313 * Tp * (1000/3600) * WS + 0.4167 * HRS
    } else
    {
      env.PETI <<- Tp
    }
    anim.a2 <<- 1 + 0.0091 * (20 - env.PETI)
    anim.a1 <<- ifelse(anim.species == "Sheep", 0.06214, ifelse(anim.indigenous == T, 0.0652, 0.0777))
    anim.NEmrBasal.rate <<- anim.a1 * anim.a2 * (exp(-0.03 * anim.age/12)) * anim.SBW_GU^0.75
    # +++++++++++++++++++++++++++++++++++++++
    # NEmr for physical activity (NEmrAct)
    # +++++++++++++++++++++++++++++++++++++++
    if (anim.species == "Sheep")
    {
      anim.NEmrAct.rate <<- (0.62 * (anim.walk.horiz.rate/1000) + 6.69 * (anim.walk.vert.rate/1000)) * anim.FBW/1000
    } else
```

```
    {
      anim.NEmrAct.rate <<- (0.836 * (anim.walk.horiz.rate/1000) + 6.69 * (anim.walk.vert.rate/1000)) * anim.FBW/1000
    }
    # ++++++++++++++++++++++++++++++
    # NEmr for cold stress (NEmrCS)
    # ++++++++++++++++++++++++++++++
    if (exists("anim.NEpr.rate") == FALSE) anim.NEpr.rate <<- 0
    if (exists("anim.NElr.rate") == FALSE) anim.NElr.rate <<- 0
    if (exists("anim.NEgr.rate") == FALSE) anim.NEgr.rate <<- 0
    anim.HE.rate <<- ME * DMI - (anim.NEmrBasal.rate + anim.NEgr.rate + anim.NEpr.rate + anim.NElr.rate)
    anim.body.SA <<- 0.09 * anim.SBW^0.67
    E <- anim.body.E_factor <<- 1.3/4.184  # Evaporative losses coefficient, Mcal/(m^2.d)
    z <- anim.body.z_factor <<- ifelse(anim.species == "Sheep", 0.141, 0.11)  # oc.m^2.d/MJ
    r <- anim.body.r_factor <<- ifelse(anim.age <= 12, 50, 120)  # Assumes lamb or kid is less than 1 yr old
    anim.body.TI <<- 4.184 * 1.3  # oC.m^2.d/Mcal
    anim.body.EI <<- 4.184 * ((r/((0.481 + 0.326 * sqrt(WS)) * (r + WD))) + r * log((r + WD)/r) * (z - 0.017 * sqrt(WS)))  # oC.m^2.d/Mcal
    anim.body.IN <<- anim.body.TI + (1 - 0.3 * (1 - exp(-1.5 * RF/WD))) * anim.body.EI
    anim.body.LCT <<- 39 + E * anim.body.EI - anim.body.IN * (anim.HE.rate/anim.body.SA)
    if (anim.body.LCT > Tc)
    {
      anim.MEmrCS.rate <<- anim.body.SA * (anim.body.LCT - Tc)/anim.body.IN
    } else anim.MEmrCS.rate <<- 0
    anim.NEmrCS.rate <<- anim.MEmrCS.rate * km
    # ++++++++++++++++++++++++++++++
    # NEmr for heat stress (NEmrHS)
    # ++++++++++++++++++++++++++++++
    anim.NEmrHS.rate <<- 0
    # +++++++++++++++++++++++++
    # NEmr for urea (NEmrUrea)
    # +++++++++++++++++++++++++
    if (exists("rum.N_balance.rate") == T) RNB <- TOkg(rum.N_balance.rate) else RNB <- 0
    if (exists("rum.Recycled_N.rate") == T) RRN <- TOkg(rum.Recycled_N.rate) else RRN <- 0
    if (exists("anim.MPe_balance.rate") == T) MPB <- TOkg(anim.MPe_balance.rate/1000)/6.25 else MPB <- 0
    anim.NEmrUrea.rate <<- max(0, (RNB - RRN + MPB)) * 1000 * 0.0073 * km
    anim.NEmr.rate <<- anim.NEmrBasal.rate + anim.NEmrAct.rate + anim.NEmrCS.rate + anim.NEmrHS.rate + anim.NEmrUrea.rate
    anim.MEmr.rate <<- anim.NEmr.rate/ratio.NEmr.MEmr
    # +++++++++++++++++++++++++++++
    # Metabolizable protein (MPmr)
    # +++++++++++++++++++++++++++++
    anim.UPA.rate <<- (0.147 * anim.FBW_GU + 3.375)/0.67
    anim.FPN.rate <<- 15.2 * DMI/0.67
    anim.SPA.rate <<- ifelse(anim.species == "Sheep", CW/(0.6 * 365), 0.1125 * anim.FBW^0.75)
    anim.MPmr.rate <<- anim.UPA.rate + anim.SPA.rate + anim.FPN.rate
    ratio.NPmr.MPmr <<- 0.67
    anim.NPmr.rate <<- anim.MPmr.rate * ratio.NPmr.MPmr
    # +++++++++++++++++++++++++++++++++
    # Metabolizable amino acids (MAA)
    # +++++++++++++++++++++++++++++++++
    # AA are Met, Lys, His, Phe, Trp, Thr, Leu, Ile, Val, Arg
    # Uses the same calculation logic for cattle
```

```
      anim.MAAmr.rate <<- anim.NPmr.rate * (anim.tissue.AA.conc/100)/anim.tissue.AA_Eff.frac  # g metabolizable AA/d
    }
    anim.FFM.rate <<- anim.NEmr.rate/NEma
    anim.DMI.L.frac <<- ifelse(anim.FFM.rate > 0, DMI/anim.FFM.rate)
    if (blnReturnNEmr == T) return(anim.NEmr.rate) else return(invisible(TRUE))
  }
```

5.3.3 Lactation requirements

```
calcLactationRequirement <- function(blnReturnNElr = FALSE, MY = NA, MkFat = NA, MkTP = NA, MkL = 4.85, NEma = NA, NEga = NA, NEla = NA)
{
  # Returns anim.NElr.rate, Mcal/d
  if (isLactating == FALSE | is.na(anim.species) | anim.diet.DMI.rate <= 0)
  {
    anim.lactation.milk.rate <<- 0
    ratio.NElr.MElr <<- 0
    anim.NElr.rate <<- 0
    anim.MElr.rate <<- 0
    ratio.NPlr.MPlr <<- 0
    anim.NPlr.rate <<- 0
    anim.MPlr.rate <<- 0
    anim.MAAlr.rate <<- rep(0, 10)
    calf.DMI_forage.rate <<- 0
    anim.FFL.rate <<- 0
    anim.lactation.milk.rate_pred <<- 0
    anim.lactation.milk.fat.conc_pred <<- 0
    anim.lactation.milk.protein.conc_pred <<- 0
    return(invisible(NULL))
  }
  if (anim.species == "Cattle" & anim.type != "Milk")
  {
    if (is.na(MY) == TRUE) PKYD <- anim.lactation.milk.peak.rate
    if (is.na(MkFat) == TRUE) MkFat <- anim.lactation.milk.peak.fat.conc
    if (is.na(MkTP) == TRUE) MkTP <- anim.lactation.milk.peak.protein.conc
  } else
  {
    if (is.na(MY) == TRUE) MY <- anim.lactation.milk.rate
    if (is.na(MkFat) == TRUE) MkFat <- anim.lactation.milk.fat.conc
    if (anim.species == "Goats")
    {
      if (is.na(MkTP) == TRUE) MkTP <- ifelse(anim.lactation.milk.protein.type == "True", anim.lactation.milk.protein.conc, anim.lactation.milk.protein.conc * 0.92)
    } else
    {
      if (is.na(MkTP) == TRUE) MkTP <- ifelse(anim.lactation.milk.protein.type == "True", anim.lactation.milk.protein.conc, anim.lactation.milk.protein.conc * 0.93)
    }
  }
  if (is.na(NEma) == TRUE) NEma <- anim.diet.NEm.frac
  if (is.na(NEla) == TRUE) NEla <- anim.diet.NEl.frac
  if (is.na(NEga) == TRUE) NEga <- anim.diet.NEg.frac
  if (anim.species == "Cattle")
  {
    DIM <- anim.lactation.days
    DG <- anim.pregnancy.days
    if (anim.type != "Milk")
```

```
    {
      # Beef and dual-purpose
      # +++ MY +++
      RelMY <- anim.lactation.milk.factor
      T <- 8.5
      MY <- (DIM * (0.125 * RelMY + 0.375) * PKYD * exp(1))/(7 * T * exp(DIM/(7 * T)))
      if ((anim.age/12) <= 2) MY <- MY * 0.74
      if ((anim.age/12) > 2 & (anim.age/12) <= 3) MY <- MY * 0.88
      anim.lactation.milk.rate <<- anim.lactation.milk.rate_pred <<- MY
    } else
    {
      # Predicted MY for dairy Uses March et al. (1988) and Skidmore (1990)
      if (anim.lactation.count == 1)
      {
        RHA <- 9000
        MY_A <- (RHA * 0.01 - lbTOkg(20))/2.96
        MY_b <- 0.08
        MY_c <- -0.002
        MY_d <- -0.001
        anim.lactation.milk.rate_pred <<- MY_A * (DIM^MY_b) * exp(MY_c * DIM) * exp(MY_d * DG)
      } else
      {
        RHA <- 10000
        MY_A <- (RHA * 0.01 + lbTOkg(14))/2.96
        if (anim.lactation.count == 2)
        {
          MY_b <- 0.12
          MY_c <- -0.004
          MY_d <- -0.002
        } else
        {
          MY_b <- 0.16
          MY_c <- -0.005
          MY_d <- -0.002
        }
        anim.lactation.milk.rate_pred <<- MY_A * (DIM^MY_b) * exp(MY_c * DIM) * exp(MY_d * DG)
      }
    }
    anim.lactation.milk.fat.conc_pred <<- (MkFat * (((DIM + 1)/7)^-0.13) * exp(0.02 * (DIM + 1)/7))/0.9922
    anim.lactation.milk.protein.conc_pred <<- (MkTP * (((DIM + 1)/7)^-0.12) * exp(0.01 * (DIM + 1)/7))/0.875
    if (flag_CurveAdjustedMkFatMkProtein == TRUE)
    {
      MkFat <- anim.lactation.milk.fat.conc_pred
      MkProt <- anim.lactation.milk.protein.conc_pred
    }
    # +++ Energy +++
    ratio.NElr.MElr <<- 0.644
    anim.NElr.rate <<- MY * (0.0929 * MkFat + 0.0547 * MkTP/0.93 + 0.0395 * MkL)
    anim.MElr.rate <<- anim.NElr.rate/ratio.NElr.MElr
    # +++ Protein +++
    ratio.NPlr.MPlr <<- 0.67
```

```
      anim.NPlr.rate <<- MY * (MkTP/100) * 1000
      anim.MPlr.rate <<- anim.NPlr.rate/ratio.NPlr.MPlr
      # +++ Amino acids +++
      # AA are Met, Lys, His, Phe, Trp, Thr, Leu, Ile, Val, Arg
      anim.MAAlr.rate <<- (anim.MPlr.rate * ratio.NPlr.MPlr) * (anim.lactation.milk.AA.conc/100)/anim.lactation.milk.AA_Eff.frac
  # g AA/d
      if (anim.type != "Milk")
      {
        # Nursing calves submodel
        PML <- PKYD
        ForageDE <- c(2.2, 2.4, 2.6, 2.8, 3, 3.2)
        CalfBW <- c(75, 100, 125, 150, 175, 200, 225, 250)
        calf.DMI_forage.rate <<- as.data.frame(expand.grid(PML, ForageDE, CalfBW))
        colnames(calf.DMI_forage.rate) <<- c("PML", "ForageDE", "CalfBW")
        calf.DMI_forage.rate$ForageDMI <<- apply(calf.DMI_forage.rate[, c("PML", "ForageDE", "CalfBW")], 1, function(x)
  calcDMINursingCalves(x[1], x[2], x[3]))
        # print(ftable(xtabs(ForageDMI~ForageDE+CalfBW,data=calf.DMI_forage.rate)),digits=2)
      }
    } else
    {
      if (anim.species == "Sheep")
      {
        # +++ Energy +++
        ratio.NElr.MElr <<- 0.644
        anim.NElr.rate <<- MY * (0.25173 + 0.08964 * MkFat + 0.03785 * MkTP/0.93)
        anim.MElr.rate <<- anim.NElr.rate/ratio.NElr.MElr
        # +++ Protein +++
        ratio.NPlr.MPlr <<- 0.58
        anim.NPlr.rate <<- MY * (MkTP/100) * 1000
        anim.MPlr.rate <<- anim.NPlr.rate/ratio.NPlr.MPlr
      } else
      {
        # Goats
        # +++ Energy +++
        ratio.NElr.MElr <<- 0.644
        anim.NElr.rate <<- MY * (0.28972 + 0.07193 * MkFat + 0.04828 * MkTP/0.92)
        anim.MElr.rate <<- anim.NElr.rate/ratio.NElr.MElr
        # +++ Protein +++
        ratio.NPlr.MPlr <<- 0.64
        anim.NPlr.rate <<- MY * (MkTP/100) * 1000
        anim.MPlr.rate <<- anim.NPlr.rate/ratio.NPlr.MPlr
      }
      # +++ Amino acids +++
      # AA are Met, Lys, His, Phe, Trp, Thr, Leu, Ile, Val, Arg
      # USes the same calculation logic for cattle
      anim.MAAlr.rate <<- (anim.MPlr.rate * ratio.NPlr.MPlr) * (anim.lactation.milk.AA.conc/100)/anim.lactation.milk.AA_Eff.frac
  # g AA/d
    }
    anim.FFL.rate <<- anim.NElr.rate/NEla
    if (blnReturnNElr == T) return(anim.NElr.rate) else return(invisible(TRUE))
  }
```

5.3.4 Pregnancy requirements

```
calcPregnancyRequirement <- function(blnReturnNEpr = FALSE, ME = NA)
{
  # Returns anim.NEpr.rate, Mcal/d
  if (isPregnant == FALSE | is.na(anim.species) | anim.diet.DMI.rate <= 0)
  {
    anim.pregnancy.uterus.weight <<- 0
    anim.pregnancy.uterus.weight.rate <<- 0
    anim.NEpr.rate <<- 0
    ratio.NEpr.MEpr <<- 0
    anim.MEpr.rate <<- 0
    anim.NPpr.rate <<- 0
    ratio.NPpr.MPpr <<- 0
    anim.MPpr.rate <<- 0
    anim.MAApr.rate <<- rep(0, 10)
    anim.FFP.rate <<- 0
    return(invisible(NULL))
  }
  if (is.na(ME) == TRUE) ME <- anim.diet.ME.frac
  DG <- anim.pregnancy.days
  if (anim.species == "Cattle")
  {
    CBW <- anim.pregnancy.calf.body.weight_birth
    if (anim.type == "Milk")
    {
      # Dairy
      # +++ Growth +++
      anim.pregnancy.uterus.weight <<- (CBW/47) * 0.1436 * exp(0.03729 * DG - 5.164e-05 * DG^2)
      anim.pregnancy.uterus.weight.rate <<- (CBW/47) * 0.1436 * (0.03729 - 0.00010328 * DG) * exp(0.03729 * DG - 5.164e-05 * DG^2)
      # +++ Energy +++
      anim.NEpr.rate <<- ifelse(DG >= 190, (CBW/47) * (0.00318 * DG - 0.0352), 0)
      ratio.NEpr.MEpr <<- 0.14
      anim.MEpr.rate <<- anim.NEpr.rate/ratio.NEpr.MEpr
      # +++ Protein +++
      anim.NPpr.rate <<- ifelse(DG >= 190, (CBW/47) * (0.69 * DG - 69.2), 0)
      ratio.NPpr.MPpr <<- 0.33
      anim.MPpr.rate <<- anim.NPpr.rate/ratio.NPpr.MPpr
    } else
    {
      # Beef
      # +++ Growth +++
      anim.pregnancy.uterus.weight <<- (CBW/41) * 0.7439 * exp(0.02 * DG - 1.43e-05 * DG^2)
      anim.pregnancy.uterus.weight.rate <<- (CBW/41) * 0.7439 * (0.02 - 2.86e-05 * DG) * exp(0.02 * DG - 1.43e-05 * DG^2)
      # +++ Energy +++
      anim.NEpr.rate <<- (CBW/41) * 69.73 * (0.0323 - 5.5e-05 * DG) * exp(0.0323 * DG - 2.75e-05 * DG^2)/1000
      ratio.NEpr.MEpr <<- 0.13
      anim.MEpr.rate <<- anim.NEpr.rate/ratio.NEpr.MEpr
      # +++ Protein +++
```

```
        anim.NPpr.rate <<- (CBW/41) * 2.312 * (0.0278 - 3.52e-05 * DG) * exp(0.0278 * DG - 1.76e-05 * DG^2)/0.16
        ratio.NPpr.MPpr <<- 0.5
        anim.MPpr.rate <<- anim.NPpr.rate/ratio.NPpr.MPpr
      }
      # +++ Amino acids +++
      # AA are Met, Lys, His, Phe, Trp, Thr, Leu, Ile, Val, Arg
      # The conceptus AA concentration is the same of tissue AA concentrations
      anim.MAApr.rate <<- (anim.MPpr.rate * ratio.NPpr.MPpr) * (anim.pregnancy.uterus.AA.conc/100)/anim.preg-
nancy.uterus.AA_Eff.frac  # g AA/d
    } else
    {
      if (anim.species == "Sheep") LBW <- anim.pregnancy.lamb.body.weight_birth
      if (anim.species == "Goats") LBW <- anim.pregnancy.kid.body.weight_birth
      # +++ Growth +++
      anim.pregnancy.uterus.weight <<- (LBW/4) * 175.915 * exp(-8.38 * exp(-0.00608 * DG))
      anim.pregnancy.uterus.weight.rate <<- (LBW/4) * 8.96293 * exp(-8.38 * exp(-0.00608 * DG) - 0.00608 * DG)
      # +++ Energy +++
      anim.NEpr.rate <<- (LBW/4) * 36.628 * exp(-11.465 * exp(-0.00643 * DG) - 0.00643 * DG)
      ratio.NEpr.MEpr <<- 0.13
      anim.MEpr.rate <<- anim.NEpr.rate/ratio.NEpr.MEpr
      # +++ Protein +++
      anim.NPpr.rate <<- (LBW/4) * 5712.24 * exp(-11.22 * exp(-0.00601 * DG) - 0.00601 * DG)
      ratio.NPpr.MPpr <<- ifelse(anim.species == "Sheep", 0.7, 0.33)
      anim.MPpr.rate <<- anim.NPpr.rate/ratio.NPpr.MPpr
      # +++ Amino acids +++
      # AA are Met, Lys, His, Phe, Trp, Thr, Leu, Ile, Val, Arg
      # The conceptus AA concentration is the same of tissue AA concentrations
      # Uses the same calculation logic for cattle
      anim.MAApr.rate <<- (anim.MPpr.rate * ratio.NPpr.MPpr) * (anim.pregnancy.uterus.AA.conc/100)/anim.preg-
nancy.uterus.AA_Eff.frac  # g AA/d
    }
    anim.FFP.rate <<- anim.MEpr.rate/ME  # Uses MEpr and diet ME to compute FFP
    calcBW()  # Adjust animal's BW to gravid uterus weight
    if (blnReturnNEpr == T) return(anim.NEpr.rate) else return(invisible(TRUE))
  }
```

5.3.5 Growth requirements

```
calcGrowthRequirement <- function(blnReturnNEgr = FALSE, DMI = NA, ME = NA, NEma = NA, NEga = NA)
{
  # Returns anim.NEgr.rate, Mcal/d
  if (is.na(DMI) == TRUE) DMI <- anim.diet.DMI.rate
  if (is.na(ME) == TRUE) ME <- anim.diet.ME.frac
  if (is.na(NEma) == TRUE) NEma <- anim.diet.NEm.frac
  if (is.na(NEga) == TRUE) NEga <- anim.diet.NEg.frac
  if (exists("anim.FFM.rate") == TRUE) FFM <- anim.FFM.rate else FFM <- 0
  if (exists("anim.FFL.rate") == TRUE) FFL <- anim.FFL.rate else FFL <- 0
  if (exists("anim.FFP.rate") == TRUE) FFP <- anim.FFP.rate else FFP <- 0
  if ((DMI - FFM - FFL - FFP <= 0) | isGrowing == FALSE)
  {
    anim.body.weight_conception <<- 0
    TCW1_factor <<- 0
    anim.TPW1 <<- 0
    anim.TPA1 <<- 0
    anim.ADG_BP <<- 0
    anim.TCW1 <<- 0
    anim.ADG_AP <<- 0
    anim.TCW2 <<- 0
    anim.ADG_AC1 <<- 0
    anim.TCW3 <<- 0
    anim.ADG_AC2 <<- 0
    anim.TCW4 <<- 0
    anim.ADG_AC3 <<- 0
    anim.pregnancy.weight_conception1 <<- 0
    anim.pregnancy.gain_conception1 <<- 0
    anim.pregnancy.age_conception1 <<- 0
    anim.pregnancy.weight_calving1 <<- 0
    anim.pregnancy.gain_precalving1 <<- 0
    anim.pregnancy.weight_calving2 <<- 0
    anim.pregnancy.gain_precalving2 <<- 0
    anim.pregnancy.weight_calving3 <<- 0
    anim.pregnancy.gain_precalving3 <<- 0
    anim.pregnancy.weight_calving4 <<- 0
    anim.pregnancy.gain_precalving4 <<- 0
    anim.SWG <<- 0
    anim.EWG <<- 0
    anim.body.weight.gain_shrunk <<- 0
    anim.body.weight.gain_empty <<- 0
    anim.body.weight.gain_target <<- 0
    anim.SRW <<- 0
    anim.EqSBW <<- 0
    anim.EqEBW <<- 0
    anim.NEgr.rate <<- 0
    ratio.NEgr.MEgr <<- 0
    anim.MEgr.rate <<- 0
    anim.body.weight.gain_protein.conc <<- 0
```

```
      anim.NPgr.rate <<- 0
      anim.RE.Protein.frac <<- 0
      anim.body.weight.gain_fat.conc <<- 0
      anim.MAAgr.rate <<- rep(0, 10)
      anim.RE.fat.frac <<- 0
      ratio.NPgr.MPgr <<- 0
      anim.MPgr.rate <<- 0
      anim.mammogenesis.NEgr.rate <<- 0
      anim.mammogenesis.MEgr.rate <<- 0
      anim.mammogenesis.NPgr.rate <<- 0
      anim.mammogenesis.MPgr.rate <<- 0
      anim.FFG.rate <<- 0
      return(invisible(NULL))
    }
    if (anim.species == "Cattle")
    {
      if (anim.sex == "Female")
      {
        # Predicts ideal and real SBW and ADG
        # Ideal target BW and ADG
        DG <- anim.pregnancy.days
        CvI <- anim.pregnancy.calving_interval
        DIM <- anim.lactation.days
        WW <- anim.body.weight_weaning
        WA <- anim.age_weaning
        anim.body.weight_conception <<- anim.MSBW * anim.body.weight_conception_frac
        breeds_dairy <- c("Ayrshire", "Braunvieh", "Brown Swiss", "Friesian", "Gelbvieh", "Guernsey", "Gir", "Holstein", "Jer-
sey", "Simmental")
        TCW1_factor <<- ifelse(length(which(breeds_dairy == anim.breed)) > 0, 0.85, 0.8)
        anim.TPW1 <<- anim.pregnancy.weight_conception1 <<- anim.body.weight_conception  # kg
        anim.TPA1 <<- anim.pregnancy.age_conception1 <<- 30.4 * anim.pregnancy.calving_age - 280  # d
        anim.ADG_BP <<- anim.pregnancy.gain_conception1 <<- (anim.TPW1 - WW)/(anim.TPA1 - WA * 30.4)  # kg/d
        anim.TCW1 <<- anim.pregnancy.weight_calving1 <<- anim.MSBW * TCW1_factor  # kg
        anim.ADG_AP <<- anim.pregnancy.gain_precalving1 <<- (anim.TCW1 - anim.TPW1)/(280 - DG)  # kg/d
        anim.TCW2 <<- anim.pregnancy.weight_calving2 <<- anim.MSBW * 0.92  # kg
        anim.ADG_AC1 <<- anim.pregnancy.gain_precalving2 <<- (anim.TCW2 - anim.TCW1)/(CvI * 30.4)  # kg/d
        anim.TCW3 <<- anim.pregnancy.weight_calving3 <<- anim.MSBW * 0.96  # kg
        anim.ADG_AC2 <<- anim.pregnancy.gain_precalving3 <<- (anim.TCW3 - anim.TCW2)/(CvI * 30.4)  # kg/d
        anim.TCW4 <<- anim.pregnancy.weight_calving4 <<- anim.MSBW  # kg
        anim.ADG_AC3 <<- anim.pregnancy.gain_precalving4 <<- (anim.TCW4 - anim.TCW3)/(CvI * 30.4)  # kg/d
        # Real target BW and ADG
        if (anim.stage_type == "Replacement")
        {
          parity <- 0
          if (anim.age * 30.4 < anim.pregnancy.age_conception1)
          {
            # Non-bred heifer
            anim.body.weight.gain_shrunk <<- (anim.TPW1 - anim.SBW)/(anim.TPA1 - anim.age * 30.4)
          } else
          {
            # Bred heifer, before first calving, DG > 0
```

```
        anim.body.weight.gain_shrunk <<- (anim.TCW1 - anim.SBW)/(280 - DG)
      }
    } else
    {
      # dry or lactating cow at which parity/calving?
      parity <- max(0, floor((anim.age - anim.pregnancy.calving_age)/anim.pregnancy.calving_interval) + 1)
      calving.age.expected <- anim.pregnancy.calving_age + parity * anim.pregnancy.calving_interval  # months
      # The (calving.age.expected - anim.age)---in days---is equal to (calving interval - days in milk) RNS uses the former
      # calculation to prevent inconsistencies with incorrect days in milk (DIM) input
      if (parity == 0)
      {
        # going to first calving? Something is wrong; it should be a replacement heifer
        anim.body.weight.gain_shrunk <<- max(0, (anim.TCW1 - anim.SBW)/((calving.age.expected - anim.age) * 30.4))
      }
      if (parity == 1)
      {
        # going to second calving
        anim.body.weight.gain_shrunk <<- max(0, (anim.TCW2 - anim.SBW)/((calving.age.expected - anim.age) * 30.4))
      }
      if (parity == 2)
      {
        # going to third calving
        anim.body.weight.gain_shrunk <<- max(0, (anim.TCW3 - anim.SBW)/((calving.age.expected - anim.age) * 30.4))
      }
      if (parity >= 3)
      {
        # going to fourth calving or more
        anim.body.weight.gain_shrunk <<- max(0, (anim.TCW4 - anim.SBW)/((calving.age.expected - anim.age) * 30.4))
      }
    }
    if (anim.stage_type == "Replacement") anim.body.weight_standard <<- 478

    if (parity == Inf | (anim.pregnancy.days == 0 & anim.lactation.days ==0))
    {
      # Assume female under growing/finishing conditions
      anim.SRW <<- anim.body.weight_standard
      anim.EqSBW <<- anim.SBW * anim.SRW/anim.MSBW
      anim.EqEBW <<- anim.EqSBW * 0.891
      # +++ Energy +++
      anim.NEgr.rate <<- max(0, (DMI - (FFM + FFL + FFP)) * NEga)
      ratio.NEgr.MEgr <<- NEga/ME
      anim.MEgr.rate <<- isz(anim.NEgr.rate,ratio.NEgr.MEgr)
      anim.EWG <<- anim.body.weight.gain_empty <<- 12.341 * (anim.EqEBW^-0.6837) * (anim.NEgr.rate^0.9116)
      anim.SWG <<- anim.body.weight.gain_shrunk <<- 13.91 * (anim.EqSBW^-0.6837) * (anim.NEgr.rate^0.9116)
      anim.body.weight.gain_target <<- anim.SWG
    } else
    {
      anim.SWG <<- anim.body.weight.gain_shrunk
      anim.EWG <<- anim.body.weight.gain_empty <<- anim.SWG * 0.956
      anim.body.weight.gain_target <<- anim.SWG + anim.pregnancy.uterus.weight.rate
      anim.SRW <<- anim.body.weight_standard
```

```
            anim.EqSBW <<- anim.SBW_GU * anim.SRW/anim.MSBW
            anim.EqEBW <<- anim.EBW_GU * anim.SRW/anim.MSBW
            # +++ Energy +++
            anim.NEgr.rate <<- 0.0625 * (anim.EqEBW^0.75) * (anim.body.weight.gain_empty^1.097)
            ratio.NEgr.MEgr <<- NEga/ME
            anim.MEgr.rate <<- isz(anim.NEgr.rate,ratio.NEgr.MEgr)
          }
          # +++ Protein +++
          PIG <- anim.body.weight.gain_protein.conc <<- 0
          if (anim.SWG > 0) PIG <- anim.body.weight.gain_protein.conc <<- (268 - 29.4 * anim.NEgr.rate/anim.SWG)/10  # %
          anim.NPgr.rate <<- anim.SWG * (PIG/100) * 1000  # g/d
          # For the sake of consistency, FIG is computed by difference rather than using an empirical equation
          anim.RE.Protein.frac <<- PIG * 5.7/100  # Mcal/kg
          FIG <- anim.body.weight.gain_fat.conc <<- 0
          if (anim.SWG > 0) FIG <- anim.body.weight.gain_fat.conc <<- 100 * ((anim.NEgr.rate - anim.NPgr.rate * 0.0057)/9.4)/anim.SWG
          anim.RE.fat.frac <<- FIG * 9.4/100  # Mcal/kg
          if (flag_NPgr_MPgr == 0) ratio.NPgr.MPgr <<- ifelse(anim.EqSBW <= 300, 0.834 - anim.EqSBW * 0.00114, 0.492)  # NRC (1996, 2000)
          if (flag_NPgr_MPgr == 1) ratio.NPgr.MPgr <<- ifelse(anim.EqSBW <= 478, 0.834 - anim.EqSBW * 0.00114, 0.289)  # Fox et al. (2004)
          if (flag_NPgr_MPgr == 2) ratio.NPgr.MPgr <<- 0.492 + 104.93 * exp(-0.0486 * anim.SBW)  # NASEM (2016)
          # Alternatively, ratio.NPgr.MPgr<<-0.49+126.017*exp(-0.06889*anim.EqSBW)
          if (flag_NPgr_MPgr == 3) ratio.NPgr.MPgr <<- 0.112 + 2.271 * exp(-0.01887 * anim.EqSBW)  # RNS
          anim.MPgr.rate <<- anim.NPgr.rate/ratio.NPgr.MPgr
          # +++ Mammogenesis +++
          anim.mammogenesis.NEgr.rate <<- 0
          anim.mammogenesis.MEgr.rate <<- 0
          anim.mammogenesis.NPgr.rate <<- 0
          anim.mammogenesis.MPgr.rate <<- 0
          if (DG > 259 & (anim.stage_type == "Replacement" | anim.stage_type == "Dry"))
          {
            # +++ Energy +++
            anim.mammogenesis.NEgr.rate <<- 1
            anim.mammogenesis.MEgr.rate <<- anim.mammogenesis.NEgr.rate/ratio.NEgr.MEgr
            # +++ Protein +++
            anim.mammogenesis.NPgr.rate <<- 80
            anim.mammogenesis.MPgr.rate <<- anim.mammogenesis.NPgr.rate/ratio.NPgr.MPgr
          }
          # +++ Amino acids +++
          # AA are Met, Lys, His, Phe, Trp, Thr, Leu, Ile, Val, Arg
          # The conceptus AA concentration is the same of tissue AA concentrations
          if (flag_UserAAGrowth == TRUE)
          {
            anim.MAAgr.rate <<- (anim.MPgr.rate * ratio.NPgr.MPgr) * (anim.growth.AA.conc/100)/anim.growth.AA_Eff.frac  # g AA/d
          } else
          {
            anim.MAAgr.rate <<- (anim.MPgr.rate * ratio.NPgr.MPgr) * (anim.growth.AA.conc/100)/ratio.NPgr.MPgr  # g AA/d
          }
        }
```

```
    if ((anim.sex != "Female" & anim.stage_type == "Growing/Finishing") | (anim.stage_type == "Replacement" & flag_RH_tar-getADG == 1))
    {
      anim.SRW <<- anim.body.weight_standard
      anim.EqSBW <<- anim.SBW * anim.SRW/anim.MSBW
      anim.EqEBW <<- anim.EqSBW * 0.891
      # +++ Energy +++
      anim.NEgr.rate <<- max(0, (DMI - (FFM + FFL + FFP)) * NEga)
      ratio.NEgr.MEgr <<- NEga/ME
      anim.MEgr.rate <<- isz(anim.NEgr.rate,ratio.NEgr.MEgr)
      anim.EWG <<- anim.body.weight.gain_empty <<- 12.341 * (anim.EqEBW^-0.6837) * (anim.NEgr.rate^0.9116)
      anim.SWG <<- anim.body.weight.gain_shrunk <<- 13.91 * (anim.EqSBW^-0.6837) * (anim.NEgr.rate^0.9116)
      # +++ Protein +++
      PIG <- anim.body.weight.gain_protein.conc <<- 0
      if (anim.SWG > 0) PIG <- anim.body.weight.gain_protein.conc <<- (268 - 29.4 * anim.NEgr.rate/anim.SWG)/10  # %
      anim.NPgr.rate <<- anim.SWG * (PIG/100) * 1000  # g/d
      # For the sake of consistency, FIG is computed by difference rather than using an empirical equation
      anim.RE.Protein.frac <<- PIG * 5.7/100  # Mcal/kg
      FIG <- anim.body.weight.gain_fat.conc <<- 0
      if (anim.SWG > 0) FIG <- anim.body.weight.gain_fat.conc <<- 100 * ((anim.NEgr.rate - anim.NPgr.rate * 0.0057)/9.4)/anim.SWG
      anim.RE.fat.frac <<- FIG * 9.4/100  # Mcal/kg
      if (flag_NPgr_MPgr == 0) ratio.NPgr.MPgr <<- ifelse(anim.EqSBW <= 300, 0.834 - anim.EqSBW * 0.00114, 0.492)  # NRC (1996, 2000)
      if (flag_NPgr_MPgr == 1) ratio.NPgr.MPgr <<- ifelse(anim.EqSBW <= 478, 0.834 - anim.EqSBW * 0.00114, 0.289)  # Fox et al. (2004)
      if (flag_NPgr_MPgr == 2) ratio.NPgr.MPgr <<- 0.492 + 104.93 * exp(-0.0486 * anim.SBW)  # NASEM (2016)
      # Alternatively, ratio.NPgr.MPgr<<-0.49+126.017*exp(-0.06889*anim.EqSBW)
      if (flag_NPgr_MPgr == 3) ratio.NPgr.MPgr <<- 0.112 + 2.271 * exp(-0.01887 * anim.EqSBW)  # RNS
      anim.MPgr.rate <<- anim.NPgr.rate/ratio.NPgr.MPgr
      anim.mammogenesis.NEgr.rate <<- 0
      anim.mammogenesis.MEgr.rate <<- 0
      anim.mammogenesis.NPgr.rate <<- 0
      anim.mammogenesis.MPgr.rate <<- 0
      # +++ Amino acids +++
      # AA are Met, Lys, His, Phe, Trp, Thr, Leu, Ile, Val, Arg
      # The conceptus AA concentration is the same of tissue AA concentrations
      if (flag_UserAAGrowth == TRUE)
      {
        anim.MAAgr.rate <<- (anim.MPgr.rate * ratio.NPgr.MPgr) * (anim.growth.AA.conc/100)/anim.growth.AA_Eff.frac  # g AA/d
      } else
      {
        anim.MAAgr.rate <<- (anim.MPgr.rate * ratio.NPgr.MPgr) * (anim.growth.AA.conc/100)/ratio.NPgr.MPgr  # g AA/d
      }
    }
  } else
  {
    # Sheep and goats
    if (anim.stage_type == "Growing/Finishing" | anim.stage_type == "Replacement")
    {
      # +++ Energy +++
```

```
    anim.MEgr.rate <<- DMI * ME - (anim.MEmr.rate + anim.MEpr.rate + anim.MElr.rate)  # Mcal/d
    L <- anim.DMI.L.frac
    P <- anim.u.frac
    R <- 2 * (L - 1)
    PIG <- anim.body.weight.gain_protein.conc <<- (212 - 4 * R - (120 - 4 * R)/(1 + exp(-6 * (P - 0.4))))/10  # %
    FIG <- anim.body.weight.gain_fat.conc <<- (43 + 28 * R + (490 - 28 * R)/(1 + exp(-6 * (P - 0.4))))/10  # %
    REProt <- anim.RE.Protein.frac <<- PIG * 5.7/100  # Mcal/kg
    REFat <- anim.RE.fat.frac <<- FIG * 9.4/100  # Mcal/kg
    REp <- anim.REp.frac <<- REProt/(REProt + REFat)
    kg <- ratio.NEgr.MEgr <<- 18.36/(27 + 41 * REp)
    anim.NEgr.rate <<- anim.MEgr.rate * kg
    EVG <- (6.7 + R + ((16.5 - R)/(1 + exp(-6 * (P - 0.4)))))/4.184  # Mcal/kg
    anim.SWG <<- anim.body.weight.gain_shrunk <<- anim.NEgr.rate/(0.92 * EVG)  # kg/d
    anim.EWG <<- anim.body.weight.gain_empty <<- 0.92 * anim.SWG  # kg/d
    # +++ Protein +++
    anim.NPgr.rate <<- 1000 * anim.EWG * (PIG/100)  # g/d
    ratio.NPgr.MPgr <<- 0.7
    anim.MPgr.rate <<- anim.NPgr.rate/ratio.NPgr.MPgr  # g/d
    anim.mammogenesis.NEgr.rate <<- 0
    anim.mammogenesis.MEgr.rate <<- 0
    anim.mammogenesis.NPgr.rate <<- 0
    anim.mammogenesis.MPgr.rate <<- 0
    # +++ Amino acids +++
    # AA are Met, Lys, His, Phe, Trp, Thr, Leu, Ile, Val, Arg
    # The conceptus AA concentration is the same of tissue AA concentrations
    # RNS uses the same calculation logic for cattle
    if (flag_UserAAGrowth == TRUE)
    {
      anim.MAAgr.rate <<- (anim.MPgr.rate * ratio.NPgr.MPgr) * (anim.growth.AA.conc/100)/anim.growth.AA_Eff.frac  # g AA/d
    } else
    {
      anim.MAAgr.rate <<- (anim.MPgr.rate * ratio.NPgr.MPgr) * (anim.growth.AA.conc/100)/ratio.NPgr.MPgr  # g AA/d
    }
  } else
  {
    anim.MEgr.rate <<- 0
    anim.body.weight.gain_protein.conc <<- 0
    anim.body.weight.gain_fat.conc <<- 0
    anim.RE.Protein.frac <<- 0
    anim.RE.fat.frac <<- 0
    anim.REp.frac <<- 0
    ratio.NEgr.MEgr <<- 0
    anim.NEgr.rate <<- 0
    anim.SWG <<- anim.body.weight.gain_shrunk <<- 0
    anim.EWG <<- anim.body.weight.gain_empty <<- 0
    # +++ Protein +++
    anim.NPgr.rate <<- 0
    ratio.NPgr.MPgr <<- 0
    anim.MPgr.rate <<- 0
    anim.mammogenesis.NEgr.rate <<- 0
    anim.mammogenesis.MEgr.rate <<- 0
```

```
            anim.mammogenesis.NPgr.rate <<- 0
            anim.mammogenesis.MPgr.rate <<- 0
            anim.MAAgr.rate <<- 0
        }
    }
    anim.FFG.rate <<- anim.MEgr.rate/ME  # Uses MEgr and diet ME to compute FFG
    if (blnReturnNEgr == T) return(anim.NEgr.rate) else return(invisible(TRUE))
}
```

5.3.6 Body reserves

```
calcBodyReserves <- function(DMI = NA, ME = NA, MEB = NA)
{
  if (isBodyReserves == FALSE | is.na(anim.species) | anim.diet.DMI.rate <= 0)
  {
    anim.diet.MEBalance.rate <<- 0
    anim.diet.NEBalance.rate <<- 0
    anim.diet.MPBalance.rate <<- 0
    anim.diet.NPBalance.rate <<- 0
    ratio.MErtoNEr.frac <<- 0
    ratio.MPrtoNPr.frac <<- 0
    dSBW_dBCS_SBW <<- 0
    anim.EB.BCSChange.time <<- 0
    anim.BCS1 <<- 0
    anim.EBW1 <<- 0
    anim.EB.Fat1.frac <<- 0
    anim.EB.Prot1.frac <<- 0
    anim.EB.Ash1.frac <<- 0
    anim.EB.Water1.frac <<- 0
    anim.EB.Fat1.amt <<- 0
    anim.EB.Prot1.amt <<- 0
    anim.EB.Ash1.amt <<- 0
    anim.EB.Water1.amt <<- 0
    anim.EB.Energy1.amt <<- 0
    anim.BCS2 <<- 0
    anim.EBW2 <<- 0
    anim.EB.Fat1.frac <<- 0
    anim.EB.Prot1.frac <<- 0
    anim.EB.Ash1.frac <<- 0
    anim.EB.Water1.frac <<- 0
    anim.EB.Fat1.amt <<- 0
    anim.EB.Prot1.amt <<- 0
    anim.EB.Ash1.amt <<- 0
    anim.EB.Water1.amt <<- 0
    anim.EB.Energy1.amt <<- 0
    anim.EB.EnergyChange.amt <<- 0
    anim.EB.ProteinChange.amt <<- 0
    anim.EB.EWG.rate <<- 0
    anim.EB.SWG.rate <<- 0
    anim.EB.FWG.rate <<- 0
    anim.FBW25 <<- 0
    anim.BCS_vector <<- 0
    anim.EBW_vector <<- 0
    anim.EB.fat.amt_vector <<- 0
    anim.EB.protein.amt_vector <<- 0
    anim.EB.energy.amt_vector <<- 0
    anim.EB.EnergyChange.amt_vector <<- 0
    return(invisible(NULL))
  }
```

```
  if (is.na(MEB) == TRUE)
  {
    if (is.na(DMI) == TRUE) DMI <- anim.diet.DMI.rate
    if (is.na(ME) == TRUE) ME <- anim.diet.ME.frac
    if (exists("anim.FFM.rate") == TRUE) FFM <- anim.FFM.rate else FFM <- 0
    if (exists("anim.FFL.rate") == TRUE) FFL <- anim.FFL.rate else FFL <- 0
    if (exists("anim.FFP.rate") == TRUE) FFP <- anim.FFP.rate else FFP <- 0
    # if (exists("anim.FFG.rate") == TRUE) FFG <- anim.FFG.rate else FFG <- 0
    FFG <- 0 # Growth requirements are not included in the body reserved
    anim.diet.MEBalance.rate <<- MEB <- (DMI - FFM - FFG - FFL - FFP) * ME
  } else anim.diet.MEBalance.rate <<- MEB
  if (anim.species == "Cattle")
  {
    dSBW_dBCS_SBW <<- 7.43/100
    if (flag_dSBW_dBCS == 0) dSBW_dBCS_SBW <<- 6.85/100
    if (flag_dSBW_dBCS == 1) dSBW_dBCS_SBW <<- 7.105/100
    if (flag_dSBW_dBCS == 3) dSBW_dBCS_SBW <<- flag_dSBW_dBCS_User/100
    if (tolower(anim.stage_option) == "mean")
    {
      # compute ME balance and assign it to body reserves (change in BCS)
      #     ME balance = MEI - (MEmr + MEpr + MElr + MEgr)
      #     MErr = ME Balance
      #     ME Residue = 0
      anim.BCS1 <<- bcs1 <- calcBCS(anim.body.condition_mean, "1-9")
      # Empty Body (EB) composiition
      anim.EBW1 <<- ifelse(flag_EB_SBWGUW == TRUE, 0.851 * anim.SBW_GU, 0.851 * anim.SBW)
      anim.EB.Fat1.frac <<- -0.040604 + 0.046814 * bcs1
      anim.EB.Prot1.frac <<- 0.218778 - 0.008893 * bcs1
      anim.EB.Ash1.frac <<- 0.068589 - 0.0035539 * bcs1
      anim.EB.Water1.frac <<- 1 - (anim.EB.Fat1.frac + anim.EB.Prot1.frac + anim.EB.Ash1.frac)
      anim.EB.Fat1.amt <<- anim.EBW1 * anim.EB.Fat1.frac
      anim.EB.Prot1.amt <<- anim.EBW1 * anim.EB.Prot1.frac
      anim.EB.Ash1.amt <<- anim.EBW1 * anim.EB.Ash1.frac
      anim.EB.Water1.amt <<- anim.EBW1 * anim.EB.Water1.frac
      anim.EB.Energy1.amt <<- 9.4 * anim.EB.Fat1.amt + 5.7 * anim.EB.Prot1.amt
      # Compute the number of days to change 1 BCS
      if (MEB < 0)
      {
        anim.BCS2 <<- bcs2 <- max(1, bcs1 - 1)  # BCS cannot be less than 1
      } else
      {
        anim.BCS2 <<- bcs2 <- min(9, bcs1 + 1)  # BCS cannot be greater than 9
      }
      # Compute the next/previous EBW If assuming constant ash amount
      if (flag_EB_ash == TRUE)
      {
        anim.EBW2 <<- anim.EB.Ash1.amt/(0.068589 - 0.0035539 * bcs2)
      } else
      {
        anim.waf1 <- 1 - dSBW_dBCS_SBW * (5 - bcs1)
        anim.waf2 <- 1 - dSBW_dBCS_SBW * (5 - bcs2)
```

```
        anim.EBW2 <<- (anim.EBW1/anim.waf1) * anim.waf2
      }
      anim.EB.Fat2.frac <<- -0.040604 + 0.046814 * bcs2
      anim.EB.Prot2.frac <<- 0.218778 - 0.008893 * bcs2
      anim.EB.Ash2.frac <<- 0.068589 - 0.0035539 * bcs2
      anim.EB.Water2.frac <<- 1 - (anim.EB.Fat2.frac + anim.EB.Prot2.frac + anim.EB.Ash2.frac)
      anim.EB.Fat2.amt <<- anim.EBW2 * anim.EB.Fat2.frac
      anim.EB.Prot2.amt <<- anim.EBW2 * anim.EB.Prot2.frac
      anim.EB.Ash2.amt <<- anim.EBW2 * anim.EB.Ash2.frac
      anim.EB.Water2.amt <<- anim.EBW2 * anim.EB.Water2.frac
      anim.EB.Energy2.amt <<- 9.4 * anim.EB.Fat2.amt + 5.7 * anim.EB.Prot2.amt
      anim.EB.EnergyChange.amt <<- anim.EB.Energy2.amt - anim.EB.Energy1.amt
      anim.EB.ProteinChange.amt <<- anim.EB.Prot2.amt - anim.EB.Prot1.amt
      anim.diet.NEBalance.rate <<- 0
      anim.EB.BCSChange.time <<- 0
      if (MEB > 0)
      {
        # Positive ME balance: cow will gain 1 BCS
        if (anim.type == "Milk" & anim.stage_type == "Lactating")
        {
          # lactating dairy cattle
          # Mcal NEl/d with efficiency of 75% of ME to NEr
          ratio.MErtoNEr.frac <<- 0.75
          anim.diet.NEBalance.rate <<- MEB * ratio.MErtoNEr.frac

        } else
        {
          # Beef cattle, dry dairy cattle
          # Mcal NEl/d with efficiency of 60% of ME to NEr
          ratio.MErtoNEr.frac <<- 0.6
          anim.diet.NEBalance.rate <<- MEB * ratio.MErtoNEr.frac
        }
      } else
      {
        # Negative ME balance: cow will lose 1 BCS
        if (anim.type == "Milk" & anim.stage_type == "Lactating")
        {
          # lactating dairy cattle
          # Mcal NEm/d with efficiency of 78.5% of ME to NEr
          ratio.MErtoNEr.frac <<- (0.644/0.82)
          anim.diet.NEBalance.rate <<- MEB * ratio.MErtoNEr.frac
        } else
        {
          # Beef cattle, dry dairy cattle
          # Mcal NEm/d with efficiency of 75%
          ratio.MErtoNEr.frac <<- (0.6/0.8)
          anim.diet.NEBalance.rate <<- MEB * ratio.MErtoNEr.frac
        }
      }
      # Days to change 1 BCS
      if (anim.diet.NEBalance.rate != 0) anim.EB.BCSChange.time <<- anim.EB.EnergyChange.amt/anim.diet.NEBalance.rate
```

```
      # kg/d
      if (anim.EB.BCSChange.time != 0)
      {
        anim.EB.EWG.rate <<- (anim.EBW2 - anim.EBW1)/anim.EB.BCSChange.time
        anim.EB.SWG.rate <<- (anim.EBW2/0.851 - anim.EBW1/0.851)/anim.EB.BCSChange.time
        anim.EB.FWG.rate <<- (anim.EBW2/0.851/0.96 - anim.EBW1/0.851/0.96)/anim.EB.BCSChange.time
      } else
      {
        anim.EB.EWG.rate <<- 0
        anim.EB.SWG.rate <<- 0
        anim.EB.FWG.rate <<- 0
      }
    } else
    {
      # If BCS type = Period, compute ME required for BCS change and show ME balance is an error
      #     ME Balance = MEI - (MEmr + MEpr + MElr + MEgr + MErr)
      #     ME Residue = ME Balance
      anim.BCS1 <<- bcs1 <- calcBCS(anim.body.condition_initial, "1-9")
      anim.BCS2 <<- bcs2 <- calcBCS(anim.body.condition_final, "1-9")
      # BCS1 to BCS2 in anim.stage.days time
      anim.EB.BCSChange.time <<- anim.stage.days
      anim.EBW1 <<- 0.851 * anim.iSBW
      # Initial empty body (EB) composiition
      anim.EB.Fat1.frac <<- -0.040604 + 0.046814 * bcs1
      anim.EB.Prot1.frac <<- 0.218778 - 0.008893 * bcs1
      anim.EB.Ash1.frac <<- 0.068589 - 0.0035539 * bcs1
      anim.EB.Water1.frac <<- 1 - (anim.EB.Fat1.frac + anim.EB.Prot1.frac + anim.EB.Ash1.frac)
      anim.EB.Fat1.amt <<- anim.EBW1 * anim.EB.Fat1.frac
      anim.EB.Prot1.amt <<- anim.EBW1 * anim.EB.Prot1.frac
      anim.EB.Ash1.amt <<- anim.EBW1 * anim.EB.Ash1.frac
      anim.EB.Water1.amt <<- anim.EBW1 * anim.EB.Water1.frac
      anim.EB.Energy1.amt <<- 9.4 * anim.EB.Fat1.amt + 5.7 * anim.EB.Prot1.amt
      if (anim.fSBW == 0)
      {
        # if final SBW is zero
        # Compute final EBW using BCS weight adjustment factors
        if (flag_EB_ash == TRUE)
        {
          anim.EBW2 <<- anim.EB.Ash1.amt/(0.068589 - 0.0035539 * bcs2)
        } else
        {
          anim.waf1 <- 1 - dSBW_dBCS_SBW * (5 - bcs1)
          anim.waf2 <- 1 - dSBW_dBCS_SBW * (5 - bcs2)
          anim.EBW2 <<- (anim.EBW1/anim.waf1) * anim.waf2
        }
      } else
      {
        # Use the user-inputted value
        anim.EBW2 <<- 0.851 * anim.fSBW
      }
      # Final empty body (EB) composiition
```

```
    anim.EB.Fat2.frac <<- -0.040604 + 0.046814 * bcs2
    anim.EB.Prot2.frac <<- 0.218778 - 0.008893 * bcs2
    anim.EB.Ash2.frac <<- 0.068589 - 0.0035539 * bcs2
    anim.EB.Water2.frac <<- 1 - (anim.EB.Fat2.frac + anim.EB.Prot2.frac + anim.EB.Ash2.frac)
    anim.EB.Fat2.amt <<- anim.EBW2 * anim.EB.Fat2.frac
    anim.EB.Prot2.amt <<- anim.EBW2 * anim.EB.Prot2.frac
    anim.EB.Ash2.amt <<- anim.EBW2 * anim.EB.Ash2.frac
    anim.EB.Water2.amt <<- anim.EBW2 * anim.EB.Water2.frac
    anim.EB.Energy2.amt <<- 9.4 * anim.EB.Fat2.amt + 5.7 * anim.EB.Prot2.amt
    # Energy and protein change
    anim.EB.EnergyChange.amt <<- anim.EB.Energy2.amt - anim.EB.Energy1.amt
    anim.EB.ProteinChange.amt <<- anim.EB.Prot2.amt - anim.EB.Prot1.amt
    # Rather than MEB, uses the energy change as an indication
    # if animals were on positive or negative energy balance
    if (anim.EB.EnergyChange.amt > 0)
    {
      # Gaining BCS, requires ME (positive)
      if (anim.type == "Milk" & anim.stage_type == "Lactating")
      {
        # lactating dairy cattle
        ratio.MErtoNEr.frac <<- 0.75
      } else
      {
        # Beef cattle, dry dairy cattle
        ratio.MErtoNEr.frac <<- 0.6
      }
      ratio.MPrtoNPr.frac <<- 0.7
    } else
    {
      # Losing BCS, provides ME (negative)
      if (anim.type == "Milk" & anim.stage_type == "Lactating")
      {
        # lactating dairy cattle
        ratio.MErtoNEr.frac <<- (0.644/0.82)
      } else
      {
        # Beef cattle, dry dairy cattle
        ratio.MErtoNEr.frac <<- (0.6/0.8)
      }
      ratio.MPrtoNPr.frac <<- (0.67/0.8)
    }
    anim.diet.MEBalance.rate <<- (anim.EB.EnergyChange.amt/ratio.MErtoNEr.frac)/anim.EB.BCSChange.time
    anim.diet.MPBalance.rate <<- (anim.EB.ProteinChange.amt/ratio.MPrtoNPr.frac)/anim.EB.BCSChange.time
    anim.diet.NEBalance.rate <<- anim.diet.MEBalance.rate * ratio.MErtoNEr.frac
    anim.diet.NPBalance.rate <<- anim.diet.MPBalance.rate * ratio.MPrtoNPr.frac
    # kg/d
    if (anim.EB.BCSChange.time != 0)
    {
      anim.EB.EWG.rate <<- (anim.EBW2 - anim.EBW1)/anim.EB.BCSChange.time
      anim.EB.SWG.rate <<- (anim.EBW2/0.851 - anim.EBW1/0.851)/anim.EB.BCSChange.time
      anim.EB.FWG.rate <<- (anim.EBW2/0.851/0.96 - anim.EBW1/0.851/0.96)/anim.EB.BCSChange.time
```

```
        } else
        {
          anim.EB.EWG.rate <<- 0
          anim.EB.SWG.rate <<- 0
          anim.EB.FWG.rate <<- 0
        }
      }
      # Compute the BCS x EBW table for each BCS
      anim.BCS_vector <<- c(1, 2, 3, 4, 5, 6, 7, 8, 9)
      if (flag_EB_ash == TRUE)
      {
        anim.EBW_vector <<- anim.EB.Ash1.amt/(0.068589 - 0.0035539 * anim.BCS_vector)
      } else
      {
        anim.waf1 <- 1 - dSBW_dBCS_SBW * (5 - bcs1)
        anim.waf2 <- 1 - dSBW_dBCS_SBW * (5 - anim.BCS_vector)
        anim.EBW_vector <<- (anim.EBW1/anim.waf1) * anim.waf2
      }
      anim.EB.fat.amt_vector <<- anim.EBW_vector * (-0.040604 + 0.046814 * anim.BCS_vector)
      anim.EB.protein.amt_vector <<- anim.EBW_vector * (0.218778 - 0.008893 * anim.BCS_vector)
      anim.EB.energy.amt_vector <<- 9.4 * anim.EB.fat.amt_vector + 5.7 * anim.EB.protein.amt_vector
      anim.EB.EnergyChange.amt_vector <<- vector("numeric", 8)
      for (i in 1:8)
      {
        anim.EB.EnergyChange.amt_vector[i] <<- anim.EB.energy.amt_vector[i + 1] - anim.EB.energy.amt_vector[i]
      }
    } else
    {
      # Sheep and goats
      if (tolower(anim.stage_option) == "mean")
      {
        # compute ME balance and assign it to body reserves (change in BCS)
        #    ME balance = MEI - (MEmr + MEpr + MElr + MEgr)
        #    MErr = ME Balance
        #    ME Residue = 0
        anim.BCS1 <<- bcs1 <- calcBCS(anim.body.condition_mean, "0-5")
        # Empty Body (EB) composiition
        if (flag_EB_SBWGUW == TRUE)
        {
          if (bcs1 == 2.5)
          {
            anim.FBW25 <<- anim.FBW_GU
          } else
          {
            anim.FBW25 <<- (anim.FBW_GU - (2.796 * bcs1 - 5.311))/(0.692 + 0.111 * bcs1)
          }
        } else
        {
          if (bcs1 == 2.5)
          {
            anim.FBW25 <<- anim.FBW
```

```
        } else
        {
          anim.FBW25 <<- (anim.FBW - (2.796 * bcs1 - 5.311))/(0.692 + 0.111 * bcs1)
        }
      }
      if (bcs1 == 2.5)
      {
        # 2.5 on scale 0-5
        anim.EBW1 <<- 0.8513 * (0.96 * anim.FBW25)
      } else
      {
        anim.EBW1 <<- 0.8513 * (0.96 * (anim.FBW25 * (0.692 + 0.111 * bcs1) + (2.795 * bcs1 - 5.311)))
      }
      if (anim.species == "Sheep") anim.EB.Fat1.frac <<- 0.0269 + 0.0868 * bcs1
      if (anim.species == "Goats") anim.EB.Fat1.frac <<- 0.0289 + 0.0708 * bcs1
      anim.EB.Prot1.frac <<- 0.1449 + 0.0279 * bcs1 - 0.0039 * bcs1^2
      anim.EB.Ash1.frac <<- NA
      anim.EB.Water1.frac <<- NA
      anim.EB.Fat1.amt <<- anim.EBW1 * anim.EB.Fat1.frac
      anim.EB.Prot1.amt <<- anim.EBW1 * anim.EB.Prot1.frac
      anim.EB.Ash1.amt <<- anim.EBW1 * anim.EB.Ash1.frac
      anim.EB.Water1.amt <<- anim.EBW1 * anim.EB.Water1.frac
      anim.EB.Energy1.amt <<- 9.4 * anim.EB.Fat1.amt + 5.7 * anim.EB.Prot1.amt
      # Compute the number of days to change 1 BCS
      if (MEB < 0)
      {
        # 1 BCS on 1-9 scale is 0.625 On 0-5 scale, using 0.5
        anim.BCS2 <<- bcs2 <- max(0, bcs1 - 0.5)  # BCS cannot be less than 0
      } else
      {
        anim.BCS2 <<- bcs2 <- min(5, bcs1 + 0.5)  # BCS cannot be greater than 5
      }
      # Compute the next/previous EBW If assuming constant ash amount
      if (bcs2 == 2.5)
      {
        # 2.5 on scale 0-5
        anim.EBW2 <<- 0.8513 * (0.96 * anim.FBW25)
      } else
      {
        anim.EBW2 <<- 0.8513 * (0.96 * (anim.FBW25 * (0.692 + 0.111 * bcs2) + (2.795 * bcs2 - 5.311)))
      }
      if (anim.species == "Sheep") anim.EB.Fat2.frac <<- 0.0269 + 0.0868 * bcs2
      if (anim.species == "Goats") anim.EB.Fat2.frac <<- 0.0289 + 0.0708 * bcs2
      anim.EB.Prot2.frac <<- 0.1449 + 0.0279 * bcs2 - 0.0039 * bcs2^2
      anim.EB.Ash2.frac <<- NA
      anim.EB.Water2.frac <<- NA
      anim.EB.Fat2.amt <<- anim.EBW2 * anim.EB.Fat2.frac
      anim.EB.Prot2.amt <<- anim.EBW2 * anim.EB.Prot2.frac
      anim.EB.Ash2.amt <<- anim.EBW2 * anim.EB.Ash2.frac
      anim.EB.Water2.amt <<- anim.EBW2 * anim.EB.Water2.frac
      anim.EB.Energy2.amt <<- 9.4 * anim.EB.Fat2.amt + 5.7 * anim.EB.Prot2.amt
```

```
      anim.EB.EnergyChange.amt <<- anim.EB.Energy2.amt - anim.EB.Energy1.amt
      anim.EB.ProteinChange.amt <<- anim.EB.Prot2.amt - anim.EB.Prot1.amt
      anim.diet.NEBalance.rate <<- 0
      anim.EB.BCSChange.time <<- 0
      if (MEB > 0)
      {
        # Positive ME balance
        ratio.MErtoNEr.frac <<- 0.6
        anim.diet.NEBalance.rate <<- MEB * ratio.MErtoNEr.frac
      } else
      {
        ratio.MErtoNEr.frac <<- (0.6/0.8)
        anim.diet.NEBalance.rate <<- MEB * ratio.MErtoNEr.frac
      }
      # Days to change 1 BCS
      if (anim.diet.NEBalance.rate != 0) anim.EB.BCSChange.time <<- anim.EB.EnergyChange.amt/anim.diet.NEBalance.rate
      # g/d
      if (anim.EB.BCSChange.time != 0)
      {
        anim.EB.EWG.rate <<- 1000 * (anim.EBW2 - anim.EBW1)/anim.EB.BCSChange.time
        anim.EB.SWG.rate <<- 1000 * (anim.EBW2/0.851 - anim.EBW1/0.851)/anim.EB.BCSChange.time
        anim.EB.FWG.rate <<- 1000 * (anim.EBW2/0.851/0.96 - anim.EBW1/0.851/0.96)/anim.EB.BCSChange.time
      } else
      {
        anim.EB.EWG.rate <<- 0
        anim.EB.SWG.rate <<- 0
        anim.EB.FWG.rate <<- 0
      }
    } else
    {
      # If BCS type = Period, compute ME required for BCS change and show ME balance is an error
      #     ME Balance = MEI - (MEmr + MEpr + MElr + MEgr + MErr)
      #     ME Residue = ME Balance
      anim.BCS1 <<- bcs1 <- calcBCS(anim.body.condition_initial, "0-5")
      anim.BCS2 <<- bcs2 <- calcBCS(anim.body.condition_final, "0-5")
      # BCS1 to BCS2 in anim.stage.days time
      anim.EB.BCSChange.time <<- anim.stage.days
      # Initial empty body (EB) composition
      if (bcs1 == 2.5)
      {
        anim.FBW25 <<- anim.iFBW
      } else
      {
        anim.FBW25 <<- (anim.iFBW - (2.796 * bcs1 - 5.311))/(0.692 + 0.111 * bcs1)
      }
      anim.reserves.bcsChange.time <- anim.stage.days
      if (anim.iSBW == 0)
      {
        # if initial SBW is zero Compute initial EBW using BCS1
        if (bcs1 == 2.5)
        {
```

```
        # 2.5 on scale 0-5
        anim.EBW1 <<- 0.8513 * (0.96 * anim.FBW25)
      } else
      {
        anim.EBW1 <<- 0.8513 * (0.96 * (anim.FBW25 * (0.692 + 0.111 * bcs1) + (2.795 * bcs1 - 5.311)))
      }
    } else
    {
      anim.EBW1 <<- 0.8513 * anim.iSBW
    }
    # Initial empty body (EB) composiition
    if (anim.species == "Sheep") anim.EB.Fat1.frac <<- 0.0269 + 0.0868 * bcs1
    if (anim.species == "Goats") anim.EB.Fat1.frac <<- 0.0289 + 0.0708 * bcs1
    anim.EB.Prot1.frac <<- 0.1449 + 0.0279 * bcs1 - 0.0039 * bcs1^2
    anim.EB.Ash1.frac <<- NA
    anim.EB.Water1.frac <<- NA
    anim.EB.Fat1.amt <<- anim.EBW1 * anim.EB.Fat1.frac
    anim.EB.Prot1.amt <<- anim.EBW1 * anim.EB.Prot1.frac
    anim.EB.Ash1.amt <<- anim.EBW1 * anim.EB.Ash1.frac
    anim.EB.Water1.amt <<- anim.EBW1 * anim.EB.Water1.frac
    anim.EB.Energy1.amt <<- 9.4 * anim.EB.Fat1.amt + 5.7 * anim.EB.Prot1.amt
    # Final empty body (EB) composiition
    if (bcs2 == 2.5)
    {
      anim.FBW25 <<- anim.fFBW
    } else
    {
      anim.FBW25 <<- (anim.fFBW - (2.796 * bcs2 - 5.311))/(0.692 + 0.111 * bcs2)
    }
    if (anim.fSBW == 0)
    {
      # if final SBW is zero Compute final EBW using BCS
      if (bcs2 == 2.5)
      {
        # 2.5 on scale 0-5
        anim.EBW2 <<- 0.8513 * (0.96 * anim.FBW25)
      } else
      {
        anim.EBW2 <<- 0.8513 * (0.96 * (anim.FBW25 * (0.692 + 0.111 * bcs2) + (2.795 * bcs2 - 5.311)))
      }
    } else
    {
      anim.EBW2 <<- 0.8513 * anim.fSBW
    }
    if (anim.species == "Sheep") anim.EB.Fat2.frac <<- 0.0269 + 0.0868 * bcs2
    if (anim.species == "Goats") anim.EB.Fat2.frac <<- 0.0289 + 0.0708 * bcs2
    anim.EB.Prot2.frac <<- 0.1449 + 0.0279 * bcs2 - 0.0039 * bcs2^2
    anim.EB.Ash2.frac <<- NA
    anim.EB.Water2.frac <<- NA
    anim.EB.Fat2.amt <<- anim.EBW2 * anim.EB.Fat2.frac
    anim.EB.Prot2.amt <<- anim.EBW2 * anim.EB.Prot2.frac
```

```
      anim.EB.Ash2.amt <<- anim.EBW2 * anim.EB.Ash2.frac
      anim.EB.Water2.amt <<- anim.EBW2 * anim.EB.Water2.frac
      anim.EB.Energy2.amt <<- 9.4 * anim.EB.Fat2.amt + 5.7 * anim.EB.Prot2.amt
      # Energy and protein change
      anim.EB.EnergyChange.amt <<- anim.EB.Energy2.amt - anim.EB.Energy1.amt
      anim.EB.ProteinChange.amt <<- anim.EB.Prot2.amt - anim.EB.Prot1.amt
      # Rather than MEB, uses the energy change as an indication
      # if animals were on positive or negative energy balance
      if (anim.EB.EnergyChange.amt > 0)
      {
        # Gaining BCS, requires ME (positive)
        ratio.MErtoNEr.frac <<- 0.6
        ratio.MPrtoNPr.frac <<- 0.7
      } else
      {
        # Losing BCS, provides ME (negative)
        ratio.MErtoNEr.frac <<- (0.6/0.8)
        ratio.MPrtoNPr.frac <<- (0.67/0.8)
      }
      # Required ME for the BCS change
      anim.diet.MEBalance.rate <<- (anim.EB.EnergyChange.amt/ratio.MErtoNEr.frac)/anim.EB.BCSChange.time
      anim.diet.MPBalance.rate <<- (anim.EB.ProteinChange.amt/ratio.MPrtoNPr.frac)/anim.EB.BCSChange.time
      anim.diet.NEBalance.rate <<- anim.diet.MEBalance.rate * ratio.MErtoNEr.frac
      anim.diet.NPBalance.rate <<- anim.diet.MPBalance.rate * ratio.MPrtoNPr.frac
      # kg/d
      if (anim.EB.BCSChange.time != 0)
      {
        anim.EB.EWG.rate <<- (anim.EBW2 - anim.EBW1)/anim.EB.BCSChange.time
        anim.EB.SWG.rate <<- (anim.EBW2/0.851 - anim.EBW1/0.851)/anim.EB.BCSChange.time
        anim.EB.FWG.rate <<- (anim.EBW2/0.851/0.96 - anim.EBW1/0.851/0.96)/anim.EB.BCSChange.time
      } else
      {
        anim.EB.EWG.rate <<- 0
        anim.EB.SWG.rate <<- 0
        anim.EB.FWG.rate <<- 0
      }
    }
    # Compute the BCS x EBW table for each BCS
    anim.BCS_vector <<- c(0, 0.5, 1, 1.5, 2, 2.5, 3, 3.5, 4, 4.5, 5)
    anim.EBW_vector <<- ifelse(anim.BCS_vector == 2.5, 0.8513 * (0.96 * anim.FBW25), 0.8513 * (0.96 * (anim.FBW25 * (0.692 +
  0.111 * anim.BCS_vector) + (2.795 * anim.BCS_vector - 5.311))))
    if (anim.species == "Sheep") anim.EB.fat.amt_vector <<- anim.EBW_vector * (0.0269 + 0.0868 * anim.BCS_vector)
    if (anim.species == "Goats") anim.EB.fat.amt_vector <<- anim.EBW_vector * (0.0289 + 0.0708 * anim.BCS_vector)
    anim.EB.protein.amt_vector <<- anim.EBW_vector * (0.1449 + 0.0279 * anim.BCS_vector - 0.0039 * anim.BCS_vector^2)
    anim.EB.energy.amt_vector <<- 9.4 * anim.EB.fat.amt_vector + 5.7 * anim.EB.protein.amt_vector
    anim.EB.EnergyChange.amt_vector <<- vector("numeric", length(anim.BCS_vector) - 1)
    for (i in 1:(length(anim.BCS_vector) - 1))
    {
      anim.EB.EnergyChange.amt_vector[i] <<- anim.EB.energy.amt_vector[i + 1] - anim.EB.energy.amt_vector[i]
    }
  }
```

```
    return(invisible(TRUE))
}
```

5.3.7 Mineral requirements

```
calcMineralRequirement <- function()
{
  DMI <- anim.diet.DMI.rate
  ADG <- anim.body.weight.gain_shrunk
  CFW <- anim.wool.rate  # Clean fleece weight
  # Litter (lamb or kids) body weight
  if (anim.species == "Sheep") LBW <- anim.pregnancy.lamb.body.weight_birth
  if (anim.species == "Goats") LBW <- anim.pregnancy.kid.body.weight_birth
  DP <- anim.pregnancy.days  # Days pregnant
  MY <- anim.lactation.milk.rate  # Milk yield
  MkF <- anim.lactation.milk.fat.conc  # Milk fat %
  conc <- anim.diet.Concentrate.frac * 100  # % of dietary concentrate
  if (DMI <= 0 | anim.SBW <= 0) return(invisible(NULL))
  # Minerals
  if (anim.species == "Cattle")
  {
    if (anim.type == "Milk")
    {
      # Dairy
      FCM <- anim.lactation.FCM.rate <<- 0.4 * MY + 0.15 * MkF * MY
      # Calcium (Ca), g/d
      anim.Ca.maintenance <<- ifelse(anim.stage_type == "Lactating", 0.031 * anim.FBW, 0.0154 * anim.FBW) + 0.0008 * anim.FBW
      anim.Ca.pregnancy <<- ifelse(DP >= 190, 0.02456 * (0.05581 - 0.00014 * DP) * exp((0.05581 - 0.00007 * DP)*DP), 0)
      if (MY > 0)
      {
        anim.Ca.lactation <<- 1.37 * FCM # All all breeds except Holstein, Shorthorn, or Jersey
        if (anim.breed == "Holstein" | anim.breed == "Shorthorn") anim.Ca.lactation <<- 1.22 * FCM
        if (anim.breed == "Jersey") anim.Ca.lactation <<- 1.45 * FCM
      } else anim.Ca.lactation <<- 0
      anim.Ca.growth <<- 9.83 * (anim.MFBW/anim.FBW)^0.22 * ADG / 0.96
      # Phosphorus (P), g/d
      anim.P.maintenance <<- ifelse(anim.stage_type == "Lactating" | anim.stage_type == "Dry", 1 * DMI, 0.8 * DMI) + 0.002 * anim.FBW
      anim.P.pregnancy <<- ifelse(DP >= 190, 0.02743 * (0.05527 - 0.00015 * DP) * exp((0.05527 - 0.000075 * DP)*DP), 0)
      anim.P.lactation <<- ifelse(MY > 0, 0.9 * FCM, 0)
      anim.P.growth <<- (1.2 + 4.635 * (anim.MFBW/anim.FBW)^0.22) * ADG / 0.96
      # Magnesium (Mg), g/d
      anim.Mg.maintenance <<- 0.003 * anim.FBW
      anim.Mg.pregnancy <<- ifelse(DP >= 190, 0.33, 0)
      anim.Mg.lactation <<- ifelse(MY > 0, 0.15 * FCM, 0)
      anim.Mg.growth <<- 0.45 * ADG / 0.96
      # Sulfur (S), g/d
      anim.S.maintenance <<- 2 * DMI
      anim.S.pregnancy <<- 0
      anim.S.lactation <<- 0
      anim.S.growth <<- 0
      # Chlorine (Cl), g/d
      anim.Cl.maintenance <<- 0.0225 * anim.FBW
```

```
      anim.Cl.pregnancy <<- ifelse(DP >= 190, 1, 0)
      anim.Cl.lactation <<- ifelse(MY > 0, 1.15 * FCM, 0)
      anim.Cl.growth <<- 1 * ADG / 0.96
      # Potassium (K), g/d
      if (anim.stage_type == "Lactating")
      {
        if (env.temp_curr <= 25) anim.K.maintenance <<- 6.1 * DMI + 0.038 * anim.FBW
        if (env.temp_curr > 25 & env.temp_curr < 30) anim.K.maintenance <<- 6.1 * DMI + 0.038 * anim.FBW + 0.0004 * anim.FBW
        if (env.temp_curr >= 30) anim.K.maintenance <<- 6.1 * DMI + 0.038 * anim.FBW + 0.004 * anim.FBW
      } else
      {
        if (env.temp_curr <= 25) anim.K.maintenance <<- 2.6 * DMI + 0.038 * anim.FBW
        if (env.temp_curr > 25 & env.temp_curr < 30) anim.K.maintenance <<- 2.6 * DMI + 0.038 * anim.FBW + 0.0004 * anim.FBW
        if (env.temp_curr >= 30) anim.K.maintenance <<- 2.6 * DMI + 0.038 * anim.FBW + 0.004 * anim.FBW
      }
      anim.K.pregnancy <<- ifelse(DP >= 190, 1.027, 0)
      anim.K.lactation <<- ifelse(MY > 0, 1.5 * FCM, 0)
      anim.K.growth <<- 1.6 * ADG / 0.96
      # Sodium (Na), g/d
      if (anim.stage_type == "Lactating")
      {
        if (env.temp_curr <= 25) anim.Na.maintenance <<- 0.038 * anim.FBW
        if (env.temp_curr > 25 & env.temp_curr < 30) anim.Na.maintenance <<- 0.038 * anim.FBW + 0.1 * anim.FBW
        if (env.temp_curr >= 30) anim.Na.maintenance <<- 0.038 * anim.FBW + 0.5 * anim.FBW
      } else
      {
        if (env.temp_curr <= 25) anim.Na.maintenance <<- 0.015 * anim.FBW
        if (env.temp_curr > 25 & env.temp_curr < 30) anim.Na.maintenance <<- 0.015 * anim.FBW + 0.1 * anim.FBW
        if (env.temp_curr >= 30) anim.Na.maintenance <<- 0.015 * anim.FBW + 0.5 * anim.FBW
      }
      anim.Na.pregnancy <<- ifelse(DP >= 190, 1.39, 0)
      anim.Na.lactation <<- ifelse(MY > 0, 0.63 * FCM, 0)
      anim.Na.growth <<- 1.4 * ADG / 0.96
      # Copper (Cu), mg/d
      anim.Cu.maintenance <<- 0.0071 * anim.FBW
      anim.Cu.pregnancy <<- ifelse(DP > 0 & DP < 100, 0.5, ifelse(DP >= 100 & DP <= 225, 1.5, ifelse(DP > 225, 2, 0)))
      anim.Cu.lactation <<- ifelse(MY > 0, 0.15 * FCM, 0)
      anim.Cu.growth <<- 1.15 * ADG / 0.96
      # Iodine (I), mg/d
      anim.I.maintenance <<- ifelse(anim.stage_type == "Lactating", 1.5, 0.6) * 0.01 * anim.FBW
      anim.I.pregnancy <<- 0
      anim.I.lactation <<- 0
      anim.I.growth <<- 0
      # Iron (Fe), mg/d
      anim.Fe.maintenance <<- 0
      anim.Fe.pregnancy <<- ifelse(DP >= 190, 18, 0)
      anim.Fe.lactation <<- ifelse(MY > 0, 1 * FCM, 0)
      anim.Fe.growth <<- 34 * ADG / 0.96
      # Manganese (Mn), mg/d
      anim.Mn.maintenance <<- 0.002 * anim.FBW
      anim.Mn.pregnancy <<- ifelse(DP >= 190, 0.3, 0)
```

```
        anim.Mn.lactation <<- ifelse(MY > 0, 0.03 * FCM, 0)
        anim.Mn.growth <<- 0.7 * ADG / 0.96
        # Zinc (Zn), mg/d
        anim.Zn.maintenance <<- 0.033 * anim.FBW + 0.012 * anim.FBW
        anim.Zn.pregnancy <<- ifelse(DP >= 190, 12, 0)
        anim.Zn.lactation <<- ifelse(MY > 0, 4 * FCM, 0)
        anim.Zn.growth <<- 24 * ADG / 0.96
        # Cobalt (Co), mg/d
        anim.Co.maintenance <<- 0.11 * DMI
        anim.Co.pregnancy <<- 0
        anim.Co.lactation <<- 0
        anim.Co.growth <<- 0
        # Selenium (Se), mg/d
        anim.Se.maintenance <<- 0.3 * DMI
        anim.Se.pregnancy <<- 0
        anim.Se.lactation <<- 0
        anim.Se.growth <<- 0
      } else
      {
        # Beef and dual-purposes
        CBW <- anim.pregnancy.calf.body.weight_birth
        PIG <- anim.NPgr.rate
        # Calcium (Ca), g/d
        anim.Ca.maintenance <<- 0.0154 * anim.SBW
        anim.Ca.pregnancy <<- ifelse (DP > 90, CBW * (11.7 / 90), 0)
        anim.Ca.lactation <<- ifelse (MY > 0, 1.23 * MY, 0)
        anim.Ca.growth <<- 0.071 * PIG
        # Phosphorus (P), g/d
        anim.P.maintenance <<- 0.016 * anim.SBW
        anim.P.pregnancy <<- ifelse (DP > 90, CBW * (7.6 / 90), 0)
        anim.P.lactation <<- ifelse (MY > 0, 0.95 * MY, 0)
        anim.P.growth <<- 0.039 * PIG
        # Magnesium (Mg), g/d
        if (anim.stage_type == "Lactating")
        {
          anim.Mg.maintenance <<- (0.2/100) * DMI * 1000
        } else
        {
          if (DP > 0)
          {
            anim.Mg.maintenance <<- (0.12/100) * DMI * 1000
          } else anim.Mg.maintenance <<- (0.1/100) * DMI * 1000
        }
        anim.Mg.pregnancy <<- 0
        anim.Mg.lactation <<- 0
        anim.Mg.growth <<- 0
        # Potassium (K), g/d
        if (anim.stage_type == "Lactating")
        {
          anim.K.maintenance <<- (0.7/100) * DMI * 1000
        } else anim.K.maintenance <<- (0.6/100) * DMI * 1000
```

```
        anim.K.pregnancy <<- 0
        anim.K.lactation <<- 0
        anim.K.growth <<- 0
        # Sodium (Na), g/d
        if (anim.stage_type == "Lactating")
        {
          anim.Na.maintenance <<- (0.07/100) * DMI * 1000
        } else anim.Na.maintenance <<- (0.1/100) * DMI * 1000
        anim.Na.pregnancy <<- 0
        anim.Na.lactation <<- 0
        anim.Na.growth <<- 0
        # Chlorine (Cl), g/d
        anim.Cl.maintenance <<- 0
        anim.Cl.pregnancy <<- 0
        anim.Cl.lactation <<- 0
        anim.Cl.growth <<- 0
        # Sulfur (S), g/d
        anim.S.maintenance <<- (0.15/100) * DMI * 1000
        anim.S.pregnancy <<- 0
        anim.S.lactation <<- 0
        anim.S.growth <<- 0
        # Cobalt (Co), mg/d
        anim.Co.maintenance <<- 0.15 * DMI
        anim.Co.pregnancy <<- 0
        anim.Co.lactation <<- 0
        anim.Co.growth <<- 0
        # Copper (Cu), mg/d
        anim.Cu.maintenance <<- 10 * DMI
        anim.Cu.pregnancy <<- 0
        anim.Cu.lactation <<- 0
        anim.Cu.growth <<- 0
        # Iodine (I), mg/d
        anim.I.maintenance <<- 0.5 * DMI
        anim.I.pregnancy <<- 0
        anim.I.lactation <<- 0
        anim.I.growth <<- 0
        # Iron (Fe), mg/d
        anim.Fe.maintenance <<- 50 * DMI
        anim.Fe.pregnancy <<- 0
        anim.Fe.lactation <<- 0
        anim.Fe.growth <<- 0
        # Manganese (Mn), mg/d
        anim.Mn.maintenance <<- ifelse(anim.stage_type == "Lactating" | DP > 0, 40, 20) * DMI
        anim.Mn.pregnancy <<- 0
        anim.Mn.lactation <<- 0
        anim.Mn.growth <<- 0
        # Selenium, mg/d
        anim.Se.maintenance <<- 0.1 * DMI
        anim.Se.pregnancy <<- 0
        anim.Se.lactation <<- 0
        anim.Se.growth <<- 0
```

```
        # Zinc (Zn), mg/d
        anim.Zn.maintenance <<- 30 * DMI
        anim.Zn.pregnancy <<- 0
        anim.Zn.lactation <<- 0
        anim.Zn.growth <<- 0
      }
      # Molybdenum (Mo), mg/d
      anim.Mo.maintenance <<- 0
      anim.Mo.growth <<- 0
      anim.Mo.pregnancy <<- 0
      anim.Mo.lactation <<- 0
      # Chromium (Cr), mg/d
      anim.Cr.maintenance <<- 0
      anim.Cr.growth <<- 0
      anim.Cr.pregnancy <<- 0
      anim.Cr.lactation <<- 0
      if (anim.stage_type != "Lactating")
      {
        anim.Cr.growth <<- 0.6
      } else
      {
        anim.Cr.lactation <<- 7.75
      }
    } else
    {
      # Sheep and Goats
      FCM <- anim.lactation.FCM.rate <<- 0.3688 * MY + 0.0971 * MkF * MY
      # Calcium (Ca), g/d
      anim.Ca.maintenance <<- ifelse(anim.age < 3, 0.3, 0.18) * anim.FBW^0.75
      anim.Ca.growth <<- 0.018 * ADG
      anim.Ca.pregnancy <<- ifelse (DP > 0, ifelse(DP >= (152/7 - 5) * 7, 0.6, 1.1) * LBW, 0)
      if (anim.stage_type == "Lactating") anim.Ca.lactation <<- 6 * FCM else anim.Ca.lactation <<- 0
      # Phosphorus (P), g/d
      anim.P.maintenance <<- ifelse(anim.age < 3, 0.175, 0.12) * anim.FBW^0.75
      anim.P.growth <<- 0.008 * ADG
      anim.P.pregnancy <<- ifelse(DP > 0, ifelse(DP >= (152/7 - 5) * 7, 0.25, 0.5) * LBW, 0)
      if (anim.stage_type == "Lactating") anim.P.lactation <<- 2.5 * FCM else anim.P.lactation <<- 0
      if (anim.species == "Sheep")
      {
        # Sheep
        # Sodium (Na), g/d
        anim.Na.maintenance <<- (0.0108/0.91) * anim.SBW
        anim.Na.growth <<- (1.1/0.91) * ADG
        anim.Na.pregnancy <<- ifelse(DP < 105, 0, ifelse(DP >= 105 & DP < 133, 0.021/0.91, 0.013/0.91)) * LBW
        if (anim.stage_type == "Lactating") anim.Na.lactation <<- (0.4/0.91) * MY else anim.Na.lactation <<- 0
        # Chlorine (Cl), g/d
        anim.Cl.maintenance <<- (0.0079/0.85) * anim.SBW
        anim.Cl.growth <<- (0.8/0.85) * ADG
        anim.Cl.pregnancy <<- ifelse(DP < 105, 0, ifelse(DP >= 105 & DP < 133, 0.015/0.85, 0.009/0.85)) * LBW
        if (anim.stage_type == "Lactating") anim.Cl.lactation <<- (1.1/0.85) * MY else anim.Cl.lactation <<- 0
        # Potassium (K), g/d
```

```
    anim.K.maintenance <<- (0.038/0.9) * anim.SBW + (2.6/0.9) * DMI
    anim.K.growth <<- (1.8/0.9) * ADG
    anim.K.pregnancy <<- ifelse(DP < 105, 0, ifelse(DP >= 105 & DP < 133, 0.029/0.9, 0.023/0.9)) * LBW
    if (anim.stage_type == "Lactating") anim.K.lactation <<- (1.4/0.9) * MY else anim.K.lactation <<- 0
    # Magnesium (Mg), g/d
    anim.Mg.maintenance <<- (0.003/0.17) * anim.SBW
    anim.Mg.growth <<- (0.41/0.17) * ADG
    anim.Mg.pregnancy <<- ifelse(DP < 105, 0, ifelse(DP >= 105 & DP < 133, 0.009/0.17, 0.013/0.17)) * LBW
    if (anim.stage_type == "Lactating") anim.Mg.lactation <<- (0.17/0.17) * MY else anim.Mg.lactation <<- 0
    # Sulfur (S), g/d
    anim.S.maintenance <<- (0.18/100) * DMI * 1000
    anim.S.growth <<- 0
    anim.S.pregnancy <<- 0
    anim.S.lactation <<- 0
    # Cobalt (Co), mg/d
    anim.Co.maintenance <<- 0.2 * DMI
    anim.Co.growth <<- 0
    anim.Co.pregnancy <<- 0
    anim.Co.lactation <<- 0
    # Copper (Cu), mg/d
    if (anim.stage_type == "Growing/Finishing")
    {
      if (anim.age < 3)
      {
        if (anim.SBW <= 5) AC <- 0.9
        if (anim.SBW > 5 & anim.SBW <= 10) AC <- 0.53
        if (anim.SBW > 10) AC <- 0.2
      } else AC <- ifelse(conc > 50, 0.06, 0.045)
    } else
    {
      if (anim.stage_type == "Lactating") AC <- 0.045 else AC <- 0.06
    }
    anim.Cu.maintenance <<- (0.004/AC) * anim.SBW
    anim.Cu.growth <<- (1.06/AC) * ADG + (0.0137/AC) * CFW
    anim.Cu.pregnancy <<- (0.05/AC) * LBW
    if (anim.stage_type == "Lactating") anim.Cu.lactation <<- (0.2/AC) * MY else anim.Cu.lactation <- 0
    # Iodine (I), mg/d
    if (anim.stage_type == "Lactating")
    {
      anim.I.maintenance <<- 0
      anim.I.growth <<- 0
      anim.I.pregnancy <<- 0
      anim.I.lactation <<- 0.8 * DMI
    } else
    {
      anim.I.maintenance <<- 0.5 * DMI
      anim.I.growth <<- 0
      anim.I.pregnancy <<- 0
      anim.I.lactation <<- 0
    }
    # Iron (Fe), mg/d
```

```
        AC <- ifelse(anim.age <= 3, 0.5, 0.19)
        anim.Fe.maintenance <<- (0.014/0.1) * anim.SBW
        anim.Fe.growth <<- (55/AC) * ADG + (30/(365 * 0.1)) * CFW
        anim.Fe.pregnancy <<- ifelse(DP < 105, 0, (0.5/0.1)) * LBW
        if (anim.stage_type == "Lactating") anim.Fe.lactation <<- (0.9/0.1) * MY else anim.Fe.lactation <<- 0
        # Manganese (Mg), mg/d
        anim.Mn.maintenance <<- (0.002/0.0075) * anim.SBW
        anim.Mn.growth <<- (0.47/0.0075) * ADG + (2.5/(365 * 0.0075)) * CFW
        anim.Mn.pregnancy <<- ifelse(DP < 105, 0, (0.02/0.0075)) * LBW
        if (anim.stage_type == "Lactating") anim.Mn.lactation <<- (0.055/0.0075) * MY else anim.Mn.lactation <<- 0
        # Molybdenum (Mo), mg/d
        anim.Mo.maintenance <<- 0.5 * DMI
        anim.Mo.growth <<- 0
        anim.Mo.pregnancy <<- 0
        anim.Mo.lactation <<- 0
        # Selenium (Se), mg/d
        AC <- ifelse(conc > 50, 0.6, 0.31)
        anim.Se.maintenance <<- (0.00025/AC) * anim.SBW
        anim.Se.growth <<- (0.5/AC) * ADG + (0.38/AC) * CFW
        anim.Se.pregnancy <<- ifelse(DP < 105, 0, (0.0025/AC)) * LBW
        if (anim.stage_type == "Lactating") anim.Se.lactation <<- (0.14/AC) * MY else anim.Se.lactation <<- 0
        # Zinc (Zn), mg/d
        if (anim.stage_type == "Growing/Finishing")
        {
          if (anim.SBW < 10) AC <- 0.55
          if (anim.SBW >= 10 & anim.SBW < 40) AC <- 0.3
          if (anim.SBW >= 40) AC <- 0.2
        } else AC <- 0.15
        anim.Zn.maintenance <<- 0.076 * anim.SBW
        anim.Zn.growth <<- (24/AC) * ADG + (115/(365 * AC)) * CFW
        anim.Zn.pregnancy <<- ifelse(DP < 105, 0, (0.375/AC)) * LBW
        if (anim.stage_type == "Lactating") anim.Zn.lactation <<- (7.4/AC) * MY else anim.Zn.lactation <<- 0
      } else
      {
        # Goats
        # Sodium (Na), g/d
        anim.Na.maintenance <<- (0.015/0.8) * anim.SBW
        anim.Na.growth <<- (1.6/0.8) * ADG
        anim.Na.pregnancy <<- ifelse(DP < 105, 0, 0.034/0.8) * LBW
        if (anim.stage_type == "Lactating") anim.Na.lactation <<- (0.4/0.8) * MY else anim.Na.lactation <<- 0
        # Chlorine (Cl), g/d
        anim.Cl.maintenance <<- (0.022/0.8) * anim.SBW
        anim.Cl.growth <<- (1/0.8) * ADG
        anim.Cl.pregnancy <<- ifelse(DP < 105, 0, 0.024/0.8) * LBW
        if (anim.stage_type == "Lactating") anim.Cl.lactation <<- (1.1/0.8) * MY else anim.Cl.lactation <<- 0
        # Potassium (K), g/d
        anim.K.maintenance <<- (0.05/0.9) * anim.SBW + (2.6/0.9) * DMI
        anim.K.growth <<- (2.4/0.9) * ADG
        anim.K.pregnancy <<- ifelse(DP < 105, 0, 0.042/0.9) * LBW
        if (anim.stage_type == "Lactating") anim.K.lactation <<- (2/0.9) * MY else anim.K.lactation <<- 0
        # Magnesium (Mg), g/d
```

```
        anim.Mg.maintenance <<- (0.0035/0.2) * anim.SBW
        anim.Mg.growth <<- (0.4/0.2) * ADG
        anim.Mg.pregnancy <<- ifelse(DP < 105, 0, 0.006/0.2) * LBW
        if (anim.stage_type == "Lactating") anim.Mg.lactation <<- (0.14/0.2) * MY else anim.Mg.lactation <<- 0
        # Sulfur (S), g/d
        if (anim.stage_type == "Lactating")
        {
          anim.S.maintenance <<- 0
          anim.S.growth <<- 0
          anim.S.pregnancy <<- 0
          anim.S.lactation <<- (0.26/100) * DMI * 1000
        } else
        {
          anim.S.maintenance <<- (0.22/100) * DMI * 1000
          anim.S.growth <<- 0
          anim.S.pregnancy <<- 0
          anim.S.lactation <<- 0
        }
        # Cobalt (Co), mg/d
        anim.Co.maintenance <<- 0.11 * DMI
        anim.Co.growth <<- 0
        anim.Co.pregnancy <<- 0
        anim.Co.lactation <<- 0
        # Copper (Cu), mg/d
        if (anim.stage_type == "Growing/Finishing")
        {
          anim.Cu.maintenance <<- 25 * DMI
          anim.Cu.growth <<- 0
          anim.Cu.pregnancy <<- 0
          anim.Cu.lactation <<- 0
        } else
        {
          if (anim.stage_type == "Lactating")
          {
            anim.Cu.maintenance <<- 0
            anim.Cu.growth <<- 0
            anim.Cu.pregnancy <<- 0
            anim.Cu.lactation <<- 15 * DMI
          } else
          {
            anim.Cu.maintenance <<- 20 * DMI
            anim.Cu.growth <<- 0
            anim.Cu.pregnancy <<- 0
            anim.Cu.lactation <<- 0
          }
        }
        # Iodine (I), mg/d
        if (anim.stage_type == "Lactating")
        {
          anim.I.maintenance <<- 0
          anim.I.growth <<- 0
```

```
    anim.I.pregnancy <<- 0
    anim.I.lactation <<- 0.8 * DMI
  } else
  {
    anim.I.maintenance <<- 0.5 * DMI
    anim.I.growth <<- 0
    anim.I.pregnancy <<- 0
    anim.I.lactation <<- 0
  }
  # Iron (Fe), mg/d
  if (anim.stage_type == "Growing/Finishing")
  {
    anim.Fe.maintenance <<- 95 * DMI
    anim.Fe.growth <<- 0
    anim.Fe.pregnancy <<- 0
    anim.Fe.lactation <<- 0
  } else
  {
    anim.Fe.maintenance <<- 35 * DMI
    anim.Fe.growth <<- 0
    anim.Fe.pregnancy <<- 0
    anim.Fe.lactation <<- 0
  }
  # Manganese (Mg), mg/d
  anim.Mn.maintenance <<- (0.002/0.0075) * anim.SBW
  anim.Mn.growth <<- (0.7/0.0075) * ADG + (2.5/(365 * 0.0075)) * CFW
  anim.Mn.pregnancy <<- ifelse(DP < 105, 0, (0.025/0.0075)) * LBW
  if (anim.stage_type == "Lactating") anim.Mn.lactation <<- (0.03/0.0075) * MY else anim.Mn.lactation <<- 0
  # Molybdenum (Mo), mg/d
  anim.Mo.maintenance <<- 1 * DMI
  anim.Mo.growth <<- 0
  anim.Mo.pregnancy <<- 0
  anim.Mo.lactation <<- 0
  # Selenium (Se), mg/d
  AC <- ifelse(conc > 50, 0.6, 0.31)
  anim.Se.maintenance <<- (0.083/AC) + 0.015 * DMI
  anim.Se.growth <<- (0.5/AC) * ADG + (0.38/AC) * CFW
  anim.Se.pregnancy <<- ifelse(DP < 105, 0, (0.0021/AC)) * LBW
  if (anim.stage_type == "Lactating") anim.Se.lactation <<- (0.1/AC) * MY else anim.Se.lactation <<- 0
  # Zinc (Zn), mg/d
  if (anim.stage_type == "Growing/Finishing")
  {
    if (anim.age < 3) AC <- 0.5 else AC <- 0.3
  } else AC <- 0.15
  anim.Zn.maintenance <<- (0.045/AC) * anim.SBW
  anim.Zn.growth <<- (25/AC) * ADG + (115/(365 * AC)) * CFW
  anim.Zn.pregnancy <<- ifelse(DP < 105, 0, (0.5/AC)) * LBW
  if (anim.stage_type == "Lactating")
    anim.Zn.lactation <<- (5.5/AC) * MY else anim.Zn.lactation <<- 0
}
# Chromium (Cr), mg/d
```

```
      anim.Cr.maintenance <<- 0
      anim.Cr.growth <<- 0
      anim.Cr.pregnancy <<- 0
      anim.Cr.lactation <<- 0
    }
    anim.Ca.requirement.rate <<- anim.Ca.maintenance + anim.Ca.growth + anim.Ca.pregnancy + anim.Ca.lactation
    anim.P.requirement.rate <<- anim.P.maintenance + anim.P.growth + anim.P.pregnancy + anim.P.lactation
    anim.Mg.requirement.rate <<- anim.Mg.maintenance + anim.Mg.growth + anim.Mg.pregnancy + anim.Mg.lactation
    anim.K.requirement.rate <<- anim.K.maintenance + anim.K.growth + anim.K.pregnancy + anim.K.lactation
    anim.S.requirement.rate <<- anim.S.maintenance + anim.S.growth + anim.S.pregnancy + anim.S.lactation
    anim.Cl.requirement.rate <<- anim.Cl.maintenance + anim.Cl.growth + anim.Cl.pregnancy + anim.Cl.lactation
    anim.Na.requirement.rate <<- anim.Na.maintenance + anim.Na.growth + anim.Na.pregnancy + anim.Na.lactation
    anim.Fe.requirement.rate <<- anim.Fe.maintenance + anim.Fe.growth + anim.Fe.pregnancy + anim.Fe.lactation
    anim.Zn.requirement.rate <<- anim.Zn.maintenance + anim.Zn.growth + anim.Zn.pregnancy + anim.Zn.lactation
    anim.Cu.requirement.rate <<- anim.Cu.maintenance + anim.Cu.growth + anim.Cu.pregnancy + anim.Cu.lactation
    anim.Mn.requirement.rate <<- anim.Mn.maintenance + anim.Mn.growth + anim.Mn.pregnancy + anim.Mn.lactation
    anim.Se.requirement.rate <<- anim.Se.maintenance + anim.Se.growth + anim.Se.pregnancy + anim.Se.lactation
    anim.Co.requirement.rate <<- anim.Co.maintenance + anim.Co.growth + anim.Co.pregnancy + anim.Co.lactation
    anim.I.requirement.rate <<- anim.I.maintenance + anim.I.growth + anim.I.pregnancy + anim.I.lactation
    anim.Mo.requirement.rate <<- anim.Mo.maintenance + anim.Mo.growth + anim.Mo.pregnancy + anim.Mo.lactation
    anim.Cr.requirement.rate <<- anim.Cr.maintenance + anim.Cr.growth + anim.Cr.pregnancy + anim.Cr.lactation
    anim.Ca.balance.rate <<- si.diet.GCa.rate * 1000 - anim.Ca.requirement.rate
    anim.P.balance.rate <<- si.diet.GP.rate * 1000 - anim.P.requirement.rate
    anim.Mg.balance.rate <<- si.diet.GMg.rate * 1000 - anim.Mg.requirement.rate
    anim.K.balance.rate <<- si.diet.GK.rate * 1000 - anim.K.requirement.rate
    anim.S.balance.rate <<- si.diet.GS.rate * 1000 - anim.S.requirement.rate
    anim.Cl.balance.rate <<- si.diet.GCl.rate * 1000 - anim.Cl.requirement.rate
    anim.Na.balance.rate <<- si.diet.GNa.rate * 1000 - anim.Na.requirement.rate
    anim.Fe.balance.rate <<- si.diet.GFe.rate * 1000000 - anim.Fe.requirement.rate
    anim.Zn.balance.rate <<- si.diet.GZn.rate * 1000000 - anim.Zn.requirement.rate
    anim.Cu.balance.rate <<- si.diet.GCu.rate * 1000000 - anim.Cu.requirement.rate
    anim.Mn.balance.rate <<- si.diet.GMn.rate * 1000000 - anim.Mn.requirement.rate
    anim.Se.balance.rate <<- si.diet.GSe.rate * 1000000 - anim.Se.requirement.rate
    anim.Co.balance.rate <<- si.diet.GCo.rate * 1000000 - anim.Co.requirement.rate
    anim.I.balance.rate <<- si.diet.GI.rate * 1000000 - anim.I.requirement.rate
    anim.Mo.balance.rate <<- - anim.Mo.requirement.rate
    anim.Cr.balance.rate <<- si.diet.GCr.rate * 1000000 - anim.Cr.requirement.rate
    # Ratios
    diet.NtoS.ratio <<- (anim.diet.CP.rate * 0.16) / anim.diet.S.rate
    diet.NPNtoS.ratio <<- (anim.diet.NPN.rate * 0.16) / anim.diet.S.rate
    diet.CatoP.ratio <<- anim.diet.Ca.rate / anim.diet.P.rate
    diet.GCatoGP.ratio <<- si.diet.GCa.rate / si.diet.GP.rate
    return(invisible(TRUE))
  }
```

5.3.8 Vitamin requirements

```
calcVitaminRequirement <- function()
{
  if (is.na(anim.species) | anim.diet.DMI.rate <= 0)
  {
    anim.VitA.requirement.rate <<- 0
    anim.VitD.requirement.rate <<- 0
    anim.VitE.requirement.rate <<- 0
    anim.VitA.balance.rate <<- 0
    anim.VitD.balance.rate <<- 0
    anim.VitE.balance.rate <<- 0
    return(invisible(NULL))
  }
  DMI <- anim.diet.DMI.rate
  ADG <- anim.body.weight.gain_shrunk
  DG <- anim.pregnancy.days   # Days pregnant
  # Vitamins
  if (anim.species == "Cattle")
  {
    if (anim.type == "Milk")
    {
      # Dairy cattle
      if (anim.stage_type == "Lactating")
      {
        anim.VitA.requirement.rate <<- 110 * anim.FBW   # IU/d
        anim.VitD.requirement.rate <<- 30 * anim.FBW   # IU/d
        anim.VitE.requirement.rate <<- 0.8 * anim.FBW   # IU/d
      } else
      {
        if (anim.stage_type == "Dry")
        {
          anim.VitA.requirement.rate <<- 110 * anim.FBW   # IU/d
          anim.VitD.requirement.rate <<- 30 * anim.FBW   # IU/d
          anim.VitE.requirement.rate <<- 1.6 * anim.FBW   # IU/d
        } else
        {
          anim.VitA.requirement.rate <<- 80 * anim.FBW   # IU/d
          anim.VitD.requirement.rate <<- 30 * anim.FBW   # IU/d
          anim.VitE.requirement.rate <<- 0.8 * anim.FBW   # IU/d
        }
      }
    } else
    {
      # Beef cattle
      if (anim.stage_type == "Lactating" | anim.sex == "Bulls")
      {
        anim.VitA.requirement.rate <<- 3900 * DMI   # IU/d
        anim.VitD.requirement.rate <<- 275 * DMI   # IU/d
        anim.VitE.requirement.rate <<- 35 * DMI   # IU/d
```

```
        } else
        {
          if (anim.stage_type == "Dry" | anim.stage_type == "Replacement")
          {
            anim.VitA.requirement.rate <<- 2800 * DMI   # IU/d
            anim.VitD.requirement.rate <<- 275 * DMI   # IU/d
            anim.VitE.requirement.rate <<- 35 * DMI   # IU/d
          } else
          {
            anim.VitA.requirement.rate <<- 2200 * DMI   # IU/d
            anim.VitD.requirement.rate <<- 275 * DMI   # IU/d
            anim.VitE.requirement.rate <<- 35 * DMI   # IU/d
          }
        }
      }
    } else
    {
      # Sheep and goats
      if (anim.stage_type == "Lactating")
      {
        anim.VitA.requirement.rate <<- 178 * anim.FBW   # IU/d
        anim.VitD.requirement.rate <<- 5.6 * anim.FBW + 716   # IU/d
        anim.VitE.requirement.rate <<- 5.6 * anim.FBW   # IU/d
      } else
      {
        if (anim.sex == "Female" & DG > 0)
        {
          if (DG < 152 * 2/3)
          {
            # Early pregnancy
            anim.VitA.requirement.rate <<- 105 * anim.FBW   # IU/d
            anim.VitD.requirement.rate <<- 5.6 * anim.FBW   # IU/d
            anim.VitE.requirement.rate <<- 5.3 * anim.FBW   # IU/d
          } else
          {
            # Late pregnancy
            anim.VitA.requirement.rate <<- 152 * anim.FBW   # IU/d
            anim.VitD.requirement.rate <<- 5.6 * anim.FBW + 213   # IU/d
            anim.VitE.requirement.rate <<- 5.6 * anim.FBW   # IU/d
          }
        } else
        {
          anim.VitA.requirement.rate <<- 333 * anim.FBW   # IU/d
          anim.VitD.requirement.rate <<- 5.6 * anim.FBW + 1.08 * ADG * 1000   # IU/d
          anim.VitD.requirement.rate <<- anim.VitD.requirement.rate * ifelse(anim.age < 4, 1.2, 1)
          anim.VitE.requirement.rate <<- 10 * anim.FBW   # IU/d
        }
      }
    }
  anim.VitA.balance.rate <<- anim.diet.VitA.rate - anim.VitA.requirement.rate/1000 # kIU/d
  anim.VitD.balance.rate <<- anim.diet.VitD.rate - anim.VitD.requirement.rate/1000 # kIU/d
```

```
    anim.VitE.balance.rate <<- anim.diet.VitE.rate - anim.VitE.requirement.rate # IU/d
    return(invisible(TRUE))
  }
```

6 Supplementary calculations

6.1 Code

6.1.1 Energy and protein balance and allowable performance

```
calcAllowable <- function()
{
  # Reset dry matter required
  anim.DMR <<- 0
  if (is.na(anim.species) | anim.diet.DMI.rate <= 0)
  {
    anim.peNDF_required.rate <<- 0
    anim.peNDF_required_acidosis.rate <<-0
    anim.peNDF_required_gain.rate <<- 0
    anim.peNDF_balance.rate <<- 0
    anim.NDF_required.rate <<- 0
    anim.NDF_balance.rate <<- 0
    anim.SWG_MEallowable <<- anim.body.weight.gain_shrunk_MEallowable <<- 0
    anim.SWG_MPallowable <<- anim.body.weight.gain_shrunk_MPallowable <<- 0
    anim.MY_MEallowable <<- anim.lactation.milk.rate_MEallowable <<- 0
    anim.MY_MPallowable <<- anim.lactation.milk.rate_MPallowable <<- 0
    anim.MEm_available.rate <<- 0
    anim.MEm_required.rate <<- 0
    anim.MEm_balance.rate <<- 0
    anim.MEp_available.rate <<- 0
    anim.MEp_required.rate <<- 0
    anim.MEp_balance.rate <<- 0
    anim.MEl_available.rate <<- 0
    anim.MEl_required.rate <<- 0
    anim.MEl_balance.rate <<- 0
    anim.MEg_available.rate <<- 0
    anim.MEg_required.rate <<- 0
    anim.MEg_balance.rate <<- 0
    anim.MEr_available.rate <<- 0
    anim.MEr_required.rate <<- 0
    anim.MEr_balance.rate <<- 0
    anim.MEe_available.rate <<- 0
    anim.MEe_required.rate <<- 0
    anim.MEe_balance.rate <<- 0
    anim.MPm_available.rate <<- 0
    anim.MPm_required.rate <<- 0
```

```
    anim.MPm_balance.rate <<- 0
    anim.MPp_available.rate <<- 0
    anim.MPp_required.rate <<- 0
    anim.MPp_balance.rate <<- 0
    anim.MPl_available.rate <<- 0
    anim.MPl_required.rate <<- 0
    anim.MPl_balance.rate <<- 0
    anim.MPg_available.rate <<- 0
    anim.MPg_required.rate <<- 0
    anim.MPg_balance.rate <<- 0
    anim.MPr_available.rate <<- 0
    anim.MPr_required.rate <<- 0
    anim.MPr_balance.rate <<- 0
    anim.MPe_available.rate <<- 0
    anim.MPe_required.rate <<- 0
    anim.MPe_balance.rate <<- 0
    anim.MY_MAAallowable.rate_vector <<- rep(0, 10)
    anim.MY_MAAallowable.label_vector <<- rep(NA, 10)
    anim.MY_MAAallowable.label_min <<- NA
    anim.MY_MAAallowable.label_max <<- NA
    anim.MY_MAAallowable.rate_min <<- 0
    anim.MY_MAAallowable.rate_max <<- 0
    anim.SWG_MAAallowable.rate_vector <<- rep(0, 10)
    anim.SWG_MAAallowable.label_vector <<- rep(NA, 10)
    anim.SWG_MAAallowable.label_min <<- NA
    anim.SWG_MAAallowable.label_max <<- NA
    anim.SWG_MAAallowable.rate_min <<- 0
    anim.SWG_MAAallowable.rate_max <<- 0
    return(invisible(NULL))
  }
  # ++++++++++++++++++++++++
  # +++ Fiber requirement +++
  # ++++++++++++++++++++++++
  if (isLactating == TRUE)
  {
    anim.peNDF_required.rate <<- 0.23 * anim.diet.DMI.rate
  } else
  {
    anim.peNDF_required.rate <<- anim.peNDF_required_acidosis.rate <<- 0.1 * anim.diet.DMI.rate
    anim.peNDF_required_gain.rate <<- 0.15 * anim.diet.DMI.rate
  }
  if (anim.species == "Cattle")
  {
    # Mertens (1985; Proc. of the 46th Minnesota Nutrition Conference, 209-224)
    anim.NDF_required.rate <<- 0.011 * anim.SBW
  } else
  {
    # Cannas et al. (2016; CJAS 96:628)
    anim.NDF_required.rate <<- 0.01 * (5.4442 * anim.SBW^(-0.25)) * anim.SBW
  }
  anim.peNDF_balance.rate <<- anim.diet.peNDF.rate - anim.peNDF_required.rate
```

```
    anim.NDF_balance.rate <<- anim.diet.NDF.rate - anim.NDF_required.rate
    # ++++++++++++++++++++
    # +++ ME allowable +++
    # ++++++++++++++++++++
    MEI <- anim.diet.ME.rate
    if (isLactating == TRUE)
    {
      if (tolower(anim.stage_option) == "mean")
      {
        # Mean BCS
        MER <- anim.MEmr.rate + (anim.MEgr.rate + anim.mammogenesis.MEgr.rate) + anim.MEpr.rate
        # ME available for lactation
        MEAL <- MEI - MER
        anim.MY_MEallowable <<- anim.lactation.milk.rate_MEallowable <<- 0
        if (MEAL > 0 & anim.lactation.milk.rate > 0) anim.MY_MEallowable <<- anim.lactation.milk.rate_MEallowable <<- MEAL/(anim.MElr.rate/anim.lactation.milk.rate)
      } else
      {
        # Period BCS
        MER <- anim.MEmr.rate + (anim.MEgr.rate + anim.mammogenesis.MEgr.rate) + anim.MEpr.rate + anim.diet.MEBalance.rate
        MEAL <- MEI - MER
        anim.MY_MEallowable <<- anim.lactation.milk.rate_MEallowable <<- 0
        if (MEAL > 0 & anim.lactation.milk.rate > 0) anim.MY_MEallowable <<- anim.lactation.milk.rate_MEallowable <<- MEAL/(anim.MElr.rate/anim.lactation.milk.rate)
      }
    } else
    {
      # Nonlactating
      MER <- anim.MEmr.rate + anim.MElr.rate + anim.MEpr.rate
      # ME available for growth
      MEAG <- MEI - MER
      anim.SWG_MEallowable <<- anim.body.weight.gain_shrunk_MEallowable <<- 0
      if (MEAG > 0 & anim.body.weight.gain_shrunk > 0) anim.SWG_MEallowable <<- anim.body.weight.gain_shrunk_MEallowable <<- MEAG/((anim.MEgr.rate + anim.mammogenesis.MEgr.rate)/anim.SWG)
    }
    # ++++++++++++++++++++
    # +++ MP allowable +++
    # ++++++++++++++++++++
    MPI <- anim.diet.MP.rate * 1000
    if (isLactating == TRUE)
    {
      if (tolower(anim.stage_option) == "mean")
      {
        # Mean BCS
        MPR <- anim.MPmr.rate + (anim.MPgr.rate + anim.mammogenesis.NPgr.rate) + anim.MPpr.rate
        # MP available for lactation
        MPAL <- MPI - MPR
        anim.MY_MPallowable <<- anim.lactation.milk.rate_MPallowable <<- 0
        if (MPAL > 0 & anim.lactation.milk.rate > 0) anim.MY_MPallowable <<- anim.lactation.milk.rate_MPallowable <<- MPAL/(anim.MPlr.rate/anim.lactation.milk.rate)
      } else
```

```
      {
        # Period BCS
        MPR <- anim.MPmr.rate + (anim.MPgr.rate + anim.mammogenesis.NPgr.rate) + anim.MPpr.rate + anim.diet.MPBalance.rate*1000
        MPAL <- MPI - MPR
        anim.MY_MPallowable <<- anim.lactation.milk.rate_MPallowable <<- 0
        if (MPAL > 0 & anim.lactation.milk.rate > 0) anim.MY_MPallowable <<- anim.lactation.milk.rate_MPallowable <<- MPAL/(anim.MPlr.rate/anim.lactation.milk.rate)
      }
    } else
    {
      # Nonlactating
      MPR <- anim.MPmr.rate + anim.MPlr.rate + anim.MPpr.rate
      # MP available for growth
      MPAG <- MPI - MPR
      anim.SWG_MPallowable <<- anim.body.weight.gain_shrunk_MPallowable <<- 0
      if (MPAG > 0 & anim.body.weight.gain_shrunk > 0) anim.SWG_MPallowable <<- anim.body.weight.gain_shrunk_MPallowable <<- MPAG/((anim.MPgr.rate + anim.mammogenesis.NPgr.rate)/anim.SWG)
    }
    # ++++++++++++++++++++++++++++
    # +++ Amino acid allowable +++
    # ++++++++++++++++++++++++++++
    if (isLactating == TRUE)
    {
      if (anim.species == "Cattle" & anim.type != "Milk")
      {
        MkTP <- anim.lactation.milk.peak.protein.conc
      } else
      {
        if (anim.species == "Goats")
        {
          MkTP <- ifelse(anim.lactation.milk.protein.type == "True", anim.lactation.milk.protein.conc, anim.lactation.milk.protein.conc * 0.92)
        } else
        {
          MkTP <- ifelse(anim.lactation.milk.protein.type == "True", anim.lactation.milk.protein.conc, anim.lactation.milk.protein.conc * 0.93)
        }
      }
      MAAAL <- rep(0, 10)
      MAAAL[1] <- si.diet.GMet.rate * 1000 - (anim.MAAmr.rate[1] + anim.MAApr.rate[1] + anim.MAAgr.rate[1])
      MAAAL[2] <- si.diet.GLys.rate * 1000 - (anim.MAAmr.rate[2] + anim.MAApr.rate[2] + anim.MAAgr.rate[2])
      MAAAL[3] <- si.diet.GHis.rate * 1000 - (anim.MAAmr.rate[3] + anim.MAApr.rate[3] + anim.MAAgr.rate[3])
      MAAAL[4] <- si.diet.GPhe.rate * 1000 - (anim.MAAmr.rate[4] + anim.MAApr.rate[4] + anim.MAAgr.rate[4])
      MAAAL[5] <- si.diet.GTrp.rate * 1000 - (anim.MAAmr.rate[5] + anim.MAApr.rate[5] + anim.MAAgr.rate[5])
      MAAAL[6] <- si.diet.GThr.rate * 1000 - (anim.MAAmr.rate[6] + anim.MAApr.rate[6] + anim.MAAgr.rate[6])
      MAAAL[7] <- si.diet.GLeu.rate * 1000 - (anim.MAAmr.rate[7] + anim.MAApr.rate[7] + anim.MAAgr.rate[7])
      MAAAL[8] <- si.diet.GIle.rate * 1000 - (anim.MAAmr.rate[8] + anim.MAApr.rate[8] + anim.MAAgr.rate[8])
      MAAAL[9] <- si.diet.GVal.rate * 1000 - (anim.MAAmr.rate[9] + anim.MAApr.rate[9] + anim.MAAgr.rate[9])
      MAAAL[10] <- si.diet.GArg.rate * 1000 - (anim.MAAmr.rate[10] + anim.MAApr.rate[10] + anim.MAAgr.rate[10])
      anim.MY_MAAallowable.rate_vector <<- rep(0,10)
```

```
      if (MkTP > 0) anim.MY_MAAallowable.rate_vector <<- (10 * MAAAL * anim.lactation.milk.AA_Eff.frac)/(MkTP * anim.lactation.milk.AA.conc)
      anim.MY_MAAallowable.label_vector <<- c("Met","Lys","His","Phe","Trp","Thr","Leu","Ile","Val","Arg")
      anim.MY_MAAallowable.label_min <<- anim.MY_MAAallowable.label_vector[which.min(anim.MY_MAAallowable.rate_vector)]
      anim.MY_MAAallowable.label_max <<- anim.MY_MAAallowable.label_vector[which.max(anim.MY_MAAallowable.rate_vector)]
      anim.MY_MAAallowable.rate_min <<- min(anim.MY_MAAallowable.rate_vector)
      anim.MY_MAAallowable.rate_max <<- max(anim.MY_MAAallowable.rate_vector)
    } else
    {
      PIG <- anim.body.weight.gain_protein.conc
      MAAAG <- rep(0, 10)
      MAAAG[1] <- si.diet.GMet.rate * 1000 - (anim.MAAmr.rate[1] + anim.MAApr.rate[1] + anim.MAAlr.rate[1])
      MAAAG[2] <- si.diet.GLys.rate * 1000 - (anim.MAAmr.rate[2] + anim.MAApr.rate[2] + anim.MAAlr.rate[2])
      MAAAG[3] <- si.diet.GHis.rate * 1000 - (anim.MAAmr.rate[3] + anim.MAApr.rate[3] + anim.MAAlr.rate[3])
      MAAAG[4] <- si.diet.GPhe.rate * 1000 - (anim.MAAmr.rate[4] + anim.MAApr.rate[4] + anim.MAAlr.rate[4])
      MAAAG[5] <- si.diet.GTrp.rate * 1000 - (anim.MAAmr.rate[5] + anim.MAApr.rate[5] + anim.MAAlr.rate[5])
      MAAAG[6] <- si.diet.GThr.rate * 1000 - (anim.MAAmr.rate[6] + anim.MAApr.rate[6] + anim.MAAlr.rate[6])
      MAAAG[7] <- si.diet.GLeu.rate * 1000 - (anim.MAAmr.rate[7] + anim.MAApr.rate[7] + anim.MAAlr.rate[7])
      MAAAG[8] <- si.diet.GIle.rate * 1000 - (anim.MAAmr.rate[8] + anim.MAApr.rate[8] + anim.MAAlr.rate[8])
      MAAAG[9] <- si.diet.GVal.rate * 1000 - (anim.MAAmr.rate[9] + anim.MAApr.rate[9] + anim.MAAlr.rate[9])
      MAAAG[10] <- si.diet.GArg.rate * 1000 - (anim.MAAmr.rate[10] + anim.MAApr.rate[10] + anim.MAAlr.rate[10])
      anim.SWG_MAAallowable.rate_vector <<- rep(0,10)
      if (PIG > 0)
      {
        if (flag_UserAAGrowth == TRUE)
        {
          if (PIG > 0) anim.SWG_MAAallowable.rate_vector <<- (10 * MAAAG * anim.growth.AA_Eff.frac)/(PIG * anim.growth.AA.conc)
        } else
        {
          if (PIG > 0) anim.SWG_MAAallowable.rate_vector <<- (10 * MAAAG * ratio.NPgr.MPgr)/(PIG * anim.growth.AA.conc)
        }
      }
      anim.SWG_MAAallowable.label_vector <<- c("Met","Lys","His","Phe","Trp","Thr","Leu","Ile","Val","Arg")
      anim.SWG_MAAallowable.label_min <<- anim.SWG_MAAallowable.label_vector[which.min(anim.SWG_MAAallowable.rate_vector)]
      anim.SWG_MAAallowable.label_max <<- anim.SWG_MAAallowable.label_vector[which.max(anim.SWG_MAAallowable.rate_vector)]
      anim.SWG_MAAallowable.rate_min <<- min(anim.SWG_MAAallowable.rate_vector)
      anim.SWG_MAAallowable.rate_max <<- max(anim.SWG_MAAallowable.rate_vector)
    }
    # ++++++++++++++++++++++++
    # +++ ME and MP balance +++
    # ++++++++++++++++++++++++
    if (isLactating == TRUE)
    {
      if (tolower(anim.stage_option) == "mean")
      {
        # ME balance
        anim.MEm_available.rate <<- anim.diet.ME.rate
        anim.MEm_required.rate <<- anim.MEmr.rate
        anim.MEm_balance.rate <<- anim.MEm_available.rate - anim.MEm_required.rate
        anim.MEp_available.rate <<- anim.MEm_balance.rate
        anim.MEp_required.rate <<- anim.MEpr.rate
```

```
        anim.MEp_balance.rate <<- anim.MEp_available.rate - anim.MEp_required.rate
        anim.MEl_available.rate <<- anim.MEp_balance.rate
        anim.MEl_required.rate <<- anim.MElr.rate
        anim.MEl_balance.rate <<- anim.MEl_available.rate - anim.MEl_required.rate
        anim.MEg_available.rate <<- anim.MEl_balance.rate
        anim.MEg_required.rate <<- (anim.MEgr.rate + anim.mammogenesis.MEgr.rate)
        anim.MEg_balance.rate <<- anim.MEg_available.rate - anim.MEg_required.rate
        anim.MEr_available.rate <<- anim.MEg_balance.rate
        anim.MEr_required.rate <<- 0
        anim.MEr_balance.rate <<- anim.MEr_available.rate - anim.MEr_required.rate
        anim.MEe_available.rate <<- anim.diet.ME.rate
        anim.MEe_required.rate <<- anim.MEm_required.rate + anim.MEp_required.rate + anim.MEl_required.rate + anim.MEg_re-
quired.rate + anim.MEr_required.rate
        anim.MEe_balance.rate <<- anim.MEe_available.rate - anim.MEe_required.rate
        # MP balance
        anim.MPm_available.rate <<- anim.diet.MP.rate * 1000
        anim.MPm_required.rate <<- anim.MPmr.rate
        anim.MPm_balance.rate <<- anim.MPm_available.rate - anim.MPm_required.rate
        anim.MPp_available.rate <<- anim.MPm_balance.rate
        anim.MPp_required.rate <<- anim.MPpr.rate
        anim.MPp_balance.rate <<- anim.MPp_available.rate - anim.MPp_required.rate
        anim.MPl_available.rate <<- anim.MPp_balance.rate
        anim.MPl_required.rate <<- anim.MPlr.rate
        anim.MPl_balance.rate <<- anim.MPl_available.rate - anim.MPl_required.rate
        anim.MPg_available.rate <<- anim.MPl_balance.rate
        anim.MPg_required.rate <<- (anim.MPgr.rate + anim.mammogenesis.NPgr.rate)
        anim.MPg_balance.rate <<- anim.MPg_available.rate - anim.MPg_required.rate
        anim.MPr_available.rate <<- anim.MPg_balance.rate
        anim.MPr_required.rate <<- 0
        anim.MPr_balance.rate <<- anim.MPr_available.rate - anim.MPr_required.rate
        anim.MPe_available.rate <<- anim.diet.MP.rate * 1000
        anim.MPe_required.rate <<- anim.MPm_required.rate + anim.MPp_required.rate + anim.MPl_required.rate + anim.MPg_re-
quired.rate + anim.MPr_required.rate
        anim.MPe_balance.rate <<- anim.MPe_available.rate - anim.MPe_required.rate
      } else
      {
        # ME balance
        anim.MEm_available.rate <<- anim.diet.ME.rate
        anim.MEm_required.rate <<- anim.MEmr.rate
        anim.MEm_balance.rate <<- anim.MEm_available.rate - anim.MEm_required.rate
        anim.MEp_available.rate <<- anim.MEm_balance.rate
        anim.MEp_required.rate <<- anim.MEpr.rate
        anim.MEp_balance.rate <<- anim.MEp_available.rate - anim.MEp_required.rate
        anim.MEl_available.rate <<- anim.MEp_balance.rate
        anim.MEl_required.rate <<- anim.MElr.rate
        anim.MEl_balance.rate <<- anim.MEl_available.rate - anim.MEl_required.rate
        anim.MEg_available.rate <<- anim.MEl_balance.rate
        anim.MEg_required.rate <<- (anim.MEgr.rate + anim.mammogenesis.MEgr.rate)
        anim.MEg_balance.rate <<- anim.MEg_available.rate - anim.MEg_required.rate
        anim.MEr_available.rate <<- anim.MEg_balance.rate
        anim.MEr_required.rate <<- anim.diet.MEBalance.rate
```

```
        anim.MEr_balance.rate <<- anim.MEr_available.rate - anim.MEr_required.rate
        anim.MEe_available.rate <<- anim.diet.ME.rate
        anim.MEe_required.rate <<- anim.MEm_required.rate + anim.MEp_required.rate + anim.MEl_required.rate + anim.MEg_required.rate + anim.MEr_required.rate
        anim.MEe_balance.rate <<- anim.MEe_available.rate - anim.MEe_required.rate
        # MP balance
        anim.MPm_available.rate <<- anim.diet.MP.rate * 1000
        anim.MPm_required.rate <<- anim.MPmr.rate
        anim.MPm_balance.rate <<- anim.MPm_available.rate - anim.MPm_required.rate
        anim.MPp_available.rate <<- anim.MPm_balance.rate
        anim.MPp_required.rate <<- anim.MPpr.rate
        anim.MPp_balance.rate <<- anim.MPp_available.rate - anim.MPp_required.rate
        anim.MPl_available.rate <<- anim.MPp_balance.rate
        anim.MPl_required.rate <<- anim.MPlr.rate
        anim.MPl_balance.rate <<- anim.MPl_available.rate - anim.MPl_required.rate
        anim.MPg_available.rate <<- anim.MPl_balance.rate
        anim.MPg_required.rate <<- (anim.MPgr.rate + anim.mammogenesis.NPgr.rate)
        anim.MPg_balance.rate <<- anim.MPg_available.rate - anim.MPg_required.rate
        anim.MPr_available.rate <<- anim.MPg_balance.rate
        anim.MPr_required.rate <<- anim.diet.MPBalance.rate*1000
        anim.MPr_balance.rate <<- anim.MPr_available.rate - anim.MPr_required.rate
        anim.MPe_available.rate <<- anim.diet.MP.rate * 1000
        anim.MPe_required.rate <<- anim.MPm_required.rate + anim.MPp_required.rate + anim.MPl_required.rate + anim.MPg_required.rate + anim.MPr_required.rate
        anim.MPe_balance.rate <<- anim.MPe_available.rate - anim.MPe_required.rate
      }
    } else
    {
      # ME balance
      anim.MEm_available.rate <<- anim.diet.ME.rate
      anim.MEm_required.rate <<- anim.MEmr.rate
      anim.MEm_balance.rate <<- anim.MEm_available.rate - anim.MEm_required.rate
      anim.MEp_available.rate <<- anim.MEm_balance.rate
      anim.MEp_required.rate <<- anim.MEpr.rate
      anim.MEp_balance.rate <<- anim.MEp_available.rate - anim.MEp_required.rate
      anim.MEl_available.rate <<- anim.MEp_balance.rate
      anim.MEl_required.rate <<- anim.MElr.rate
      anim.MEl_balance.rate <<- anim.MEl_available.rate - anim.MEl_required.rate
      anim.MEg_available.rate <<- anim.MEl_balance.rate
      # ME required for growth is a function of MP allowable gain
      anim.MEg_required.rate <<- 0
      if (anim.SWG>0) anim.MEg_required.rate <<- anim.body.weight.gain_shrunk_MPallowable * ((anim.MEgr.rate + anim.mammogenesis.MEgr.rate)/anim.SWG)
      anim.MEg_balance.rate <<- anim.MEg_available.rate - anim.MEg_required.rate
      anim.MEr_available.rate <<- ifelse(anim.MEg_balance.rate > 0, anim.MEg_balance.rate, 0)
      anim.MEr_required.rate <<- 0
      anim.MEr_balance.rate <<- anim.MEr_available.rate - anim.MEr_required.rate
      anim.MEe_available.rate <<- anim.diet.ME.rate
      anim.MEe_required.rate <<- anim.MEm_required.rate + anim.MEp_required.rate + anim.MEl_required.rate + anim.MEg_required.rate + anim.MEr_required.rate
      anim.MEe_balance.rate <<- anim.MEe_available.rate - anim.MEe_required.rate
```

```
    # MP balance
    anim.MPm_available.rate <<- anim.diet.MP.rate * 1000
    anim.MPm_required.rate <<- anim.MPmr.rate
    anim.MPm_balance.rate <<- anim.MPm_available.rate - anim.MPm_required.rate
    anim.MPp_available.rate <<- anim.MPm_balance.rate
    anim.MPp_required.rate <<- anim.MPpr.rate
    anim.MPp_balance.rate <<- anim.MPp_available.rate - anim.MPp_required.rate
    anim.MPl_available.rate <<- anim.MPp_balance.rate
    anim.MPl_required.rate <<- anim.MPlr.rate
    anim.MPl_balance.rate <<- anim.MPl_available.rate - anim.MPl_required.rate
    anim.MPg_available.rate <<- anim.MPl_balance.rate
    # MP required for growth is a function of ME allowable gain
    anim.MPg_required.rate <<- 0
    if (anim.SWG>0) anim.MPg_required.rate <<- anim.body.weight.gain_shrunk_MEallowable * ((anim.MPgr.rate + anim.mammogene-
sis.NPgr.rate)/anim.SWG)
    anim.MPg_balance.rate <<- anim.MPg_available.rate - anim.MPg_required.rate
    anim.MPr_available.rate <<- ifelse(anim.MPg_balance.rate>0,anim.MPg_balance.rate,0)
    anim.MPr_required.rate <<- 0
    anim.MPr_balance.rate <<- anim.MPr_available.rate - anim.MPr_required.rate
    anim.MPe_available.rate <<- anim.diet.MP.rate * 1000
    anim.MPe_required.rate <<- anim.MPm_required.rate + anim.MPp_required.rate + anim.MPl_required.rate + anim.MPg_re-
quired.rate + anim.MPr_required.rate
    anim.MPe_balance.rate <<- anim.MPe_available.rate - anim.MPe_required.rate
  }
  return(invisible(TRUE))
}
```

6.1.2 Summary report

```
displaySummary <- function()
{
  if (SolutionLevel == 0 | SolutionLevel == 1)
  {
    if (is.na(anim.species) | anim.diet.DMI.rate <= 0) return(invisible(NULL))
    cat("#Title/Inv#Summary Report\n")
    if (existsnonNA("granst.selected") != FALSE & exists("granst.list2") != FALSE)
    {
      title <- granst.list2[granst.selected]
      if (nchar(title) > 102)
      {
        title <- substr(title, 1, 102)
      }
      cat(paste(string(" ", floor((102 - nchar(title))/2)), title,"\n", sep=""))
      #cat(paste(string(" ", floor((102 - nchar(title))/2)), string(".", nchar(title)), "\n", sep=""))
    }
    # One line info
    heading <- paste("Species:", anim.species, " | Type:", anim.type, " | Sex:", anim.sex,  sep = "")
    if (anim.stage_type == "Lactating")
    {
      if (anim.type == "Milk")
      {
        heading <- paste(heading, " | MY:", trimws(formatC(ifelse(tolower(Unit) == "metric", anim.lactation.milk.rate, kgTOlb(anim.lactation.milk.rate)), format = "f", digits = 1, width = 5)),
                          " | DIM:", trimws(anim.lactation.days), sep = "")
      } else
      {
        heading <- paste(heading, " | MY:", trimws(formatC(ifelse(tolower(Unit) == "metric", anim.lactation.milk.peak.rate, kgTOlb(anim.lactation.milk.peak.rate)), format = "f", digits = 1, width = 5)),
                          " | DIM:", trimws(anim.lactation.days), sep = "")
      }
      heading <- paste(heading, " | DG:", trimws(anim.pregnancy.days), sep = "")
    }
    if (anim.stage_type == "Dry" | anim.stage_type == "Replacement")
      heading <- paste(heading, " | DG:", trimws(anim.pregnancy.days), sep = "")
    if (anim.stage_type == "Growing/Finishing" & anim.species == "Cattle")
      heading <- paste(heading," | SRW:", trimws(formatC(ifelse(tolower(Unit) == "metric", anim.body.weight_standard, kgTOlb(anim.body.weight_standard)), format = "f", digits = 0, width = 4)),
                        " | MBW:", trimws(formatC(ifelse(tolower(Unit) == "metric", anim.body.weight_mature, kgTOlb(anim.body.weight_mature)), format = "f", digits = 0, width = 4)), sep = "")
    if (tolower(anim.stage_option) == "mean")
    {
      heading <- paste(heading, " | BW:", formatC(ifelse(tolower(Unit) == "metric", anim.body.weight_mean, kgTOlb(anim.body.weight_mean)), format = "f", digits = 0, width = 4),
                        " | BCS:", formatC(anim.body.condition_mean, format = "f", digits = 1, width = 3), sep = "")
    } else
    {
```

```
        heading <- paste(heading, " | BW:{", trimws(formatC(ifelse(tolower(Unit) == "metric", anim.body.weight_initial,
kgTOlb(anim.body.weight_initial)), format = "f", digits = 0, width = 4)), "-",
                                trimws(formatC(ifelse(tolower(Unit) == "metric", anim.body.weight_final, kgTOlb(anim.body.weight_fi-
nal)), format = "f", digits = 0, width = 4)), "}",
                                " | BCS:{", trimws(formatC(anim.body.condition_initial, format = "f", digits = 1, width = 3)), "-",
                                trimws(formatC(anim.body.condition_final, format = "f", digits = 1, width = 3)), "}", sep="")
    }
    cat(paste(string(" ", floor((102 - nchar(heading))/2)), heading, "\n", sep=""))
    cat(paste(string(" ", floor((102 - nchar(heading))/2)), string("=", nchar(heading)), "\n\n", sep=""))
    #cat("\n")
    #title <- "Summary Report"
    #cat(paste(title, "\n", string("=", nchar(title)), "\n\n", sep = ""))
    subtitle1 <- "Metabolizable Energy (ME) Balance"
    subtitle1 <- paste(subtitle1, string(" ", 34 - nchar(subtitle1)), sep = "")
    subtitle2 <- "Metabolizable Protein (MP) Balance"
    subtitle2 <- paste(subtitle2, string(" ", 34 - nchar(subtitle2)), sep = "")
    cat(paste("Items", string(" ", 13 - 5), " ", subtitle1, " ", subtitle2, " ", "  Ca  ", " ", "   P","\n",
              string("-", 13), " ", string("-", nchar(subtitle1)), "  ", string("-", nchar(subtitle2)), "  ", string("-", 7),
"  ", string("-", 7), "\n", sep = ""))
    cat(paste(string(" ", 13), " Available    Required     Balance   Available    Required     Balance      g/d
g/d","\n", sep = ""))
    cat(paste(string(" ", 13), "    Mcal/d      Mcal/d      Mcal/d         g/d         g/d         g/d","\n", sep = ""))
    cat(paste(string(" ", 13), " ", string("-", nchar(subtitle1)), "  ", string("-", nchar(subtitle2)), "  ", string("-", 7),
"  ", string("-", 7), "\n", sep = ""))
    cat(paste("Supplied      ", formatC(anim.diet.ME.rate, format = "f", digits = 3, width = 10), string(" ", 2 + 10 + 2 + 10
+ 2),
              formatC(anim.diet.MP.rate*1000, format = "f", digits = 2, width = 10), string(" ", 2 + 10 + 2 + 10 + 2),
              formatC(si.diet.GCa.rate*1000, format = "f", digits = 2, width = 7), string(" ", 2),
              formatC(si.diet.GP.rate*1000, format = "f", digits = 2, width = 7), "\n", sep=""))
    cat(paste(string("-", 13 + 1 + 34 + 2 + 34 + 2 + 7 + 2 + 7), "\n", sep = ""))
    cat(paste("Required\n"))
    cat(paste("  Maintenance  ",
              formatC(anim.MEm_available.rate, format = "f", digits = 3, width = 10), string(" ", 2),
              formatC(anim.MEm_required.rate, format = "f", digits = 3, width = 10), string(" ", 2),
              formatC(anim.MEm_balance.rate, format = "f", digits = 3, width = 10), string(" ", 2),
              formatC(anim.MPm_available.rate, format = "f", digits = 2, width = 10), string(" ", 2),
              formatC(anim.MPm_required.rate, format = "f", digits = 2, width = 10), string(" ", 2),
              formatC(anim.MPm_balance.rate, format = "f", digits = 2, width = 10), string(" ", 2),
              formatC(anim.Ca.maintenance, format = "f", digits = 2, width = 7), string(" ", 2),
              formatC(anim.P.maintenance, format = "f", digits = 2, width = 7), "\n", sep=""))
    cat(paste("  Pregnancy    ",
              formatC(anim.MEp_available.rate, format = "f", digits = 3, width = 10), string(" ", 2),
              formatC(anim.MEp_required.rate, format = "f", digits = 3, width = 10), string(" ", 2),
              formatC(anim.MEp_balance.rate, format = "f", digits = 3, width = 10), string(" ", 2),
              formatC(anim.MPp_available.rate, format = "f", digits = 2, width = 10), string(" ", 2),
              formatC(anim.MPp_required.rate, format = "f", digits = 2, width = 10), string(" ", 2),
              formatC(anim.MPp_balance.rate, format = "f", digits = 2, width = 10), string(" ", 2),
              formatC(anim.Ca.pregnancy, format = "f", digits = 2, width = 7), string(" ", 2),
              formatC(anim.P.pregnancy, format = "f", digits = 2, width = 7), "\n", sep=""))
    cat(paste("  Lactation    ",
              formatC(anim.MEl_available.rate, format = "f", digits = 3, width = 10), string(" ", 2),
```

```
                formatC(anim.MEl_required.rate, format = "f", digits = 3, width = 10), string(" ", 2),
                formatC(anim.MEl_balance.rate, format = "f", digits = 3, width = 10), string(" ", 2),
                formatC(anim.MPl_available.rate, format = "f", digits = 2, width = 10), string(" ", 2),
                formatC(anim.MPl_required.rate, format = "f", digits = 2, width = 10), string(" ", 2),
                formatC(anim.MPl_balance.rate, format = "f", digits = 2, width = 10), string(" ", 2),
                formatC(anim.Ca.lactation, format = "f", digits = 2, width = 7), string(" ", 2),
                formatC(anim.P.lactation, format = "f", digits = 2, width = 7), "\n", sep=""))
    cat(paste("  Growth        ",
                formatC(anim.MEg_available.rate, format = "f", digits = 3, width = 10), string(" ", 2),
                formatC(anim.MEg_required.rate, format = "f", digits = 3, width = 10), string(" ", 2),
                formatC(anim.MEg_balance.rate, format = "f", digits = 3, width = 10), string(" ", 2),
                formatC(anim.MPg_available.rate, format = "f", digits = 2, width = 10), string(" ", 2),
                formatC(anim.MPg_required.rate, format = "f", digits = 2, width = 10), string(" ", 2),
                formatC(anim.MPg_balance.rate, format = "f", digits = 2, width = 10), string(" ", 2),
                formatC(anim.Ca.growth, format = "f", digits = 2, width = 7), string(" ", 2),
                formatC(anim.P.growth, format = "f", digits = 2, width = 7), "\n", sep=""))
    cat(paste("  Reserves     ",
                formatC(anim.MEr_available.rate, format = "f", digits = 3, width = 10), string(" ", 2),
                formatC(anim.MEr_required.rate, format = "f", digits = 3, width = 10), string(" ", 2),
                formatC(anim.MEr_balance.rate, format = "f", digits = 3, width = 10), string(" ", 2),
                formatC(anim.MPr_available.rate, format = "f", digits = 2, width = 10), string(" ", 2),
                formatC(anim.MPr_required.rate, format = "f", digits = 2, width = 10), string(" ", 2),
                formatC(anim.MPr_balance.rate, format = "f", digits = 2, width = 10), string(" ", 2),
                "  ---   ", string(" ", 2), "  ---   ", "\n", sep=""))
    cat(paste(string("-", 13 + 1 + 34 + 2 + 34 + 2 + 7 + 2 + 7), "\n", sep = ""))
    cat(paste("Balance          ",
                formatC(anim.MEe_available.rate, format = "f", digits = 3, width = 10), string(" ", 2),
                formatC(anim.MEe_required.rate, format = "f", digits = 3, width = 10), string(" ", 2),
                formatC(anim.MEe_balance.rate, format = "f", digits = 3, width = 10), string(" ", 2),
                formatC(anim.MPe_available.rate, format = "f", digits = 2, width = 10), string(" ", 2),
                formatC(anim.MPe_required.rate, format = "f", digits = 2, width = 10), string(" ", 2),
                formatC(anim.MPe_balance.rate, format = "f", digits = 2, width = 10), string(" ", 2),
                formatC(anim.Ca.balance.rate, format = "f", digits = 2, width = 7), string(" ", 2),
                formatC(anim.P.balance.rate, format = "f", digits = 2, width = 7), "\n", sep=""))
    cat("\n\n")
    subtitle1 <- "Animal Intake & Performance"
    subtitle1 <- paste(subtitle1, string(" ", 50 - nchar(subtitle1)), sep = "")
    subtitle2 <- "Diet Summary & Diet Evaluation"
    subtitle2 <- paste(subtitle2, string(" ", 50 - nchar(subtitle2)), sep = "")
    cat(paste(subtitle1, "  ", subtitle2, "\n", string("-", nchar(subtitle1)), "  ", string("-", nchar(subtitle2)), "\n", sep = ""))
    cat(paste(ifelse(tolower(Unit) == "metric", "Dry matter intake, kg/d", "Dry matter intake, lb/d"), string(" ", 50 - 23), "  ",
                "DM, % AF          : ", formatC(anim.diet.DM.conc, format = "f", digits = 3, width = 7), "  ",
                "NDF, % DM         : ", formatC(isz(anim.diet.NDF.rate * 100,anim.diet.DMI.rate), format = "f", digits = 3, width = 7), "\n", sep = ""))
    if (anim.diet.DMI.rate>0)
    {
      cat(paste("    Predicted [", formatC(ifelse(tolower(Unit) == "metric", anim.DMI.rate_min, kgTOlb(anim.DMI.rate_min)), format = "f", digits = 2, width = 5), "; ",
```

```
                     formatC(ifelse(tolower(Unit) == "metric", anim.DMI.rate_max, kgTOlb(anim.DMI.rate_max)), format = "f", digits = 2, width = 5), "](",
                     formatC(100 * anim.DMI.rate_avg/anim.diet.DMI.rate, format = "f", digits = 2, width = 7), "% obs): ", formatC(ifelse(tolower(Unit) == "metric", anim.DMI.rate_avg, kgTOlb(anim.DMI.rate_avg)), format = "f", digits = 3, width = 7), "  ",
                     "Forage, %       : ", formatC(anim.diet.Forage.frac * 100, format = "f", digits = 3, width = 7), "  ",
                     "ADF, % DM       : ", formatC(isz(anim.diet.ADF.rate * 100,anim.diet.DMI.rate), format = "f", digits = 3, width = 7), "\n", sep = ""))
      } else
      {
        cat(paste("   Predicted [", formatC(ifelse(tolower(Unit) == "metric", anim.DMI.rate_min, kgTOlb(anim.DMI.rate_min)), format = "f", digits = 2, width = 5), "; ",
                     formatC(ifelse(tolower(Unit) == "metric", anim.DMI.rate_max, kgTOlb(anim.DMI.rate_max)), format = "f", digits = 2, width = 5),
                     "]               : ", formatC(anim.DMI.rate_avg, format = "f", digits = 3, width = 7), "  ",
                     "Forage, %       : ", formatC(anim.diet.Forage.frac * 100, format = "f", digits = 3, width = 7), "  ",
                     "ADF, % DM       : ", formatC(isz(anim.diet.ADF.rate * 100,anim.diet.DMI.rate), format = "f", digits = 3, width = 7), "\n", sep = ""))
      }
      if (flag_DMRType==0)
      {
        cat(paste("   Required                             : ", "  NA    ", "  ",
                     "CP, % DM        : ", formatC(anim.diet.CP.conc, format = "f", digits = 3, width = 7), "  ",
                     "Lignin, % NDF   : ", formatC(isz(anim.diet.lignin.rate * 100,anim.diet.NDF.rate), format = "f", digits = 3, width = 7), "\n", sep = ""))
      } else
      {
        if (anim.diet.DMI.rate>0)
        {

          if (flag_DMRType==1)
          {
            cat(paste("   Required (ME basis, ", formatC(anim.DMR * 100/anim.diet.DMI.rate, format = "f", digits = 2, width = 6), "% obs)        : ",
                         formatC(ifelse(tolower(Unit) == "metric", anim.DMR, kgTOlb(anim.DMR)), format = "f", digits = 3, width = 7), "  ",
                         "CP, % DM        : ", formatC(anim.diet.CP.conc, format = "f", digits = 3, width = 7), "  ",
                         "Lignin, % NDF   : ", formatC(isz(anim.diet.lignin.rate * 100,anim.diet.NDF.rate), format = "f", digits = 3, width = 7), "\n", sep = ""))
          }
          if (flag_DMRType==2)
          {
            cat(paste("   Required (MP basis, ", formatC(anim.DMR * 100/anim.diet.DMI.rate, format = "f", digits = 2, width = 6), "% obs)        : ",
                         formatC(ifelse(tolower(Unit) == "metric", anim.DMR, kgTOlb(anim.DMR)), format = "f", digits = 3, width = 7), "  ",
                         "CP, % DM        : ", formatC(anim.diet.CP.conc, format = "f", digits = 3, width = 7), "  ",
                         "Lignin, % NDF   : ", formatC(isz(anim.diet.lignin.rate * 100,anim.diet.NDF.rate), format = "f", digits = 3, width = 7), "\n", sep = ""))
          }
          if (flag_DMRType==3)
```

```
        {
          if (isLactating==TRUE)
          {
            cat(paste("   Required (", anim.MY_MAAallowable.label_min," basis,  ", formatC(anim.DMR * 100/anim.diet.DMI.rate, format = "f", digits = 2, width = 6), "% obs)      : ",
                      formatC(ifelse(tolower(Unit) == "metric", anim.DMR, kgTOlb(anim.DMR)), format = "f", digits = 3, width = 7), "  ",
                      "CP, % DM        : ", formatC(anim.diet.CP.conc, format = "f", digits = 3, width = 7), "  ",
                      "Lignin, % NDF   : ", formatC(isz(anim.diet.lignin.rate * 100,anim.diet.NDF.rate), format = "f", digits = 3, width = 7), "\n", sep = ""))
          } else
          {
            cat(paste("   Required (", anim.SWG_MAAallowable.label_min," basis,  ", formatC(anim.DMR * 100/anim.diet.DMI.rate, format = "f", digits = 2, width = 6), "% obs)      : ",
                      formatC(ifelse(tolower(Unit) == "metric", anim.DMR, kgTOlb(anim.DMR)), format = "f", digits = 3, width = 7), "  ",
                      "CP, % DM        : ", formatC(anim.diet.CP.conc, format = "f", digits = 3, width = 7), "  ",
                      "Lignin, % NDF   : ", formatC(isz(anim.diet.lignin.rate * 100,anim.diet.NDF.rate), format = "f", digits = 3, width = 7), "\n", sep = ""))
          }
        }
        if (flag_DMRType==4)
        {
          cat(paste("   Required (ME & MP bases, ", formatC(anim.DMR * 100/anim.diet.DMI.rate, format = "f", digits = 2, width = 6), "% obs) : ",
                    formatC(ifelse(tolower(Unit) == "metric", anim.DMR, kgTOlb(anim.DMR)), format = "f", digits = 3, width = 7), "  ",
                    "CP, % DM        : ", formatC(anim.diet.CP.conc, format = "f", digits = 3, width = 7), "  ",
                    "Lignin, % NDF   : ", formatC(isz(anim.diet.lignin.rate * 100,anim.diet.NDF.rate), format = "f", digits = 3, width = 7), "\n", sep = ""))
        }
        if (flag_DMRType==5)
        {
          if (isLactating==TRUE)
          {
            cat(paste("   Required (ME,MP,", anim.MY_MAAallowable.label_min, " bases,", formatC(anim.DMR * 100/anim.diet.DMI.rate, format = "f", digits = 2, width = 6), "% obs): ",
                      formatC(ifelse(tolower(Unit) == "metric", anim.DMR, kgTOlb(anim.DMR)), format = "f", digits = 3, width = 7), "  ",
                      "CP, % DM        : ", formatC(anim.diet.CP.conc, format = "f", digits = 3, width = 7), "  ",
                      "Lignin, % NDF   : ", formatC(isz(anim.diet.lignin.rate * 100,anim.diet.NDF.rate), format = "f", digits = 3, width = 7), "\n", sep = ""))
          } else
          {
            cat(paste("   Required (ME,MP,", anim.SWG_MAAallowable.label_min, " bases,", formatC(anim.DMR * 100/anim.diet.DMI.rate, format = "f", digits = 2, width = 6), "% obs): ",
                      formatC(ifelse(tolower(Unit) == "metric", anim.DMR, kgTOlb(anim.DMR)), format = "f", digits = 3, width = 7), "  ",
                      "CP, % DM        : ", formatC(anim.diet.CP.conc, format = "f", digits = 3, width = 7), "  ",
                      "Lignin, % NDF   : ", formatC(isz(anim.diet.lignin.rate * 100,anim.diet.NDF.rate), format = "f", digits = 3, width = 7), "\n", sep = ""))
```

```
                }
            }
            if (flag_DMRType==6)
            {
                if (isLactating==TRUE)
                {
                    cat(paste("    Required (ME,MP,", anim.MY_MAAallowable.label_min, " bases,", formatC(anim.DMR * 100/anim.diet.DMI.rate, format = "f", digits = 2, width = 6), "% obs): ",
                                    formatC(ifelse(tolower(Unit) == "metric", max(anim.DMR), kgTOlb(max(anim.DMR))), format = "f", digits = 3, width = 7), "  ",
                                    "CP, % DM           : ", formatC(anim.diet.CP.conc, format = "f", digits = 3, width = 7), "  ",
                                    "Lignin, % NDF   : ", formatC(isz(anim.diet.lignin.rate * 100,anim.diet.NDF.rate), format = "f", digits = 3, width = 7), "\n", sep = ""))
                } else
                {
                    cat(paste("    Required (ME,MP,", anim.SWG_MAAallowable.label_min, "bases,", formatC(anim.DMR * 100/anim.diet.DMI.rate, format = "f", digits = 2, width = 6), "% obs): ",
                                    formatC(ifelse(tolower(Unit) == "metric", max(anim.DMR), kgTOlb(max(anim.DMR))), format = "f", digits = 3, width = 7), "  ",
                                    "CP, % DM           : ", formatC(anim.diet.CP.conc, format = "f", digits = 3, width = 7), "  ",
                                    "Lignin, % NDF   : ", formatC(isz(anim.diet.lignin.rate * 100,anim.diet.NDF.rate), format = "f", digits = 3, width = 7), "\n", sep = ""))
                }
            }
        } else
        {
            if (flag_DMRType==1)
            {
                cat(paste("    Required (ME basis)                    : ",
                                formatC(ifelse(tolower(Unit) == "metric", anim.DMR, kgTOlb(anim.DMR)), format = "f", digits = 3, width = 7), "  ",
                                "CP, % DM           : ", formatC(anim.diet.CP.conc, format = "f", digits = 3, width = 7), "  ",
                                "Lignin, % NDF   : ", formatC(isz(anim.diet.lignin.rate * 100,anim.diet.NDF.rate), format = "f", digits = 3, width = 7), "\n", sep = ""))
            }
            if (flag_DMRType==2)
            {
                cat(paste("    Required (MP basis)                    : ",
                                formatC(ifelse(tolower(Unit) == "metric", anim.DMR, kgTOlb(anim.DMR)), format = "f", digits = 3, width = 7), "  ",
                                "CP, % DM           : ", formatC(anim.diet.CP.conc, format = "f", digits = 3, width = 7), "  ",
                                "Lignin, % NDF   : ", formatC(isz(anim.diet.lignin.rate * 100,anim.diet.NDF.rate), format = "f", digits = 3, width = 7), "\n", sep = ""))
            }
            if (flag_DMRType==3)
            {
                if (isLactating==TRUE)
                {
                    cat(paste("    Required (", anim.MY_MAAallowable.label_min," basis)                    : ",
                                    formatC(ifelse(tolower(Unit) == "metric", anim.DMR, kgTOlb(anim.DMR)), format = "f", digits = 3, width = 7), "  ",
```

```
                    "CP, % DM         : ", formatC(anim.diet.CP.conc, format = "f", digits = 3, width = 7), "  ",
                    "Lignin, % NDF  : ", formatC(isz(anim.diet.lignin.rate * 100,anim.diet.NDF.rate), format = "f", digits = 3, width = 7), "\n", sep = ""))
            } else
            {
             cat(paste("   Required (", anim.SWG_MAAallowable.label_min," basis)                    : ",
                    formatC(ifelse(tolower(Unit) == "metric", anim.DMR, kgTOlb(anim.DMR)), format = "f", digits = 3, width = 7), "  ",
                    "CP, % DM         : ", formatC(anim.diet.CP.conc, format = "f", digits = 3, width = 7), "  ",
                    "Lignin, % NDF  : ", formatC(isz(anim.diet.lignin.rate * 100,anim.diet.NDF.rate), format = "f", digits = 3, width = 7), "\n", sep = ""))
            }
          }
          if (flag_DMRType==4)
          {
            cat(paste("   Required (ME & MP bases)                : ",
                   formatC(ifelse(tolower(Unit) == "metric", anim.DMR, kgTOlb(anim.DMR)), format = "f", digits = 3, width = 7), "  ",
                   "CP, % DM         : ", formatC(anim.diet.CP.conc, format = "f", digits = 3, width = 7), "  ",
                   "Lignin, % NDF  : ", formatC(isz(anim.diet.lignin.rate * 100,anim.diet.NDF.rate), format = "f", digits = 3, width = 7), "\n", sep = ""))
          }
          if (flag_DMRType==5)
          {
            if (isLactating==TRUE)
            {
             cat(paste("   Required (ME,MP,", anim.MY_MAAallowable.label_min, " bases)             : ",
                    formatC(ifelse(tolower(Unit) == "metric", anim.DMR, kgTOlb(anim.DMR)), format = "f", digits = 3, width = 7), "  ",
                    "CP, % DM         : ", formatC(anim.diet.CP.conc, format = "f", digits = 3, width = 7), "  ",
                    "Lignin, % NDF  : ", formatC(isz(anim.diet.lignin.rate * 100,anim.diet.NDF.rate), format = "f", digits = 3, width = 7), "\n", sep = ""))
            } else
            {
             cat(paste("   Required (ME,MP,", anim.SWG_MAAallowable.label_min, " bases)             : ",
                    formatC(ifelse(tolower(Unit) == "metric", anim.DMR, kgTOlb(anim.DMR)), format = "f", digits = 3, width = 7), "  ",
                    "CP, % DM         : ", formatC(anim.diet.CP.conc, format = "f", digits = 3, width = 7), "  ",
                    "Lignin, % NDF  : ", formatC(isz(anim.diet.lignin.rate * 100,anim.diet.NDF.rate), format = "f", digits = 3, width = 7), "\n", sep = ""))
            }
          }
          if (flag_DMRType==6)
          {
            if (isLactating==TRUE)
            {
             cat(paste("   Required (ME,MP,", anim.MY_MAAallowable.label_min, " bases)             : ",
                    formatC(ifelse(tolower(Unit) == "metric", max(anim.DMR), kgTOlb(max(anim.DMR))), format = "f", digits = 3, width = 7), "  ",
                    "CP, % DM         : ", formatC(anim.diet.CP.conc, format = "f", digits = 3, width = 7), "  ",
```

```
                        "Lignin, % NDF  : ", formatC(isz(anim.diet.lignin.rate * 100,anim.diet.NDF.rate), format = "f", digits = 3, width = 7), "\n", sep = ""))
            } else
            {
                cat(paste("   Required (ME,MP,", anim.SWG_MAAallowable.label_min, "bases)          : ",
                        formatC(ifelse(tolower(Unit) == "metric", max(anim.DMR), kgTOlb(max(anim.DMR))), format = "f", digits = 3, width = 7), "  ",
                        "CP, % DM       : ", formatC(anim.diet.CP.conc, format = "f", digits = 3, width = 7), "  ",
                        "Lignin, % NDF  : ", formatC(isz(anim.diet.lignin.rate * 100,anim.diet.NDF.rate), format = "f", digits = 3, width = 7), "\n", sep = ""))
            }
        }
    }
  }
  cat(paste("   User-inputted (obs)  (",formatC(isz(anim.diet.DMI.rate * 100, anim.body.weight_mean), format = "f", digits = 2, width = 4),"% BW)         : ", formatC(ifelse(tolower(Unit) == "metric", anim.diet.DMI.rate, kgTOlb(anim.diet.DMI.rate)), format = "f", digits = 3, width = 7), "  ",
                "NDIN, % DM     : ", formatC(isz(anim.diet.NDIP.rate * 100,anim.diet.DMI.rate), format = "f", digits = 3, width = 7), "  ",
                "peNDF, % NDF   : ", formatC(isz(anim.diet.peNDF.rate * 100,anim.diet.NDF.rate), format = "f", digits = 3, width = 7), "\n", sep = ""))

  cat(paste(ifelse(tolower(Unit) == "metric", "Predicted water intake, kg/d             : ", "Predicted water intake, lb/d : "), formatC(ifelse(tolower(Unit) == "metric", anim.WI.rate, kgTOlb(anim.WI.rate)), format = "f", digits = 3, width = 7)," ",
                "ADIN, % DM     : ", formatC(isz(anim.diet.ADIP.rate * 100,anim.diet.DMI.rate), format = "f", digits = 3, width = 7), "  ",
                "EE, % DM       : ", formatC(isz(anim.diet.EE.rate * 100,anim.diet.DMI.rate), format = "f", digits = 3, width = 7), "\n", sep = ""))

  if (isLactating == TRUE)
  {
    cat(paste(ifelse(tolower(Unit) == "metric", "Milk production, kg/d", "Milk production, lb/d"), string(" ", 50 - 21), " ",
                "NFC, % DM      : ", formatC(isz(anim.diet.NFC.rate * 100,anim.diet.DMI.rate), format = "f", digits = 3, width = 7), "  ",
                "Ash, % DM      : ", formatC(isz(anim.diet.ash.rate * 100,anim.diet.DMI.rate), format = "f", digits = 3, width = 7), "\n", sep = ""))
    if (anim.lactation.milk.rate>0)
    {
      cat(paste("   ME allowable milk  (", formatC(100 * anim.MY_MEallowable/anim.lactation.milk.rate, format = "f", digits = 2, width = 7),
                "% obs)       : ", formatC(ifelse(tolower(Unit) == "metric", anim.MY_MEallowable, kgTOlb(anim.MY_MEallowable)), format = "f", digits = 3, width = 7), "  ",
                string("-", nchar(subtitle2)), "\n", sep = ""))
      cat(paste("   MP allowable milk  (", formatC(100 * anim.MY_MPallowable/anim.lactation.milk.rate, format = "f", digits = 2, width = 7),
                "% obs)       : ", formatC(ifelse(tolower(Unit) == "metric", anim.MY_MPallowable, kgTOlb(anim.MY_MPallowable)), format = "f", digits = 3, width = 7), "  ",
                "tTDN, % DM     : ", formatC(anim.diet.tTDN.conc, format = "f", digits = 3, width = 7), "  ",
```

```
                    "RDP, % CP         : ", formatC(isz((anim.diet.CP.rate - rum.diet.RUCP.rate) * 100, anim.diet.CP.rate), format = "f", digits = 3, width = 7), "\n", sep = ""))
            cat(paste("    ", anim.MY_MAAallowable.label_min, " allowable milk (", formatC(100 * anim.MY_MAAallowable.rate_min/anim.lactation.milk.rate, format = "f", digits = 2, width = 7),
                    "% obs)       : ", formatC(ifelse(tolower(Unit) == "metric", anim.MY_MAAallowable.rate_min, kgTOlb(anim.MY_MAAallowable.rate_min)), format = "f", digits = 3, width = 7), "  ",
                    "aTDN, % DM        : ", formatC(anim.diet.aTDN.conc, format = "f", digits = 3, width = 7), "  ",
                    "RDP, % DM         : ", formatC(isz((anim.diet.CP.rate - rum.diet.RUCP.rate) * 100, anim.diet.DMI.rate), format = "f", digits = 3, width = 7), "\n", sep = ""))
        } else
        {
            cat(paste("    ME allowable milk                   : ", formatC(ifelse(tolower(Unit) == "metric", anim.MY_MEallowable, kgTOlb(anim.MY_MEallwable)), format = "f", digits = 3, width = 7), "  ",
                    string("-", nchar(subtitle2)), "\n", sep = ""))
            cat(paste("    MP allowable milk                   : ", formatC(ifelse(tolower(Unit) == "metric", anim.MY_MPallowable, kgTOlb(anim.MY_MPallowable)), format = "f", digits = 3, width = 7), "  ",
                    "tTDN, % DM        : ", formatC(anim.diet.tTDN.conc, format = "f", digits = 3, width = 7), "  ",
                    "RDP, % CP         : ", formatC(isz((anim.diet.CP.rate - rum.diet.RUCP.rate) * 100, anim.diet.CP.rate), format = "f", digits = 3, width = 7), "\n", sep = ""))
            cat(paste("    ", anim.MY_MAAallowable.label_min, " allowable milk                 : ", formatC(ifelse(tolower(Unit) == "metric", anim.MY_MAAallowable.rate_min, kgTOlb(anim.MY_MAAallowable.rate_min)), format = "f", digits = 3, width = 7), "  ",
                    "aTDN, % DM        : ", formatC(anim.diet.aTDN.conc, format = "f", digits = 3, width = 7), "  ",
                    "RDP, % DM         : ", formatC(isz((anim.diet.CP.rate - rum.diet.RUCP.rate) * 100, anim.diet.DMI.rate), format = "f", digits = 3, width = 7), "\n", sep = ""))
        }
        cat(paste("    User-inputted (obs)                 : ", formatC(ifelse(tolower(Unit) == "metric", anim.lactation.milk.rate, kgTOlb(anim.lactation.milk.rate)), format = "f", digits = 3, width = 7), "  ",
                  ifelse(tolower(Unit) == "metric", "GE, Mcal/kg     : ", "GE, Mcal/lb     : "), formatC(ifelse(tolower(Unit) == "metric", anim.diet.GE.frac, PERkgTOPERlb(anim.diet.GE.frac)), format = "f", digits = 3, width = 7), "  ",
                  "RUP, % CP         : ", formatC(isz(rum.diet.RUCP.rate * 100, anim.diet.CP.rate), format = "f", digits = 3, width = 7), "\n", sep = ""))
        cat(paste(string(" ", 50), "  ",
                  ifelse(tolower(Unit) == "metric", "DE, Mcal/kg     : ", "DE, Mcal/lb     : "), formatC(ifelse(tolower(Unit) == "metric", anim.diet.DE.frac, PERkgTOPERlb(anim.diet.DE.frac)), format = "f", digits = 3, width = 7), "  ",
                  "RUP, % DM         : ", formatC(isz(rum.diet.RUCP.rate * 100, anim.diet.DMI.rate), format = "f", digits = 3, width = 7), "\n", sep = ""))
        subtitle1 <- "Efficiency of use, %                  Energy    Protein"
        cat(paste(subtitle1, "  ",
                  ifelse(tolower(Unit) == "metric", "ME, Mcal/kg     : ", "ME, Mcal/lb     : "), formatC(ifelse(tolower(Unit) == "metric", anim.diet.ME.frac, PERkgTOPERlb(anim.diet.ME.frac)), format = "f", digits = 3, width = 7), "  ",
                  ifelse(tolower(Unit) == "metric", "MP, kg/d        : ", "MP, lb/d        : "), formatC(ifelse(tolower(Unit) == "metric", anim.diet.MP.rate, kgTOlb(anim.diet.MP.rate)), format = "f", digits = 3, width = 7), "\n", sep = ""))
        cat(paste(string("-", 50), "  ",
                  ifelse(tolower(Unit) == "metric", "NEm, Mcal/kg    : ", "NEm, Mcal/lb    : "), formatC(ifelse(tolower(Unit) == "metric", anim.diet.NEm.frac, PERkgTOPERlb(anim.diet.NEm.frac)), format = "f", digits = 3, width = 7), "  ",
                  " MP bact, %     : ", formatC(isz(anim.diet.bact.MP.rate * 100, anim.diet.MP.rate) , format = "f", digits = 3, width = 7), "\n", sep = ""))
        cat(paste("Maintenance                          : ", formatC(ratio.NEmr.MEmr * 100, format = "f", digits = 3, width = 7), "  ", formatC(ratio.NPmr.MPmr * 100, format = "f", digits = 3, width = 7), "  ",
```

```
                 ifelse(tolower(Unit) == "metric", "NEg, Mcal/kg   : ", "NEg, Mcal/lb   : "), formatC(ifelse(tolower(Unit) == "metric", anim.diet.NEg.frac, PERkgTOPERlb(anim.diet.NEg.frac)), format = "f", digits = 3, width = 7), "  ",
                 "  MP feeds, %  : ", formatC(isz(anim.diet.fd.MP.rate * 100, anim.diet.MP.rate) , format = "f", digits = 3, width = 7), "\n", sep = ""))
      cat(paste("Pregnancy                        : ", formatC(ratio.NEpr.MEpr * 100, format = "f", digits = 3, width = 7), "  ", formatC(ratio.NPpr.MPpr * 100, format = "f", digits = 3, width = 7), "  ",
                 ifelse(tolower(Unit) == "metric", "NEl, Mcal/kg   : ", "NEl, Mcal/lb   : "), formatC(ifelse(tolower(Unit) == "metric", anim.diet.NEl.frac, PERkgTOPERlb(anim.diet.NEl.frac)), format = "f", digits = 3, width = 7), "  ",
                 "DCAB1, meq/100g: ", formatC(anim.DCAB1.rate, format = "f", digits = 2, width = 7), "\n", sep = ""))
      cat(paste("Lactation                        : ", formatC(ratio.NElr.MElr * 100, format = "f", digits = 3, width = 7), "  ", formatC(ratio.NPlr.MPlr * 100, format = "f", digits = 3, width = 7), "  ",
                 "CH4, g/d       : ", formatC(rum.diet.methane.rate * 1000, format = "f", digits = 3, width = 7), "  ",
                 "DCAB2, meq/100g: ", formatC(anim.DCAB3.rate, format = "f", digits = 2, width = 7), "\n", sep = ""))
    } else
    {
      cat(paste(ifelse(tolower(Unit) == "metric", "Average daily gain, kg/d", "Average daily gain, lb/d"), string(" ", 50 - 24), "  ",
                 "NFC, % DM      : ", formatC(isz(anim.diet.NFC.rate * 100,anim.diet.DMI.rate), format = "f", digits = 3, width = 7), "  ",
                 "Ash, % DM      : ", formatC(isz(anim.diet.ash.rate * 100,anim.diet.DMI.rate), format = "f", digits = 3, width = 7), "\n", sep = ""))
      if (anim.body.ADG>0)
      {
        cat(paste("   ME allowable gain (", formatC(100*anim.SWG_MEallowable/anim.body.ADG,format = "f", digits=2, width = 7),
                  "% obs)      : ", formatC(ifelse(tolower(Unit) == "metric", anim.SWG_MEallowable, kgTOlb(anim.SWG_MEallowable)), format = "f", digits = 3, width = 7), "  ",
                  string("-", nchar(subtitle2)), "\n", sep = ""))
        cat(paste("   MP allowable gain (",formatC(100*anim.SWG_MPallowable/anim.body.ADG,format = "f", digits=2, width = 7),
                  "% obs)      : ", formatC(ifelse(tolower(Unit) == "metric", anim.SWG_MPallowable, kgTOlb(anim.SWG_MPallowable)), format = "f", digits = 3, width = 7), "  ",
                  "tTDN, % DM      : ", formatC(anim.diet.tTDN.conc, format = "f", digits = 3, width = 7), "  ",
                  "RDP, % CP       : ", formatC(isz((anim.diet.CP.rate - rum.diet.RUCP.rate) * 100, anim.diet.CP.rate), format = "f", digits = 3, width = 7), "\n", sep = ""))
        cat(paste("   ", anim.SWG_MAAallowable.label_min, " allowable gain (", formatC(100*anim.SWG_MAAallowable.rate_min/anim.body.ADG,format = "f", digits=2, width = 7),
                  "% obs)     : ", formatC(ifelse(tolower(Unit) == "metric", anim.SWG_MAAallowable.rate_min, kgTOlb(anim.SWG_MAAallowable.rate_min)), format = "f", digits = 3, width = 7), "  ",
                  "aTDN, % DM      : ", formatC(anim.diet.aTDN.conc, format = "f", digits = 3, width = 7), "  ",
                  "RDP, % DM       : ", formatC(isz((anim.diet.CP.rate - rum.diet.RUCP.rate) * 100, anim.diet.DMI.rate), format = "f", digits = 3, width = 7), "\n", sep = ""))
      } else
      {
        cat(paste("   ME allowable gain                        : ", formatC(ifelse(tolower(Unit) == "metric", anim.SWG_MEallowable, kgTOlb(anim.SWG_MEallowable)), format = "f", digits = 3, width = 7), "  ",
                  string("-", nchar(subtitle2)), "\n", sep = ""))
        cat(paste("   MP allowable gain                        : ", formatC(ifelse(tolower(Unit) == "metric", anim.SWG_MPallowable,kgTOlb(anim.SWG_MPallowable)), format = "f", digits = 3, width = 7), "  ",
                  "tTDN, % DM      : ", formatC(anim.diet.tTDN.conc, format = "f", digits = 3, width = 7), "  ",
                  "RDP, % CP        : ", formatC(isz((anim.diet.CP.rate - rum.diet.RUCP.rate) * 100, anim.diet.CP.rate), format = "f", digits = 3, width = 7), "\n", sep = ""))
```

```
        cat(paste("    ", anim.SWG_MAAallowable.label_min, " allowable gain                  : ",
formatC(ifelse(tolower(Unit) == "metric", anim.SWG_MAAallowable.rate_min, kgTOlb(anim.SWG_MAAallowable.rate_min)), format =
"f", digits = 3, width = 7), "   ",
                        "aTDN, % DM      : ", formatC(anim.diet.aTDN.conc, format = "f", digits = 3, width = 7), "   ",
                        "RDP, % DM       : ", formatC(isz((anim.diet.CP.rate - rum.diet.RUCP.rate) * 100, anim.diet.DMI.rate), for-
mat = "f", digits = 3, width = 7), "\n", sep = ""))
        }
        cat(paste("   User-inputted (obs)                        : ", formatC(ifelse(tolower(Unit) == "metric", anim.body.ADG,
kgTOlb(anim.body.ADG)), format = "f", digits = 3, width = 7), "   ",
                     ifelse(tolower(Unit) == "metric", "GE, Mcal/kg     : ", "GE, Mcal/lb     : "), formatC(ifelse(tolower(Unit) ==
"metric", anim.diet.GE.frac, PERkgTOPERlb(anim.diet.GE.frac)), format = "f", digits = 3, width = 7), "   ",
                     "RUP, % CP       : ", formatC(isz(rum.diet.RUCP.rate * 100, anim.diet.CP.rate), format = "f", digits = 3, width
= 7), "\n", sep = ""))
        cat(paste(string(" ", 50), "   ",
                     "DE, Mcal/kg     : ", formatC(anim.diet.DE.frac, format = "f", digits = 3, width = 7), "   ",
                     "RUP, % DM       : ", formatC(isz(rum.diet.RUCP.rate * 100, anim.diet.DMI.rate), format = "f", digits = 3,
width = 7), "\n", sep = ""))
        subtitle1 <- "Efficiency of use, %                Energy   Protein"
        cat(paste(subtitle1, "   ",
                     ifelse(tolower(Unit) == "metric", "ME, Mcal/kg     : ", "ME, Mcal/lb     : "), formatC(ifelse(tolower(Unit) ==
"metric", anim.diet.ME.frac, PERkgTOPERlb(anim.diet.ME.frac)), format = "f", digits = 3, width = 7), "   ",
                     ifelse(tolower(Unit) == "metric", "MP, kg/d        : ", "MP, lb/d        : "), formatC(ifelse(tolower(Unit) ==
"metric", anim.diet.MP.rate, kgTOlb(anim.diet.MP.rate)), format = "f", digits = 3, width = 7), "\n", sep = ""))
        cat(paste(string("-", 50), "   ",
                     ifelse(tolower(Unit) == "metric", "NEm, Mcal/kg    : ", "NEm, Mcal/lb    : "), formatC(ifelse(tolower(Unit) ==
"metric", anim.diet.NEm.frac, PERkgTOPERlb(anim.diet.NEm.frac)), format = "f", digits = 3, width = 7), "   ",
                     "  MP bact,   %  : ", formatC(isz(anim.diet.bact.MP.rate * 100, anim.diet.MP.rate) , format = "f", digits = 3,
width = 7), "\n", sep = ""))
        cat(paste("Maintenance                       : ", formatC(ratio.NEmr.MEmr * 100, format = "f", digits = 3, width = 7), "
", formatC(ratio.NPmr.MPmr * 100, format = "f", digits = 3, width = 7), "   ",
                     ifelse(tolower(Unit) == "metric", "NEg, Mcal/kg    : ", "NEg, Mcal/lb    : "), formatC(ifelse(tolower(Unit) ==
"metric", anim.diet.NEg.frac, PERkgTOPERlb(anim.diet.NEg.frac)), format = "f", digits = 3, width = 7), "   ",
                     "  MP feeds, %   : ", formatC(isz(anim.diet.fd.MP.rate * 100, anim.diet.MP.rate) , format = "f", digits = 3,
width = 7), "\n", sep = ""))
        cat(paste("Pregnancy                         : ", formatC(ratio.NEpr.MEpr * 100, format = "f", digits = 3, width = 7), "
", formatC(ratio.NPpr.MPpr * 100, format = "f", digits = 3, width = 7), "   ",
                     ifelse(tolower(Unit) == "metric", "NEl, Mcal/kg    : ", "NEl, Mcal/lb    : "), formatC(ifelse(tolower(Unit) ==
"metric", anim.diet.NEl.frac, PERkgTOPERlb(anim.diet.NEl.frac)), format = "f", digits = 3, width = 7), "   ",
                     "DCAB1, meq/100g: ", formatC(anim.DCAB1.rate, format = "f", digits = 2, width = 7), "\n", sep = ""))
        cat(paste("Growth                            : ", formatC(ratio.NEgr.MEgr * 100, format = "f", digits = 3, width = 7), "
", formatC(ratio.NPgr.MPgr * 100, format = "f", digits = 3, width = 7), "   ",
                     "CH4, g/d        : ", formatC(rum.diet.methane.rate * 1000, format = "f", digits = 3, width = 7), "   ",
                     "DCAB2, meq/100g: ", formatC(anim.DCAB3.rate, format = "f", digits = 2, width = 7), "\n", sep = ""))
      }

      # Ration summary
      if (length(anim.fd.DMI.rate)>=10)
      {
        newpage()
        if (existsnonNA("granst.selected") != FALSE & exists("granst.list2") != FALSE)
        {
```

```
          title <- granst.list2[granst.selected]
          if (nchar(title) > 102)
          {
            title <- substr(title, 1, 102)
          }
          cat(paste(string(" ", floor((102 - nchar(title))/2)), title,"\n", sep=""))
          #cat(paste(string(" ", floor((102 - nchar(title))/2)), string(".", nchar(title)), "\n", sep=""))
        }
        cat(paste(string(" ", floor((102 - nchar(heading))/2)), heading,"\n", sep=""))
        cat(paste(string(" ", floor((102 - nchar(heading))/2)), string("=", nchar(heading)), "\n\n", sep=""))
      } else
      {
        cat("\n\n")
      }
      cat(paste("Feed name (ID)", string(" ", 50 - 14), "  ", "Dry Matter", string(" ", 24 - 10), "  ", "As-fed", "\n", sep = ""))
      cat(paste(string("-", 50), "  ", string("-", 24), "  ", string("-", 24), "\n", sep = ""))
      if (tolower(Unit) == "metric")
      {
        cat(paste(string(" ", 50), "  ", "   $/kg", "  ", "   kg/d", "  ", "      %", "  ", "   $/kg", "  ", "   kg/d", "  ", "      %", "\n", sep = ""))
        cat(paste(string("-", 50), "  ", string("-", 24), "  ", string("-", 24), "\n", sep = ""))
        for (i in 1:length(anim.fd.DMI.rate))
        {
          fdDM <- as.numeric(feeds3[, "DM"])/100
          fdtxt <- substr(paste(feeds3[i, "FeedName.x"], " (", feeds3[i,"FeedID"], ")", sep = ""), 1, 50)
          cat(paste(fdtxt, string(" ", 50 - nchar(fdtxt)), "  ",
                    formatC(anim.fd.Price.amt[i], format = "f", digits = 3, width = 7), "  ",
                    formatC(anim.fd.DMI.rate[i], format = "f", digits = 3, width = 7), "  ",
                    formatC(isz(anim.fd.DMI.rate[i] * 100, anim.diet.DMI.rate), format = "f", digits = 3, width = 7), "  ",
                    formatC(anim.fd.Price.amt[i] * fdDM[i], format = "f", digits = 3, width = 7), "  ",
                    formatC(isz(anim.fd.DMI.rate[i], fdDM[i]), format = "f", digits = 3, width = 7), "  ",
                    formatC(isz(anim.fd.AFI.rate[i] * 100, anim.diet.AFI.rate) , format = "f", digits = 3, width = 7), "\n", sep = ""))
        }
        cat(paste(string("-", 50), "  ", string("-", 24), "  ", string("-", 24), "\n", sep = ""))
        cat(paste("Total", string(" ", 50 - 5), "  ",
                  formatC(anim.diet.Price.amt, format = "f", digits = 3, width = 7), "  ",
                  formatC(anim.diet.DMI.rate, format = "f", digits = 3, width = 7), "  ",
                  formatC(100, format = "f", digits = 0, width = 6), "  ",
                  formatC(isz(anim.diet.Price.amt * anim.diet.DMI.rate, anim.diet.AFI.rate), format = "f", digits = 3, width = 7), "  ",
                  formatC(anim.diet.AFI.rate, format = "f", digits = 3, width = 7), "  ",
                  formatC(100, format = "f", digits = 0, width = 6), "\n", sep = ""))
        cat("\n\n")

        # Costs
        cat("Costs\n")
        cat(paste(string("-", 102), "\n", sep = ""))
        cat(paste(frmttxt("Ration:", 34), frmttxt("Production:", 34), frmttxt("Environmental:", 34), "\n", sep=""))
```

```
        cat(paste(frmttxt(paste("  $", format(anim.diet.Price.rate, format = "f", digits = 2, width = 6, justify = "right", nsmall = 2), "/day", sep=""), 34),
                  frmttxt(paste("  $", ifelse(isLactating==TRUE,
                                paste(format(isz(anim.diet.Price.rate, pmin.positive(c(anim.MY_MEallowable, anim.MY_MPallowable, anim.MY_MAAallowable.rate_min))), format = "f", digits = 2, width = 6, justify = "right", nsmall = 2), "/kg milk", sep=""),
                                paste(format(isz(anim.diet.Price.rate, pmin.positive(c(anim.SWG_MEallowable, anim.SWG_MPallowable, anim.SWG_MAAallowable.rate_min))), format = "f", digits = 2, width = 6, justify = "right", nsmall = 2), "/kg gain", sep = "")), sep=""), 34),
                  frmttxt(paste("  $", format(isz(anim.diet.Price.rate, rum.diet.methane.rate), format = "f", digits = 2, width = 6, justify = "right", nsmall = 2), "/kg of methane", sep=""), 34), "\n", sep=""))
        cat(paste(frmttxt(paste("  $", format(anim.diet.Price.amt * 1000, format = "f", digits = 2, width = 6, justify = "right", nsmall = 2), "/Metric Ton (DM Basis)", sep=""), 34),
                  frmttxt(paste("  $", format(isz(anim.diet.Price.rate*100, anim.diet.aTDN.rate), format = "f", digits = 2, width = 6, justify = "right", nsmall = 2), "/100 kg aTDN", sep=""), 34),
                  frmttxt(paste("  $", format(isz(anim.diet.Price.rate*100, rum.diet.methane.rate * 1000/0.6556), format = "f", digits = 2, width = 6, justify = "right", nsmall = 2), "/100 L of methane", sep=""), 34), "\n", sep=""))
        cat(paste(frmttxt(paste("  $", format(anim.diet.Price.amt * 1000 * (anim.diet.DM.conc/100), format = "f", digits = 2, width = 6, justify = "right", nsmall = 2), "/Metric Ton (AF Basis)", sep=""), 34),
                  frmttxt(paste("  $", format(isz(anim.diet.Price.rate*100, anim.diet.ME.rate), format = "f", digits = 2, width = 6, justify = "right", nsmall = 2), "/100 kg ME", sep=""), 34),
                  frmttxt("", 34), "\n", sep=""))
        cat(paste(frmttxt("", 34),
                  frmttxt(paste("  $", format(isz(anim.diet.Price.rate*100, anim.diet.NEg.rate), format = "f", digits = 2, width = 6, justify = "right", nsmall = 2), "/100 kg NEg", sep=""), 34),
                  frmttxt("", 34), "\n", sep=""))
        cat(paste(frmttxt("", 34),
                  frmttxt(paste("  $", format(isz(anim.diet.Price.rate*100, anim.diet.MP.rate), format = "f", digits = 2, width = 6, justify = "right", nsmall = 2), "/100 kg MP", sep=""), 34),
                  frmttxt("", 34), "\n", sep=""))
        cat(paste(string("-", 102), "\n", sep = ""))
      } else
      {
        cat(paste(string(" ", 50), "  ", "  $/lb", "  ", "   lb/d", "  ", "     %", "  ", "  $/lb", "  ", "   lb/d", "  ", "     %", "\n", sep = ""))
        cat(paste(string("-", 50), "  ", string("-", 24), "  ", string("-", 24), "\n", sep = ""))
        for (i in 1:length(anim.fd.DMI.rate))
        {
          fdDM <- as.numeric(feeds3[, "DM"])/100
          fdtxt <- substr(paste(feeds3[i, "FeedName.x"], " (", feeds3[i,"FeedID"], ")", sep = ""), 1, 50)
          cat(paste(fdtxt, string(" ", 50 - nchar(fdtxt)), "  ",
                    formatC(PERlb(anim.fd.Price.amt[i], T), format = "f", digits = 3, width = 7), "  ",
                    formatC(kgTOlb(anim.fd.DMI.rate[i]), format = "f", digits = 3, width = 7), "  ",
                    formatC(isz(anim.fd.DMI.rate[i] * 100, anim.diet.DMI.rate), format = "f", digits = 3, width = 7), "  ",
                    formatC(PERlb(anim.fd.Price.amt[i], T) * fdDM[i], format = "f", digits = 3, width = 7), "  ",
                    formatC(isz(kgTOlb(anim.fd.DMI.rate[i]), fdDM[i]), format = "f", digits = 3, width = 7), "  ",
                    formatC(isz(anim.fd.AFI.rate[i] * 100, anim.diet.AFI.rate) , format = "f", digits = 3, width = 7), "\n", sep = ""))
        }
        cat(paste(string("-", 50), "  ", string("-", 24), "  ", string("-", 24), "\n", sep = ""))
        cat(paste("Total", string(" ", 50 - 5), "  ",
```

```
                    formatC(PERlb(anim.diet.Price.amt, T), format = "f", digits = 3, width = 7), "  ",
                    formatC(kgTOlb(anim.diet.DMI.rate), format = "f", digits = 3, width = 7), "  ",
                    formatC(100, format = "f", digits = 0, width = 6), "  ",
                    formatC(isz(PERlb(anim.diet.Price.amt, T) * anim.diet.DMI.rate, anim.diet.AFI.rate), format = "f", digits = 3, width = 7), "  ",
                    formatC(kgTOlb(anim.diet.AFI.rate), format = "f", digits = 3, width = 7), "  ",
                    formatC(100, format = "f", digits = 0, width = 6), "\n", sep = ""))
        cat("\n\n")

        # Costs
        cat("Costs\n")
        cat(paste(string("-", 102), "\n", sep = ""))
        cat(paste(frmttxt("Ration:", 34), frmttxt("Production:", 34), frmttxt("Environmental:", 34), "\n", sep=""))
        cat(paste(frmttxt(paste("  $", format(anim.diet.Price.rate, format = "f", digits = 2, width = 6, justify = "right", nsmall = 2), "/day", sep=""), 34),
                    frmttxt(paste("  $", ifelse(isLactating==TRUE,
                                        paste(format(isz(anim.diet.Price.rate, kgTOlb(pmin.positive(c(anim.MY_MEallowable, anim.MY_MPallowable, anim.MY_MAAallowable.rate_min)))), format = "f", digits = 2, width = 6, justify = "right", nsmall = 2), "/lb milk", sep=""),
                                        paste(format(isz(anim.diet.Price.rate, kgTOlb(pmin.positive(c(anim.SWG_MEallowable, anim.SWG_MPallowable, anim.SWG_MAAallowable.rate_min)))), format = "f", digits = 2, width = 6, justify = "right", nsmall = 2), "/lb gain", sep = "")), sep=""), 34),
                    frmttxt(paste("  $", format(isz(anim.diet.Price.rate, kgTOlb(rum.diet.methane.rate)), format = "f", digits = 2, width = 6, justify = "right", nsmall = 2), "/lb of methane", sep=""), 34), "\n", sep=""))
        cat(paste(frmttxt(paste("  $", format(PERlb(anim.diet.Price.amt, T) * 2000, format = "f", digits = 2, width = 6, justify = "right", nsmall = 2), "/English Ton (DM Basis)", sep=""), 34),
                    frmttxt(paste("  $", format(isz(anim.diet.Price.rate*100, kgTOlb(anim.diet.aTDN.rate)), format = "f", digits = 2, width = 6, justify = "right", nsmall = 2), "/100 lb aTDN", sep=""), 34),
                    frmttxt(paste("  $", format(isz(anim.diet.Price.rate*100, rum.diet.methane.rate * 1000/0.6556), format = "f", digits = 2, width = 6, justify = "right", nsmall = 2), "/100 L of methane", sep=""), 34), "\n", sep=""))
        cat(paste(frmttxt(paste("  $", format(PERlb(anim.diet.Price.amt, T) * 2000 * (anim.diet.DM.conc/100), format = "f", digits = 2, width = 6, justify = "right", nsmall = 2), "/English Ton (AF Basis)", sep=""), 34),
                    frmttxt(paste("  $", format(isz(anim.diet.Price.rate*100, kgTOlb(anim.diet.ME.rate)), format = "f", digits = 2, width = 6, justify = "right", nsmall = 2), "/100 lb ME", sep=""), 34),
                    frmttxt("", 34), "\n", sep=""))
        cat(paste(frmttxt("", 34),
                    frmttxt(paste("  $", format(isz(anim.diet.Price.rate*100, kgTOlb(anim.diet.NEg.rate)), format = "f", digits = 2, width = 6, justify = "right", nsmall = 2), "/100 lb NEg", sep=""), 34),
                    frmttxt("", 34), "\n", sep=""))
        cat(paste(frmttxt("", 34),
                    frmttxt(paste("  $", format(isz(anim.diet.Price.rate*100, kgTOlb(anim.diet.MP.rate)), format = "f", digits = 2, width = 6, justify = "right", nsmall = 2), "/100 lb MP", sep=""), 34),
                    frmttxt("", 34), "\n", sep=""))
        cat(paste(string("-", 102), "\n", sep = ""))
      }
    }

    if (SolutionLevel == 2)
    {
      if (is.na(anim.species) | anim.diet.DMI.rate <= 0) return(invisible(NULL))
      cat("#Title/Inv#Summary Report\n")
```

```
    if (existsnonNA("granst.selected") != FALSE & exists("granst.list2") != FALSE)
    {
      title <- granst.list2[granst.selected]
      if (nchar(title) > 102)
      {
        title <- substr(title, 1, 102)
      }
      cat(paste(string(" ", floor((102 - nchar(title))/2)), title,"\n", sep=""))
      #cat(paste(string(" ", floor((102 - nchar(title))/2)), string(".", nchar(title)), "\n", sep=""))
    }
    # One line info
    heading <- paste("Species:", anim.species, " | Type:", anim.type, " | Sex:", anim.sex,  sep = "")
    if (anim.stage_type == "Lactating")
    {
      if (anim.type == "Milk")
      {
        heading <- paste(heading, " | MY:", trimws(formatC(ifelse(tolower(Unit) == "metric", anim.lactation.milk.rate, kgTOlb(anim.lactation.milk.rate)), format = "f", digits = 1, width = 5)),
                         " | DIM:", trimws(anim.lactation.days), sep = "")
      } else
      {
        heading <- paste(heading, " | MY:", trimws(formatC(ifelse(tolower(Unit) == "metric", anim.lactation.milk.peak.rate, kgTOlb(anim.lactation.milk.peak.rate)), format = "f", digits = 1, width = 5)),
                         " | DIM:", trimws(anim.lactation.days), sep = "")
      }
      heading <- paste(heading, " | DG:", trimws(anim.pregnancy.days), sep = "")
    }
    if (anim.stage_type == "Dry" | anim.stage_type == "Replacement")
      heading <- paste(heading, " | DG:", trimws(anim.pregnancy.days), sep = "")
    if (anim.stage_type == "Growing/Finishing" & anim.species == "Cattle")
      heading <- paste(heading," | SRW:", trimws(formatC(ifelse(tolower(Unit) == "metric", anim.body.weight_standard, kgTOlb(anim.body.weight_standard)), format = "f", digits = 0, width = 4)),
                       " | MBW:", trimws(formatC(ifelse(tolower(Unit) == "metric", anim.body.weight_mature, kgTOlb(anim.body.weight_mature)), format = "f", digits = 0, width = 4)), sep = "")
    if (tolower(anim.stage_option) == "mean")
    {
      heading <- paste(heading, " | BW:", formatC(ifelse(tolower(Unit) == "metric", anim.body.weight_mean, kgTOlb(anim.body.weight_mean)), format = "f", digits = 0, width = 4),
                       " | BCS:", formatC(anim.body.condition_mean, format = "f", digits = 1, width = 3), sep = "")
    } else
    {
      heading <- paste(heading, " | BW:(", trimws(formatC(ifelse(tolower(Unit) == "metric", anim.body.weight_initial, kgTOlb(anim.body.weight_initial)), format = "f", digits = 0, width = 4)), "-",
                       trimws(formatC(ifelse(tolower(Unit) == "metric", anim.body.weight_final, kgTOlb(anim.body.weight_final)), format = "f", digits = 0, width = 4)), ")",
                       " | BCS:(", trimws(formatC(anim.body.condition_initial, format = "f", digits = 1, width = 3)), "-",
                       trimws(formatC(anim.body.condition_final, format = "f", digits = 1, width = 3)), ")", sep="")
    }
    cat(paste(string(" ", floor((102 - nchar(heading))/2)), heading, "\n", sep=""))
    cat(paste(string(" ", floor((102 - nchar(heading))/2)), string("=", nchar(heading)), "\n\n", sep=""))
    #cat("\n")
```

```
    #title <- "Summary Report"
    #cat(paste(title, "\n", string("=", nchar(title)), "\n\n", sep = ""))
    subtitle1 <- "Metabolizable Energy (ME) Balance"
    subtitle1 <- paste(subtitle1, string(" ", 34 - nchar(subtitle1)), sep = "")
    subtitle2 <- "Metabolizable Protein (MP) Balance"
    subtitle2 <- paste(subtitle2, string(" ", 34 - nchar(subtitle2)), sep = "")
    cat(paste("Items", string(" ", 13 - 5), " ", subtitle1, "  ", subtitle2, "  ", "   Ca   ", "  ", "    P","\n",
              string("-", 13), " ", string("-", nchar(subtitle1)), "  ", string("-", nchar(subtitle2)), "  ", string("-", 7),
"  ", string("-", 7), "\n", sep = ""))
    cat(paste(string(" ", 13), " Available    Required     Balance   Available    Required     Balance       g/d
g/d","\n", sep = ""))
    cat(paste(string(" ", 13), "    Mcal/d      Mcal/d      Mcal/d         g/d         g/d         g/d","\n", sep = ""))
    cat(paste(string(" ", 13), " ", string("-", nchar(subtitle1)), "  ", string("-", nchar(subtitle2)), "  ", string("-", 7),
"  ", string("-", 7), "\n", sep = ""))
    cat(paste("Supplied      ", formatC(anim.diet.ME.rate, format = "f", digits = 3, width = 10), string(" ", 2 + 10 + 2 + 10
+ 2),
              formatC(anim.diet.MP.rate*1000, format = "f", digits = 2, width = 10), string(" ", 2 + 10 + 2 + 10 + 2),
              formatC(si.diet.GCa.rate*1000, format = "f", digits = 2, width = 7), string(" ", 2),
              formatC(si.diet.GP.rate*1000, format = "f", digits = 2, width = 7), "\n", sep=""))
    cat(paste(string("-", 13 + 1 + 34 + 2 + 34 + 2 + 7 + 2 + 7), "\n", sep = ""))
    cat(paste("Required\n"))
    cat(paste("  Maintenance ",
              formatC(anim.MEm_available.rate, format = "f", digits = 3, width = 10), string(" ", 2),
              formatC(anim.MEm_required.rate, format = "f", digits = 3, width = 10), string(" ", 2),
              formatC(anim.MEm_balance.rate, format = "f", digits = 3, width = 10), string(" ", 2),
              formatC(anim.MPm_available.rate, format = "f", digits = 2, width = 10), string(" ", 2),
              formatC(anim.MPm_required.rate, format = "f", digits = 2, width = 10), string(" ", 2),
              formatC(anim.MPm_balance.rate, format = "f", digits = 2, width = 10), string(" ", 2),
              formatC(anim.Ca.maintenance, format = "f", digits = 2, width = 7), string(" ", 2),
              formatC(anim.P.maintenance, format = "f", digits = 2, width = 7), "\n", sep=""))
    cat(paste("  Pregnancy   ",
              formatC(anim.MEp_available.rate, format = "f", digits = 3, width = 10), string(" ", 2),
              formatC(anim.MEp_required.rate, format = "f", digits = 3, width = 10), string(" ", 2),
              formatC(anim.MEp_balance.rate, format = "f", digits = 3, width = 10), string(" ", 2),
              formatC(anim.MPp_available.rate, format = "f", digits = 2, width = 10), string(" ", 2),
              formatC(anim.MPp_required.rate, format = "f", digits = 2, width = 10), string(" ", 2),
              formatC(anim.MPp_balance.rate, format = "f", digits = 2, width = 10), string(" ", 2),
              formatC(anim.Ca.pregnancy, format = "f", digits = 2, width = 7), string(" ", 2),
              formatC(anim.P.pregnancy, format = "f", digits = 2, width = 7), "\n", sep=""))
    cat(paste("  Lactation   ",
              formatC(anim.MEl_available.rate, format = "f", digits = 3, width = 10), string(" ", 2),
              formatC(anim.MEl_required.rate, format = "f", digits = 3, width = 10), string(" ", 2),
              formatC(anim.MEl_balance.rate, format = "f", digits = 3, width = 10), string(" ", 2),
              formatC(anim.MPl_available.rate, format = "f", digits = 2, width = 10), string(" ", 2),
              formatC(anim.MPl_required.rate, format = "f", digits = 2, width = 10), string(" ", 2),
              formatC(anim.MPl_balance.rate, format = "f", digits = 2, width = 10), string(" ", 2),
              formatC(anim.Ca.lactation, format = "f", digits = 2, width = 7), string(" ", 2),
              formatC(anim.P.lactation, format = "f", digits = 2, width = 7), "\n", sep=""))
    cat(paste("  Growth      ",
              formatC(anim.MEg_available.rate, format = "f", digits = 3, width = 10), string(" ", 2),
              formatC(anim.MEg_required.rate, format = "f", digits = 3, width = 10), string(" ", 2),
```

```
                    formatC(anim.MEg_balance.rate, format = "f", digits = 3, width = 10), string(" ", 2),
                    formatC(anim.MPg_available.rate, format = "f", digits = 2, width = 10), string(" ", 2),
                    formatC(anim.MPg_required.rate, format = "f", digits = 2, width = 10), string(" ", 2),
                    formatC(anim.MPg_balance.rate, format = "f", digits = 2, width = 10), string(" ", 2),
                    formatC(anim.Ca.growth, format = "f", digits = 2, width = 7), string(" ", 2),
                    formatC(anim.P.growth, format = "f", digits = 2, width = 7), "\n", sep=""))
        cat(paste("  Reserves     ",
                    formatC(anim.MEr_available.rate, format = "f", digits = 3, width = 10), string(" ", 2),
                    formatC(anim.MEr_required.rate, format = "f", digits = 3, width = 10), string(" ", 2),
                    formatC(anim.MEr_balance.rate, format = "f", digits = 3, width = 10), string(" ", 2),
                    formatC(anim.MPr_available.rate, format = "f", digits = 2, width = 10), string(" ", 2),
                    formatC(anim.MPr_required.rate, format = "f", digits = 2, width = 10), string(" ", 2),
                    formatC(anim.MPr_balance.rate, format = "f", digits = 2, width = 10), string(" ", 2),
                    "  ---   ", string(" ", 2), "  ---   ", "\n", sep=""))
        cat(paste(string("-", 13 + 1 + 34 + 2 + 34 + 2 + 7 + 2 + 7), "\n", sep = ""))
        cat(paste("Balance          ",
                    formatC(anim.MEe_available.rate, format = "f", digits = 3, width = 10), string(" ", 2),
                    formatC(anim.MEe_required.rate, format = "f", digits = 3, width = 10), string(" ", 2),
                    formatC(anim.MEe_balance.rate, format = "f", digits = 3, width = 10), string(" ", 2),
                    formatC(anim.MPe_available.rate, format = "f", digits = 2, width = 10), string(" ", 2),
                    formatC(anim.MPe_required.rate, format = "f", digits = 2, width = 10), string(" ", 2),
                    formatC(anim.MPe_balance.rate, format = "f", digits = 2, width = 10), string(" ", 2),
                    formatC(anim.Ca.balance.rate, format = "f", digits = 2, width = 7), string(" ", 2),
                    formatC(anim.P.balance.rate, format = "f", digits = 2, width = 7), "\n", sep=""))
        cat("\n\n")
        subtitle1 <- "Animal Intake & Performance"
        subtitle1 <- paste(subtitle1, string(" ", 50 - nchar(subtitle1)), sep = "")
        subtitle2 <- "Diet Summary & Nutrient Fractionation"
        subtitle2 <- paste(subtitle2, string(" ", 50 - nchar(subtitle2)), sep = "")
        cat(paste(subtitle1, "  ", subtitle2, "\n", string("-", nchar(subtitle1)), "  ", string("-", nchar(subtitle2)), "\n", sep
= ""))
        cat(paste(ifelse(tolower(Unit) == "metric", "Dry matter intake, kg/d", "Dry matter intake, lb/d"), string(" ", 50 - 23), "
",
                    "DM, % AF        : ", formatC(anim.diet.DM.conc, format = "f", digits = 3, width = 7), "  ",
                    "CHO fractions, % DM\n", sep = ""))

        if (anim.diet.DMI.rate>0)
        {
          cat(paste("   Predicted [", formatC(ifelse(tolower(Unit) == "metric", anim.DMI.rate_min, kgTOlb(anim.DMI.rate_min)),
format = "f", digits = 2, width = 5), "; ",
                      formatC(ifelse(tolower(Unit) == "metric", anim.DMI.rate_max, kgTOlb(anim.DMI.rate_max)), format = "f", digits
= 2, width = 5), "](",
                      formatC(100 * anim.DMI.rate_avg/anim.diet.DMI.rate, format = "f", digits = 2, width = 7), "% obs): ",
formatC(ifelse(tolower(Unit) == "metric", anim.DMI.rate_avg, kgTOlb(anim.DMI.rate_avg)), format = "f", digits = 3, width = 7),
"  ",
                      "Forage, %       : ", formatC(anim.diet.Forage.frac * 100, format = "f", digits = 3, width = 7), "  ",
                      "  A1|VFA          : ", formatC(isz(anim.diet.CHOA1.rate * 100, anim.diet.DMI.rate), format = "f", digits = 3,
width = 6), "\n", sep = ""))
        } else
        {
```

```
      cat(paste("    Predicted [", formatC(ifelse(tolower(Unit) == "metric", anim.DMI.rate_min, kgTOlb(anim.DMI.rate_min)), format = "f", digits = 2, width = 5), "; ",
                 formatC(ifelse(tolower(Unit) == "metric", anim.DMI.rate_max, kgTOlb(anim.DMI.rate_max)), format = "f", digits = 2, width = 5),
                 "]                : ", formatC(anim.DMI.rate_avg, format = "f", digits = 3, width = 7), "  ",
                 "Forage, %        : ", formatC(anim.diet.Forage.frac * 100, format = "f", digits = 3, width = 7), "  ",
                 "  A1|VFA          : ", formatC(isz(anim.diet.CHOA1.rate * 100, anim.diet.DMI.rate), format = "f", digits = 3, width = 6), "\n", sep = ""))
    }

    if (flag_DMRType==0)
    {
      cat(paste("    Required                                    : ", "  NA    ", "  ",
                 "CP, % DM         : ", formatC(anim.diet.CP.conc, format = "f", digits = 3, width = 7), "  ",
                 "  A2|Lactate      : ", formatC(isz(anim.diet.CHOA2.rate * 100, anim.diet.DMI.rate), format = "f", digits = 3, width = 6), "\n", sep = ""))
    } else
    {
      if (anim.diet.DMI.rate>0)
      {

        if (flag_DMRType==1)
        {
          cat(paste("    Required (ME basis, ", formatC(anim.DMR * 100/anim.diet.DMI.rate, format = "f", digits = 2, width = 6), "% obs)          : ",
                     formatC(ifelse(tolower(Unit) == "metric", anim.DMR, kgTOlb(anim.DMR)), format = "f", digits = 3, width = 7), "  ",
                     "CP, % DM         : ", formatC(anim.diet.CP.conc, format = "f", digits = 3, width = 7), "  ",
                     "  A2|Lactate      : ", formatC(isz(anim.diet.CHOA2.rate * 100, anim.diet.DMI.rate), format = "f", digits = 3, width = 6), "\n", sep = ""))
        }
        if (flag_DMRType==2)
        {
          cat(paste("    Required (MP basis, ", formatC(anim.DMR * 100/anim.diet.DMI.rate, format = "f", digits = 2, width = 6), "% obs)          : ",
                     formatC(ifelse(tolower(Unit) == "metric", anim.DMR, kgTOlb(anim.DMR)), format = "f", digits = 3, width = 7), "  ",
                     "CP, % DM         : ", formatC(anim.diet.CP.conc, format = "f", digits = 3, width = 7), "  ",
                     "  A2|Lactate      : ", formatC(isz(anim.diet.CHOA2.rate * 100, anim.diet.DMI.rate), format = "f", digits = 3, width = 6), "\n", sep = ""))
        }
        if (flag_DMRType==3)
        {
          if (isLactating==TRUE)
          {
            cat(paste("    Required (", anim.MY_MAAallowable.label_min," basis, ", formatC(anim.DMR * 100/anim.diet.DMI.rate, format = "f", digits = 2, width = 6), "% obs)      : ",
                       formatC(ifelse(tolower(Unit) == "metric", anim.DMR, kgTOlb(anim.DMR)), format = "f", digits = 3, width = 7), "  ",
                       "CP, % DM         : ", formatC(anim.diet.CP.conc, format = "f", digits = 3, width = 7), "  ",
```

```
                    "  A2|Lactate     : ", formatC(isz(anim.diet.CHOA2.rate * 100, anim.diet.DMI.rate), format = "f", digits = 3, width = 6), "\n", sep = ""))
          } else
          {
            cat(paste("   Required (", anim.SWG_MAAallowable.label_min," basis, ", formatC(anim.DMR * 100/anim.diet.DMI.rate, format = "f", digits = 2, width = 6), "% obs)      : ",
                    formatC(ifelse(tolower(Unit) == "metric", anim.DMR, kgTOlb(anim.DMR)), format = "f", digits = 3, width = 7), "  ",
                    "CP, % DM         : ", formatC(anim.diet.CP.conc, format = "f", digits = 3, width = 7), "  ",
                    "  A2|Lactate     : ", formatC(isz(anim.diet.CHOA2.rate * 100, anim.diet.DMI.rate), format = "f", digits = 3, width = 6), "\n", sep = ""))
          }
        }
        if (flag_DMRType==4)
        {
          cat(paste("   Required (ME & MP bases, ", formatC(anim.DMR * 100/anim.diet.DMI.rate, format = "f", digits = 2, width = 6), "% obs) : ",
                  formatC(ifelse(tolower(Unit) == "metric", anim.DMR, kgTOlb(anim.DMR)), format = "f", digits = 3, width = 7), "  ",
                  "CP, % DM         : ", formatC(anim.diet.CP.conc, format = "f", digits = 3, width = 7), "  ",
                  "  A2|Lactate     : ", formatC(isz(anim.diet.CHOA2.rate * 100, anim.diet.DMI.rate), format = "f", digits = 3, width = 6), "\n", sep = ""))
        }
        if (flag_DMRType==5)
        {
          if (isLactating==TRUE)
          {
            cat(paste("   Required (ME,MP,", anim.MY_MAAallowable.label_min, " bases,", formatC(anim.DMR * 100/anim.diet.DMI.rate, format = "f", digits = 2, width = 6), "% obs): ",
                    formatC(ifelse(tolower(Unit) == "metric", anim.DMR, kgTOlb(anim.DMR)), format = "f", digits = 3, width = 7), "  ",
                    "CP, % DM         : ", formatC(anim.diet.CP.conc, format = "f", digits = 3, width = 7), "  ",
                    "  A2|Lactate     : ", formatC(isz(anim.diet.CHOA2.rate * 100, anim.diet.DMI.rate), format = "f", digits = 3, width = 6), "\n", sep = ""))
          } else
          {
            cat(paste("   Required (ME,MP,", anim.SWG_MAAallowable.label_min, " bases,", formatC(anim.DMR * 100/anim.diet.DMI.rate, format = "f", digits = 2, width = 6), "% obs): ",
                    formatC(ifelse(tolower(Unit) == "metric", anim.DMR, kgTOlb(anim.DMR)), format = "f", digits = 3, width = 7), "  ",
                    "CP, % DM         : ", formatC(anim.diet.CP.conc, format = "f", digits = 3, width = 7), "  ",
                    "  A2|Lactate     : ", formatC(isz(anim.diet.CHOA2.rate * 100, anim.diet.DMI.rate), format = "f", digits = 3, width = 6), "\n", sep = ""))
          }
        }
        if (flag_DMRType==6)
        {
          if (isLactating==TRUE)
          {
            cat(paste("   Required (ME,MP,", anim.MY_MAAallowable.label_min, " bases,", formatC(anim.DMR * 100/anim.diet.DMI.rate, format = "f", digits = 2, width = 6), "% obs): ",
```

```
                    formatC(ifelse(tolower(Unit) == "metric", max(anim.DMR), kgTOlb(max(anim.DMR))), format = "f", digits = 3, width = 7), "  ",
                    "CP, % DM          : ", formatC(anim.diet.CP.conc, format = "f", digits = 3, width = 7), "  ",
                    "  A2|Lactate     : ", formatC(isz(anim.diet.CHOA2.rate * 100, anim.diet.DMI.rate), format = "f", digits = 3, width = 6), "\n", sep = ""))
            } else
            {
                cat(paste("   Required (ME,MP,", anim.SWG_MAAallowable.label_min, "bases,", formatC(anim.DMR * 100/anim.diet.DMI.rate, format = "f", digits = 2, width = 6), "% obs): ",
                    formatC(ifelse(tolower(Unit) == "metric", max(anim.DMR), kgTOlb(max(anim.DMR))), format = "f", digits = 3, width = 7), "  ",
                    "CP, % DM          : ", formatC(anim.diet.CP.conc, format = "f", digits = 3, width = 7), "  ",
                    "  A2|Lactate     : ", formatC(isz(anim.diet.CHOA2.rate * 100, anim.diet.DMI.rate), format = "f", digits = 3, width = 6), "\n", sep = ""))
            }
          }
        } else
        {
          if (flag_DMRType==1)
          {
            cat(paste("   Required (ME basis)                    : ",
                  formatC(ifelse(tolower(Unit) == "metric", anim.DMR, kgTOlb(anim.DMR)), format = "f", digits = 3, width = 7), "  ",
                  "CP, % DM          : ", formatC(anim.diet.CP.conc, format = "f", digits = 3, width = 7), "  ",
                  "  A2|Lactate     : ", formatC(isz(anim.diet.CHOA2.rate * 100, anim.diet.DMI.rate), format = "f", digits = 3, width = 6), "\n", sep = ""))
          }
          if (flag_DMRType==2)
          {
            cat(paste("   Required (MP basis)                    : ",
                  formatC(ifelse(tolower(Unit) == "metric", anim.DMR, kgTOlb(anim.DMR)), format = "f", digits = 3, width = 7), "  ",
                  "CP, % DM          : ", formatC(anim.diet.CP.conc, format = "f", digits = 3, width = 7), "  ",
                  "  A2|Lactate     : ", formatC(isz(anim.diet.CHOA2.rate * 100, anim.diet.DMI.rate), format = "f", digits = 3, width = 6), "\n", sep = ""))
          }
          if (flag_DMRType==3)
          {
            if (isLactating==TRUE)
            {
              cat(paste("   Required (", anim.MY_MAAallowable.label_min," basis)                    : ",
                    formatC(ifelse(tolower(Unit) == "metric", anim.DMR, kgTOlb(anim.DMR)), format = "f", digits = 3, width = 7), "  ",
                    "CP, % DM          : ", formatC(anim.diet.CP.conc, format = "f", digits = 3, width = 7), "  ",
                    "  A2|Lactate     : ", formatC(isz(anim.diet.CHOA2.rate * 100, anim.diet.DMI.rate), format = "f", digits = 3, width = 6), "\n", sep = ""))
            } else
            {
              cat(paste("   Required (", anim.SWG_MAAallowable.label_min," basis)                    : ",
                    formatC(ifelse(tolower(Unit) == "metric", anim.DMR, kgTOlb(anim.DMR)), format = "f", digits = 3, width = 7), "  ",
```

```
                              "CP, % DM          : ", formatC(anim.diet.CP.conc, format = "f", digits = 3, width = 7), "  ",
                              "  A2|Lactate     : ", formatC(isz(anim.diet.CHOA2.rate * 100, anim.diet.DMI.rate), format = "f", digits = 3, width = 6), "\n", sep = ""))
          }
        }
        if (flag_DMRType==4)
        {
          cat(paste("   Required (ME & MP bases)                    : ",
                        formatC(ifelse(tolower(Unit) == "metric", anim.DMR, kgTOlb(anim.DMR)), format = "f", digits = 3, width = 7), "  ",
                        "CP, % DM          : ", formatC(anim.diet.CP.conc, format = "f", digits = 3, width = 7), "  ",
                        "  A2|Lactate     : ", formatC(isz(anim.diet.CHOA2.rate * 100, anim.diet.DMI.rate), format = "f", digits = 3, width = 6), "\n", sep = ""))
        }
        if (flag_DMRType==5)
        {
          if (isLactating==TRUE)
          {
            cat(paste("   Required (ME,MP,", anim.MY_MAAallowable.label_min, " bases)             : ",
                          formatC(ifelse(tolower(Unit) == "metric", anim.DMR, kgTOlb(anim.DMR)), format = "f", digits = 3, width = 7), "  ",
                          "CP, % DM          : ", formatC(anim.diet.CP.conc, format = "f", digits = 3, width = 7), "  ",
                          "  A2|Lactate     : ", formatC(isz(anim.diet.CHOA2.rate * 100, anim.diet.DMI.rate), format = "f", digits = 3, width = 6), "\n", sep = ""))
          } else
          {
            cat(paste("   Required (ME,MP,", anim.SWG_MAAallowable.label_min, " bases)            : ",
                          formatC(ifelse(tolower(Unit) == "metric", anim.DMR, kgTOlb(anim.DMR)), format = "f", digits = 3, width = 7), "  ",
                          "CP, % DM          : ", formatC(anim.diet.CP.conc, format = "f", digits = 3, width = 7), "  ",
                          "  A2|Lactate     : ", formatC(isz(anim.diet.CHOA2.rate * 100, anim.diet.DMI.rate), format = "f", digits = 3, width = 6), "\n", sep = ""))
          }
        }
        if (flag_DMRType==6)
        {
          if (isLactating==TRUE)
          {
            cat(paste("   Required (ME,MP,", anim.MY_MAAallowable.label_min, " bases)             : ",
                          formatC(ifelse(tolower(Unit) == "metric", max(anim.DMR), kgTOlb(max(anim.DMR))), format = "f", digits = 3, width = 7), "  ",
                          "CP, % DM          : ", formatC(anim.diet.CP.conc, format = "f", digits = 3, width = 7), "  ",
                          "  A2|Lactate     : ", formatC(isz(anim.diet.CHOA2.rate * 100, anim.diet.DMI.rate), format = "f", digits = 3, width = 6), "\n", sep = ""))
          } else
          {
            cat(paste("   Required (ME,MP,", anim.SWG_MAAallowable.label_min, "bases)             : ",
                          formatC(ifelse(tolower(Unit) == "metric", max(anim.DMR), kgTOlb(max(anim.DMR))), format = "f", digits = 3, width = 7), "  ",
                          "CP, % DM          : ", formatC(anim.diet.CP.conc, format = "f", digits = 3, width = 7), "  ",
```

```
                        "  A2|Lactate     : ", formatC(isz(anim.diet.CHOA2.rate * 100, anim.diet.DMI.rate), format = "f", digits
= 3, width = 6), "\n", sep = ""))
              }
            }
          }
        }
        cat(paste("   User-inputted (obs)  (",formatC(isz(anim.diet.DMI.rate * 100, anim.body.weight_mean), format = "f", digits =
2, width = 4),"% BW)          : ", formatC(ifelse(tolower(Unit) == "metric", anim.diet.DMI.rate, kgTOlb(anim.diet.DMI.rate)),
format = "f", digits = 3, width = 7), "  ",
                        "Soluble CP, %CP: ", formatC(isz(anim.diet.SP.rate * 100,anim.diet.CP.rate), format = "f", digits = 3, width =
7), "  ",
                        "  A3|Organic Ac.: ", formatC(isz(anim.diet.CHOA3.rate * 100, anim.diet.DMI.rate), format = "f", digits = 3,
width = 6), "\n", sep = ""))
        cat(paste(ifelse(tolower(Unit) == "metric", "Predicted water intake, kg/d            : ", "Predicted water intake, lb/d
: "), formatC(ifelse(tolower(Unit) == "metric", anim.WI.rate, kgTOlb(anim.WI.rate)), format = "f", digits = 3, width = 7),"
",
                        "NPN, % CP      : ", formatC(isz(anim.diet.NPN.rate * 100, anim.diet.CP.rate), format = "f", digits = 3, width =
7), "  ",
                        "  A4|Sugars      : ", formatC(isz(anim.diet.CHOA4.rate * 100,anim.diet.DMI.rate), format = "f", digits = 3,
width = 6), "\n", sep = ""))
        if (isLactating == TRUE)
        {
          cat(paste(ifelse(tolower(Unit) == "metric", "Milk production, kg/d", "Milk production, lb/d"), string(" ", 50 - 21), "
",
                          "NDF, % DM      : ", formatC(isz(anim.diet.NDF.rate * 100,anim.diet.DMI.rate), format = "f", digits = 3, width
= 7), "  ",
                          "  B1|Starch      : ", formatC(isz(anim.diet.CHOB1.rate * 100,anim.diet.DMI.rate), format = "f", digits = 3,
width = 6), "\n", sep = ""))
          if (anim.lactation.milk.rate>0)
          {
            cat(paste("   ME allowable milk  (", formatC(100 * anim.MY_MEallowable/anim.lactation.milk.rate, format = "f", digits =
2, width = 7),
                            "% obs)       : ", formatC(ifelse(tolower(Unit) == "metric", anim.MY_MEallowable, kgTOlb(anim.MY_MEallowa-
ble)), format = "f", digits = 3, width = 7), "  ",
                            "ADF, % DM      : ", formatC(isz(anim.diet.ADF.rate * 100,anim.diet.DMI.rate), format = "f", digits = 3,
width = 7), "  ",
                            "  B2|Pectin      : ", formatC(isz(anim.diet.CHOB2.rate * 100,anim.diet.DMI.rate), format = "f", digits = 3,
width = 6), "\n", sep = ""))
            cat(paste("   MP allowable milk  (", formatC(100 * anim.MY_MPallowable/anim.lactation.milk.rate, format = "f", digits =
2, width = 7),
                            "% obs)       : ", formatC(ifelse(tolower(Unit) == "metric", anim.MY_MPallowable, kgTOlb(anim.MY_MPallowa-
ble)), format = "f", digits = 3, width = 7), "  ",
                            "Lignin, % NDF  : ", formatC(isz(anim.diet.lignin.rate * 100,anim.diet.NDF.rate), format = "f", digits = 3,
width = 7), "  ",
                            "  B3|Fiber       : ", formatC(isz(anim.diet.CHOB3.rate * 100,anim.diet.DMI.rate), format = "f", digits = 3,
width = 6), "\n", sep = ""))
            cat(paste("    ", anim.MY_MAAallowable.label_min, " allowable milk  (", formatC(100 * anim.MY_MAAallowa-
ble.rate_min/anim.lactation.milk.rate, format = "f", digits = 2, width = 7),
                            "% obs)      : ", formatC(ifelse(tolower(Unit) == "metric", anim.MY_MAAallowable.rate_min,
kgTOlb(anim.MY_MAAallwable.rate_min)), format = "f", digits = 3, width = 7), "  ",
```

```
                         "peNDF, % NDF    : ", formatC(isz(anim.diet.peNDF.rate * 100,anim.diet.NDF.rate), format = "f", digits = 3, width = 7), "  ",
                         "  C |Unavailable: ", formatC(isz(anim.diet.CHOC.rate * 100,anim.diet.DMI.rate), format = "f", digits = 3, width = 6), "\n", sep = ""))
        } else
        {
          cat(paste("   ME allowable milk                          : ", formatC(ifelse(tolower(Unit) == "metric", anim.MY_MEallowable, kgTOlb(anim.MY_MEallwable)), format = "f", digits = 3, width = 7), "  ",
                         "ADF, % DM       : ", formatC(isz(anim.diet.ADF.rate * 100,anim.diet.DMI.rate), format = "f", digits = 3, width = 7), "  ",
                         "  B2|Pectin      : ", formatC(isz(anim.diet.CHOB2.rate * 100,anim.diet.DMI.rate), format = "f", digits = 3, width = 6), "\n", sep = ""))
          cat(paste("   MP allowable milk                          : ", formatC(ifelse(tolower(Unit) == "metric", anim.MY_MPallowable, kgTOlb(anim.MY_MPallowable)), format = "f", digits = 3, width = 7), "  ",
                         "Lignin, % NDF  : ", formatC(isz(anim.diet.lignin.rate * 100,anim.diet.NDF.rate), format = "f", digits = 3, width = 7), "  ",
                         "  B3|Fiber       : ", formatC(isz(anim.diet.CHOB3.rate * 100,anim.diet.DMI.rate), format = "f", digits = 3, width = 6), "\n", sep = ""))
          cat(paste("   ", anim.MY_MAAallowable.label_min, " allowable milk                    : ", formatC(ifelse(tolower(Unit) == "metric", anim.MY_MAAallowable.rate_min, kgTOlb(anim.MY_MAAallowable.rate_min)), format = "f", digits = 3, width = 7), "  ",
                         "peNDF, % NDF    : ", formatC(isz(anim.diet.peNDF.rate * 100,anim.diet.NDF.rate), format = "f", digits = 3, width = 7), "  ",
                         "  C |Unavailable: ", formatC(isz(anim.diet.CHOC.rate * 100,anim.diet.DMI.rate), format = "f", digits = 3, width = 6), "\n", sep = ""))
        }
        cat(paste("   User-inputted (obs)                          : ", formatC(ifelse(tolower(Unit) == "metric", anim.lactation.milk.rate, kgTOlb(anim.lactation.milk.rate)), format = "f", digits = 3, width = 7), "  ",
                       "NDIN, % DM      : ", formatC(isz(anim.diet.NDIP.rate * 100,anim.diet.DMI.rate), format = "f", digits = 3, width = 7), "  ",
                       "PROT fractions, % DM\n", sep = ""))
        cat(paste(string(" ", 50), "  ",
                       "ADIN, % DM      : ", formatC(isz(anim.diet.ADIP.rate * 100,anim.diet.DMI.rate), format = "f", digits = 3, width = 7), "  ",
                       "  A |Nonamino N : ", formatC(isz(anim.diet.ProtA.rate * 100,anim.diet.DMI.rate), format = "f", digits = 3, width = 6), "\n", sep = ""))
        subtitle1 <- "Efficiency of use, %                   Energy   Protein"
        cat(paste(subtitle1, "  ",
                       "NFC, % DM       : ", formatC(isz(anim.diet.NFC.rate * 100,anim.diet.DMI.rate), format = "f", digits = 3, width = 7), "  ",
                       "  B1|TP fast kd : ", formatC(isz(anim.diet.ProtB1.rate * 100,anim.diet.DMI.rate), format = "f", digits = 3, width = 6), "\n", sep = ""))
        cat(paste(string("-", 50), "  ",
                       "EE, % DM        : ", formatC(isz(anim.diet.EE.rate * 100,anim.diet.DMI.rate), format = "f", digits = 3, width = 7), "  ",
                       "  B2|TP med. kd : ", formatC(isz(anim.diet.ProtB2.rate * 100,anim.diet.DMI.rate), format = "f", digits = 3, width = 6), "\n", sep = ""))
        cat(paste("Maintenance                          : ", formatC(ratio.NEmr.MEmr * 100, format = "f", digits = 3, width = 7), "  ", formatC(ratio.NPmr.MPmr * 100, format = "f", digits = 3, width = 7), "  ",
                       "TDC, % DM       : ", formatC(isz(anim.diet.TDC.rate * 100,anim.diet.DMI.rate), format = "f", digits = 3, width = 7), "  ",
```

```
                     "  B3|TP slow kd : ", formatC(isz(anim.diet.ProtB3.rate * 100,anim.diet.DMI.rate), format = "f", digits = 3, width = 6), "\n", sep = ""))
              cat(paste("Pregnancy                              : ", formatC(ratio.NEpr.MEpr * 100, format = "f", digits = 3, width = 7), " ", formatC(ratio.NPpr.MPpr * 100, format = "f", digits = 3, width = 7), "  ",
                     "Ash, % DM        : ", formatC(isz(anim.diet.ash.rate * 100,anim.diet.DMI.rate), format = "f", digits = 3, width = 7), "  ",
                     "  C |Unavailable: ", formatC(isz(anim.diet.ProtC.rate * 100,anim.diet.DMI.rate), format = "f", digits = 3, width = 6), "\n", sep = ""))
              cat(paste("Lactation                              : ", formatC(ratio.NElr.MElr * 100, format = "f", digits = 3, width = 7), " ", formatC(ratio.NPlr.MPlr * 100, format = "f", digits = 3, width = 7), "  ",
                     "Diet Ca:P        : ", formatC(diet.CatoP.ratio, format = "f", digits = 3, width = 7), "  ",
                     "Diet N:S          : ", formatC(diet.NtoS.ratio, format = "f", digits = 3, width = 6), "\n", sep=""))
         } else
         {
              cat(paste(ifelse(tolower(Unit) == "metric", "Average daily gain, kg/d", "Average daily gain, lb/d"), string(" ", 50 - 24), "  ",
                     "NDF, % DM        : ", formatC(isz(anim.diet.NDF.rate * 100,anim.diet.DMI.rate), format = "f", digits = 3, width = 7), "  ",
                     "  B1|Starch       : ", formatC(isz(anim.diet.CHOB1.rate * 100,anim.diet.DMI.rate), format = "f", digits = 3, width = 6), "\n", sep = ""))
              if (anim.body.ADG>0)
              {
                cat(paste("   ME allowable gain (", formatC(100*anim.SWG_MEallowable/anim.body.ADG,format = "f", digits=2, width = 7),
                       "% obs)          : ", formatC(ifelse(tolower(Unit) == "metric", anim.SWG_MEallowable, kgTOlb(anim.SWG_MEallowable)), format = "f", digits = 3, width = 7), "  ",
                       "ADF, % DM        : ", formatC(isz(anim.diet.ADF.rate * 100,anim.diet.DMI.rate), format = "f", digits = 3, width = 7), "  ",
                       "  B2|Pectin       : ", formatC(isz(anim.diet.CHOB2.rate * 100,anim.diet.DMI.rate), format = "f", digits = 3, width = 6), "\n", sep = ""))
                cat(paste("   MP allowable gain (",formatC(100*anim.SWG_MPallowable/anim.body.ADG,format = "f", digits=2, width = 7),
                       "% obs)          : ", formatC(ifelse(tolower(Unit) == "metric", anim.SWG_MPallowable, kgTOlb(anim.SWG_MPallowable)), format = "f", digits = 3, width = 7), "  ",
                       "Lignin, % NDF   : ", formatC(isz(anim.diet.lignin.rate * 100,anim.diet.NDF.rate), format = "f", digits = 3, width = 7), "  ",
                       "  B3|Fiber        : ", formatC(isz(anim.diet.CHOB3.rate * 100,anim.diet.DMI.rate), format = "f", digits = 3, width = 6), "\n", sep = ""))
                cat(paste("   ", anim.SWG_MAAallowable.label_min, " allowable gain (", formatC(100*anim.SWG_MAAallowable.rate_min/anim.body.ADG,format = "f", digits=2, width = 7),
                       "% obs)         : ", formatC(ifelse(tolower(Unit) == "metric", anim.SWG_MAAallowable.rate_min, kgTOlb(anim.SWG_MAAallowable.rate_min)), format = "f", digits = 3, width = 7), "  ",
                       "peNDF, % NDF    : ", formatC(isz(anim.diet.peNDF.rate * 100,anim.diet.NDF.rate), format = "f", digits = 3, width = 7), "  ",
                       "  C |Unavailable: " , formatC(isz(anim.diet.CHOC.rate * 100,anim.diet.DMI.rate), format = "f", digits = 3, width = 6), "\n", sep = ""))
              } else
              {
                cat(paste("   ME allowable gain                          : ", formatC(ifelse(tolower(Unit) == "metric", anim.SWG_MEallowable, kgTOlb(anim.SWG_MEallowable)), format = "f", digits = 3, width = 7), "  ",
                       "ADF, % DM        : ", formatC(isz(anim.diet.ADF.rate * 100,anim.diet.DMI.rate), format = "f", digits = 3, width = 7), "  ",
```

```
                        "  B2|Pectin      : ", formatC(isz(anim.diet.CHOB2.rate * 100,anim.diet.DMI.rate), format = "f", digits = 3, width = 6), "\n", sep = ""))
            cat(paste("   MP allowable gain                           : ", formatC(ifelse(tolower(Unit) == "metric", anim.SWG_MPallowable,kgTOlb(anim.SWG_MPallowable)), format = "f", digits = 3, width = 7), "   ",
                        "Lignin, % NDF   : ", formatC(isz(anim.diet.lignin.rate * 100,anim.diet.NDF.rate), format = "f", digits = 3, width = 7), "   ",
                        "  B3|Fiber       : ", formatC(isz(anim.diet.CHOB3.rate * 100,anim.diet.DMI.rate), format = "f", digits = 3, width = 6), "\n", sep = ""))
            cat(paste("   ", anim.SWG_MAAallowable.label_min, " allowable gain                   : ", formatC(ifelse(tolower(Unit) == "metric", anim.SWG_MAAallowable.rate_min, kgTOlb(anim.SWG_MAAallowable.rate_min)), format = "f", digits = 3, width = 7), "   ",
                        "peNDF, % NDF    : ", formatC(isz(anim.diet.peNDF.rate * 100,anim.diet.NDF.rate), format = "f", digits = 3, width = 7), "   ",
                        "  C |Unavailable: " , formatC(isz(anim.diet.CHOC.rate * 100,anim.diet.DMI.rate), format = "f", digits = 3, width = 6), "\n", sep = ""))
          }
          cat(paste("   User-inputted                              : ", formatC(ifelse(tolower(Unit) == "metric", anim.body.ADG, kgTOlb(anim.body.ADG)), format = "f", digits = 3, width = 7), "   ",
                      "NDIN, % DM      : ", formatC(isz(anim.diet.NDIP.rate * 100,anim.diet.DMI.rate), format = "f", digits = 3, width = 7), "   ",
                      "Protein fractions, % DM\n", sep = ""))
          cat(paste(string(" ", 50), "   ",
                      "ADIN, % DM      : ", formatC(isz(anim.diet.ADIP.rate * 100,anim.diet.DMI.rate), format = "f", digits = 3, width = 7), "   ",
                      "  A |Nonamino N : ", formatC(isz(anim.diet.ProtA.rate * 100,anim.diet.DMI.rate), format = "f", digits = 3, width = 6), "\n", sep = ""))
          subtitle1 <- "Efficiency of use, %                    Energy    Protein"
          cat(paste(subtitle1, "   ",
                      "NFC, % DM       : ", formatC(isz(anim.diet.NFC.rate * 100,anim.diet.DMI.rate), format = "f", digits = 3, width = 7), "   ",
                      "  B1|TP fast kd : ", formatC(isz(anim.diet.ProtB1.rate * 100,anim.diet.DMI.rate), format = "f", digits = 3, width = 6), "\n", sep = ""))
          cat(paste(string("-", 50), "   ",
                      "EE, % DM        : ", formatC(isz(anim.diet.EE.rate * 100,anim.diet.DMI.rate), format = "f", digits = 3, width = 7), "   ",
                      "  B2|TP med. kd : ", formatC(isz(anim.diet.ProtB2.rate * 100,anim.diet.DMI.rate), format = "f", digits = 3, width = 6), "\n", sep = ""))
          cat(paste("Maintenance                            : ", formatC(ratio.NEmr.MEmr * 100, format = "f", digits = 3, width = 7), "   ", formatC(ratio.NPmr.MPmr * 100, format = "f", digits = 3, width = 7), "   ",
                      "TDC, % DM       : ", formatC(isz(anim.diet.TDC.rate * 100,anim.diet.DMI.rate), format = "f", digits = 3, width = 7), "   ",
                      "  B3|TP slow kd : ", formatC(isz(anim.diet.ProtB3.rate * 100,anim.diet.DMI.rate), format = "f", digits = 3, width = 6), "\n", sep = ""))
          cat(paste("Pregnancy                              : ", formatC(ratio.NEpr.MEpr * 100, format = "f", digits = 3, width = 7), "   ", formatC(ratio.NPpr.MPpr * 100, format = "f", digits = 3, width = 7), "   ",
                      "Ash, % DM       : ", formatC(isz(anim.diet.ash.rate * 100,anim.diet.DMI.rate), format = "f", digits = 3, width = 7), "   ",
                      "  C |Unavailable: ", formatC(isz(anim.diet.ProtC.rate * 100,anim.diet.DMI.rate), format = "f", digits = 3, width = 6), "\n", sep = ""))
          cat(paste("Growth                                 : ", formatC(ratio.NEgr.MEgr * 100, format = "f", digits = 3, width = 7), "   ", formatC(ratio.NPgr.MPgr * 100, format = "f", digits = 3, width = 7), "   ",
```

```
                  "Diet Ca:P          : ", formatC(diet.CatoP.ratio, format = "f", digits = 3, width = 7), "  ",
                  "Diet N:S           : ", formatC(diet.NtoS.ratio, format = "f", digits = 3, width = 6), "\n", sep=""))
    }
    cat("\n")
    # BCAA balance in the rumen
    bcaa_bal <- c(rum.diet.BCAA_Leu.rate,rum.diet.BCAA_Ile.rate,rum.diet.BCAA_Val.rate)*1000
    bcaa_req <- c(rum.diet.bact.Leu.rate,rum.diet.bact.Ile.rate,rum.diet.bact.Val.rate)*1000
    bcaa_idx <- which.min(bcaa_bal/bcaa_req)
    bcaa_min <- 100 + (bcaa_bal*100/bcaa_req)[bcaa_idx]
    bcaa_txt <- c("Leu", "Ile", "Val")[bcaa_idx]
    subtitle1 <- "Ruminal Parameters & Balances"
    subtitle1 <- paste(subtitle1, string(" ", 50 - nchar(subtitle1)), sep = "")
    subtitle2 <- "Diet Evaluation & Biological Values"
    subtitle2 <- paste(subtitle2, string(" ", 50 - nchar(subtitle2)), sep = "")
    cat(paste(subtitle1, "  ", subtitle2, "\n", string("-", nchar(subtitle1)), "  ", string("-", nchar(subtitle2)), "\n", sep = ""))
    cat(paste("pH|dietary peNDF (peNDF: ",formatC(anim.diet.peNDF.conc, format = "f", digits = 2, width = 5)," % DM)      : ", formatC(rum.pH_peNDF, format = "f", digits = 3, width = 7), "  ",
              ifelse(tolower(Unit) == "metric", "GE, Mcal/kg    : ", "GE, Mcal/lb    : "), formatC(ifelse(tolower(Unit) == "metric", anim.diet.GE.frac, PERkgTOPERlb(anim.diet.GE.frac)), format = "f", digits = 3, width = 7), "  ",
              ifelse(tolower(Unit) == "metric", "DE, Mcal/kg    : ", "DE, Mcal/lb    : "), formatC(ifelse(tolower(Unit) == "metric", anim.diet.DE.frac, PERkgTOPERlb(anim.diet.DE.frac)), format = "f", digits = 3, width = 7), "\n", sep = ""))
    cat(paste("pH|VFA balance (Eq. peNDF: ", ifelse(existsnonNA("rum.pH_VFA"), formatC(optimize(function(x) abs(calcRumenpH_peNDF(flag_ph, x) - rum.pH_VFA),
                                                                            interval=c(1, 40),maximum=F)$minimum, format="f", digits=2, width=5), "   NA")," % DM)     : ",
              formatC(rum.pH_VFA, format = "f", digits = 3, width = 7), "  ",
              ifelse(tolower(Unit) == "metric", "ME, Mcal/kg    : ", "ME, Mcal/lb    : "), formatC(ifelse(tolower(Unit) == "metric", anim.diet.ME.frac, PERkgTOPERlb(anim.diet.ME.frac)), format = "f", digits = 3, width = 7), "  ",
              ifelse(tolower(Unit) == "metric", "NEm, Mcal/kg   : ", "NEm, Mcal/lb   : "), formatC(ifelse(tolower(Unit) == "metric", anim.diet.NEm.frac, PERkgTOPERlb(anim.diet.NEm.frac)), format = "f", digits = 3, width = 7), "\n", sep = ""))
    cat(paste("Fermentability, % DM", string(" ", 30), "  ",
              ifelse(tolower(Unit) == "metric", "NEg, Mcal/kg   : ", "NEg, Mcal/lb   : "), formatC(ifelse(tolower(Unit) == "metric", anim.diet.NEg.frac, PERkgTOPERlb(anim.diet.NEg.frac)), format = "f", digits = 3, width = 7), "  ",
              ifelse(tolower(Unit) == "metric", "NEl, Mcal/kg   : ", "NEl, Mcal/lb   : "), formatC(ifelse(tolower(Unit) == "metric", anim.diet.NEl.frac, PERkgTOPERlb(anim.diet.NEl.frac)), format = "f", digits = 3, width = 7), "\n", sep = ""))
    cat(paste("   Sugar (CHOA4)                             : ", formatC(isz(rum.diet.DCHOA4.rate * 100, anim.diet.DMI.rate), format = "f", digits = 3, width = 7), "  ",
              "aDMD, % DM     : ", formatC(anim.diet.aDMD.conc, format = "f", digits = 3, width = 7), "  ",
              "tDMD, % DM     : ", formatC(anim.diet.tDMD.conc, format = "f", digits = 3, width = 7), "\n", sep = ""))
    cat(paste("   Starch (CHOB1)                            : ", formatC(isz(rum.diet.DCHOB1.rate * 100, anim.diet.DMI.rate), format = "f", digits = 3, width = 7), "  ",
              "aOMD, % DM     : ", formatC(anim.diet.aOMD.conc, format = "f", digits = 3, width = 7), "  ",
              "tOMD, % DM     : ", formatC(anim.diet.tOMD.conc, format = "f", digits = 3, width = 7), "\n", sep = ""))
    cat(paste("   Soluble fiber, pectin (CHOB2)             : ", formatC(isz(rum.diet.DCHOB2.rate * 100, anim.diet.DMI.rate), format = "f", digits = 3, width = 7), "  ",
              "FOM, % DM      : ", formatC(isz(anim.diet.FOMI.rate * 100, anim.diet.DMI.rate), format = "f", digits = 3, width = 7), "  ",
              "FOM, % OM      : ", formatC(isz(anim.diet.FOMI.rate * 100, anim.diet.OMI.rate), format = "f", digits = 3, width = 7), "\n", sep = ""))
```

```
    cat(paste("   Fiber, NDF (CHOB3)                    : ", formatC(isz(rum.diet.DCHOB3.rate * 100, anim.diet.DMI.rate), format = "f", digits = 3, width = 7), "  ",
              ifelse(tolower(Unit) == "metric", "IDM, kg/d      : ", "IDM, lb/d      : "), formatC(ifelse(tolower(Unit) == "metric", fc.diet.IDM.rate, kgTOlb(fc.diet.IDM.rate)), format = "f", digits = 3, width = 7), "  ",
              "IDM, % DM       : ", formatC(isz(fc.diet.IDM.rate * 100, anim.diet.DMI.rate), format = "f", digits = 3, width = 7), "\n", sep = ""))
    cat(paste("Recycled N, g/d (",  formatC(isz(rum.Recycled_N.rate * 100, anim.diet.CP.rate/6.25), format = "f", digits = 1, width = 5),
              "% N intake)          : ", formatC(rum.Recycled_N.rate * 1000, format = "f", digits = 2, width = 7), "  ",
              "aTDN, %         : ", formatC(anim.diet.aTDN.conc, format = "f", digits = 3, width = 7), "  ",
              "tTDN, %         : ", formatC(anim.diet.tTDN.conc, format = "f", digits = 3, width = 7), "\n", sep = ""))
    cat(paste("Nitrogen balance, g/d (", formatC(100 + rum.N_balance.rate * 100/(rum.diet.bact.NFC_AminoN.rate + rum.diet.bact.NFC_AmmoniaN.rate + rum.diet.bact.FC_AmmoniaN.rate), format = "f", digits = 1, width = 5),
              "% req)          : ", formatC(rum.N_balance.rate * 1000, format = "f", digits = 2, width = 7), "  ",
              "RDP, % DM       : ", formatC(isz((anim.diet.CP.rate - rum.diet.RUCP.rate) * 100, anim.diet.DMI.rate), format = "f", digits = 3, width = 7), "  ",
              "RDP, % CP       : ", formatC(isz((anim.diet.CP.rate - rum.diet.RUCP.rate) * 100, anim.diet.CP.rate), format = "f", digits = 3, width = 7), "\n", sep = ""))
    cat(paste("   Urea cost, Mcal/d (", formatC(isz(anim.NEmrUrea.rate * 100, anim.MEm_required.rate), format = "f", digits = 2, width = 5),
              "% MEm)          : " , formatC(anim.NEmrUrea.rate, format = "f", digits = 3, width = 7), "  ",
              "RUP, % DM       : ", formatC(isz(rum.diet.RUCP.rate * 100, anim.diet.DMI.rate), format = "f", digits = 3, width = 7), "  ",
              "RUP, % CP       : ", formatC(isz(rum.diet.RUCP.rate * 100, anim.diet.CP.rate), format = "f", digits = 3, width = 7), "\n", sep = ""))
    cat(paste("Amino-N balance, g/d (", formatC(100 + rum.AminoN_balance.rate * 100/rum.diet.bact.NFC_AminoN.rate, format = "f", digits = 1, width = 5),
              "% req)          : ", formatC(rum.AminoN_balance.rate * 1000, format = "f", digits = 2, width = 7), "  ",
              ifelse(tolower(Unit) == "metric", "MP, kg/d       : ", "MP, lb/d       : "), formatC(ifelse(tolower(Unit) == "metric", anim.diet.MP.rate, kgTOlb(anim.diet.MP.rate)), format = "f", digits = 3, width = 7), "  ",
              "MP, % CP        : ", formatC(isz(anim.diet.MP.rate * 100, anim.diet.CP.rate), format = "f", digits = 3, width = 7), "\n", sep = ""))
    cat(paste("BCAA (", bcaa_txt, ") balance, g/d (", formatC(bcaa_min, format = "f", digits = 1, width = 5),
              "% req)      : ", formatC(bcaa_bal[bcaa_idx], format = "f", digits = 2, width = 7), "  ",
              ifelse(tolower(Unit) == "metric", "  MP bact, kg/d: ", "  MP bact, lb/d: "), formatC(ifelse(tolower(Unit) == "metric", anim.diet.bact.MP.rate, kgTOlb(anim.diet.bact.MP.rate)), format = "f", digits = 3, width = 7), "  ",
              "MP bact, % MP  : ", formatC(isz(anim.diet.bact.MP.rate * 100, anim.diet.MP.rate) , format = "f", digits = 3, width = 7), "\n", sep = ""))
    if (isLactating == TRUE)
    {
      cat(paste(ifelse(tolower(Unit) == "metric", "peNDF balance, kg/d (", "peNDF balance, lb/d ("), formatC(100 + anim.peNDF_balance.rate * 100/anim.peNDF_required.rate, format = "f", digits = 1, width = 5),
                "% req)          : ", formatC(ifelse(tolower(Unit) == "metric", anim.peNDF_balance.rate, kgTOlb(anim.peNDF_balance.rate)), format = "f", digits = 3, width = 7), "  ",
                ifelse(tolower(Unit) == "metric", "  MP feed, kg/d: ", "  MP feed, lb/d: "), formatC(ifelse(tolower(Unit) == "metric", anim.diet.fd.MP.rate, kgTOlb(anim.diet.fd.MP.rate)), format = "f", digits = 3, width = 7), "  ",
                "MP feed, % MP  : ", formatC(isz(anim.diet.fd.MP.rate * 100, anim.diet.MP.rate) , format = "f", digits = 3, width = 7), "\n", sep = ""))
      cat(paste(ifelse(tolower(Unit) == "metric", "NDF balance, kg/d (", "NDF balance, lb/d ("), formatC(100 + anim.NDF_balance.rate * 100/anim.NDF_required.rate, format = "f", digits = 1, width = 5),
```

```
                    "% req)             : ", formatC(ifelse(tolower(Unit) == "metric", anim.NDF_balance.rate, kgTOlb(anim.NDF_balance.rate)), format = "f", digits = 3, width = 7), "  ",
                    "DCAB1, meq/100g: ", formatC(anim.DCAB1.rate, format = "f", digits = 2, width = 7), "  ",
                    "DCAB3, meq/100g: ", formatC(anim.DCAB3.rate, format = "f", digits = 2, width = 7), "\n", sep=""))
      } else
      {
        cat(paste(ifelse(tolower(Unit) == "metric", "peNDF min acidosis, kg/d (", "peNDF min acidosis, lb/d ("), formatC(100 + (anim.diet.peNDF.rate - anim.peNDF_required_acidosis.rate) * 100/anim.peNDF_required.rate, format = "f", digits = 1, width = 5),
                    "% req)     : ", formatC(ifelse(tolower(Unit) == "metric", anim.diet.peNDF.rate - anim.peNDF_required_acidosis.rate, kgTOlb(anim.diet.peNDF.rate - anim.peNDF_required_acidosis.rate)), format = "f", digits = 3, width = 7), "  ",
                    ifelse(tolower(Unit) == "metric", "  MP Feed, kg/d: ", "  MP Feed, lb/d: "), formatC(ifelse(tolower(Unit) == "metric", anim.diet.fd.MP.rate, kgTOlb(anim.diet.fd.MP.rate)), format = "f", digits = 3, width = 7), "  ",
                    "MP Feed, % MP  : ", formatC(isz(anim.diet.fd.MP.rate * 100, anim.diet.MP.rate) , format = "f", digits = 3, width = 7), "\n", sep = ""))
        cat(paste(ifelse(tolower(Unit) == "metric", "peNDF max gain, kg/d (", "peNDF max gain, lb/d ("), formatC(100 + (anim.diet.peNDF.rate - anim.peNDF_required_gain.rate) * 100/anim.NDF_required.rate, format = "f", digits = 1, width = 5),
                    "% req)          : ", formatC(ifelse(tolower(Unit) == "metric", anim.diet.peNDF.rate - anim.peNDF_required_gain.rate, kgTOlb(anim.diet.peNDF.rate - anim.peNDF_required_gain.rate)), format = "f", digits = 3, width = 7), "  ",
                    "DCAB1, meq/100g: ", formatC(anim.DCAB1.rate, format = "f", digits = 2, width = 7), "  ",
                    "DCAB3, meq/100g: ", formatC(anim.DCAB3.rate, format = "f", digits = 2, width = 7), "\n", sep=""))
      }

      cat("\n")
      if (!existsnonNA("fc.diet.IDM.rate")) fc.diet.IDM.rate <- 0
      if (!existsnonNA("fc.diet.CP.rate")) fc.diet.CP.rate <- 0
      if (!existsnonNA("rum.acetate.conc")) rum.acetate.conc <- 0
      if (!existsnonNA("rum.diet.methane.rate")) rum.diet.methane.rate <- 0
      if (!existsnonNA("fc.diet.fd_IOM.rate")) fc.diet.fd_IOM.rate <- 0
      if (!existsnonNA("fc.diet.CHO.rate")) fc.diet.CHO.rate <- 0
      if (!existsnonNA("rum.propionate.conc")) rum.propionate.conc <- 0
      if (!existsnonNA("fc.diet.Endogenous.CP.rate")) fc.diet.Endogenous.CP.rate <- 0
      if (!existsnonNA("fc.diet.Endogenous.fat.rate")) fc.diet.Endogenous.fat.rate <- 0
      if (!existsnonNA("fc.diet.Endogenous.ash.rate")) fc.diet.Endogenous.ash.rate <- 0
      if (!existsnonNA("fc.diet.EE.rate")) fc.diet.EE.rate <- 0
      if (!existsnonNA("rum.butyrate.conc")) rum.butyrate.conc <- 0
      if (!existsnonNA("fc.diet.bact.CP.rate")) fc.diet.bact.CP.rate <- 0
      if (!existsnonNA("fc.diet.bact.CHO.rate")) fc.diet.bact.CHO.rate <- 0
      if (!existsnonNA("fc.diet.bact.EE.rate")) fc.diet.bact.EE.rate <- 0
      if (!existsnonNA("fc.diet.bact.ash.rate")) fc.diet.bact.ash.rate <- 0
      if (!existsnonNA("fc.diet.ash.rate")) fc.diet.ash.rate <- 0
      if (!existsnonNA("rum.lactate.conc")) rum.lactate.conc <- 0
      subtitle1 <- "Excretions & Emissions"
      subtitle1 <- paste(subtitle1, string(" ", 102 - nchar(subtitle1)), sep = "")
      cat(paste(subtitle1, "\n", string("-", nchar(subtitle1)), "\n", sep = ""))
      cat(paste(ifelse(tolower(Unit) == "metric", "Fecal, kg/d", "Fecal, lb/d"), string(" ", 50 - 11), "  ", "Ruminal VFA, Lactate, and Methane (CH4)\n", sep = ""))
      cat(paste(" Dry matter    : ", formatC(ifelse(tolower(Unit) == "metric", fc.diet.IDM.rate, kgTOlb(fc.diet.IDM.rate)), format = "f", digits = 3, width = 7), "  ",
                  " Crude protein : ", formatC(ifelse(tolower(Unit) == "metric", fc.diet.CP.rate, kgTOlb(fc.diet.CP.rate)), format = "f", digits = 3, width = 7), "  ",
```

```
                   " Acetate, mM    : ", formatC(rum.acetate.conc, format = "f", digits = 3, width = 7), "  ",
                   " CH4, g/d       : ", formatC(rum.diet.methane.rate * 1000, format = "f", digits = 3, width = 7), "\n", sep = ""))
    cat(paste(" Organic matter: ", formatC(ifelse(tolower(Unit) == "metric", fc.diet.fd_IOM.rate, kgTOlb(fc.diet.fd_IOM.rate)), format = "f", digits = 3, width = 7), "  ",
                   " Carbohydrate   : ", formatC(ifelse(tolower(Unit) == "metric", fc.diet.CHO.rate, kgTOlb(fc.diet.CHO.rate)), format = "f", digits = 3, width = 7), "  ",
                   " Propionate, mM: ", formatC(rum.propionate.conc, format = "f", digits = 3, width = 7), "  ",
                   " CH4, L/d       : ", formatC(rum.diet.methane.rate * 1000/0.6556, format = "f", digits = 3, width = 7), "\n", sep = ""))
    cat(paste(" Endogenous     : ", formatC(ifelse(tolower(Unit) == "metric", fc.diet.Endogenous.CP.rate + fc.diet.Endogenous.fat.rate + fc.diet.Endogenous.ash.rate,
                                                  kgTOlb(fc.diet.Endogenous.CP.rate + fc.diet.Endogenous.fat.rate + fc.diet.Endogenous.ash.rate)), format = "f", digits = 3, width = 7), "  ",
                   " Fat            : ", formatC(ifelse(tolower(Unit) == "metric", fc.diet.EE.rate, kgTOlb(fc.diet.EE.rate)), format = "f", digits = 3, width = 7), "  ",
                   " Butyrate, mM   : ", formatC(rum.butyrate.conc, format = "f", digits = 3, width = 7), "  ",
                   " CH4, g/kg FOM : ", formatC(isz(rum.diet.methane.rate * 1000, anim.diet.FOMI.rate), format = "f", digits = 3, width = 7), "\n", sep = ""))
    cat(paste(" Microbial      : ", formatC(ifelse(tolower(Unit) == "metric", fc.diet.bact.CP.rate + fc.diet.bact.CHO.rate + fc.diet.bact.EE.rate + fc.diet.bact.ash.rate,
                                                  kgTOlb(fc.diet.bact.CP.rate + fc.diet.bact.CHO.rate + fc.diet.bact.EE.rate + fc.diet.bact.ash.rate)), format = "f", digits = 3, width = 7), "  ",
                   " Ash            : ", formatC(ifelse(tolower(Unit) == "metric", fc.diet.ash.rate, kgTOlb(fc.diet.ash.rate)), format = "f", digits = 3, width = 7), "  ",
                   " Lactate, mM    : ", formatC(rum.lactate.conc, format = "f", digits = 3, width = 7), "  ",
                   " CH4, g/kg DM   : ", formatC(isz(rum.diet.methane.rate * 1000, anim.diet.DMI.rate), format = "f", digits = 3, width = 7), "\n", sep = ""))
    newpage()
    # Ration summary
    if (existsnonNA("granst.selected") != FALSE & exists("granst.list2") != FALSE)
    {
      title <- granst.list2[granst.selected]
      if (nchar(title) > 102)
      {
        title <- substr(title, 1, 102)
      }
      cat(paste(string(" ", floor((102 - nchar(title))/2)), title,"\n", sep=""))
      #cat(paste(string(" ", floor((102 - nchar(title))/2)), string(".", nchar(title)), "\n", sep=""))
    }
    cat(paste(string(" ", floor((102 - nchar(heading))/2)), heading,"\n", sep=""))
    cat(paste(string(" ", floor((102 - nchar(heading))/2)), string("=", nchar(heading)), "\n\n", sep=""))
    #cat("\n")
    #title <- "Ration Formulation"
    #cat(paste(title, "\n", string("=", nchar(title)), "\n\n", sep = ""))
    cat(paste("Feed name (ID)", string(" ", 50 - 14), "  ", "Dry Matter", string(" ", 24 - 10), "  ", "As-fed", "\n", sep = ""))
    cat(paste(string("-", 50), "  ", string("-", 24), "  ", string("-", 24), "\n", sep = ""))
    if (tolower(Unit) == "metric")
    {
```

```
    cat(paste(string(" ", 50), "  ", "   $/kg", "  ", "   kg/d", "  ", "      %", "  ", "   $/kg", "  ", "   kg/d", "  ", "
%", "\n", sep = ""))
    cat(paste(string("-", 50), "  ", string("-", 24), "  ", string("-", 24), "\n", sep = ""))
    for (i in 1:length(anim.fd.DMI.rate))
    {
      fdDM <- as.numeric(feeds3[, "DM"])/100
      fdtxt <- substr(paste(feeds3[i, "FeedName.x"], " (", feeds3[i,"FeedID"], ")", sep = ""), 1, 50)
      cat(paste(fdtxt, string(" ", 50 - nchar(fdtxt)), "  ",
                formatC(anim.fd.Price.amt[i], format = "f", digits = 3, width = 7), "  ",
                formatC(anim.fd.DMI.rate[i], format = "f", digits = 3, width = 7), " ",
                formatC(isz(anim.fd.DMI.rate[i] * 100, anim.diet.DMI.rate), format = "f", digits = 3, width = 7), "  ",
                formatC(anim.fd.Price.amt[i] * fdDM[i], format = "f", digits = 3, width = 7), "  ",
                formatC(isz(anim.fd.DMI.rate[i], fdDM[i]), format = "f", digits = 3, width = 7), " ",
                formatC(isz(anim.fd.AFI.rate[i] * 100, anim.diet.AFI.rate) , format = "f", digits = 3, width = 7), "\n", sep
= ""))
    }
    cat(paste(string("-", 50), "  ", string("-", 24), "  ", string("-", 24), "\n", sep = ""))
    cat(paste("Total", string(" ", 50 - 5), "  ",
              formatC(anim.diet.Price.amt, format = "f", digits = 3, width = 7), "  ",
              formatC(anim.diet.DMI.rate, format = "f", digits = 3, width = 7), "  ",
              formatC(100, format = "f", digits = 0, width = 6), "  ",
              formatC(isz(anim.diet.Price.amt * anim.diet.DMI.rate, anim.diet.AFI.rate), format = "f", digits = 3, width =
7), "  ",
              formatC(anim.diet.AFI.rate, format = "f", digits = 3, width = 7), "  ",
              formatC(100, format = "f", digits = 0, width = 6), "\n", sep = ""))
    cat("\n\n")

    # Costs
    cat("Costs\n")
    cat(paste(string("-", 102), "\n", sep = ""))
    cat(paste(frmttxt("Ration:", 34), frmttxt("Production:", 34), frmttxt("Environmental:", 34), "\n", sep=""))
    cat(paste(frmttxt(paste("  $", format(anim.diet.Price.rate, format = "f", digits = 2, width = 6, justify = "right",
nsmall = 2), "/day", sep=""), 34),
              frmttxt(paste("  $", ifelse(isLactating==TRUE,
                                          paste(format(isz(anim.diet.Price.rate, pmin.positive(c(anim.MY_MEallowable,
anim.MY_MPallowable, anim.MY_MAAallowable.rate_min))), format = "f", digits = 2, width = 6, justify = "right", nsmall = 2),
"/kg milk", sep=""),
                                          paste(format(isz(anim.diet.Price.rate, pmin.positive(c(anim.SWG_MEallowable,
anim.SWG_MPallowable, anim.SWG_MAAallowable.rate_min))), format = "f", digits = 2, width = 6, justify = "right", nsmall = 2),
"/kg gain", sep = "")), sep=""), 34),
              frmttxt(paste("  $", format(isz(anim.diet.Price.rate*100, fc.diet.IDM.rate), format = "f", digits = 2, width =
6, justify = "right", nsmall = 2), "/100 kg feces (DM Basis)", sep=""), 34), "\n", sep=""))
    cat(paste(frmttxt(paste("  $", format(anim.diet.Price.amt * 1000, format = "f", digits = 2, width = 6, justify =
"right", nsmall = 2), "/Metric Ton (DM Basis)", sep=""), 34),
              frmttxt(paste("  $", format(isz(anim.diet.Price.rate*100, anim.diet.aTDN.rate), format = "f", digits = 2,
width = 6, justify = "right", nsmall = 2), "/100 kg aTDN", sep=""), 34),
              frmttxt(paste("  $", format(isz(anim.diet.Price.rate, rum.diet.methane.rate), format = "f", digits = 2, width
= 6, justify = "right", nsmall = 2), "/kg of methane", sep=""), 34), "\n", sep=""))
    cat(paste(frmttxt(paste("  $", format(anim.diet.Price.amt * 1000 * (anim.diet.DM.conc/100), format = "f", digits = 2,
width = 6, justify = "right", nsmall = 2), "/Metric Ton (AF Basis)", sep=""), 34),
```

```
                frmttxt(paste("  $", format(isz(anim.diet.Price.rate*100, anim.diet.ME.rate), format = "f", digits = 2, width = 6, justify = "right", nsmall = 2), "/100 kg ME", sep=""), 34),
                frmttxt(paste("  $", format(isz(anim.diet.Price.rate*100, rum.diet.methane.rate * 1000/0.6556), format = "f", digits = 2, width = 6, justify = "right", nsmall = 2), "/100 L of methane", sep=""), 34), "\n", sep=""))
          cat(paste(frmttxt("", 34),
                frmttxt(paste("  $", format(isz(anim.diet.Price.rate*100, anim.diet.NEg.rate), format = "f", digits = 2, width = 6, justify = "right", nsmall = 2), "/100 kg NEg", sep=""), 34),
                frmttxt("", 34), "\n", sep=""))
          cat(paste(frmttxt("", 34),
                frmttxt(paste("  $", format(isz(anim.diet.Price.rate*100, anim.diet.MP.rate), format = "f", digits = 2, width = 6, justify = "right", nsmall = 2), "/100 kg MP", sep=""), 34),
                frmttxt("", 34), "\n", sep=""))
          cat(paste(string("-", 102), "\n", sep = ""))
        } else
        {
          cat(paste(string(" ", 50), "  ", "   $/lb", "  ", "    lb/d", "  ", "      %", "  ", "   $/lb", "  ", "    lb/d", "  ", "      %", "\n", sep = ""))
          cat(paste(string("-", 50), "  ", string("-", 24), "  ", string("-", 24), "\n", sep = ""))
          for (i in 1:length(anim.fd.DMI.rate))
          {
            fdDM <- as.numeric(feeds3[, "DM"])/100
            fdtxt <- substr(paste(feeds3[i, "FeedName.x"], " (", feeds3[i,"FeedID"], ")", sep = ""), 1, 50)
            cat(paste(fdtxt, string(" ", 50 - nchar(fdtxt)), "  ",
                      formatC(PERlb(anim.fd.Price.amt[i], T), format = "f", digits = 3, width = 7), "  ",
                      formatC(kgTOlb(anim.fd.DMI.rate[i]), format = "f", digits = 3, width = 7), " ",
                      formatC(isz(anim.fd.DMI.rate[i] * 100, anim.diet.DMI.rate), format = "f", digits = 3, width = 7), "  ",
                      formatC(PERlb(anim.fd.Price.amt[i], T) * fdDM[i], format = "f", digits = 3, width = 7), "  ",
                      formatC(isz(kgTOlb(anim.fd.DMI.rate[i]), fdDM[i]), format = "f", digits = 3, width = 7), " ",
                      formatC(isz(anim.fd.AFI.rate[i] * 100, anim.diet.AFI.rate) , format = "f", digits = 3, width = 7), "\n", sep = ""))
          }
          cat(paste(string("-", 50), "  ", string("-", 24), "  ", string("-", 24), "\n", sep = ""))
          cat(paste("Total", string(" ", 50 - 5), "  ",
                    formatC(PERlb(anim.diet.Price.amt, T), format = "f", digits = 3, width = 7), "  ",
                    formatC(kgTOlb(anim.diet.DMI.rate), format = "f", digits = 3, width = 7), "  ",
                    formatC(100, format = "f", digits = 0, width = 6), "  ",
                    formatC(isz(PERlb(anim.diet.Price.amt, T) * anim.diet.DMI.rate, anim.diet.AFI.rate), format = "f", digits = 3, width = 7), "  ",
                    formatC(kgTOlb(anim.diet.AFI.rate), format = "f", digits = 3, width = 7), "  ",
                    formatC(100, format = "f", digits = 0, width = 6), "\n", sep = ""))
          cat("\n\n")

          # Costs
          cat("Costs\n")
          cat(paste(string("-", 102), "\n", sep = ""))
          cat(paste(frmttxt("Ration:", 34), frmttxt("Production:", 34), frmttxt("Environmental:", 34), "\n", sep=""))
          cat(paste(frmttxt(paste("  $", format(anim.diet.Price.rate, format = "f", digits = 2, width = 6, justify = "right", nsmall = 2), "/day", sep=""), 34),
                    frmttxt(paste("  $", ifelse(isLactating==TRUE,
```

```
                   paste(format(isz(anim.diet.Price.rate, kgTOlb(pmin.positive(c(anim.MY_MEallowable, anim.MY_MPallowable, anim.MY_MAAallowable.rate_min)))), format = "f", digits = 2, width = 6, justify = "right", nsmall = 2), "/lb milk", sep=""),
                   paste(format(isz(anim.diet.Price.rate, kgTOlb(pmin.positive(c(anim.SWG_MEallowable, anim.SWG_MPallowable, anim.SWG_MAAallowable.rate_min)))), format = "f", digits = 2, width = 6, justify = "right", nsmall = 2), "/lb gain", sep = "")), sep=""), 34),
          frmttxt(paste("  $", format(isz(anim.diet.Price.rate*100, kgTOlb(fc.diet.IDM.rate)), format = "f", digits = 2, width = 6, justify = "right", nsmall = 2), "/100 lb feces (DM Basis)", sep=""), 34), "\n", sep=""))
    cat(paste(frmttxt(paste("  $", format(PERlb(anim.diet.Price.amt, T) * 2000, format = "f", digits = 2, width = 6, justify = "right", nsmall = 2), "/English Ton (DM Basis)", sep=""), 34),
          frmttxt(paste("  $", format(isz(anim.diet.Price.rate*100, kgTOlb(anim.diet.aTDN.rate)), format = "f", digits = 2, width = 6, justify = "right", nsmall = 2), "/100 lb aTDN", sep=""), 34),
          frmttxt(paste("  $", format(isz(anim.diet.Price.rate, kgTOlb(rum.diet.methane.rate)), format = "f", digits = 2, width = 6, justify = "right", nsmall = 2), "/lb of methane", sep=""), 34), "\n", sep=""))
    cat(paste(frmttxt(paste("  $", format(PERlb(anim.diet.Price.amt, T) * 2000 * (anim.diet.DM.conc/100), format = "f", digits = 2, width = 6, justify = "right", nsmall = 2), "/English Ton (AF Basis)", sep=""), 34),
          frmttxt(paste("  $", format(isz(anim.diet.Price.rate*100, kgTOlb(anim.diet.ME.rate)), format = "f", digits = 2, width = 6, justify = "right", nsmall = 2), "/100 lb ME", sep=""), 34),
          frmttxt(paste("  $", format(isz(anim.diet.Price.rate*100, rum.diet.methane.rate * 1000/0.6556), format = "f", digits = 2, width = 6, justify = "right", nsmall = 2), "/100 L of methane", sep=""), 34), "\n", sep=""))
    cat(paste(frmttxt("", 34),
          frmttxt(paste("  $", format(isz(anim.diet.Price.rate*100, kgTOlb(anim.diet.NEg.rate)), format = "f", digits = 2, width = 6, justify = "right", nsmall = 2), "/100 lb NEg", sep=""), 34),
          frmttxt("", 34), "\n", sep=""))
    cat(paste(frmttxt("", 34),
          frmttxt(paste("  $", format(isz(anim.diet.Price.rate*100, kgTOlb(anim.diet.MP.rate)), format = "f", digits = 2, width = 6, justify = "right", nsmall = 2), "/100 lb MP", sep=""), 34),
          frmttxt("", 34), "\n", sep=""))
    cat(paste(string("-", 102), "\n", sep = ""))
  }

  cat("\n\n")
  # Biological indices
  CH4_VFA_Mcal <- (sum(rum.fd.methane.rate * 1000)/1000)*13.3
  CH4_VFA_GE <- isz(CH4_VFA_Mcal*100, anim.diet.GE.rate)
  Vr <- rum.volume/1000 # m^3
  kl <- rum.kp_liquid.fracprate*24 # %/d
  NH3mM <- rum.N_balance.rate*1000/((kl/100)*Vr*14) # mM
  subtitle1 <- "Biological Indices                               Value    Ideal/Range          Comments (References)"
  subtitle2 <- "------------------------------------------------- ------- --------------- -----------------------------------"
  cat(paste(subtitle1, "\n", subtitle2, "\n", sep = ""))
  cat(paste("Ruminal Methane\n", sep = ""))
  if(anim.diet.ionophore==TRUE)
  {
    if(anim.type=="Milk")
    {
      cat(paste("   Methane, Mcal/d                              : ",
                formatC(CH4_VFA_Mcal, format = "f", digits = 3, width = 7), " ",
                "[2.10 to 6.25] ", " ", "Dairy animal with ionophore (1)     ", "\n", sep = ""))
      cat(paste("   Methane, % GE                                : ",
                formatC(CH4_VFA_GE, format = "f", digits = 3, width = 7), " ",
```

```
                    " [2.7 to 7.7]   ", " ", "Dairy animal with ionophore (1)     ", "\n", sep = ""))
        } else
        {
          cat(paste("   Methane, Mcal/d                             : ",
                    formatC(CH4_VFA_Mcal, format = "f", digits = 3, width = 7), " ",
                    "[0.77 to 2.27] ", " ", "Beef animal with ionophore (1)      ", "\n", sep = ""))
          cat(paste("   Methane, % GE                               : ",
                    formatC(CH4_VFA_GE, format = "f", digits = 3, width = 7), " ",
                    " [2.0 to 9.3]   ", " ", "Beef animal with ionophore (1)      ", "\n", sep = ""))
        }
      } else
      {
        if(anim.type=="Milk")
        {
          cat(paste("   Methane, Mcal/d                             : ",
                    formatC(CH4_VFA_Mcal, format = "f", digits = 3, width = 7), " ",
                    "[2.38 to 6.20] ", " ", "Dairy animal without ionophore (1) ", "\n", sep = ""))
          cat(paste("   Methane, % GE                               : ",
                    formatC(CH4_VFA_GE, format = "f", digits = 3, width = 7), " ",
                    " [2.5 to 7.3]   ", " ", "Dairy animal without ionophore (1) ", "\n", sep = ""))
        } else
        {
          cat(paste("   Methane, Mcal/d                             : ",
                    formatC(CH4_VFA_Mcal, format = "f", digits = 3, width = 7), " ",
                    "[0.93 to 2.85] ", " ", "Beef animal without ionophore (1)  ", "\n", sep = ""))
          cat(paste("   Methane, % GE                               : ",
                    formatC(CH4_VFA_GE, format = "f", digits = 3, width = 7), " ",
                    " [2.4 to 9.2]   ", " ", "Beef animal without ionophore (1)  ", "\n", sep = ""))
        }
      }
      cat(paste("Ruminal Nitrogen\n", sep = ""))
      cat(paste("   Ruminally degradable protein, % BW    : ",
                formatC(isz(rum.diet.RDP.rate*100, anim.FBW), format = "f", digits = 3, width = 7), " ",
                "[0.08 to 0.12] ", " ", "Grazing low-quality forage (4,5,6) ", "\n", sep = ""))
      cat(paste("   Ruminal ammonia-N, mM                 : ",
                formatC(NH3mM, format = "f", digits = 3, width = 7), " ",
                "     > 3.6      ", " ", "Increase MCP and NDFD (9)           ", "\n", sep = ""))
      cat(paste("Ruminal Bacteria\n", sep = ""))
      if (anim.species=="Cattle" & anim.type=="Milk")
      {
        cat(paste("   Bacterial N/degraded CHO and CP, g/kg : ",
                  formatC((rum.diet.bact.NFC.rate + rum.diet.bact.FC.rate) *(Parm_rum.bact.CP/100/6.25) *
    1000/(rum.diet.DCHO.rate + rum.diet.DProt.rate), format = "f", digits = 3, width = 7), " ",
                  "      ~ 29      ", " ", "Maximum N use efficiency (2)        ", "\n", sep = ""))
        cat(paste("   Bacterial N/degraded CHO and TP, g/kg : ",
                  formatC((rum.diet.bact.NFC.rate + rum.diet.bact.FC.rate) * (Parm_rum.bact.CP/100/6.25) *
    1000/(rum.diet.DCHO.rate + rum.diet.DPep.rate), format = "f", digits = 3, width = 7), " ",
                  "      ~ 29      ", " ", "Maximum N use efficiency (2)        ", "\n", sep = ""))
        cat(paste("   Efficiency of amino-N use, %               : ",
```

```
              formatC(isz(((rum.diet.bact.NFC_AminoN.rate + rum.diet.bact.NFC_AmmoniaN.rate + rum.diet.bact.FC_Ammo-
niaN.rate)) * 100, (rum.bact.AminoN_Uptake.rate + rum.diet.Ammonia.rate + rum.Recycled_N.rate)), format = "f", digits = 3,
width = 7), " ",
              "       ~ 69        ", " ", "Maximum g bacterianl N/kg FOM (2)     ", "\n", sep = ""))
        cat(paste("   Bacterial CP/FOM, g/100 g  .              : ",
              formatC((rum.diet.bact.NFC.rate + rum.diet.bact.FC.rate) *(Parm_rum.bact.CP/100) * 100/(rum.diet.DCHO.rate +
rum.diet.DPep.rate), format = "f", digits = 3, width = 7), " ",
              "[14.9 to 18.1] ", " ", "Empirical determination (2,8)          ", "\n", sep = ""))
      } else
      {
        cat(paste("   Bacterial CP/FOM, g/100 g                 : ",
              formatC((rum.diet.bact.NFC.rate + rum.diet.bact.FC.rate) *(Parm_rum.bact.CP/100) * 100/(rum.diet.DCHO.rate +
rum.diet.DPep.rate), format = "f", digits = 3, width = 7), " ",
              "[9.81 to 16.3] ", " ", "Empirical determination (3)          ", "\n", sep = ""))
      }
      cat(paste("Total Digestible Nutrients\n", sep = ""))
      cat(paste("   TDN, % BW                                 : ",
            formatC(isz(anim.diet.aTDN.rate*100,anim.FBW), format = "f", digits = 3, width = 7), " ",
            "                 ", " ", "                                    ", "\n", sep = ""))
      cat(paste("   TDN-to-CP ratio                           : ",
            formatC(isz(anim.diet.aTDN.conc,anim.diet.CP.conc), format = "f", digits = 3, width = 7), " ",
            "      < 7        ", " ", "Increase suppl. DMI in grazing (6)   ", "\n", sep = ""))
      cat(paste(string("-", 102), "\n", sep = ""))
      cat(paste(
        "(1) Appuhamy et al. 2013; J. Dairy Sci. 96 (8):5161-5173\n",
        "(2) Bach et al. 2005. J. Dairy Sci. 88 (E. Suppl.):E9-E21\n",
        "(3) Galyean and Tedeschi, 2014. J. Anim. Sci. 92(11):5099-5111\n",
        "(4) Klevesahl et al., 2003; Anim. Feed Sci. Technol. 105 (1-4):5-20\n",
        "(5) Koster et al., 1996; J. Anim. Sci. 74 (10):2473-2481\n",
        "(6) Mathis et al., 2000; J. Anim. Sci. 78 (1):224-232\n",
        "(7) Moore et al., 1999; J. Anim. Sci. 77 (2):123-135\n",
        "(8) Oba and Allen, 2003. J. Dairy Sci. 86(1):195-207\n",
        "(9) Satter and Slyter, 1974; Br. J. Nutr. 32 (2):199-208\n",
        sep=""))
    }
    return(invisible(TRUE))
  }
```

(This page intentionally left blank)

Part III. Using the Ruminant Nutrition System for R

"Measuring programming progress by lines of code is like measuring aircraft building progress by weight."
Bill Gates

(This page intentionally left blank)

7 The Ruminant Nutrition System for R

7.1 Working with the RNS for R within the RNS

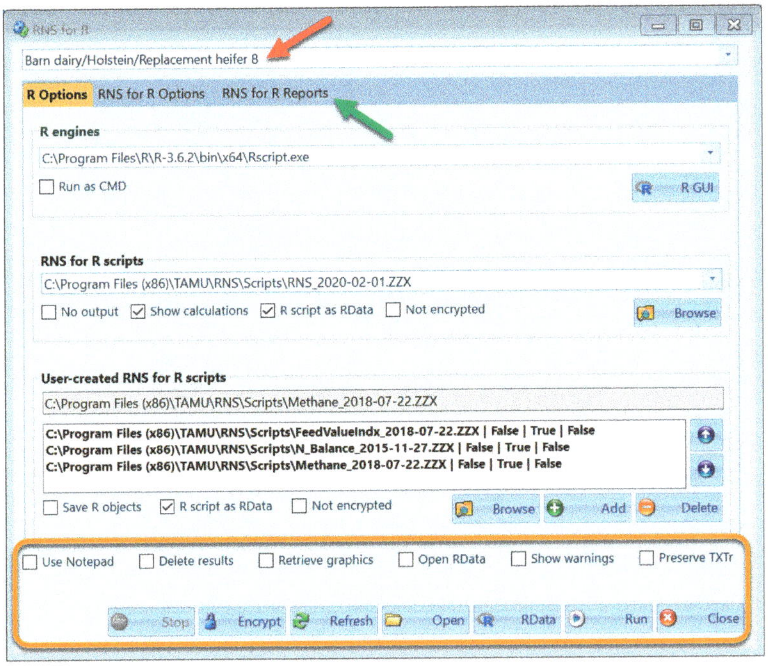

Figure 7.1. Ruminant Nutrition System (RNS) for R form.

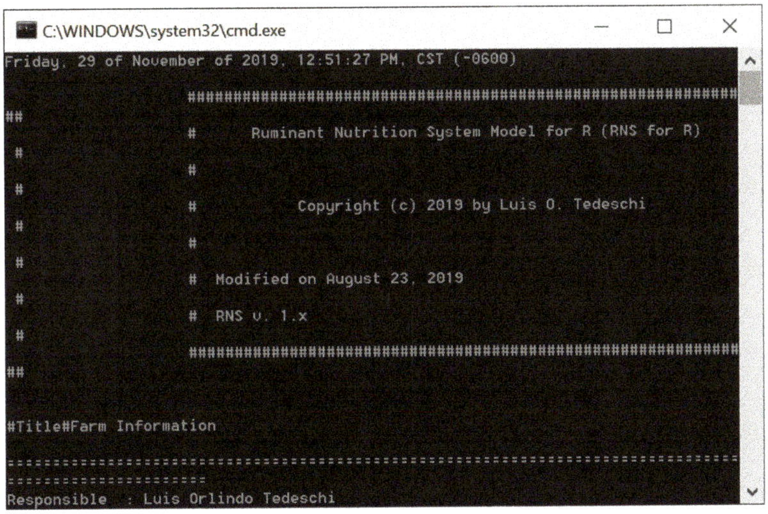

Figure 7.2. Command prompt showing RNS for R calculations.

The RNS for R provides a versatile alternative to performing the calculations described in the RNS book and listed above. A minimum understanding of the R environment is required, and there are many basic and applied publications[6] free of charge. Figure 7.1 has the form view of the RNS for R interface. There are three main sections in this form. The top portion (shown by the red arrow in Figure 7.1) has the name of the simulation file in a *drop-down listbox*. The middle portion (shown by green arrow Figure 7.1) has three tabs (*R Options*, *RNS for R Options*, and *RNS for R Reports*). The bottom portion (shown by the yellow rounded rectangle in Figure 7.1) has general settings and command buttons to set the RNS for R execution.

The ***R Options*** shown in Figure 7.1, has three parts in the top, middle, and bottom. The top part of this tab has a list of installed R engines on the user's computer. Click on the drop-down button to select which engine to use. If this is the first time using an engine version, R may take longer to execute to code because it will update the packages needed to perform the calculations. The middle part of this tab has a list of RNS for R script installed with the RNS software. The RNS for R scripts are located in the *"Documents/TAMU/RNS Files/Scripts"* and *"Program Files (x86)/TAMU/RNS/Scripts"* folders and users can add other RNS for R scripts. The checkbox No output will execute the RNS for R scripts without generating output, but creating the RData file. The checkbox Show calculations will open

(6) https://cran.r-project.org/manuals.html

a command prompt to show the progress of the RNS for R calculations (Figure 7.2). The checkbox R script as RData informs RNS for R that the R script is an object RData not a text (ASCII) file. When not encrypted, the extension of the RData file is *.RData*. Otherwise, when not encrypted, the extension of the R script is *.R*. The checkbox Not encrypted informs RNS for R that the R script is not encrypted. When encrypted, the extension of the R scripts is *.ZZX*, when not encrypted it is *.ZZZ*. The bottom part of this tab has the user-created scripts section. Users can develop R scripts to be executed with RNS for R after the main R script is executed. The *Browse* option allows users to select the R script to be used. Then, select the Save R objects is you want the R script objects to be saved with the R object, choose the R script as RData or Not encrypted as described in the previous bullet. Then, click on the *Add* button to add the user-created script and options in the list box, or click on the *Remove* button to delete a previously saved user-created script included in the list box. The arrow up/down assigns a priority in the execution of the selected user-created script.

The bottom portion in Figure 7.1 (shown in yellow rounded rectangle) has general settings and command buttons to set the RNS for R execution. The Use Notepad will open Notepad at the end of the RNS for R execution with the calculation results. The Delete results do not save the calculations results automatically. The Retrieve graphics add graphics or pictures generated during the calculation to the RNS for R file. The Open RData opens the *.RData* file generated after the calculation is finished. The Show warnings will display the warnings obtained during the execution of the RNS for R. The Preseve TXTr will keep the *.TXTr* file created during the execution of the RNS for R. The *Stop* bottom stops an active execution. The *Encrypt* button encrypts a user-created script to prevent others from changing it. The *Refresh* button refreshes the fields in the RNS for R form. The *Open* button opens an RNS for R (extension *.RNSr* or *.TXTr*) previously executed and saved. The *RData* button opens an *.RData* file previously executed and saved. The *Run* button initiates the execution of the RNS for R. The *Close* button closes the RNS for R form. Both Open RData option and the *RData* button will open the R Console with the RData (R object) generated by the RNS for R (see Section 7.2).

The ***RNS for R Options*** (Figure 7.3) allow the user to select specific procedures/calculations to be executed by the RNS for R code. This is how the user can interact with the RNS for R program indirectly. Alternative calculations and submodels are provided in this section. Each option (also referred to as *flags*) will select specific functions or submodels to be used. Some are experimental, and users are responsible for the output given different combinations of these options. These options are thoroughly discussed in the RNS book.

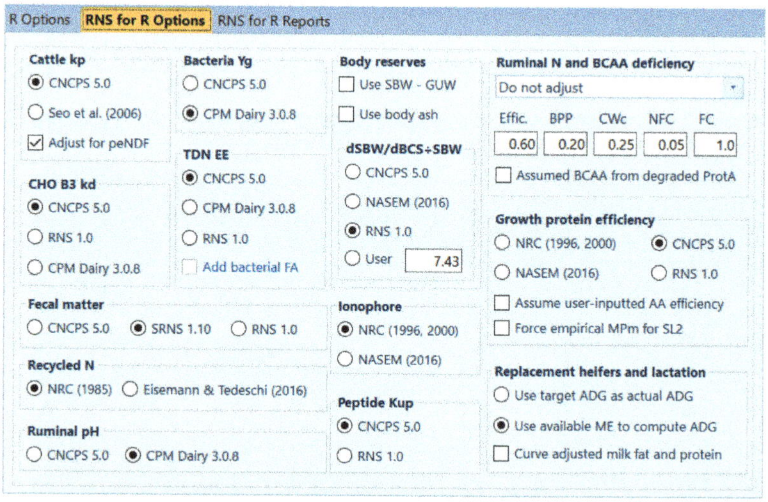

Figure 7.3. The RNS for R Options.

The ***RNS for R Reports*** (Figure 7.4) has the types of reports generated by the RNS for R calculations. The *Summary report only* will create a 2-page summary report, containing important input variables and main output variables needed to evaluate animal performance, diet composition, and nutrient excretions.

Otherwise, a complete report will be generated (usually more than 50 pages). The *Create Table of Contents (TOC)* will add a table of contents in the beginning of the report, making it easier to move around the report through hyperlinks in the PDF file. The *Dry matter required (DMR)* section allows the RNS for R to compute the dry matter required iteratively based on the individual allowable animal performance (average daily gain or milk yield) given the dietary metabolizable energy, metabolizable protein, or metabolizable amino acids. The *Optimizer engine* has different optimization options for finding the solution during the calculation of the DMR. During the optimization a command prompt will be shown to display the progress of the convergence process (Figure 7.5).

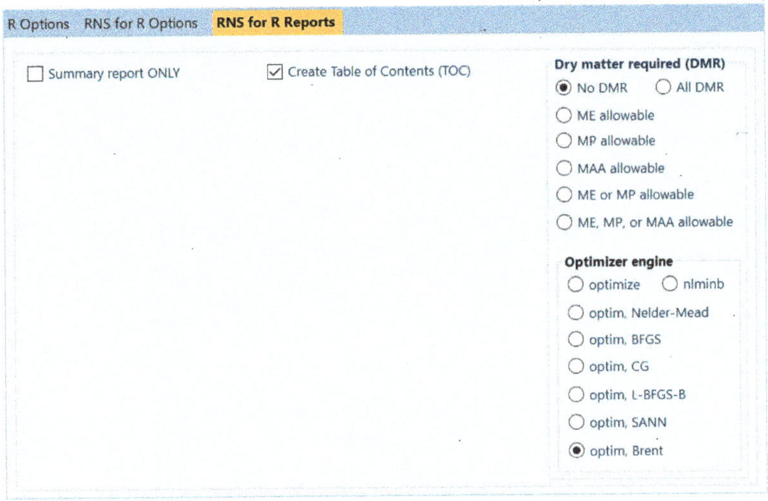

Figure 7.4. The RNS for Reports.

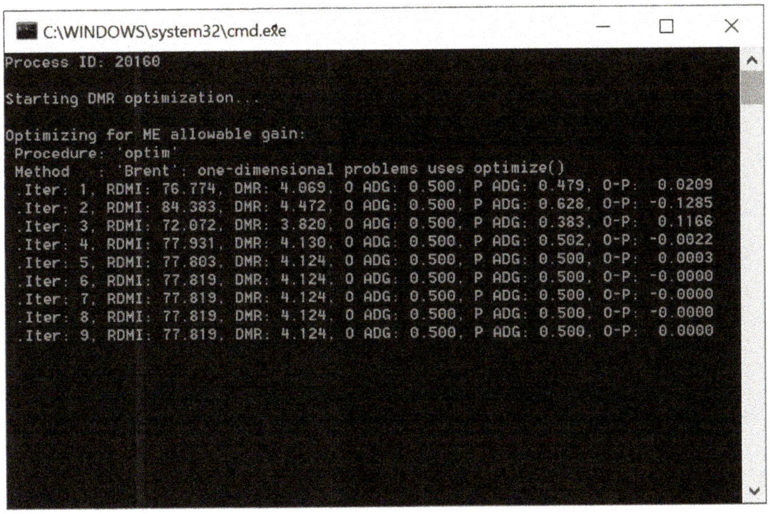

Figure 7.5. Optimization process for dry matter required calculation.

Once the execution of the RNS for R is finished, a message box similar to that shown in Figure 7.6 is displayed. If *"Quit successfully"* is not shown, the user can check the root of the problem/error by locating a file called *"warmings.txt"* that should be in the *"Documents/TAMU/RNS Files/Simulations"* folder and make necessary adjustments.

All output files will be saved in a subfolder where the simulation file resides, with a suffix *"_Output"* added. Output files created during the execution of the RNS for R script include *.TIF* files for graphics and images, *.RNSr* and *.TXTr* files containing output text, *.TXT* files containing warnings and calculation log information, and *.RData* file containing the RNS for R script codes, variables, and functions. This file can be opened with R, as discussed next. Multiple files with the same name may exist, depending on how many RNS for R executions are done. Thus, a sequential numeric suffix is added to each file. The last execution has the greatest suffix number.

7.2 Working with the RNS for R without the RNS

One of the most powerful features of the RNS for R is the creation of an R object that can be manipulated after the RNS for R execution is completed and it does not require RNS or RNS for R. All successful RNS for R executions save an R object called *"image (x).RData"* and it is located in the subfolder where the simulation file resides, with an suffix *"_Output"* added. The *"x"* is a sequential number for multiple runs of the same group/animal/stage. Figure 7.7 shows the message box that is displayed after the successful execution of an RNS for R script if the Open RData option is checked or if the user clicks on the *RData* button and select a valid RNS for R output *.RData* file.

This process will open an R Console with the selected *.RData* automatically. Figure 7.8 depicts the standard R Console using an RNS for R objects (*.RData*). The screen is self-explatory, and users can assess that informational screen by typing *"usage()"* in the prompt of the R Console. Through the R Console, users can add, modify, and execute most of the RNS calculations described in this publication and in the RNS book.

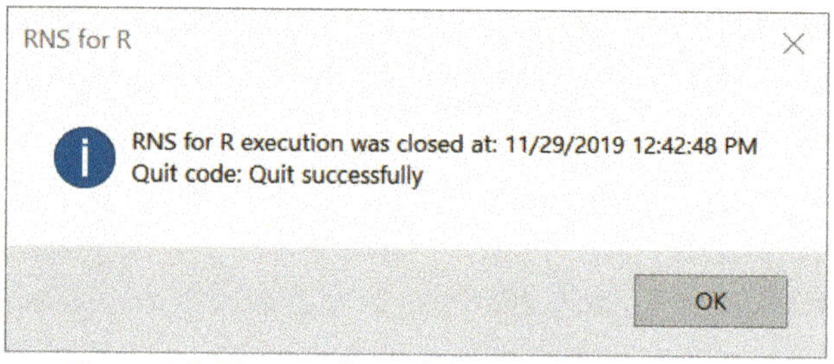

Figure 7.6. Message box of the RNS for R execution.

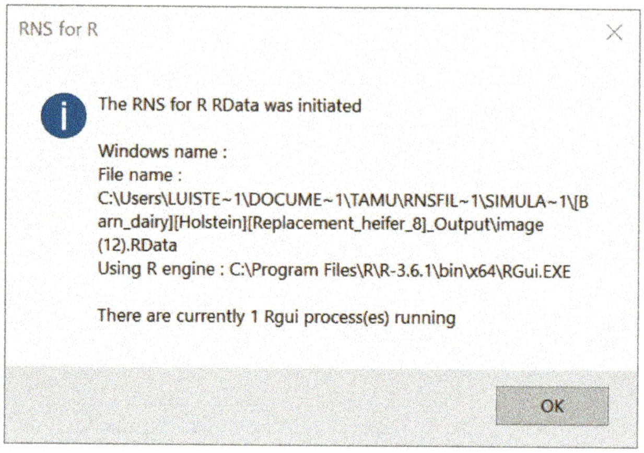

Figure 7.7. R Console informational message box.

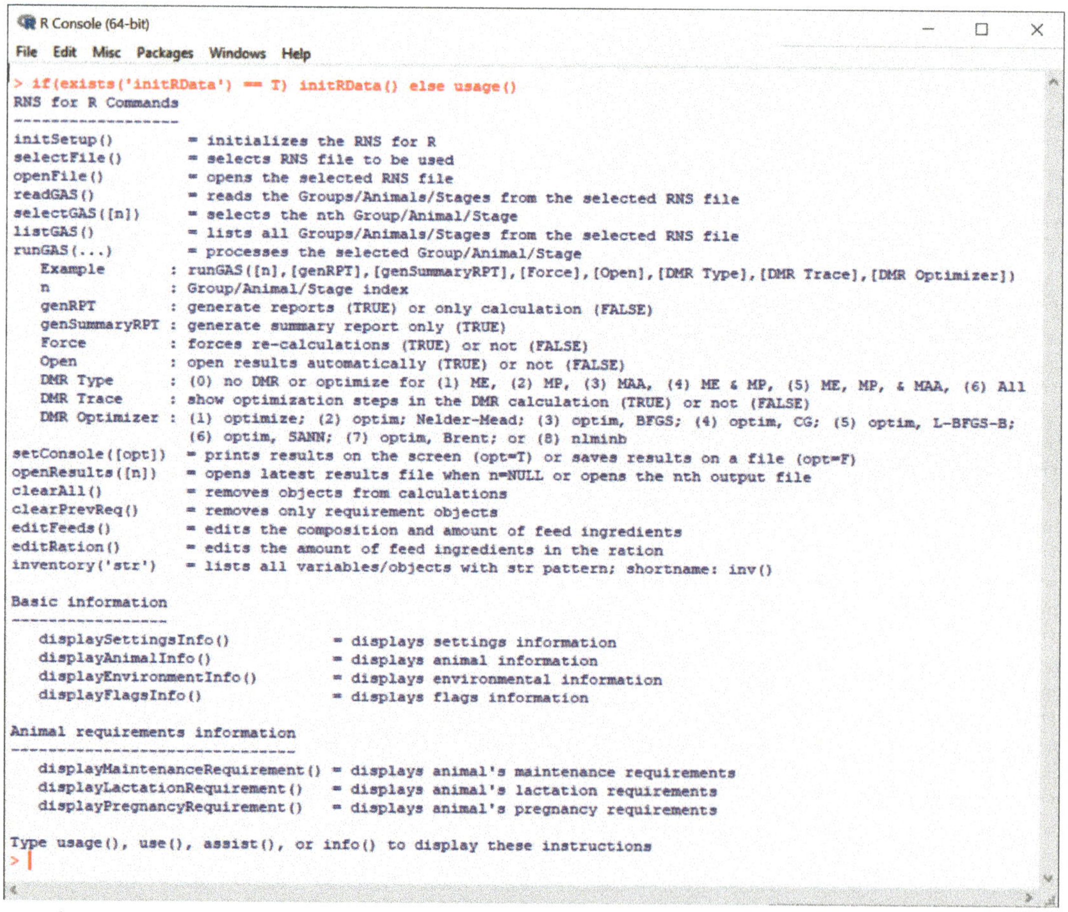

Figure 7.8. R Console of an RNS for R object (.RData). The green arrow shows the cursor (prompt).

Part IV. Interpreting the Calculations of the Ruminant Nutrition System

"... when you have eliminated the impossible, what-
ever remains, *however improbable*, must be the
truth"
Sherlock Holmes, The Sign of the Four
Sir Arthur Conan Doyle (1890).

(This page intentionally left blank)

8 Nutrient Balances and Biological Indices

8.1 Calculating the ideal levels of fiber and effective fiber in the rumen

Sections 8.1.1.4 and 11.1 of Tedeschi and Fox (2020) highlighted central biological concepts of the effectiveness of fiber for ruminants. Thought fiber is not an essential nutrient for animal survivability, both non-fermentable and fermentable dietary fibers in the diet of ruminants have beneficial properties to the gut microbiota and rumen health. Dietary fiber **(1)** promotes rumination activity and saliva production, **(2)** forms the rumen mat, **(3)** stimulates ruminal motility and the passage of material through the gastro-intestinal tract, **(4)** protects the rumen wall by maintaining the buffering capacity as volatile fatty acids are produced and accumulated in the rumen, and **(5)** prevents ruminal acidosis and the depression of cell wall digestion in cattle fed high-grain diets (Tedeschi and Fox, 2020). The effectiveness of the fiber (i.e., physically effective neutral detergent fiber; **peNDF**) of a feedstuff is related only to the physical properties of its fiber (neutral detergent fiber; **NDF**) that stimulates chewing and rumination. The establishment of a fiber requirement for ruminants has been somewhat elusive, but Mertens (1985a) reported a high correlation of NDF with rumination and rumen fill, suggesting the need to maintain a minimum amount of fiber in the rumen.

When diet energy is the first limiting factor, rumen fill limits the intake. Conversely, when diet energy is not limiting, intake is regulated by physiological feedback signals that control satiety and hunger, such as amount and site of starch digestion, and ruminal propionate production (Allen and Bradford, 2006). The optimum level of dietary NDF to maximize intake decreases as the level of milk yield increases (Mertens, 1987). Mertens (1985b) found that milk yield from several experiments was maximized when NDF intake was 1.2% ± 0.1% of body weight (**BW**). Subsequently, Mertens (1987) proposed the minimum intake of NDF (percentage of BW) to be 1.1% of BW (i.e., 1.2% minus 1 SD). The RNS uses Equations [8.1] and [8.2] to compute the requirements of NDF and peNDF intakes for different species. Williams (1988) developed different equations.

$$NDFI = \begin{cases} 1.1 \times BW / 100 & \text{Cattle} \\ \left[\left(5.4442 \times BW^{-0.25}\right) / 100\right] \times BW & \text{Sheep and goats} \end{cases} \quad [8.1]$$

$$peNDFI = \begin{cases} 0.23 \times DMI & \text{Dairy cows} \\ 0.15 \times DMI & \text{Feedlot cattle} \end{cases} \quad [8.2]$$

Where *DMI* is dry matter intake, kg/d; and *peNDFI* is physically effective neutral detergent fiber intake, kg/d.

Though successfully applied for more than two decades by consultants using CNCPS-based models, the peNDF concept has not proliferated because of a lack of practical equations to account for its interactions with multiple processes: amount and rate of rapidly fermentable carbohydrate (i.e., grain) intake, fractional degradation and passage rates of CHO fractions, and absorption of VFA. The development of routine commercial laboratory assays that satisfactorily determine peNDF has been limited, likely because of disagreement on what to measure and how to effectively do it. Farms most commonly use methods based on the sieving technique to measure peNDF. Current technologies for determining pef and peNDF include the Penn State Particle Separator (**PSPS**) (Lammers et al., 1996) and the ZBox (Cotanch and Grant, 2006). The PSPS is based on the separation of particles according to size: greater than 19 mm, between 19 mm and 8 mm, and smaller than 8 mm. The ZBox (21 cm x 21 cm x 11 cm) has an open side for insertion of interchangeable sieves with apertures of 1.14 mm, 2.38 mm, 3.18 mm, 4.76 mm, and 9.53 mm (Cotanch and Grant, 2006), which are similar to the apertures of the sieves used in the dry sieving procedure proposed by Mertens (1997). Several researchers have recommended ways to improve the on-farm applicability of the PSPS (Beauchemin and Yang, 2005; Kononoff and Heinrichs, 2003; Yang and Beauchemin, 2005, 2006). Such improvements include combining the particles retained on the 19- and 8-mm screens or by using a 1.18-mm screen modified PSPS. As concluded by Grant and Cotanch (2005), the search continues for a tool to successfully measure peNDF on the farm, though some advancements have been made in the last decade.

Tedeschi and Fox (2020, Section 11.1) recommended a minimum peNDF requirement of 7% to 10% in the DM of high-energy rations fed to growing and finishing beef cattle. With good feed-bunk management, this requirement minimizes the risk of acidosis when high-grain rations and an ionophore are fed to growing and finishing beef cattle (Fox and Tedeschi, 2002). This recommendation is based on the peNDF that was required to keep rumen pH above 5.7, which was itself based on a pH equation developed by Pitt et al. (1996). Fox and Tedeschi's (2002) recommendation agreed with the conclusions of Strasia and Gill (1990): finishing rations for cattle should contain at least 7% "high roughage" factor. However, Fox and Tedeschi (2002) also recommended at least 20% peNDF in the diet DM if the goal is to optimize forage utilization by maximizing cell wall digestibility. As Fox and Tedeschi (2002) indicated, a number of feed characteristics other than peNDF can influence both rumen pH and milk fat content, such as NFC source and intake and rates of digestion, and a safety factor should be added to the minimum peNDF requirement as needed based on experience and field observations. These peNDF requirements may be inadequate for rations with high levels of processed grain because peNDF will exert increasingly limited control over ruminal pH as the ration's effective fiber diminishes. The production rate of acids (i.e., VFA) from rapidly fermentable carbohydrates (e.g., sugar and starch) may surpass the peNDF ability to maintain an adequate ruminal pH. This is one of the reasons that the correlation between ration peNDF and ruminal pH in high-concentrate rations, those typically used for feedlot cattle, is small or non-existent. In these cases, fractional passage and absorption rates of VFA become the most important factors in controlling ruminal pH (Fox and Tedeschi, 2002), suggesting that prediction of ruminal pH in cattle fed high-grain diets will require more complex models.

8.2 Calculating the adequate balance of energy and protein in the rumen

In 1991, Moore et al. (1991) discussed the need to supplement the protein and energy of grazing animals when their forage alone would not meet their demands. They analyzed the chemical composition data of 637 samples of grass and estimated total digestible nutrients (**TDN**). The authors concluded that supplemental protein would increase forage dry matter intake (**DMI**) and average daily gain (**ADG**) for forages containing less than 7% crude protein (**CP**; dry matter basis), but that supplemental protein is unlikely to increase forage DMI when TDN-to-CP ratio is less than 8. In contrast, forage DMI and animal ADG are likely to increase for forages with TDN-to-CP ratio greater than 8.5. Subsequently, Moore et al. (1999) developed a database containing 66 publications of 126 forages (73 harvested and 53 grazed) to evaluate the forage DMI and ADG of grazing animals under different types and levels of supplementation (n = 444 comparisons of unsupplemented and supplemented treatments). The database assumed TDN to be equivalent to digestible organic matter (**DOM**), which was computed from DM digestibility when available or from tabular values assigned to the forage and supplements. Moore et al. (1999) reported that supplementation decreased forage DMI when the TDN intake of the supplement was greater than 0.7% of BW or when forage TDN-to-CP ratio was less than 7, not 8 as previously suggested by Moore et al. (1991).

We hypothesized that a TDN-to-CP ratio less than 7, which represents an adequate N diet, would trigger selective behavior of grazing animals because energy (i.e., TDN) seems to be the first limiting factor. While animals may consume less forage, they might attempt to meet their energy requirement by increasing the intake of the more energy-dense supplement, at the risk of further increasing the excess N in the rumen. Conversely, when the TDN-to-CP ratio is greater than 7, which represents an N-deficient diet, animals may increase supplement and forage intakes as N from the supplement balances out the requirement of ruminal bacteria N, increasing fiber fermentation and alleviating the rumen fill. Moore et al. (1999) proposed an empirical, nonlinear equation to predict forage-plus-supplement intake based on forage intake (percentage of BW), forage CP and TDN concentrations (percentage of OM), supplement intake (percentage of BW), and supplement CP and TDN concentrations (percentage of OM). Upon further analysis of their proposed equation using a 3D graphic (y = forage-plus-supplement intake, % of BW; x_1 = forage CP concentration, % of OM; and x_2 = forage TDN concentration, % of OM), supplement TDN shows a peculiar behavior: increased supplement TDN not only decreases the forage-plus-supplement intake, but it also changes the correlation of forage TDN and CP concentrations on forage-plus-supplement intake, with an inflection point at around 80% of supplement TDN (OM basis). DelCurto et al. (1990) reached a similar conclusion that supplemental energy without adequate protein availability was associated with reduced intake and feed digestibility. Nonetheless, the ratio of TDN-to-CP might not be the ideal target, and its generalization is prone to failure because the adequate ratio may vary depending on several factors in the production scenario. For example, CP and ruminally degraded protein (**RDP**) are not necessarily correlated, and TDN may not reflect fermentable OM (**FOM**). Bodine and Purvis II (2003) found that steers grazing dormant tallgrass prairie increased ADG when RDP-rich supplement was added to the animals' grain-based supplement.

The RNS computes the TDN-to-CP ratio and indicates that values below 7 might trigger an animal's selective behavior, leading to increased consumption of energy-based feedstuffs alongside a probable decrease in consumption of forage (i.e., roughage), but the forage-plus-supplement energy content needs to be considered. When the TDN-to-CP ratio is greater than 7, the shortage of dietary CP may also trigger increased consumption of supplement as long as it is proteinaceous, and a subsequent increase in forage consumption is an indirect effect of meeting ruminal bacteria N requirement and increased fiber fermentability in the rumen. These behaviors may not occur if the appropriate supplement (energy-dense or protein-dense) is not available to the animal.

The TDN-to-CP ratio is just one among many other indices. The search for a single, generalized index that reflects the nutritive value of feeds (more specifically, forages) likely started in the 1950s (Crampton et al., 1960; Lee et al., 2017), and, in many instances it has been disappointing (Crampton, 1957). We may never find this Holy Grail. Instead, multiple variables (e.g., ratios, balances, residues) have to be analyzed simultaneously, and diets and supplements have to be optimized for specific objectives or multi-objective optimization approaches specific to each specific production condition. These multiple objectives certainly have competing goals and often they are negatively correlated. Crampton et al. (1960) proposed the nutritive value index (**NVI**), which is the multiplication of the relative intake of forage by the forage digestibility of energy. The relative intake of forage is computed as the actual forage intake divided by $0.8 \times BW^{0.75}$. Later, Rohweder et al. (1978) developed the relative forage value (**RFV**), which is the product of the predicted DMI (as percentage of BW, assuming 120÷NDF) multiplied by predicted digestible DM (as percentage of DM, based on ADF), divided by 1.29. For example, the forage value of full-bloom alfalfa is 129, so dividing the forage value by 1.29 would yield an RFV of 100. The NVI and RFV likely provided the field's initial impetus to find other feedstuffs nutritive value indices, including quality index, relative forage quality, and feed unit and fill (INRA, Institut National de la Recherche Agronomique, 1989; Moore, 1994; Moore and Undersander, 2002). However, many of these indices rely on the empiricism of regressions to estimate biological values that are not readily available or are expensive to determine (e.g., TDN). The question then becomes, how reliable are nutritive value indices that use empirical values, which are inherently biased and may have a great degree of uncertainty?

8.3 Ruminal nitrogen balance and bacterial growth

As a general rule of thumb, improving the efficiency of ruminal bacterial growth will increase the animal's retention of N. Many comprehensive reviews of N metabolism in the rumen have been published (Bach et al., 2005; Leng and Nolan, 1984; Nolan and Dobos, 2005; Schwab et al., 2005; Smith, 1969; Stern and Hoover, 1979; Waldo, 1968; Walker et al., 2005). Stern and Hoover (1979) concluded that about 16.9 g of microbial CP (**MCP**) is obtained for every 100 g of OM apparently fermented in the rumen (i.e., FOM), but it varies largely from 6.3 to 31.6 g/100 g (i.e., 63 to 316 g/kg), depending on the diet constituents. For dairy cattle, the maximum efficiency of N use (**ENU**) by the ruminal bacteria is about 69%, achieved when the efficiency of microbial protein synthesis (**EMPS**) is 29 g of bacterial N per kilogram of FOM (Bach et al.,

2005), approximately 18.1 g MCP/100 g FOM (assuming MCP has 16% N) or 181 g MCP/kg FOM[(7)]. Because these authors indicated the relationship between ENU (*y*) and EMPS (*x*) followed a quadratic pattern, the ENU decreases at EMPS below or above 29 g/kg. Similarly, Oba and Allen (2003) reported an EMPS of 23.8 g of bacterial N per kilogram of FOM, which is equivalent to 14.875 g MCP/100 g FOM (assuming MCP has 16% N). These authors derived the theoretical maximum microbial efficiency of 39.0977 g MCP/100 g FOM that is about 31.27 or 62.55 g bacteria N per kilogram of FOM, assuming MCP has 8% or 16% N, respectively. The 39.0977 g MCP/g FOM is, however, approx. 74% greater than previously computed theoretical maximum EMPS of 22.5 g MCP/g FOM, assuming stoichiometric relationships of ruminal fermentation in grazing ruminants (Corbett et al., 1982; Corbett 1987). Values above 17 g MCP/100 FOM are rarely observed for beef cattle, though recently Bowen et al. (2017) reported 20.9 g MCP/100 FOM with cattle grazing ryegrass. Galyean and Tedeschi (2014) reported an empirical average of 8.2 g of MCP/100 g FOM, but because their equation had an intercept the average MCP efficiency (assuming an average of 5 kg of FOM/d) is closer to 11.4 g of MCP/100 g of FOM, about 18.2 g bacterial N per kilogram of FOM (assuming MCP is 16% N), which is about 30% less than that empirically obtained by Oba and Allen (2003) for lactating dairy animals (11.4 g MCP/g FOM versus 14.875 g MCP/g FOM, respectively). Based on the Galyean and Tedeschi (2014) equation, the MCP efficiency likely ranges from 9.81 to 16.3 g MCP/100 g FOM, assuming that FOM varies from 10 to 2 kg/d, respectively. This range is similar to 13 to 17 g MCP/100 g digestible organic matter intake (**DOMI**)[(8)] reported by the Agricultural and Food Research Council (AFRC, 1993) and the Commonwealth Scientific and Industrial Research Organization (CSIRO, 2007). A possible reason for the discrepancies between lactating dairy cows and beef cattle might be that shorter ruminal retention time of FOM in the lactating dairy cow is associated with a greater OM intake, yielding a greater ruminal microbial growth efficiency, compared to growing beef cattle that have a longer ruminal retention time of FOM, therefore, yielding a lower microbial growth efficiency (Leng and Nolan, 1984). Bowen et al. (2018) reported that for Brahman steers grazing pangola grass (*Digitaria eriantha*) and supplemented with urea or casein to provide 150 g RDP/kg DOMI up to 300 g RDP/kg DOMI (i.e., 15% to 30% RDP), the EMPS of 16.7 g MCP/100 g DOMI was only obtained when 29.3% of RDP was fed in the form of true protein. But in order to achieve the 16.7 g MCP/100 g DOMI, when compared to the control group, there was a 4-fold increase in ruminal NH_3-N concentration (277 mg/L versus 73 mg/L, respectively) and branched-chain volatile fatty acids (**BCVFA**: isobutyric, isovaleric, and 2-methylbutyric) concentration (44 versus 10 mmol/mol of total volatile fatty acids—**VFA**). The authors concluded that "... only high amounts of RDP supply to the rumen, in the form of true protein, resulted in increased EMPS whereas at the lower intakes of RDP formulated to achieve EMPS in the range suggested in the feeding standards (130–170 g MCP/kg DOMI) there was no difference in providing the RDP as non-protein N or degradable-protein".

In addition to the ratio of protein to energy in the rumen, the EMPS is strongly associated with the maintenance requirements of ruminal bacteria (Leng and Nolan, 1984). Typical ruminal concentration of ammonia-N in beef cattle diets ranges from 2 to 10 mM (30 to 160 mg ammonia-N/L), but can be greater than 30 mM (500 mg ammonia-N/L) for diets containing high levels of RDP (National Academies of Sciences, Engineering, and Medicine; NASEM, 2016). Previously, Satter and Slyter (1974) established that a ruminal

---

[(7)] 29 g N/kg FOM = (29 ÷1,000)×(1/0.16) = 0.181 g CP/g FOM or 18.1 g CP/100 g FOM or 181 g CP/kg FOM.

[(8)] Assuming that digestible organic matter intake (DOMI) is equal to fermentable organic matter (FOM) intake.

concentration at least 50 mg ammonia-N/L (about 3.6 mM) is needed to ensure ideal bacterial growth, but this threshold is likely to vary from 50 to 290 mg ammonia-N/L (3.6 to 20.7 mM) and it does not ensure maximal microbial protein synthesis (Stern and Hoover, 1979). Schwab et al. (2005) recommended values between 80 and 180 mg ammonia-N/L (5 to 11 mM) to maximize MCP outflow from the rumen.

The RNS model computes the net rate of ruminal N flux as the difference between supply of amino-N plus ammonia-N and the requirement of N by fiber carbohydrate (**FC**) and nonfiber carbohydrate (**NFC**) bacteria. Tedeschi and Fox (2020, Section 8.2.4.3) discussed the fundamentals of ammonia-N and amino-N balances in the rumen to meet FC and NFC bacteria requirements for growth. The inflows of ammonia-N are dietary ammonia-N, dietary amino-N (i.e., peptides) converted to ammonia-N, and ruminal recycled ammonia-N. The bacterial N removed by protozoa predation of bacteria may increase the ammonia-N in the rumen, but this is not considered as an inflow for two reasons: **(1)** the bacterial growth already accounts for predation (i.e., it assumes less bacterial update of N), so the predated bacterial N stays in the ruminal N balance, and **(2)** the *recycled* bacterial N was already accounted for upon its initial entrance into the rumen. The outflows are bacterial uptake of ammonia-N and ammonia-N escape of the rumen with the liquid phase. Figure 8.1 shows the graphical representation of the inflows and outflows of ruminal ammonia-N.

The amount of ammonia-N in the rumen can be computed by assuming a steady-state condition (i.e., inflows = outflows). To maintain the steady-state condition, the ruminal N balance would have to escape the rumen at the fractional liquid passage rate, based on Figure 8.1. Dividing the ruminal N balance (g/h)[9] by the fractional liquid passage rate (1/h) would provide the amount of ammonia-N in the rumen. Subsequently, the concentration of ruminal ammonia-N is computed assuming the molar mass of ammonia-N is 14 g/mol and calculating the ruminal volume based on BW, as shown in Equations [8.3] and [8.4]. For example, assuming ruminal N balance of 134 g/d and fractional liquid passage rate of 2.799 1/d (i.e., 0.116 1/h), the amount of ammonia-N in the rumen is 47.9 g. Figure 8.1 shows the same value. Based on the simulations in Figure 8.1, ruminal ammonia-N in the rumen reaches this level after 33 h of simulation

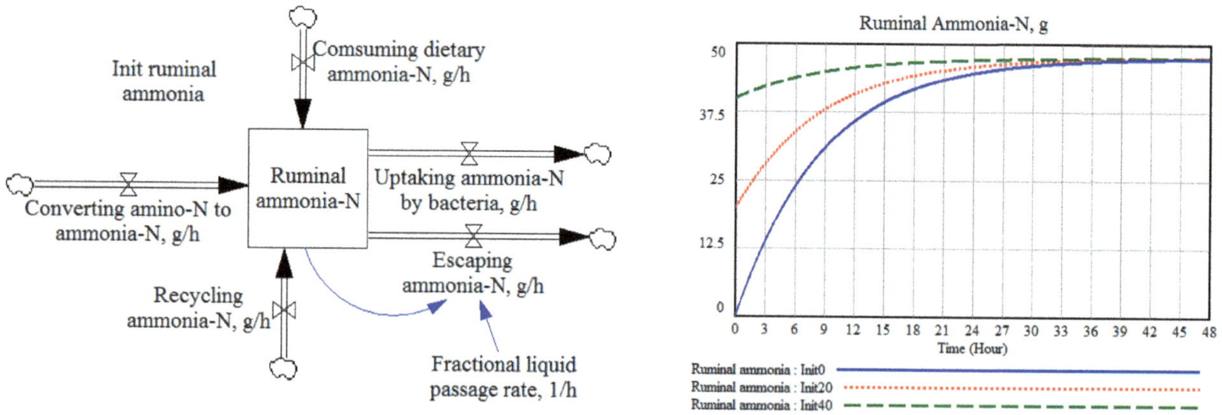

Figure 8.1. Schematic representation of ammonia-N dynamics in the rumen assuming a steady-state condition and three initial values of ammonia-N in the rumen (0, 20, and 40 g).

[9] Technically, the ruminal N balance expressed as grams per hour is, in fact, a *rate or flow*; the ruminal N balance should be expressed as grams.

regardless of the initial value of ruminal ammonia-N. Then, assuming an animal with BW of 646 kg (Equation [8.4] produces a rumen volume of 0.0715 m^3) and the molar weight of N of 14 g/mol, the concentration of ruminal ammonia-N is 47.9 mM. This value is well above the 3.6-mM threshold for ammonia-N recommended by Satter and Slyter (1974). In fact, using Equations [8.3] and [8.4], and the sketch shown in Figure 8.1, the backward calculation indicates that 3.6 mM for this same animal is equivalent to approximately 10 g/d of ammonia-N in the rumen.

$$[\mathrm{NH_3\text{-}N}] = RNB / (kl \times Vr \times 14) \quad [8.3]$$

$$Vr = 0.0888 \times FBW^{1.034} / 1000 \quad [8.4]$$

Where *[NH₃-N]* is ammonia-N, mM; *FBW* is full body weight, kg; *Kl* is fractional liquid passage rate, 1/d; *RNB* is rumen nitrogen balance, g/d; and *Vr* is rumen volume, m^3.

The flux of N across the rumen epithelium is a significant source of N to ruminants, capable of more than doubling the N intake (Lapierre and Lobley, 2001). Most CNCPS-based models compute the net flux of recycled ruminal N, and Tedeschi and Fox (2020, Section 8.2.2.2.1) discussed the recycled N and urea-N used for anabolism (**UUA**) extensively. The RNS uses the UUA as a proxy for ruminal recycled N, following the work of Eisemann and Tedeschi (2016). In general, the estimates of UUA follow a quadratic shape in regards to dietary CP (percentage of DM), and they can be lower than those estimates obtained with the equation recommended by the NRC (1985). Consequently, the concentration of ammonia-N depends on the methods used to estimate the ruminal recycled N.

Perhaps a more important question is whether the approach delineated in Figure 8.1 and Equations [8.3] and [8.4] is still valid when the ammonia-N concentration in the rumen exceeds a certain threshold. For instance, the average concentration of plasma urea-N (**PUN**) is approximately 12 mg/dL. If the concentration of ruminal ammonia-N or ruminal urea-N (**RUN**) exceeds this value, one would expect a transfer of N from the rumen into the plasma via simple diffusion. Consequently, the net recycled N (i.e., UUA) should be zero or negative. Possible ways to address this issue include **(1)** setting recycled N to zero when RUN is greater than 12 mg/dL, **(2)** including transfer rate of N from the rumen into the plasma based on the ruminal pH and RUN concentration level, and **(3)** predicting PUN given RUN levels. These approaches would require the addition of a simple diffusion submodel into the sketch shown in Figure 8.1.

8.4 Empirical calculations of nitrogen excretion

The predictability of nitrogen excretion (urinary, fecal) or secretion (milk) varies considerably. Nitrogen excretion is the result of many consecutive biological processes, from the transformation of dietary crude protein (**CP**) (i.e., nitrogen intake, **NI**) into amino acids (**AA**) by the ruminal microbes to the absorption of AA of the resultant protein escaping the rumen (i.e., ruminally undegraded protein, **RUP**) in the intestine and their metabolism by the liver, kidneys, tissues, and mammary gland. Main factors that can negatively affect nitrogen excretion include an incorrect balance between ruminally degradable protein (**RDP**) and RUP (Santos et al., 1998), and synchronization between carbohydrate and protein degradation in the rumen (Sinclair et al., 1993; Tamminga, 1991). In the end, increased excretion of nitrogen either via urine or via feces reflects a poor efficiency in capturing the nitrogen consumed by the animal.

8.4.1 Dairy cattle

Several studies (Jonker et al., 1998; Kohn et al., 2002; Nennich et al., 2005; Nennich et al., 2006; Spek et al., 2013; Wilkerson et al., 1997; Zhai et al., 2007) have developed empirical systems to predict manure production and the partition of N between feces and urine. Some models exclusively used large sets of data readily available from farms to determine empirical relationships among variables, and other models were more mechanistic in their attempt to understand the fluxes of N and possible routes for its excretion.

8.4.1.1 Predicting urinary nitrogen from milk urea nitrogen content

Wilkerson et al. (1997), for instance, compiled N balance data from 56 experiments (n = 1801 observations), conducted at the USDA Energy Metabolism Unit in Beltsville, Maryland, between from 1960 and 1990, to develop empirical regressions to estimate manure (wet feces and urine, without bedding material) and N excretion of Holstein cattle. The dataset contained dietary information (DM, CP, EE, ash, GE, OM, NDF, ADF, hemicellulose, cellulose, and ADL) and animal characteristics (age, BW, MY, milk composition, DIM and DG) of 334 lactating and dry cows and 75 growing steers and replacement heifers. The multiple quadratic regression provided the best fit with R^2 varying from 0.446 (manure production for growing and replacement cattle) to 0.944 (excreted N for growing and replacement cattle).

By contrast, Jonker et al. (1998) developed a simple mechanistic model of N fluxes to partition N among milk, feces, and urine of lactating dairy cows. Their model was based on three N balance studies (10 diets, 40 cows, and 70 observations) and required milk urea N (**MUN**, mg/dL), milk production (**MY**, kg/d), milk protein (percentage of milk DM), and dietary CP (percentage of DM) to predict urinary N (**UN**), NI, fecal N (**FN**), and DMI, as shown in Equations [8.5] to [8.8]. The relationship between UN and MUN was devised empirically. The 97 g/d is the metabolic N (endogenous and microbial fecal N), and the 0.83 is the true digestibility of protein, both determined using the Lucas test by regressing N disappearance on N intake. On the other hand, when DMI is known, one could back calculate urinary N and milk urea N by re-arranging Equations [8.6] and [8.8].

$$UN = 12.54 \times MUN \qquad [8.5]$$

$$NI = \left(UN + MN + 97\right) / 0.83 \qquad [8.6]$$

$$FN = NI - UN - MN \qquad [8.7]$$

$$DMI = \left(NI \times 6.25 / CP \times 0.01\right) / 1000 \qquad [8.8]$$

Where *CP* is crude protein, % DM; *DMI* is dry matter intake, kg/d; *FN* is fecal N, g/d; *MN* is milk N, g/d; *MUN* is milk urea N, mg/dL; *NI* is N intake, g/d; and *UN* is urinary N, g/d.

The prediction adequacy of UN from MUN has been inconsistent despite their high correlation (Kohn et al., 2002; Nennich et al., 2006). Urinary N, g/d, varies from 10×MUN (Zhai et al., 2007) to 17.6×MUN (Kauffman and St-Pierre, 2001). Kauffman and St-Pierre (2001) developed Equation [8.9] (R^2 = 0.98, σ^2 = 74.1 g^2/d^2) using Holstein and Jersey lactating cows fed four different diets (13% or 17% CP, and 30% or 40% NDF). Zhai et al. (2007) indicated that existing equations to predict urinary N (Jonker et al., 1998; Kauffman and St-Pierre, 2001) did not satisfactorily predict urinary N from Chinese Holstein cows, so they developed Equation [8.10] (r^2 = 0.82). Nennich et al. (2006) used the data of 372 lactating Holstein cows (cow x period data points) and concluded that in addition to predicting UN (Equation [8.11]), MUN can be used to predict the daily amount (kg/d) of urine excretion ($17.1 + 0.563 \times MUN$). In part, the inconsistencies in predicting UN from MUN is due to the changes in the methodology used to measure MUN concentrations. Prior to 1998, MUN values (approximately 12 mg/dL to 16 mg/dL) were artificially high due to a glitch in the hardware used by DHIA laboratories across the United States (Kohn et al., 2002). Since then, MUN values have been 8 mg/dL to 12 mg/dL. Equation [8.12] should provide more reliable values for UN given the current methodology to measure MUN, and it should be used instead of Equation [8.5]. Nousiainen et al. (2004) developed Equation [8.13] based on 50 trials with 306 different diets from Finland and Sweden.

$$UN = 0.0259 \times BW \times MUN \quad [8.9]$$

$$UN = 10.07 \times MUN + 47.29 \quad [8.10]$$

$$UN = 0.254 \times BW - 1.03 \times MY + 0.2101 \times NI + 5.09 \times MUN + 21.8 \times MTP - 6.5 \times MF - 138.8 \quad [8.11]$$

$$UN = 15.1 \times MUN + 27.8 \quad [8.12]$$

$$NI = 34 + 13.4 \times MUN \quad [8.13]$$

Where *BW* is body weight, kg; *MF* is milk fat, %; *MTP* is milk true protein, %; *MUN* is milk urea nitrogen, mg/dL; *MY* is milk yield, kg/d; and *UN* is urinary N, g/d.

More recently, Spek et al. (2013) conducted a meta-analysis with 47 trials carried out in North America and Europe to develop predictive equations of UN and urinary urea-N (**UUN**), as shown in Equations [8.14] and [8.15]. In their analysis, MUN, dietary CP, and DMI were the best predictors of UN, and for UUN, only MUN and dietary CP were significant.

$$UN = \begin{cases} \begin{cases} 29.3 + 14.08 \times MUN & \text{North America} \\ 36.4 + 11.92 \times MUN & \text{Europe} \end{cases} \\ \begin{cases} -132.2 + 7.52 \times MUN + 14.42 \times CP & \text{North America} \\ -66.4 + 7.73 \times MUN + 9.63 \times CP & \text{Europe} \end{cases} \\ \begin{cases} -168.9 + 7.84 \times MUN + 13.37 \times CP + 2.17 \times DMI & \text{North America} \\ -149.8 + 7.55 \times MUN + 9.64 \times CP + 4.55 \times DMI & \text{Europe} \end{cases} \end{cases} \quad [8.14]$$

$$UUN = \begin{cases} \begin{cases} -20.8 + 14.4 \times MUN & \text{North America} \\ -47.4 + 14.09 \times MUN & \text{Europe} \end{cases} \\ \begin{cases} -380.7 + 32 \times CP & \text{North America} \\ -324.5 + 28.7 \times CP & \text{Europe} \end{cases} \\ \begin{cases} -197.6 + 8.77 \times MUN + 14.62 \times CP & \text{North America} \\ -123.3 + 10.97 \times MUN + 7.19 \times CP & \text{Europe} \end{cases} \end{cases} \quad [8.15]$$

Where *CP* is crude protein, g/d; *DMI* is dry matter intake, kg/d; *MUN* is milk urea nitrogen, mg/dL; *UN* is urinary N, g/d; and *UUN* is urinary urea N, g/d.

Figure 8.2 shows the relationship between UN and MUN or NI for selected empirical equations listed in Table 8.1. Clearly, Equation [8.5] *underpredicts* UN (Figure 8.2A), and the equation developed by Schuba et al. (2017) *overpredicts* UN (Figure 8.2B). As shown by Spek et al. (2013), these predictive equations behave similarly, though with greater differences at high MUN values. It is not clear how much the datasets used by these studies are independent from each other, so some of the data may overlap. Consequently, their predictions can be, to some degree, correlated by design.

8.4.1.2 *Predicting urinary and fecal nitrogen from nitrogen intake*

Though NI may be accepted as the predictive variables in common practice, its prediction of UN and FN still exhibit large variation and bias. Table 8.1 lists different publications' empirical equations for predicting nitrogen excretion. Castillo et al. (2000) analyzed 91 diets from 580 lactating dairy cows from studies conducted in many parts of the world, and they reported that while FN and MUN followed a linear trend with NI (200 g/d to 750 g/d), UN had an exponential shape.

Huhtanen et al. (2008) evaluated 207 studies, encompassing 998 treatment means, of nitrogen utilization for milk protein production, UN, FN, and total manure N excretion by lactating dairy cows (Table 8.1). They indicated that nitrogen efficiency was poorly correlated with milk yield, but dietary concentration of crude protein and protein balance in the rumen were the best predictors of milk nitrogen (**MN**) with an

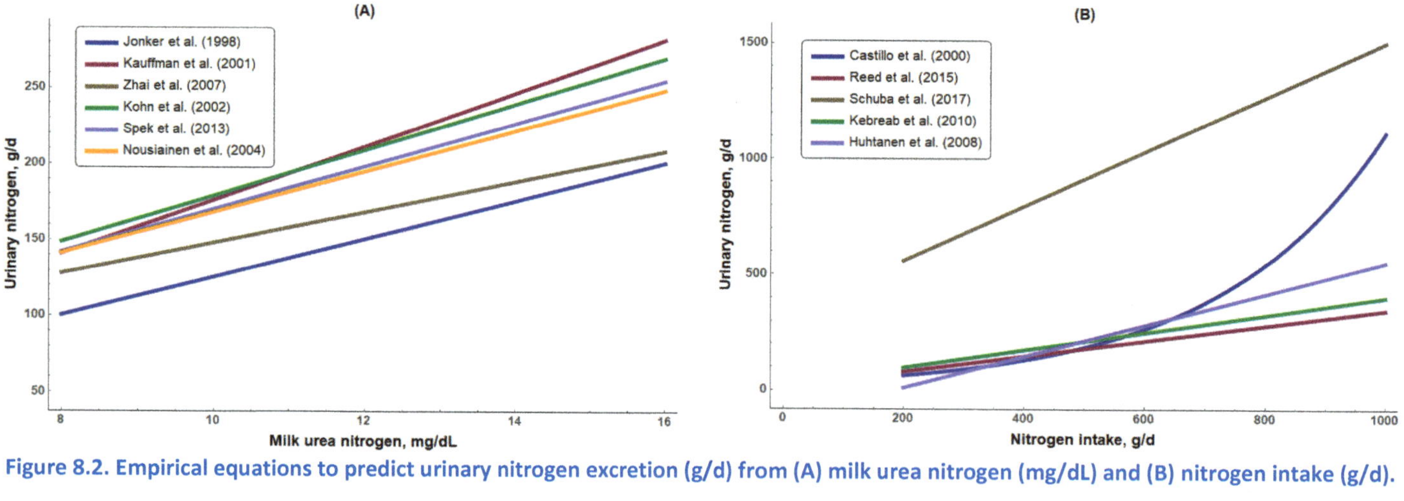

Figure 8.2. Empirical equations to predict urinary nitrogen excretion (g/d) from (A) milk urea nitrogen (mg/dL) and (B) nitrogen intake (g/d).

efficiency of 0.277 g MN/g NI, or about 28%. The authors confirmed that DMI and NI were better predictors of UN and FN than NI alone. Kebreab et al. (2010) used 470 dairy cow observations obtained from calorimetry studies conducted at the University of Reading (Kebreab et al., 2003) to develop empirical equations to predict UN, FN, and MN (Table 8.1). The authors indicated that the nitrogen correlated highly with NI but that metabolizable energy intake had the opposite effect on UN and FN, as shown in Equations [8.16] and [8.17].

$$UN = 47.8 + 0.56 \times NI - 71.4 \times ME \quad [8.16]$$

$$FN = 2.04 + 0.1 \times NI + 45.9 \times ME \quad [8.17]$$

Where NI is nitrogen intake, g/d; ME is metabolizable energy intake, MJ/kg$^{0.75}$ BW/d; and UN is urinary nitrogen, g/d.

Reed et al. (2015) developed empirical equations (Table 8.1) to predict UN (123 to 350 g/d), FN (105 to 334 g/d), total nitrogen (**TN**, 230 to 641 g/d), and MN (47.9 to 267 g/d) from NI (294 to 932 g/d). They used 1,047 records of lactating Holstein and Jersey cows from 59 indirect calorimetry studies conducted over 30 years at the Beltsville USDA Energy and Metabolism laboratory. They based their empirical equations on NI and other dietary components. The authors did not predict UN from MUN, but they compared their empirical equations with extant empirical equations that were developed in a similar way. They indicated that, compared to other equations, their UN and FN equations provided lower prediction errors and their MN equation provided similar prediction errors.

Table 8.1. Empirical equations of selected publications to predict urinary nitrogen (UN, g/d), fecal nitrogen (FN, g/d), milk nitrogen (MN, g/d), and total nitrogen (TN, g/d) excretions of lactating dairy cattle from nitrogen intake (NI, g/d), dietary crude protein (CP, % of DM), and dry matter intake (DMI, kg/d).

UN, g/d	FN, g/d	MN, g/d	TN, g/d	NI, g/d	CP, % DM	DMI, kg/d	Equations	Ref.[1]
34–437	62–201	36–161	—	182–726	—	—	$UN = 30.4 \times e^{0.0036 \times NI}$	(A)
							$FN = 0.21 \times NI + 52.3$	
							$MN = 0.17 \times NI + 41$	
—	—	57.4–231.8	—	212.6–807.4	10.1–25.2	9.9–25.2	$UN = 0.676 \times NI - 126$	(B)
							$FN = 0.197 \times NI + 54$	
—	—	—	—	—	—	6.61–27.7	$UN = 20 + 0.38 \times NI$	(C)
							$FN = 10 + 0.28 \times NI$	
							$MN = 30 + 0.2 \times NI$	
							$TN = 30 + 0.67 \times NI$	
22.3–350	35.1–334	0.85–267	80.9–641	79.9–932	5.17–23.5	3.94–29.4	$UN = 12 + 0.333 \times NI$	(D)
							$FN = 10.1 \times DMI - 18.5$	
							$TN = 20.3 + 0.654 \times NI$	
							$MN = 8.13 \times DMI - 19$	
41–342	51–386	—	—	104.8–827	—	—	$UN = 322.2 + 1.18 \times NI$	(E)
							$FN = 117.3 + 3.24 \times NI$	

[1] References: (A) = Castillo et al. (2000), (B) = Huhtanen et al. (2008), (C) = Kebreab et al. (2010) (D) = Reed et al. (2015), and (E) = Schuba et al. (2017).

Similarly, Schuba et al. (2017) performed a meta-analysis of 50 studies—27 on dairy cattle, 6 on growing cattle, 10 on sheep, and 7 on goats—to develop equations predicting UN and FN excretions (Table 8.1). They concluded that NI may influence UN and FN differently across the different species studied and that the urinary non-urea-N was not influenced by NI. The authors did not provide empirical equations for UN based on MUN because their main objective was to use NI as the independent variable. Their UN prediction for lactating dairy cows was greater than predictions of other published equations. Similarly, their UN predictive equation for growing cattle overestimates UN compared to other published equations for beef cattle, likely because the studies Schuba et al. (2017) used included replacement heifers and growing beef cattle under different treatments of protein supplements and intake levels.

8.4.2 Beef cattle

Systems for predicting manure and urinary nitrogen partitioning for beef cattle (Dong et al., 2014; Waldrip et al., 2013; Yan et al., 2007) are more recent and, in many ways, simpler than those developed for dairy cattle. Most of them use NI, dietary CP concentration, or DMI to predict NI and FN excretions. Some models were developed based on the NASEM's (2016) model (Guo et al., 2004; Guo and Zoccarato, 2005). Waldrip et al. (2013) used a meta-analysis of 12 studies conducted in the United States, Belgium, and Brazil to develop equations predicting UN and FN excretions. Dong et al. (2014) gathered 50 publications, encompassing 206 observations from 872 cattle in research trials or commercial feedyards. Reed et al. (2015) developed equations to predict UN, FN, and TN using data from 458 steers (Holstein, Angus, Hereford, and Angus x Hereford crossbreds). Reed et al. (2015) also provided other equations containing additional dietary variables. Table 8.2 lists selected publications' empirical equations for predicting UN and FN, and Figure 8.3 depicts these relationships.

Table 8.2. Empirical equations of selected publications to predict urinary nitrogen (UN, g/d), fecal nitrogen (FN, g/d), and total nitrogen (TN, g/d) excretions of beef cattle from nitrogen intake (NI, g/d), dietary crude protein (CP, % DM), and dry matter intake (DMI, kg/d).

UN, g/d	FN, g/d	TN, g/d	NI, g/d	CP, % DM	DMI, kg/d	Equations	Ref.[1]
11.5–154	35.1–80.7	47.5–217	51.2–309	7–25	4.4–10.2	$UN = 0.56 \times NI - 21.18$	(A)
						$UN = 0.61 \times NI - 3.72 \times DMI - 3.93$	
						$UN = 5.91 \times CP - 21.52$	
						$FN = 0.154 \times NI + 24.28$	
						$FN = 1.165 \times CP + 30.91$	
13.7–201.3	15.1–101.9	41.5–303	52–350	5.5–23.5	2.92–10.7	$UN = 0.51 \times NI - 14.12$	(B)
						$UN = 6.04 \times CP - 22$	
						$FN = 0.2 \times NI + 15.82$	
						$FN = 1.81 \times CP + 19.68$	
11.9–190	11–117	26.9–280	43.4–307	10.8–25.4	2.09–11.1	$UN = 6.8 + 0.405 \times NI$	(C)
						$FN = 0.506 + 0.352 \times NI$	
						$TN = 6.91 + 0.759 \times NI$	

[1] References: (A) = Waldrip et al. (2013), (B) = Dong et al. (2014), and (C) = (Reed et al., 2015).

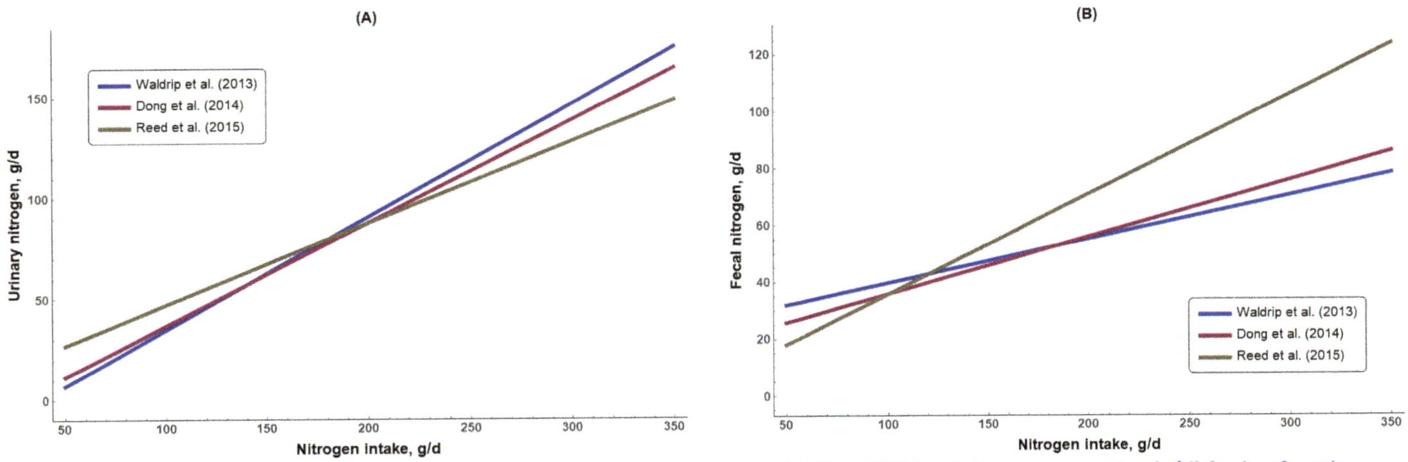

Figure 8.3. Empirical equations to predict (A) urinary nitrogen excretion (g/d) and (B) fecal nitrogen excretion (g/d) for beef cattle.

(This page intentionally left blank)

Appendices

"Programs must be written for people to read, and only incidentally for machines to execute."

Harold Abelson (Structure and Interpretation of Computer Programs, 1996)

(This page intentionally left blank)

List of Appendices

Appendix 1. R Script for Empirical Calculations of Methane

```r
main<-function()
{
  f_ <- function(a, GEI, DMI)
  {
    if (is.na(a))
    {
      d <- paste(formatC(as.character(a), format = "s", width = 9, digits = 2), " ", formatC(as.character(a), format = "s", width = 9, digits = 2), " ", formatC(as.character(a), format = "s", width = 9, digits = 2), " ", formatC(as.character(a), format = "s", width = 9, digits = 2), " ", formatC(as.character(a), format = "s", width = 9, digits = 2), sep = "")
    } else
    {
      if (is.numeric(a) == TRUE)
      {
        if (a <= 0)
        {
          a <- "#NEG#"
          d <- paste(formatC(as.character(a), format = "s", width = 9, digits = 2), " ", formatC(as.character(a), format = "s", width = 9, digits = 2), " ", formatC(as.character(a), format = "s", width = 9, digits = 2), " ", formatC(as.character(a), format = "s", width = 9, digits = 2), " ", formatC(as.character(a), format = "s", width = 9, digits = 2), sep = "")

        } else
        {
          b <- isz(isz(a, L_Mcal) * 100, GEI)
          c <- isz(a * Kg_L * 1000, DMI)
          d <- paste(formatC(a, format = "f", width = 9, digits = 2), " ", formatC(a * Kg_L * 1000, format = "f", width = 9, digits = 2), " ", formatC(a/L_Mcal, format = "f", width = 9, digits = 2), " ", formatC(a/L_MJ, format = "f", width = 9, digits = 2), " ", formatC(b, format = "f", width = 9, digits = 2), " ", formatC(c, format = "f", width = 9, digits = 2), sep = "")
        }
      } else
      {
        d <- paste(formatC(as.character(a), format = "s", width = 9, digits = 2), " ", formatC(as.character(a), format = "s", width = 9, digits = 2), " ", formatC(as.character(a), format = "s", width = 9, digits = 2), " ", formatC(as.character(a), format = "s", width = 9, digits = 2), " ", formatC(as.character(a), format = "s", width = 9, digits = 2), sep = "")
      }
    }
    return(d)
  }

  g_ <- function(a)
  {
    if (is.numeric(a))
    {
      return(formatC(a, format = "f", width = 9, digits = 2))
    } else
    {
      return(formatC(as.character(a), format = "s", width = 9, digits = 2))
```

```
        }
    }

    newpage(T)
    header <- paste("Prediction of Methane Emissions using Empirical Equations", sep = "")
    headersize <- nchar(header)
    cat(paste("#Title#", header, "\n", string("=", headersize), sep = ""), "\n\n")

    # Conversion for methane (1.013 bar, 15°C)
    # http://en.wikipedia.org/wiki/Energy_density
    # http://en.wikipedia.org/wiki/Methane

    # 55.65 MJ/kg
    # 13.3 Mcal/kg
    # 890 kJ/mol
    # 16 g/mol
    # 0.6556 g/L (kg/m^3) at 25 oC and 1 atm
    # 0.716 g/L (kg/m^3) at 0 oC and 1 atm
    MJ_Mcal <- 4.184
    Kg_MJ <- 1/55.65
    Kg_Mcal <- Kg_MJ * MJ_Mcal
    L_MJ <- 1000 * Kg_MJ/0.6556  # 25 oC and 1 atm
    L_Mcal <- 1000 * Kg_Mcal/0.6556
    Kg_L <- 0.6556/1000
    g_L <- 0.6556

    # Compatibility with different levels of solutions
    if (exists("rum.diet.DCHO.rate") & exists("si.diet.GCHO.rate")) DCHO <- (rum.diet.DCHO.rate + si.diet.GCHO.rate) else DCHO
  <- NA
    if (exists("anim.diet.CHOB1.rate") == FALSE) anim.diet.CHOB1.rate <- NA
    if (exists("anim.diet.Forage.frac") == FALSE) anim.diet.Forage.frac <- isz(anim.diet.Forage.rate, anim.diet.DMI.rate)
    if (exists("anim.diet.DE.rate") == FALSE) anim.diet.DE.rate <- NA
    if (exists("anim.diet.CHOA4.rate") == FALSE) anim.diet.CHOA4.rate <- NA
    if (exists("anim.diet.CP.conc") == FALSE) anim.diet.CP.conc <- isz(anim.diet.CP.rate * 100, anim.diet.DMI.rate)
    if (exists("si.diet.GCHO.rate") == FALSE) si.diet.GCHO.rate <- NA
    if (exists("anim.diet.aDMD.conc") == FALSE) anim.diet.aDMD.conc <- NA

    GEI <- anim.diet.GE.rate  #Mcal/d
    DEI <- anim.diet.DE.rate  #Mcal/d
    MEI <- anim.diet.ME.rate  #Mcal/d
    CPI <- anim.diet.CP.rate  #kg/d
    DMI <- anim.diet.DMI.rate #Kg/d

    # +++++
    # DAIRY
    # +++++
    #Axelsson, J. 1949. The amount of produced methane energy in the European metabolic experiments with adult cattle. Annals of
  the Royal Agricultural College of Sweden. 16:404-419.
    #Digested CHO (Rumen + SI)
    CH4_Axelsson1949_DMI <- NA
    CH4_Axelsson1949_DCHO <- NA
```

```
  if (DMI < 13) CH4_Axelsson1949_DMI <- ((-494 + 629 * DMI - 25 * (DMI^2))/1000) * L_Mcal  #MCal/d --> L/d
  if (is.na(DCHO) == FALSE & DCHO < 8.4) CH4_Axelsson1949_DCHO <- ((-213 + 984 * DCHO - 64.2 * (DCHO^2))/1000) * L_Mcal #MCal/d --> L/d

  # Moe, P. W., and H. F. Tyrrell. 1979. Methane production in dairy cows. J. Dairy Sci. 62:1583-1586.
  if (anim.diet.ADF.rate > 0)
  {
    anim.diet.HC.rate <- anim.diet.NDF.rate - anim.diet.ADF.rate
    anim.diet.C.rate <- anim.diet.ADF.rate - anim.diet.lignin.rate
    CH4_MoeTyrrell1979 <- (0.814 + 0.122 * (anim.diet.NFC.rate) + 0.415 * anim.diet.HC.rate + 0.633 * anim.diet.C.rate) * L_Mcal  #Mcal/d --> L/d
  } else
  {
    CH4_MoeTyrrell1979 <- NA
  }

  # Mills, J. A. N., E. Kebreab, C. M. Yates, L. A. Crompton, S. B. Cammell, M. S. Dhanoa, R. E. Agnew, and J. France. 2003. Alternative approaches to predicting methane emissions from dairy cows. J. Anim. Sci. 81:3141-3150.
  CH4_Millsetal2003_linear1 <- (5.93 + 0.92 * DMI) * L_MJ  #MJ/d --> L/d
  CH4_Millsetal2003_linear2 <- (8.25 + 0.07 * (MEI * MJ_Mcal)) * L_MJ  #MJ/d --> L/d
  CH4_Millsetal2003_linear3 <- (7.3 + 13.13 * (CPI/6.25) + 2.04 * anim.diet.ADF.rate + 0.33 * anim.diet.CHOB1.rate) * L_MJ #MJ/d --> L/d
  CH4_Millsetal2003_linear4 <- (1.06 + 10.27 * anim.diet.Forage.frac + 0.87 * DMI) * L_MJ  #MJ/d --> L/d
  CH4_Millsetal2003_nonlinear1 <- (56.27 - 56.27 * exp(-0.028 * DMI)) * L_MJ  #MJ/d --> L/d
  CH4_Millsetal2003_nonlinear2 <- (45.98 - 45.98 * exp(-0.003 * (MEI * MJ_Mcal))) * L_MJ  #MJ/d --> L/d
  CH4_Millsetal2003_nonlinear3 <- ifelse(anim.diet.ADF.rate > 0, (45.98 - 45.98 * exp(-(-0.0011 * (anim.diet.CHOB1.rate/anim.diet.ADF.rate) + 0.0045) * (MEI * MJ_Mcal))) * L_MJ, NA)  #MJ/d --> L/d

  # Ellis, J. L., E. Kebreab, N. E. Odongo, B. W. McBride, E. K. Okine, and J. France. 2007. Prediction of methane production from dairy and beef cattle. J. Dairy Sci. 90:3456-3467.
  CH4_Ellisetal2007_Eq1d <- (4.08 + 0.0678 * (MEI * MJ_Mcal)) * L_MJ  #MJ/d --> L/d
  CH4_Ellisetal2007_Eq2d <- (3.23 + 0.809 * DMI) * L_MJ  #MJ/d --> L/d
  CH4_Ellisetal2007_Eq3d <- (8.56 + 0.139 * (anim.diet.Forage.frac * 100)) * L_MJ  #MJ/d --> L/d
  CH4_Ellisetal2007_Eq4d <- (3.14 + 2.11 * anim.diet.NDF.rate) * L_MJ  #MJ/d --> L/d
  CH4_Ellisetal2007_Eq5d <- (5.87 + 2.43 * anim.diet.ADF.rate) * L_MJ  #MJ/d --> L/d
  CH4_Ellisetal2007_Eq6d <- (1.21 + 0.0588 * (MEI * MJ_Mcal) + 0.0926 * (anim.diet.Forage.frac * 100)) * L_MJ  #MJ/d --> L/d
  # (1.64+0.396*(MEI*MJ_Mcal)+1.45*anim.diet.NDF.rate)*L_MJ #MJ/d --> L/d
  CH4_Ellisetal2007_Eq7d <- (1.64 + 0.396 * DMI + 1.45 * anim.diet.NDF.rate) * L_MJ  #MJ/d --> L/d
  CH4_Ellisetal2007_Eq8d <- (2.16 + 0.493 * DMI - 1.36 * anim.diet.ADF.rate + 1.97 * anim.diet.NDF.rate) * L_MJ  #MJ/d --> L/d

  # Ramin, M., and P. Huhtanen. 2013. Development of equations for predicting methane emissions from ruminants. J. Dairy Sci. 96:2476-2493.
  CH4_RaminHuhtanen2013_Linear <- 62 + 25 * DMI  #L/d
  CH4_RaminHuhtanen2013_Quad <- 20 + 35.8 * DMI - 0.5 * (DMI^2)  #L/d

  # Moraes, L. E., A. B. Strathe, J. G. Fadel, D. P. Casper, and E. Kebreab. 2014. Prediction of enteric methane emissions from cattle. Global Change Biology. 20:2140-2148.
  if (anim.stage_type == "Lactating")
  {
    MkF <- as.numeric(anim.lactation.milk.fat.conc)  #milk fat, %
    CH4_Moraesetal2014_GE <- (3.247 + 0.043 * GEI * MJ_Mcal) * L_MJ  #MJ/d --> L/d
```

```
    CH4_Moraesetal2014_diet <- (0.225 + 0.042 * GEI * MJ_Mcal + 0.125 * (anim.diet.NDF.rate * 100/DMI) - 0.329 * (anim.diet.EE.rate * 100/DMI)) * L_MJ  #MJ/d --> L/d
    CH4_Moraesetal2014_animal <- (-9.311 + 0.042 * GEI * MJ_Mcal + 0.094 * (anim.diet.NDF.rate * 100/DMI) - 0.381 * (anim.diet.EE.rate * 100/DMI) + 0.008 * anim.SBW + 1.621 * MkF) * L_MJ  #MJ/d --> L/d
  } else
  {
    CH4_Moraesetal2014_GE <- (2.381 + 0.053 * GEI * MJ_Mcal) * L_MJ  #MJ/d --> L/d
    CH4_Moraesetal2014_diet <- (2.88 + 0.053 * GEI * MJ_Mcal - 0.19 * (anim.diet.EE.rate * 100/DMI)) * L_MJ  #MJ/d --> L/d
    CH4_Moraesetal2014_animal <- (2.88 + 0.053 * GEI * MJ_Mcal - 0.19 * (anim.diet.EE.rate * 100/DMI)) * L_MJ  #MJ/d --> L/d
  }

  # Mutian, N., E. Kebreab, A. N. Hristov, J. Oh, C. Arndt, A. Bannink, A. R. Bayat, A. F. Brito, T. Boland, D. Casper, L. A. Crompton, J. Dijkstra, M. A. Eugène, P. C. Garnsworthy, M. N. Haque, A. L. F. Hellwing, P. Huhtanen, M. Kreuzer, B. Kuhla, P. Lund, J. Madsen, C. Martin, S. C. McClelland, M. McGee, P. J. Moate, S. Muetzel, C. Muñoz, P. O'Kiely, N. Peiren, C. K. Reynolds, A. Schwarm, K. J. Shingfield, T. M. Storlien, M. R. Weisbjerg, D. R. Yáñez-Ruiz, and Z. Yu. 2018. Prediction of enteric methane production, yield, and intensity in dairy cattle using an intercontinental database. Global Change Biol. 24 (8):3368-3389. doi: doi:10.1111/gcb.14094
  if (anim.species == "Cattle" & anim.stage_type == "Lactating")
  {
    NDFc <- anim.diet.NDF.rate * 100/DMI
    EEc <- anim.diet.EE.rate * 100/DMI
    MY <- anim.lactation.milk.rate
    MkTP <- ifelse(anim.lactation.milk.protein.type == "True", anim.lactation.milk.protein.conc, anim.lactation.milk.protein.conc * 0.93)
    MkCP <- ifelse(anim.lactation.milk.protein.type == "True", anim.lactation.milk.protein.conc/0.93, anim.lactation.milk.protein.conc)
    ECMY <- 12.05 * (anim.lactation.milk.rate * anim.lactation.milk.fat.conc/100) +
      7.65 * (anim.lactation.milk.rate * MkTP/100) + 0.327 * anim.lactation.milk.rate
    CH4_Mutianetal2018_Eq1 <- ((7.13 + 0.0391 * GEI * MJ_Mcal)/0.05565) / g_L
    CH4_Mutianetal2018_Eq2 <- (124 + 13.3 * DMI) / g_L
    CH4_Mutianetal2018_Eq3 <- (33.2 + 13.6 * DMI + 2.43 * NDFc) / g_L
    CH4_Mutianetal2018_Eq4 <- (163 + 13.3 * DMI - 11 * EEc) / g_L
    CH4_Mutianetal2018_Eq5 <- (76.0 + 13.5 * DMI - 9.55 * EEc + 2.24 * NDFc) / g_L
    CH4_Mutianetal2018_Eq6 <- (369 - 14.7 * EEc + 1.67 * NDFc) / g_L
    CH4_Mutianetal2018_Eq7 <- (299 + 2.73 * MY) / g_L
    CH4_Mutianetal2018_Eq8 <- (259+ 3.86 * ECMY) / g_L
    CH4_Mutianetal2018_Eq9 <- (150 + 4.31* ECMY + 28.3 * MkCP) / g_L
    CH4_Mutianetal2018_Eq10 <- (-60.5 + 12.4 * DMI - 8.78 * EEc + 2.10 * NDFc + 16.1 * anim.lactation.milk.fat.conc + 0.148 * anim.FBW) / g_L
    CH4_Mutianetal2018_Eq11 <- (-37.0 - 12.3 * EEc + 2.24 * NDFc + 3.68 * ECMY + 7.81 * anim.lactation.milk.fat.conc + 17.7 * MkCP + 0.284 * anim.FBW) / g_L
  } else
  {
    CH4_Mutianetal2018_Eq1 <- NA
    CH4_Mutianetal2018_Eq2 <- NA
    CH4_Mutianetal2018_Eq3 <- NA
    CH4_Mutianetal2018_Eq4 <- NA
    CH4_Mutianetal2018_Eq5 <- NA
    CH4_Mutianetal2018_Eq6 <- NA
    CH4_Mutianetal2018_Eq7 <- NA
    CH4_Mutianetal2018_Eq8 <- NA
```

```
    CH4_Mutianetal2018_Eq9 <- NA
    CH4_Mutianetal2018_Eq10 <- NA
    CH4_Mutianetal2018_Eq11 <- NA
  }

  cat(paste("Source                        Equation          L/d       g/d     Mcal/d      MJ/d      % GEI    g/kg DM\n", string("=", 102), "\n", sep = ""))
  if (anim.species == "Cattle" & anim.type == "Milk") cat(paste("Dairy*\n", sep = "")) else cat(paste("Dairy\n", sep = ""))
  cat(paste(" Axelsoon (1949)             DMI Eq.        ", f_(CH4_Axelsson1949_DMI, GEI, DMI), "\n", sep = ""))
  cat(paste(" Axelsoon (1949)             DCHO Eq.       ", f_(CH4_Axelsson1949_DCHO, GEI, DMI), "\n", sep = ""))
  cat(paste(" Moe and Tyrrell (1979)      Eq. kg/d       ", f_(CH4_MoeTyrrell1979, GEI, DMI), "\n", sep = ""))
  cat(paste(" Mills et al. (2003)         Linear 1       ", f_(CH4_Millsetal2003_linear1, GEI, DMI), "\n", sep = ""))
  cat(paste(" Mills et al. (2003)         Linear 2       ", f_(CH4_Millsetal2003_linear2, GEI, DMI), "\n", sep = ""))
  cat(paste(" Mills et al. (2003)         Linear 3       ", f_(CH4_Millsetal2003_linear3, GEI, DMI), "\n", sep = ""))
  cat(paste(" Mills et al. (2003)         Linear 4       ", f_(CH4_Millsetal2003_linear4, GEI, DMI), "\n", sep = ""))
  cat(paste(" Mills et al. (2003)         Nonlinear 1    ", f_(CH4_Millsetal2003_nonlinear1, GEI, DMI), "\n", sep = ""))
  cat(paste(" Mills et al. (2003)         Nonlinear 2    ", f_(CH4_Millsetal2003_nonlinear2, GEI, DMI), "\n", sep = ""))
  cat(paste(" Mills et al. (2003)         Nonlinear 3*   ", f_(CH4_Millsetal2003_nonlinear3, GEI, DMI), "\n", sep = ""))
  cat(paste(" Ellis et al. (2007)         Eq. 1d         ", f_(CH4_Elliseta12007_Eq1d, GEI, DMI), "\n", sep = ""))
  cat(paste(" Ellis et al. (2007)         Eq. 2d         ", f_(CH4_Elliseta12007_Eq2d, GEI, DMI), "\n", sep = ""))
  cat(paste(" Ellis et al. (2007)         Eq. 3d*        ", f_(CH4_Elliseta12007_Eq3d, GEI, DMI), "\n", sep = ""))
  cat(paste(" Ellis et al. (2007)         Eq. 4d         ", f_(CH4_Elliseta12007_Eq4d, GEI, DMI), "\n", sep = ""))
  cat(paste(" Ellis et al. (2007)         Eq. 5d         ", f_(CH4_Elliseta12007_Eq5d, GEI, DMI), "\n", sep = ""))
  cat(paste(" Ellis et al. (2007)         Eq. 6d         ", f_(CH4_Elliseta12007_Eq6d, GEI, DMI), "\n", sep = ""))
  cat(paste(" Ellis et al. (2007)         Eq. 7d         ", f_(CH4_Elliseta12007_Eq7d, GEI, DMI), "\n", sep = ""))
  cat(paste(" Ellis et al. (2007)         Eq. 8d         ", f_(CH4_Elliseta12007_Eq8d, GEI, DMI), "\n", sep = ""))
  cat(paste(" Ramin and Huhtanen (2013)   Linear         ", f_(CH4_RaminHuhtanen2013_Linear, GEI, DMI), "\n", sep = ""))
  cat(paste(" Ramin and Huhtanen (2013)   Quadratic      ", f_(CH4_RaminHuhtanen2013_Quad, GEI, DMI), "\n", sep = ""))
  cat(paste(" Moraes et al. (2014)        GE level       ", f_(CH4_Moraesetal2014_GE, GEI, DMI), "\n", sep = ""))
  cat(paste(" Moraes et al. (2014)        Diet level     ", f_(CH4_Moraesetal2014_diet, GEI, DMI), "\n", sep = ""))
  cat(paste(" Moraes et al. (2014)        Animal level   ", f_(CH4_Moraesetal2014_animal, GEI, DMI), "\n", sep = ""))
  cat(paste(" Mutian et al. (2018)        Eq.  1 US+EU   ", f_(CH4_Mutianetal2018_Eq1, GEI, DMI), "\n", sep = ""))
  cat(paste(" Mutian et al. (2018)        Eq.  2 US+EU*  ", f_(CH4_Mutianetal2018_Eq2, GEI, DMI), "\n", sep = ""))
  cat(paste(" Mutian et al. (2018)        Eq.  3 US+EU   ", f_(CH4_Mutianetal2018_Eq3, GEI, DMI), "\n", sep = ""))
  cat(paste(" Mutian et al. (2018)        Eq.  4 US+EU   ", f_(CH4_Mutianetal2018_Eq4, GEI, DMI), "\n", sep = ""))
  cat(paste(" Mutian et al. (2018)        Eq.  5 US+EU   ", f_(CH4_Mutianetal2018_Eq5, GEI, DMI), "\n", sep = ""))
  cat(paste(" Mutian et al. (2018)        Eq.  6 US+EU   ", f_(CH4_Mutianetal2018_Eq6, GEI, DMI), "\n", sep = ""))
  cat(paste(" Mutian et al. (2018)        Eq.  7 US+EU   ", f_(CH4_Mutianetal2018_Eq7, GEI, DMI), "\n", sep = ""))
  cat(paste(" Mutian et al. (2018)        Eq.  8 US+EU   ", f_(CH4_Mutianetal2018_Eq8, GEI, DMI), "\n", sep = ""))
  cat(paste(" Mutian et al. (2018)        Eq.  9 US+EU   ", f_(CH4_Mutianetal2018_Eq9, GEI, DMI), "\n", sep = ""))
  cat(paste(" Mutian et al. (2018)        Eq. 10 US+EU   ", f_(CH4_Mutianetal2018_Eq10, GEI, DMI), "\n", sep = ""))
  cat(paste(" Mutian et al. (2018)        Eq. 11 US+EU   ", f_(CH4_Mutianetal2018_Eq11, GEI, DMI), "\n", sep = ""))

  # Statistics for dairy
  dairy_L_d <- c(CH4_Axelsson1949_DMI, CH4_Axelsson1949_DCHO, CH4_MoeTyrrell1979, CH4_Millsetal2003_linear1,
                 CH4_Millsetal2003_linear2, CH4_Millsetal2003_linear3, CH4_Millsetal2003_linear4, CH4_Millsetal2003_nonlin-
ear1,
                 CH4_Millsetal2003_nonlinear2, CH4_Millsetal2003_nonlinear3, CH4_Elliseta12007_Eq1d, CH4_Elliseta12007_Eq2d,
                 CH4_Elliseta12007_Eq3d, CH4_Elliseta12007_Eq4d, CH4_Elliseta12007_Eq5d, CH4_Elliseta12007_Eq6d,
                 CH4_Elliseta12007_Eq7d, CH4_Elliseta12007_Eq8d, CH4_RaminHuhtanen2013_Linear, CH4_RaminHuhtanen2013_Quad,
                 CH4_Moraesetal2014_GE, CH4_Moraesetal2014_diet, CH4_Moraesetal2014_animal, CH4_Mutianetal2018_Eq1,
```

```
                              CH4_Mutianetal2018_Eq2, CH4_Mutianetal2018_Eq3, CH4_Mutianetal2018_Eq4, CH4_Mutianetal2018_Eq5,
                              CH4_Mutianetal2018_Eq6, CH4_Mutianetal2018_Eq7, CH4_Mutianetal2018_Eq8, CH4_Mutianetal2018_Eq9,
                              CH4_Mutianetal2018_Eq10, CH4_Mutianetal2018_Eq11)

    dairy_L_d[dairy_L_d < 0] <- NA
    dairy_g_d <- dairy_L_d * Kg_L * 1000
    dairy_Mcal_d <- dairy_L_d/L_Mcal
    dairy_MJ_d <- dairy_L_d/L_MJ
    dairy_pGEI <- isz(dairy_Mcal_d * 100, GEI)
    dairy_g_kg <- isz(dairy_g_d, DMI)

    avg_dairy_L_d <- mean(dairy_L_d, na.rm = TRUE)
    med_dairy_L_d <- median(dairy_L_d, na.rm = TRUE)
    min_dairy_L_d <- min(dairy_L_d, na.rm = TRUE)
    max_dairy_L_d <- max(dairy_L_d, na.rm = TRUE)
    sd_dairy_L_d <- sd(dairy_L_d, na.rm = TRUE)

    avg_dairy_g_d <- mean(dairy_g_d, na.rm = TRUE)
    med_dairy_g_d <- median(dairy_g_d, na.rm = TRUE)
    min_dairy_g_d <- min(dairy_g_d, na.rm = TRUE)
    max_dairy_g_d <- max(dairy_g_d, na.rm = TRUE)
    sd_dairy_g_d <- sd(dairy_g_d, na.rm = TRUE)

    avg_dairy_Mcal_d <- mean(dairy_Mcal_d, na.rm = TRUE)
    med_dairy_Mcal_d <- median(dairy_Mcal_d, na.rm = TRUE)
    min_dairy_Mcal_d <- min(dairy_Mcal_d, na.rm = TRUE)
    max_dairy_Mcal_d <- max(dairy_Mcal_d, na.rm = TRUE)
    sd_dairy_Mcal_d <- sd(dairy_Mcal_d, na.rm = TRUE)

    avg_dairy_MJ_d <- mean(dairy_MJ_d, na.rm = TRUE)
    med_dairy_MJ_d <- median(dairy_MJ_d, na.rm = TRUE)
    min_dairy_MJ_d <- min(dairy_MJ_d, na.rm = TRUE)
    max_dairy_MJ_d <- max(dairy_MJ_d, na.rm = TRUE)
    sd_dairy_MJ_d <- sd(dairy_MJ_d, na.rm = TRUE)

    avg_dairy_pGEI <- mean(dairy_pGEI, na.rm = TRUE)
    med_dairy_pGEI <- median(dairy_pGEI, na.rm = TRUE)
    min_dairy_pGEI <- min(dairy_pGEI, na.rm = TRUE)
    max_dairy_pGEI <- max(dairy_pGEI, na.rm = TRUE)
    sd_dairy_pGEI <- sd(dairy_pGEI, na.rm = TRUE)

    avg_dairy_g_kg <- mean(dairy_g_kg, na.rm = TRUE)
    med_dairy_g_kg <- median(dairy_g_kg, na.rm = TRUE)
    min_dairy_g_kg <- min(dairy_g_kg, na.rm = TRUE)
    max_dairy_g_kg <- max(dairy_g_kg, na.rm = TRUE)
    sd_dairy_g_kg <- sd(dairy_g_kg, na.rm = TRUE)

    cat(paste(string("-", 102), "\n", sep = ""))
    cat(paste(" Statistics                    Average       ", g_(avg_dairy_L_d), " ", g_(avg_dairy_g_d), " ",
  g_(avg_dairy_Mcal_d), " ", g_(avg_dairy_MJ_d), " ", g_(avg_dairy_pGEI), " ", g_(avg_dairy_g_kg), "\n", sep = ""))
```

```
  cat(paste("                              Median        ", g_(med_dairy_L_d), " ", g_(med_dairy_g_d), " ", g_(med_dairy_Mcal_d), " ", g_(med_dairy_MJ_d), " ", g_(med_dairy_pGEI), " ", g_(med_dairy_g_kg), "\n", sep = ""))
  cat(paste("                              Std. Dev.     ", g_(sd_dairy_L_d), " ", g_(sd_dairy_g_d), " ", g_(sd_dairy_Mcal_d), " ", g_(sd_dairy_MJ_d), " ", g_(sd_dairy_pGEI), " ", g_(sd_dairy_g_kg), "\n", sep = ""))
  cat(paste("                              CV (%)        ", g_(isz(sd_dairy_L_d * 100, avg_dairy_L_d)), " ", g_(isz(sd_dairy_g_d * 100, avg_dairy_g_d)), " ", g_(isz(sd_dairy_Mcal_d * 100, avg_dairy_Mcal_d)), " ", g_(isz(sd_dairy_MJ_d * 100, avg_dairy_MJ_d)), " ", g_(isz(sd_dairy_pGEI * 100, avg_dairy_pGEI)), " ", g_(isz(sd_dairy_g_kg * 100, avg_dairy_g_kg)), "\n", sep = ""))
  cat(paste("                              Minimum       ", g_(min_dairy_L_d), " ", g_(min_dairy_g_d), " ", g_(min_dairy_Mcal_d), " ", g_(min_dairy_MJ_d), " ", g_(min_dairy_pGEI), " ", g_(min_dairy_g_kg), "\n", sep = ""))
  cat(paste("                              Maximum       ", g_(max_dairy_L_d), " ", g_(max_dairy_g_d), " ", g_(max_dairy_Mcal_d), " ", g_(max_dairy_MJ_d), " ", g_(max_dairy_pGEI), " ", g_(max_dairy_g_kg), "\n", sep = ""))

  # ++++
  # BEEF
  # ++++
  # FL<-DMI/(calcMaintenanceRequirement(TRUE)-1
  FL <- (DMI * anim.diet.ME.frac * MJ_Mcal)/(anim.FBW^0.75 * 0.46)  # as per Dr. Yan's email and paper
  q1 <- MEI/GEI
  q2 <- DEI/GEI

  # Blaxter, K. L., and J. L. Clapperton. 1965. Prediction of the amount of methane produced by ruminants. Br. J. Nutr. 19:511-522.
  CH4_BlaxterClapperton1965 <- ((1.3 + 11.2 * q2 + FL * (2.37 - 5 * q2))/100) * GEI * MJ_Mcal * L_MJ  #MJ/d --> L/d

  # Ellis, J. L., E. Kebreab, N. E. Odongo, B. W. McBride, E. K. Okine, and J. France. 2007. Prediction of methane production from dairy and beef cattle. J. Dairy Sci. 90:3456-3467.
  CH4_Ellisetal2007_Eq1b <- (4.38 + 0.0586 * (MEI * MJ_Mcal)) * L_MJ  #MJ/d --> L/d
  CH4_Ellisetal2007_Eq2b <- (3.96 + 0.561 * DMI) * L_MJ  #MJ/d --> L/d
  CH4_Ellisetal2007_Eq3b <- (4.79 + 0.0492 * (anim.diet.Forage.frac * 100)) * L_MJ  #MJ/d --> L/d
  CH4_Ellisetal2007_Eq4b <- (5.263 + 6.93 * anim.diet.lignin.rate) * L_MJ  #MJ/d --> L/d
  CH4_Ellisetal2007_Eq5b <- (5.58 + 0.848 * anim.diet.NDF.rate) * L_MJ  #MJ/d --> L/d
  CH4_Ellisetal2007_Eq6b <- (5.7 + 1.41 * anim.diet.ADF.rate) * L_MJ  #MJ/d --> L/d
  CH4_Ellisetal2007_Eq7b <- (3.05 + 0.0371 * (MEI * MJ_Mcal) + 0.801 * anim.diet.NDF.rate) * L_MJ  #MJ/d --> L/d
  CH4_Ellisetal2007_Eq8b <- (3.31 + 0.0382 * (MEI * MJ_Mcal) + 1.05 * anim.diet.ADF.rate) * L_MJ  #MJ/d --> L/d
  CH4_Ellisetal2007_Eq9b <- (0.357 + 0.0591 * (MEI * MJ_Mcal) + 0.05 * (anim.diet.Forage.frac * 100)) * L_MJ  #MJ/d --> L/d
  CH4_Ellisetal2007_Eq10b <- (-1.02 + 0.681 * DMI + 0.0481 * (anim.diet.Forage.frac * 100)) * L_MJ  #MJ/d --> L/d
  CH4_Ellisetal2007_Eq11b <- (2.3 + 1.12 * DMI - 6.26 * anim.diet.lignin.rate) * L_MJ  #MJ/d --> L/d
  CH4_Ellisetal2007_Eq12b <- (2.7 + 1.16 * DMI - 15.8 * anim.diet.EE.rate) * L_MJ  #MJ/d --> L/d
  CH4_Ellisetal2007_Eq13b <- (0.183 + 0.0433 * (MEI * MJ_Mcal) + 0.647 * anim.diet.NDF.rate + 0.0372 * (anim.diet.Forage.frac * 100)) * L_MJ  #MJ/d --> L/d
  CH4_Ellisetal2007_Eq14b <- (2.94 + 0.0585 * (MEI * MJ_Mcal) + 1.44 * anim.diet.ADF.rate - 4.16 * anim.diet.lignin.rate) * L_MJ  #MJ/d --> L/d

  # Ellis, J. L., E. Kebreab, N. E. Odongo, K. Beauchemin, S. McGinn, J. D. Nkrumah, S. S. Moore, R. Christopherson, G. K. Murdoch, B. W. McBride, E. K. Okine, and J. France. 2009. Modeling methane production from beef cattle using linear and non-linear approaches. J. Anim. Sci. 87:1334-1345.
  Cellulose <- (anim.diet.ADF.rate - anim.diet.lignin.rate)
  HemiCellulose <- (anim.diet.NDF.rate - anim.diet.ADF.rate)
  CH4_Ellisetal2009_EqA <- (2.29 + 0.67 * DMI) * L_MJ  #MJ/d --> L/d
  CH4_Ellisetal2009_EqB <- (3.05 + 3.71 * Cellulose) * L_MJ  #MJ/d --> L/d
```

```
CH4_Elliseta12009_EqC <- (4.72 + 1.13 * anim.diet.CHOB1.rate) * L_MJ  #MJ/d --> L/d
CH4_Elliseta12009_EqD <- (6.01 + 0.345 * anim.diet.NFC.rate) * L_MJ  #MJ/d --> L/d
CH4_Elliseta12009_EqE <- (3.46 + 5.06 * anim.diet.CHOA4.rate) * L_MJ  #MJ/d --> L/d
CH4_Elliseta12009_EqF <- (3.32 - 1.23 * anim.diet.CHOB1.rate + 9.48 * anim.diet.CHOA4.rate) * L_MJ  #MJ/d --> L/d
CH4_Elliseta12009_EqG <- (-1.01 + 2.76 * anim.diet.NDF.rate + 0.722 * anim.diet.CHOB1.rate) * L_MJ  #MJ/d --> L/d
CH4_Elliseta12009_EqH <- (2.26 + 5.02 * anim.diet.CHOB1.rate + 0.0236 * anim.diet.Forage.frac * 100) * L_MJ  #MJ/d --> L/d
CH4_Elliseta12009_EqI <- (2.72 + 0.0937 * MEI * MJ_Mcal + 4.31 * Cellulose - 6.49 * HemiCellulose - 7.44 *
anim.diet.EE.rate) * L_MJ  #MJ/d --> L/d
CH4_Elliseta12009_EqJ <- (0.31 + 2.88 * Cellulose + 4.15 * CPI - 3.97 * anim.diet.EE.rate) * L_MJ  #MJ/d --> L/d
CH4_Elliseta12009_EqK <- (0.561 + 5.86 * Cellulose + 0.526 * anim.diet.NFC.rate) * L_MJ  #MJ/d --> L/d
CH4_Elliseta12009_EqL <- (2.61 + 0.0687 * MEI * MJ_Mcal + 5.99 * anim.diet.CHOA4.rate - 2.15 * anim.diet.CHOB1.rate) * L_MJ
#MJ/d --> L/d
CH4_Elliseta12009_EqM <- (2.79 - 1.04 * (anim.diet.NFC.rate/anim.diet.NDF.rate) + 0.798 * DMI) * L_MJ  #MJ/d --> L/d
CH4_Elliseta12009_EqN <- (2.68 - 1.14 * (anim.diet.CHOB1.rate/anim.diet.NDF.rate) + 0.786 * DMI) * L_MJ  #MJ/d --> L/d
CH4_Elliseta12009_EqO <- (2.58 - 0.339 * (anim.diet.NFC.rate/anim.diet.ADF.rate) + 0.774 * DMI) * L_MJ  #MJ/d --> L/d
CH4_Elliseta12009_EqP <- (2.5 - 0.367 * (anim.diet.CHOB1.rate/anim.diet.ADF.rate) + 0.766 * DMI) * L_MJ  #MJ/d --> L/d
CH4_Elliseta12009_EqQ <- (7.09 * (1 - exp(-18.9 * anim.diet.EE.rate))) * L_MJ  #MJ/d --> L/d
CH4_Elliseta12009_EqR <- (8.53 * (1 - exp(-0.637 * anim.diet.NDF.rate))) * L_MJ  #MJ/d --> L/d
CH4_Elliseta12009_EqS <- (8.76 * (1 - exp(-1.86 * HemiCellulose))) * L_MJ  #MJ/d --> L/d
CH4_Elliseta12009_EqT <- (8.51 * (1 - exp(-5.5 * anim.diet.lignin.rate))) * L_MJ  #MJ/d --> L/d
CH4_Elliseta12009_EqU <- (8.23 * (1 - exp(-1.68 * anim.diet.ADF.rate))) * L_MJ  #MJ/d --> L/d
CH4_Elliseta12009_EqV <- (8.48 * (1 - exp(-0.023 * MEI * MJ_Mcal))) * L_MJ  #MJ/d --> L/d
CH4_Elliseta12009_EqW <- (10.8 * (1 - exp(-0.141 * DMI))) * L_MJ  #MJ/d --> L/d
# (9.44*exp(-0.5*(anim.diet.Forage.frac*100-48.7)/(33.3^2)))*L_MJ #MJ/d --> L/d
CH4_Elliseta12009_EqX <- (9.44 * exp(-0.5 * ((anim.diet.Forage.frac * 100 - 48.7)/33.3)^2)) * L_MJ  #MJ/d --> L/d
CH4_Elliseta12009_EqW1 <- (10.8 * (1 - exp(-(-0.0127 * (anim.diet.NFC.rate/anim.diet.ADF.rate) + 0.22) * DMI))) * L_MJ
#MJ/d --> L/d
CH4_Elliseta12009_EqW2 <- (10.8 * (1 - exp(-(-0.0138 * (anim.diet.CHOB1.rate/anim.diet.ADF.rate) + 0.211) * DMI))) * L_MJ
#MJ/d --> L/d
CH4_Elliseta12009_EqW3 <- (10.8 * (1 - exp(-(-0.034 * (anim.diet.NFC.rate/anim.diet.NDF.rate) + 0.228) * DMI))) * L_MJ
#MJ/d --> L/d

#Yan, T., M. G. Porter, and C. S. Mayne. 2009. Prediction of methane emission from beef cattle using data measured in indi-
rect open-circuit respiration calorimeters. Animal. 3:1455-1462.
#FL<-DMI/(calcMaintenanceRequirement(TRUE)-1
#q1<-MEI/GEI
#q2<-DEI/GEI
#Variables  Value   Units
#BW, kg         500   Kg
#DMI        7.61    Kg/d
#GEI        143.5   MJ/d
#MEI         88.1   MJ/d
#FL           1.81  ME intake (MJ/d)/ME requirement for maintenance (MJ/d)
#Forage     0.802   kg/kg DM
#ME         11.6    MJ/kg DM
#DE/GE      0.725   MJ/MJ
#ME/GE      0.614   MJ/MJ
#CP         136     g/kg DM
#ADF        0.329   kg/kg DM
#NDF        0.542   kg/kg DM
CH4_Yaneta12009_Eq1a <- 0.378 * anim.FBW + 64.8  #L/d
```

```
    CH4_Yanetal2009_Eq1b <- (-0.325 + 0.43 * (anim.diet.NDF.rate/DMI) + 0.044 * ((anim.diet.CP.conc * 10)/(anim.diet.ME.frac * MJ_Mcal))) * anim.FBW + 130 * FL - 172.4  #L/d
    CH4_Yanetal2009_Eq1c <- (0.964 - 4.078 * q1 + 2.623 * q2) * anim.FBW + 166.9 * FL - 194.7  #L/d
    CH4_Yanetal2009_Eq2a <- 35.1 * DMI + 14.7  #L/d
    CH4_Yanetal2009_Eq2b <- (31 - 311.5 * q1 + 206.8 * q2 + 4.3 * (anim.diet.ME.frac * MJ_Mcal)) * DMI - 13.7  #L/d
    CH4_Yanetal2009_Eq3a <- 1.959 * (anim.diet.GE.frac * MJ_Mcal * DMI) + 8.8  #L/d
    CH4_Yanetal2009_Eq3b <- (1.635 - 12.62 * q1 + 11.26 * q2) * (anim.diet.GE.frac * MJ_Mcal * DMI) - 13.8  #L/d
    CH4_Yanetal2009_Eq3c <- (0.877 - 14.66 * q1 + 13.55 * q2 + 0.457 * anim.diet.Forage.frac + 4.153 * (anim.diet.NDF.rate/DMI) - 7.47 * (anim.diet.ADF.rate/DMI)) * (GEI * MJ_Mcal) + 0.8

    # Moraes, L. E., A. B. Strathe, J. G. Fadel, D. P. Casper, and E. Kebreab. 2014. Prediction of enteric methane emissions from cattle. Global Change Biology. 20:2140-2148.
    if (anim.sex == "Female")
    {
      # Heifer
      CH4_Moraesetal2014_GE <- (1.289 + 0.051 * GEI * MJ_Mcal) * L_MJ  #MJ/d --> L/d
      CH4_Moraesetal2014_diet <- (-0.163 + 0.051 * GEI * MJ_Mcal + 0.038 * (anim.diet.NDF.rate * 100/DMI)) * L_MJ  #MJ/d --> L/d
      CH4_Moraesetal2014_animal <- (-1.487 + 0.046 * GEI * MJ_Mcal + 0.032 * (anim.diet.NDF.rate * 100/DMI) + 0.006 * anim.SBW) * L_MJ  #MJ/d --> L/d
    } else
    {
      # Steer
      CH4_Moraesetal2014_GE <- (0.743 + 0.054 * GEI * MJ_Mcal) * L_MJ  #MJ/d --> L/d
      CH4_Moraesetal2014_diet <- (0.743 + 0.054 * GEI * MJ_Mcal) * L_MJ  #MJ/d --> L/d
      CH4_Moraesetal2014_animal <- (-0.221 + 0.048 * GEI * MJ_Mcal + 0.005 * anim.SBW) * L_MJ  #MJ/d --> L/d
    }

    newpage(T)
    cat(paste("Source                        Equation            L/d       g/d     Mcal/d      MJ/d      % GEI    g/kg DM\n", string("=", 102), "\n", sep = ""))
    if (anim.species == "Cattle" & anim.type != "Milk") cat(paste("Beef*\n", sep = "")) else cat(paste("Beef\n", sep = ""))
    cat(paste(" Blaxter & Clapperton (1965)  Page 517(1)   ", f_(CH4_BlaxterClapperton1965, GEI, DMI), "\n", sep = ""))
    cat(paste(" Ellis et al. (2007)          Eq. 1b        ", f_(CH4_Ellisetal2007_Eq1b, GEI, DMI), "\n", sep = ""))
    cat(paste(" Ellis et al. (2007)          Eq. 2b        ", f_(CH4_Ellisetal2007_Eq2b, GEI, DMI), "\n", sep = ""))
    cat(paste(" Ellis et al. (2007)          Eq. 3b        ", f_(CH4_Ellisetal2007_Eq3b, GEI, DMI), "\n", sep = ""))
    cat(paste(" Ellis et al. (2007)          Eq. 4b        ", f_(CH4_Ellisetal2007_Eq4b, GEI, DMI), "\n", sep = ""))
    cat(paste(" Ellis et al. (2007)          Eq. 5b        ", f_(CH4_Ellisetal2007_Eq5b, GEI, DMI), "\n", sep = ""))
    cat(paste(" Ellis et al. (2007)          Eq. 6b        ", f_(CH4_Ellisetal2007_Eq6b, GEI, DMI), "\n", sep = ""))
    cat(paste(" Ellis et al. (2007)          Eq. 7b        ", f_(CH4_Ellisetal2007_Eq7b, GEI, DMI), "\n", sep = ""))
    cat(paste(" Ellis et al. (2007)          Eq. 8b        ", f_(CH4_Ellisetal2007_Eq8b, GEI, DMI), "\n", sep = ""))
    cat(paste(" Ellis et al. (2007)          Eq. 9b        ", f_(CH4_Ellisetal2007_Eq9b, GEI, DMI), "\n", sep = ""))
    cat(paste(" Ellis et al. (2007)          Eq. 10b       ", f_(CH4_Ellisetal2007_Eq10b, GEI, DMI), "\n", sep = ""))
    cat(paste(" Ellis et al. (2007)          Eq. 11b       ", f_(CH4_Ellisetal2007_Eq11b, GEI, DMI), "\n", sep = ""))
    cat(paste(" Ellis et al. (2007)          Eq. 12b       ", f_(CH4_Ellisetal2007_Eq12b, GEI, DMI), "\n", sep = ""))
    cat(paste(" Ellis et al. (2007)          Eq. 13b       ", f_(CH4_Ellisetal2007_Eq13b, GEI, DMI), "\n", sep = ""))
    cat(paste(" Ellis et al. (2007)          Eq. 14b*      ", f_(CH4_Ellisetal2007_Eq14b, GEI, DMI), "\n", sep = ""))
    cat(paste(" Ellis et al. (2009)          Eq. A         ", f_(CH4_Ellisetal2009_EqA, GEI, DMI), "\n", sep = ""))
    cat(paste(" Ellis et al. (2009)          Eq. B         ", f_(CH4_Ellisetal2009_EqB, GEI, DMI), "\n", sep = ""))
    cat(paste(" Ellis et al. (2009)          Eq. C         ", f_(CH4_Ellisetal2009_EqC, GEI, DMI), "\n", sep = ""))
    cat(paste(" Ellis et al. (2009)          Eq. D         ", f_(CH4_Ellisetal2009_EqD, GEI, DMI), "\n", sep = ""))
    cat(paste(" Ellis et al. (2009)          Eq. E         ", f_(CH4_Ellisetal2009_EqE, GEI, DMI), "\n", sep = ""))
```

```
cat(paste(" Ellis et al. (2009)            Eq. F          ", f_(CH4_Ellisetal2009_EqF, GEI, DMI), "\n", sep = ""))
cat(paste(" Ellis et al. (2009)            Eq. G          ", f_(CH4_Ellisetal2009_EqG, GEI, DMI), "\n", sep = ""))
cat(paste(" Ellis et al. (2009)            Eq. H          ", f_(CH4_Ellisetal2009_EqH, GEI, DMI), "\n", sep = ""))
cat(paste(" Ellis et al. (2009)            Eq. I*         ", f_(CH4_Ellisetal2009_EqI, GEI, DMI), "\n", sep = ""))
cat(paste(" Ellis et al. (2009)            Eq. J          ", f_(CH4_Ellisetal2009_EqJ, GEI, DMI), "\n", sep = ""))
cat(paste(" Ellis et al. (2009)            Eq. K          ", f_(CH4_Ellisetal2009_EqK, GEI, DMI), "\n", sep = ""))
cat(paste(" Ellis et al. (2009)            Eq. L          ", f_(CH4_Ellisetal2009_EqL, GEI, DMI), "\n", sep = ""))
cat(paste(" Ellis et al. (2009)            Eq. M          ", f_(CH4_Ellisetal2009_EqM, GEI, DMI), "\n", sep = ""))
cat(paste(" Ellis et al. (2009)            Eq. N          ", f_(CH4_Ellisetal2009_EqN, GEI, DMI), "\n", sep = ""))
cat(paste(" Ellis et al. (2009)            Eq. O          ", f_(CH4_Ellisetal2009_EqO, GEI, DMI), "\n", sep = ""))
cat(paste(" Ellis et al. (2009)            Eq. P*         ", f_(CH4_Ellisetal2009_EqP, GEI, DMI), "\n", sep = ""))
cat(paste(" Ellis et al. (2009)            Eq. Q          ", f_(CH4_Ellisetal2009_EqQ, GEI, DMI), "\n", sep = ""))
cat(paste(" Ellis et al. (2009)            Eq. R          ", f_(CH4_Ellisetal2009_EqR, GEI, DMI), "\n", sep = ""))
cat(paste(" Ellis et al. (2009)            Eq. S          ", f_(CH4_Ellisetal2009_EqS, GEI, DMI), "\n", sep = ""))
cat(paste(" Ellis et al. (2009)            Eq. T          ", f_(CH4_Ellisetal2009_EqT, GEI, DMI), "\n", sep = ""))
cat(paste(" Ellis et al. (2009)            Eq. U          ", f_(CH4_Ellisetal2009_EqU, GEI, DMI), "\n", sep = ""))
cat(paste(" Ellis et al. (2009)            Eq. V          ", f_(CH4_Ellisetal2009_EqV, GEI, DMI), "\n", sep = ""))
cat(paste(" Ellis et al. (2009)            Eq. W*         ", f_(CH4_Ellisetal2009_EqW, GEI, DMI), "\n", sep = ""))
cat(paste(" Ellis et al. (2009)            Eq. X          ", f_(CH4_Ellisetal2009_EqX, GEI, DMI), "\n", sep = ""))
cat(paste(" Ellis et al. (2009)            Eq. W1         ", f_(CH4_Ellisetal2009_EqW1, GEI, DMI), "\n", sep = ""))
cat(paste(" Ellis et al. (2009)            Eq. W2         ", f_(CH4_Ellisetal2009_EqW2, GEI, DMI), "\n", sep = ""))
cat(paste(" Ellis et al. (2009)            Eq. W3*        ", f_(CH4_Ellisetal2009_EqW3, GEI, DMI), "\n", sep = ""))
cat(paste(" Yan et al. (2009)              Eq. 1a         ", f_(CH4_Yanetal2009_Eq1a, GEI, DMI), "\n", sep = ""))
cat(paste(" Yan et al. (2009)              Eq. 1b         ", f_(CH4_Yanetal2009_Eq1b, GEI, DMI), "\n", sep = ""))
cat(paste(" Yan et al. (2009)              Eq. 1c         ", f_(CH4_Yanetal2009_Eq1c, GEI, DMI), "\n", sep = ""))
cat(paste(" Yan et al. (2009)              Eq. 2a         ", f_(CH4_Yanetal2009_Eq2a, GEI, DMI), "\n", sep = ""))
cat(paste(" Yan et al. (2009)              Eq. 2b         ", f_(CH4_Yanetal2009_Eq2b, GEI, DMI), "\n", sep = ""))
cat(paste(" Yan et al. (2009)              Eq. 3a         ", f_(CH4_Yanetal2009_Eq3a, GEI, DMI), "\n", sep = ""))
cat(paste(" Yan et al. (2009)              Eq. 3b         ", f_(CH4_Yanetal2009_Eq3b, GEI, DMI), "\n", sep = ""))
cat(paste(" Yan et al. (2009)              Eq. 3c         ", f_(CH4_Yanetal2009_Eq3c, GEI, DMI), "\n", sep = ""))
cat(paste(" Moraes et al. (2014)           GE level       ", f_(CH4_Moraesetal2014_GE, GEI, DMI), "\n", sep = ""))
cat(paste(" Moraes et al. (2014)           Diet level     ", f_(CH4_Moraesetal2014_diet, GEI, DMI), "\n", sep = ""))
cat(paste(" Moraes et al. (2014)           Animal level ", f_(CH4_Moraesetal2014_animal, GEI, DMI), "\n", sep = ""))

 # Statistics for beef
 beef_L_d <- c(CH4_BlaxterClapperton1965, CH4_Ellisetal2007_Eq1b, CH4_Ellisetal2007_Eq2b, CH4_Ellisetal2007_Eq3b, CH4_Ellisetal2007_Eq4b, CH4_Ellisetal2007_Eq5b, CH4_Ellisetal2007_Eq6b, CH4_Ellisetal2007_Eq7b, CH4_Ellisetal2007_Eq8b, CH4_Ellisetal2007_Eq9b, CH4_Ellisetal2007_Eq10b, CH4_Ellisetal2007_Eq11b, CH4_Ellisetal2007_Eq12b, CH4_Ellisetal2007_Eq13b, CH4_Ellisetal2007_Eq14b, CH4_Ellisetal2009_EqA, CH4_Ellisetal2009_EqB, CH4_Ellisetal2009_EqC, CH4_Ellisetal2009_EqD, CH4_Ellisetal2009_EqE, CH4_Ellisetal2009_EqF,
          CH4_Ellisetal2009_EqG, CH4_Ellisetal2009_EqH, CH4_Ellisetal2009_EqI, CH4_Ellisetal2009_EqJ, CH4_Ellisetal2009_EqK, CH4_Ellisetal2009_EqL, CH4_Ellisetal2009_EqM, CH4_Ellisetal2009_EqN, CH4_Ellisetal2009_EqO, CH4_Ellisetal2009_EqP, CH4_Ellisetal2009_EqQ, CH4_Ellisetal2009_EqR, CH4_Ellisetal2009_EqS, CH4_Ellisetal2009_EqT, CH4_Ellisetal2009_EqU, CH4_Ellisetal2009_EqV, CH4_Ellisetal2009_EqW, CH4_Ellisetal2009_EqX, CH4_Ellisetal2009_EqW1, CH4_Ellisetal2009_EqW2, CH4_Ellisetal2009_EqW3, CH4_Yanetal2009_Eq1a,
          CH4_Yanetal2009_Eq1b, CH4_Yanetal2009_Eq1c, CH4_Yanetal2009_Eq2a, CH4_Yanetal2009_Eq2b, CH4_Yanetal2009_Eq3a, CH4_Yanetal2009_Eq3b, CH4_Yanetal2009_Eq3c, CH4_Moraesetal2014_GE, CH4_Moraesetal2014_diet, CH4_Moraesetal2014_animal)

 beef_L_d[beef_L_d < 0] <- NA
 beef_g_d <- beef_L_d * Kg_L * 1000
 beef_Mcal_d <- beef_L_d/L_Mcal
```

```
    beef_MJ_d <- beef_L_d/L_MJ
    beef_pGEI <- isz(beef_Mcal_d * 100, GEI)
    beef_g_kg <- isz(beef_g_d, DMI)

    avg_beef_L_d <- mean(beef_L_d, na.rm = TRUE)
    med_beef_L_d <- median(beef_L_d, na.rm = TRUE)
    min_beef_L_d <- min(beef_L_d, na.rm = TRUE)
    max_beef_L_d <- max(beef_L_d, na.rm = TRUE)
    sd_beef_L_d <- sd(beef_L_d, na.rm = TRUE)

    avg_beef_g_d <- mean(beef_g_d, na.rm = TRUE)
    med_beef_g_d <- median(beef_g_d, na.rm = TRUE)
    min_beef_g_d <- min(beef_g_d, na.rm = TRUE)
    max_beef_g_d <- max(beef_g_d, na.rm = TRUE)
    sd_beef_g_d <- sd(beef_g_d, na.rm = TRUE)

    avg_beef_Mcal_d <- mean(beef_Mcal_d, na.rm = TRUE)
    med_beef_Mcal_d <- median(beef_Mcal_d, na.rm = TRUE)
    min_beef_Mcal_d <- min(beef_Mcal_d, na.rm = TRUE)
    max_beef_Mcal_d <- max(beef_Mcal_d, na.rm = TRUE)
    sd_beef_Mcal_d <- sd(beef_Mcal_d, na.rm = TRUE)

    avg_beef_MJ_d <- mean(beef_MJ_d, na.rm = TRUE)
    med_beef_MJ_d <- median(beef_MJ_d, na.rm = TRUE)
    min_beef_MJ_d <- min(beef_MJ_d, na.rm = TRUE)
    max_beef_MJ_d <- max(beef_MJ_d, na.rm = TRUE)
    sd_beef_MJ_d <- sd(beef_MJ_d, na.rm = TRUE)

    avg_beef_pGEI <- mean(beef_pGEI, na.rm = TRUE)
    med_beef_pGEI <- median(beef_pGEI, na.rm = TRUE)
    min_beef_pGEI <- min(beef_pGEI, na.rm = TRUE)
    max_beef_pGEI <- max(beef_pGEI, na.rm = TRUE)
    sd_beef_pGEI <- sd(beef_pGEI, na.rm = TRUE)

    avg_beef_g_kg <- mean(beef_g_kg, na.rm = TRUE)
    med_beef_g_kg <- median(beef_g_kg, na.rm = TRUE)
    min_beef_g_kg <- min(beef_g_kg, na.rm = TRUE)
    max_beef_g_kg <- max(beef_g_kg, na.rm = TRUE)
    sd_beef_g_kg <- sd(beef_g_kg, na.rm = TRUE)

    cat(paste(string("-", 102), "\n", sep = ""))
    cat(paste(" Statistics                    Average      ", g_(avg_beef_L_d), " ", g_(avg_beef_g_d), " ", g_(avg_beef_Mcal_d), " ", g_(avg_beef_MJ_d), " ", g_(avg_beef_pGEI), " ", g_(avg_beef_g_kg), "\n", sep = ""))
    cat(paste("                               Median       ", g_(med_beef_L_d), " ", g_(med_beef_g_d), " ", g_(med_beef_Mcal_d), " ", g_(med_beef_MJ_d), " ", g_(med_beef_pGEI), " ", g_(med_beef_g_kg), "\n", sep = ""))
    cat(paste("                               Std. Dev.    ", g_(sd_beef_L_d), " ", g_(sd_beef_g_d), " ", g_(sd_beef_Mcal_d), " ", g_(sd_beef_MJ_d), " ", g_(sd_beef_pGEI), " ", g_(sd_beef_g_kg), "\n", sep = ""))
    cat(paste("                               CV (%)       ", g_(isz(sd_beef_L_d * 100, avg_beef_L_d)), " ", g_(isz(sd_beef_g_d * 100, avg_beef_g_d)), " ", g_(isz(sd_beef_Mcal_d * 100, avg_beef_Mcal_d)), " ", g_(isz(sd_beef_MJ_d * 100, avg_beef_MJ_d)), " ", g_(isz(sd_beef_pGEI * 100, avg_beef_pGEI)), " ", g_(isz(sd_beef_g_kg * 100, avg_beef_g_kg)), "\n", sep = ""))
```

```
  cat(paste("                    Minimum          ", g_(min_beef_L_d), " ", g_(min_beef_g_d), " ", g_(min_beef_Mcal_d), " ", g_(min_beef_MJ_d), " ", g_(min_beef_pGEI), " ", g_(min_beef_g_kg), "\n", sep = ""))
  cat(paste("                    Maximum          ", g_(max_beef_L_d), " ", g_(max_beef_g_d), " ", g_(max_beef_Mcal_d), " ", g_(max_beef_MJ_d), " ", g_(max_beef_pGEI), " ", g_(max_beef_g_kg), "\n", sep = ""))

  # +++++++++++++
  # BEEF or DAIRY
  # +++++++++++++
  # Kriss, M. 1930. Quantitative relations of the dry matter of the food consumed, the heat production, the gaseous outgo, and the insensible loss in body weight of cattle. J. Agric. Res. 40:283\u0096295.
  CH4_Kriss1930 <- ((18 + 22.5 * DMI)/1000) * (1/Kg_L)  #g/d --> L/d

  # Bratzler, J. W., and E. B. Forbes. 1940. The estimation of methane production by cattle. J. Nutr. 19:611-613.
  DigestedCHO <- (DCHO + si.diet.GCHO.rate) * 1000
  CH4_BratzlerForbes1940 <- ((17.68 + 0.04012 * DigestedCHO)/1000) * (1/Kg_L)  #g/d --> L/d

  # Ellis, J. L., E. Kebreab, N. E. Odongo, B. W. McBride, E. K. Okine, and J. France. 2007. Prediction of methane production from dairy and beef cattle. J. Dairy Sci. 90:3456-3467.
  CH4_Elliseta12007_Eq1c <- (4.12 + 0.0657 * (MEI * MJ_Mcal)) * L_MJ  #MJ/d --> L/d
  CH4_Elliseta12007_Eq2c <- (3.272 + 0.736 * DMI) * L_MJ  #MJ/d --> L/d
  # (7.27+6.49*anim.diet.lignin.rate)*L_MJ #MJ/d --> L/d
  CH4_Elliseta12007_Eq3c <- (8.27 + 6.49 * anim.diet.lignin.rate) * L_MJ  #MJ/d --> L/d
  CH4_Elliseta12007_Eq4c <- (4.42 + 1.58 * anim.diet.NDF.rate) * L_MJ  #MJ/d --> L/d
  CH4_Elliseta12007_Eq5c <- (1.7 + 0.0667 * (MEI * MJ_Mcal) + 0.0314 * (anim.diet.Forage.frac * 100)) * L_MJ  #MJ/d --> L/d
  CH4_Elliseta12007_Eq6c <- (3.44 + 0.502 * DMI + 0.506 * anim.diet.NDF.rate) * L_MJ  #MJ/d --> L/d
  CH4_Elliseta12007_Eq7c <- (3.63 + 0.0549 * (MEI * MJ_Mcal) + 0.606 * anim.diet.ADF.rate) * L_MJ  #MJ/d --> L/d
  CH4_Elliseta12007_Eq8c <- (4.41 + 0.0224 * (MEI * MJ_Mcal) + 0.98 * anim.diet.NDF.rate) * L_MJ  #MJ/d --> L/d
  CH4_Elliseta12007_Eq9c <- (3.69 + 0.543 * DMI + 0.698 * anim.diet.NDF.rate - 3.26 * anim.diet.lignin.rate) * L_MJ  #MJ/d --> L/d
  CH4_Elliseta12007_Eq10c <- (3.41 + 0.52 * DMI - 0.996 * anim.diet.ADF.rate + 1.15 * anim.diet.NDF.rate) * L_MJ  #MJ/d --> L/d

  # Intergovernmental Panel on Climate Change. 2006. 2006 IPCC Guidelines for National Greenhouse Gas Inventories: Agriculture, Forestry and Other Land Use. H. S. Eggleston, L. Buendia, K. Miwa, T. Ngara and K. Tanabe, eds. vol. 4. Institute for Global Environmental Strategies (IGES), Hayama, Hanagawa, Japan. 678 p. Available at: http://www.ipcc-nggip.iges.or.jp/public/2006gl/vol4.html.
  if (anim.diet.Forage.frac <= 0.1)
  {
    Ym <- 3/100
  } else
  {
    Ym <- 6.5/100
  }
  CH4_IPCC_Tier2 <- (GEI * Ym) * L_Mcal  #Mcal/d --> L/d

  # Ricci, P., J. A. Rooke, I. Nevison, and A. Waterhouse. 2013. Methane emissions from beef and dairy cattle: Quantifying the effect of physiological stage and diet characteristics. J. Anim. Sci. 91:5379-5389.
  if (anim.diet.Forage.frac <= 0.5) Riccietal2013_Feed <- 0 else Riccietal2013_Feed <- 1
  if (anim.stage_type == "Lactating") Riccietal2013_Stage <- 1 else Riccietal2013_Stage <- 0
  CH4_Riccietal2013_GEI <- (74.34 + 0.57 * GEI * MJ_Mcal - 10.61 * Riccietal2013_Feed - 69.67 * Riccietal2013_Stage - 0.22 * GEI * MJ_Mcal * Riccietal2013_Feed + 0.57 * GEI * MJ_Mcal * Riccietal2013_Stage)/g_L  #g/d --> L/d
```

```
    CH4_Riccietal2013_DMI <- (79.87 + 9.95 * DMI - 15.15 * Riccietal2013_Feed - 74.48 * Riccietal2013_Stage - 3.67 * DMI * Riccietal2013_Feed + 10.19 * DMI * Riccietal2013_Stage)/g_L  #g/d --> L/d
    CH4_Riccietal2013_DEI <- (88.41 + 0.75 * DEI - 19.28 * Riccietal2013_Feed - 39.19 * Riccietal2013_Stage - 0.29 * DEI * Riccietal2013_Feed + 0.69 * DEI * Riccietal2013_Stage)/g_L  #g/d --> L/d
    Riccietal2013_DMD <- anim.diet.aDMD.conc/100
    if (is.na(Riccietal2013_DMD) == FALSE)
    {
     CH4_Riccietal2013_MEI <- (98.56 + 1.19 * MEI - 44.8 * Riccietal2013_DMD + 133.06 * Riccietal2013_Feed + 52.16 * Riccietal2013_Stage - 287.57 * Riccietal2013_DMD * Riccietal2013_Feed)/g_L  #g/d --> L/d
    } else CH4_Riccietal2013_MEI <- NA

    newpage(T)
    cat(paste("Source                          Equation          L/d       g/d     Mcal/d      MJ/d      % GEI    g/kg DM\n", string("=", 102), "\n", sep = ""))
    if (anim.species == "Cattle") cat(paste("Dairy or Beef*\n", sep = "")) else cat(paste("Dairy or Beef\n", sep = ""))
    cat(paste(" Kriss (1930)                   All (n=77)      ", f_(CH4_Kriss1930, GEI, DMI), "\n", sep = ""))
    cat(paste(" Bratzler & Forbes (1940)       Eq. 1           ", f_(CH4_BratzlerForbes1940, GEI, DMI), "\n", sep = ""))
    cat(paste(" IPCC (2006)                    Tier 2          ", f_(CH4_IPCC_Tier2, GEI, DMI), "\n", sep = ""))
    cat(paste(" Ellis et al. (2007)            Eq. 1c          ", f_(CH4_Ellisetal2007_Eq1c, GEI, DMI), "\n", sep = ""))
    cat(paste(" Ellis et al. (2007)            Eq. 2c*         ", f_(CH4_Ellisetal2007_Eq2c, GEI, DMI), "\n", sep = ""))
    cat(paste(" Ellis et al. (2007)            Eq. 3c          ", f_(CH4_Ellisetal2007_Eq3c, GEI, DMI), "\n", sep = ""))
    cat(paste(" Ellis et al. (2007)            Eq. 4c          ", f_(CH4_Ellisetal2007_Eq4c, GEI, DMI), "\n", sep = ""))
    cat(paste(" Ellis et al. (2007)            Eq. 5c          ", f_(CH4_Ellisetal2007_Eq5c, GEI, DMI), "\n", sep = ""))
    cat(paste(" Ellis et al. (2007)            Eq. 6c          ", f_(CH4_Ellisetal2007_Eq6c, GEI, DMI), "\n", sep = ""))
    cat(paste(" Ellis et al. (2007)            Eq. 7c          ", f_(CH4_Ellisetal2007_Eq7c, GEI, DMI), "\n", sep = ""))
    cat(paste(" Ellis et al. (2007)            Eq. 8c          ", f_(CH4_Ellisetal2007_Eq8c, GEI, DMI), "\n", sep = ""))
    cat(paste(" Ellis et al. (2007)            Eq. 9c          ", f_(CH4_Ellisetal2007_Eq9c, GEI, DMI), "\n", sep = ""))
    cat(paste(" Ellis et al. (2007)            Eq. 10c         ", f_(CH4_Ellisetal2007_Eq10c, GEI, DMI), "\n", sep = ""))
    cat(paste(" Ricci et al. (2013)            Eq. GEI         ", f_(CH4_Riccietal2013_GEI, GEI, DMI), "\n", sep = ""))
    cat(paste(" Ricci et al. (2013)            Eq. DMI         ", f_(CH4_Riccietal2013_DMI, GEI, DMI), "\n", sep = ""))
    cat(paste(" Ricci et al. (2013)            Eq. DEI         ", f_(CH4_Riccietal2013_DEI, GEI, DMI), "\n", sep = ""))
    cat(paste(" Ricci et al. (2013)            Eq. MEI         ", f_(CH4_Riccietal2013_MEI, GEI, DMI), "\n", sep = ""))

    # Statistics for dairy or beef
    dairy_beef_L_d <- c(CH4_Kriss1930, CH4_BratzlerForbes1940, CH4_IPCC_Tier2, CH4_Ellisetal2007_Eq1c, CH4_Ellisetal2007_Eq2c, CH4_Ellisetal2007_Eq3c, CH4_Ellisetal2007_Eq4c, CH4_Ellisetal2007_Eq5c, CH4_Ellisetal2007_Eq6c, CH4_Ellisetal2007_Eq7c, CH4_Ellisetal2007_Eq8c, CH4_Ellisetal2007_Eq9c, CH4_Ellisetal2007_Eq10c, CH4_Riccietal2013_GEI, CH4_Riccietal2013_DMI, CH4_Riccietal2013_DEI, CH4_Riccietal2013_MEI)

    dairy_beef_L_d[dairy_beef_L_d < 0] <- NA
    dairy_beef_g_d <- dairy_beef_L_d * Kg_L * 1000
    dairy_beef_Mcal_d <- dairy_beef_L_d/L_Mcal
    dairy_beef_MJ_d <- dairy_beef_L_d/L_MJ
    dairy_beef_pGEI <- isz(dairy_beef_Mcal_d * 100, GEI)
    dairy_beef_g_kg <- isz(dairy_beef_g_d, DMI)

    avg_dairy_beef_L_d <- mean(dairy_beef_L_d, na.rm = TRUE)
    med_dairy_beef_L_d <- median(dairy_beef_L_d, na.rm = TRUE)
    min_dairy_beef_L_d <- min(dairy_beef_L_d, na.rm = TRUE)
    max_dairy_beef_L_d <- max(dairy_beef_L_d, na.rm = TRUE)
    sd_dairy_beef_L_d <- sd(dairy_beef_L_d, na.rm = TRUE)
```

```
    avg_dairy_beef_g_d <- mean(dairy_beef_g_d, na.rm = TRUE)
    med_dairy_beef_g_d <- median(dairy_beef_g_d, na.rm = TRUE)
    min_dairy_beef_g_d <- min(dairy_beef_g_d, na.rm = TRUE)
    max_dairy_beef_g_d <- max(dairy_beef_g_d, na.rm = TRUE)
    sd_dairy_beef_g_d <- sd(dairy_beef_g_d, na.rm = TRUE)

    avg_dairy_beef_Mcal_d <- mean(dairy_beef_Mcal_d, na.rm = TRUE)
    med_dairy_beef_Mcal_d <- median(dairy_beef_Mcal_d, na.rm = TRUE)
    min_dairy_beef_Mcal_d <- min(dairy_beef_Mcal_d, na.rm = TRUE)
    max_dairy_beef_Mcal_d <- max(dairy_beef_Mcal_d, na.rm = TRUE)
    sd_dairy_beef_Mcal_d <- sd(dairy_beef_Mcal_d, na.rm = TRUE)

    avg_dairy_beef_MJ_d <- mean(dairy_beef_MJ_d, na.rm = TRUE)
    med_dairy_beef_MJ_d <- median(dairy_beef_MJ_d, na.rm = TRUE)
    min_dairy_beef_MJ_d <- min(dairy_beef_MJ_d, na.rm = TRUE)
    max_dairy_beef_MJ_d <- max(dairy_beef_MJ_d, na.rm = TRUE)
    sd_dairy_beef_MJ_d <- sd(dairy_beef_MJ_d, na.rm = TRUE)

    avg_dairy_beef_pGEI <- mean(dairy_beef_pGEI, na.rm = TRUE)
    med_dairy_beef_pGEI <- median(dairy_beef_pGEI, na.rm = TRUE)
    min_dairy_beef_pGEI <- min(dairy_beef_pGEI, na.rm = TRUE)
    max_dairy_beef_pGEI <- max(dairy_beef_pGEI, na.rm = TRUE)
    sd_dairy_beef_pGEI <- sd(dairy_beef_pGEI, na.rm = TRUE)

    avg_dairy_beef_g_kg <- mean(dairy_beef_g_kg, na.rm = TRUE)
    med_dairy_beef_g_kg <- median(dairy_beef_g_kg, na.rm = TRUE)
    min_dairy_beef_g_kg <- min(dairy_beef_g_kg, na.rm = TRUE)
    max_dairy_beef_g_kg <- max(dairy_beef_g_kg, na.rm = TRUE)
    sd_dairy_beef_g_kg <- sd(dairy_beef_g_kg, na.rm = TRUE)

    cat(paste(string("-", 102), "\n", sep = ""))
    cat(paste(" Statistics               Average      ", g_(avg_dairy_beef_L_d), " ", g_(avg_dairy_beef_g_d), " ", g_(avg_dairy_beef_Mcal_d), " ", g_(avg_dairy_beef_MJ_d), " ", g_(avg_dairy_beef_pGEI), " ", g_(avg_dairy_beef_g_kg), "\n", sep = ""))
    cat(paste("                          Median       ", g_(med_dairy_beef_L_d), " ", g_(med_dairy_beef_g_d), " ", g_(med_dairy_beef_Mcal_d), " ", g_(med_dairy_beef_MJ_d), " ", g_(med_dairy_beef_pGEI), " ", g_(med_dairy_beef_g_kg), "\n", sep = ""))
    cat(paste("                          Std. Dev.    ", g_(sd_dairy_beef_L_d), " ", g_(sd_dairy_beef_g_d), " ", g_(sd_dairy_beef_Mcal_d), " ", g_(sd_dairy_beef_MJ_d), " ", g_(sd_dairy_beef_pGEI), " ", g_(sd_dairy_beef_g_kg), "\n", sep = ""))
    cat(paste("                          CV (%)       ", g_(isz(sd_dairy_beef_L_d * 100, avg_dairy_beef_L_d)), " ", g_(isz(sd_dairy_beef_g_d * 100, avg_dairy_beef_g_d)), " ", g_(isz(sd_dairy_beef_Mcal_d * 100, avg_dairy_beef_Mcal_d)), " ", g_(isz(sd_dairy_beef_MJ_d * 100, avg_dairy_beef_MJ_d)), " ", g_(isz(sd_dairy_beef_pGEI * 100, avg_dairy_beef_pGEI)), " ", g_(isz(sd_dairy_beef_g_kg * 100, avg_dairy_beef_g_kg)), "\n", sep = ""))
    cat(paste("                          Minimum      ", g_(min_dairy_beef_L_d), " ", g_(min_dairy_beef_g_d), " ", g_(min_dairy_beef_Mcal_d), " ", g_(min_dairy_beef_MJ_d), " ", g_(min_dairy_beef_pGEI), " ", g_(min_dairy_beef_g_kg), "\n", sep = ""))
    cat(paste("                          Maximum      ", g_(max_dairy_beef_L_d), " ", g_(max_dairy_beef_g_d), " ", g_(max_dairy_beef_Mcal_d), " ", g_(max_dairy_beef_MJ_d), " ", g_(max_dairy_beef_pGEI), " ", g_(max_dairy_beef_g_kg), "\n", sep = ""))
```

```
    cat(paste(string("=", 102), "\n", sep = ""))

    cat(paste("*     = Recommended equations.\n", "GEI = Gross energy intake, Mcal/d.\n", "(1) = Digestibility predicted at production level of intake, not at maintenance level of\n", "        intake as recommended. Dataset included beef cattle and sheep.\n", sep = ""))


    # +++++++
    # BoxPlot
    # +++++++
    ok <- check.necessary.packages(c("ggplot2","gridExtra","RColorBrewer","grid"), FALSE, FALSE)
    if (ok==TRUE)
    {
      d1 <- dairy_L_d[!is.na(dairy_L_d)]
      d2 <- beef_L_d[!is.na(beef_L_d)]
      d3 <- dairy_beef_L_d[!is.na(dairy_beef_L_d)]
      d<-as.data.frame(rbind(cbind(d1,rep("Dairy only",length(d1))),
                             cbind(d2,rep("Beef only",length(d2))),
                             cbind(d3,rep("Dairy or Beef",length(d3)))))
      colnames(d)<-(c("CH4","Class"))
      d$CH4<-as.numeric(as.character(d$CH4))
      CH4_Boxplot <- createfilename(outputpath, "/BoxPlot_Methane", "TIF")
      g1<-metaboxplot2(varData=d,varXName="Class",varYName="CH4",varClass1Name=NA,varClass2Name=NA,blnViolin=F,
                       varTitle="(A)",varXLbl="Classes of Animals",varYLbl="Predicted methane emissions, L/d",
                       varXVal=NULL,varClass1Lbl=NULL,varClass2Lbl=NULL,footnote="\n*** The red values are means, and the top, center, and bottom black values are 25%, 50% (median), and 75% quantiles, respectively ***",stamptime=F,fontfamily="sans",
                       varxaxisangle=0,varyaxisangle=0, fontsizeratio=1,symbolsize=4,strPalette="Dark2",
                       blnShowVarXLegend=F,blnShowClass1Legend=F,varClass1LegendLabels=NA,blnShowClass2Legend=F,varClass2LegendLabels=NA,
                       blnSavePlot=F,fn=NA,figwidth=4000,figheight=4000,figres=400,blnReturnPlot=T,varFacetgrid=NA,
                       blnShowMean=T,blnLinkMean=T,LinkMeanLineType="dotdash",MeanColor="red",
                       ShapeValues=NA,LegendWidth=NA,LegendHeight=NA,LegendLineSize=NA,
                       annLabel=NA,annX=0,annY=0,annHJust=0,annSize=7,annColor="black",
                       blnShowBoxPlotValues=T,bxplotDigits=3,bxplotWidth=5,bxplotVjust=-0.3,bxplotHjust=-0.3,bxplotSize=5,bxplotColor="black")

      d1 <- dairy_pGEI[!is.na(dairy_pGEI)]
      d2 <- beef_pGEI[!is.na(beef_pGEI)]
      d3 <- dairy_beef_pGEI[!is.na(dairy_beef_pGEI)]
      d<-as.data.frame(rbind(cbind(d1,rep("Dairy only",length(d1))),
                             cbind(d2,rep("Beef only",length(d2))),
                             cbind(d3,rep("Dairy or Beef",length(d3)))))
      colnames(d)<-(c("CH4","Class"))
      d$CH4<-as.numeric(as.character(d$CH4))
      g2<-metaboxplot2(varData=d,varXName="Class",varYName="CH4",varClass1Name=NA,varClass2Name=NA,blnViolin=F,
                       varTitle="(B)",varXLbl="Classes of Animals",varYLbl="Predicted methane emissions, % of gross energy",
                       varXVal=NULL,varClass1Lbl=NULL,varClass2Lbl=NULL,footnote="\n*** The red values are means, and the top, center, and bottom black values are 25%, 50% (median), and 75% quantiles, respectively ***",stamptime=F,fontfamily="sans",
                       varxaxisangle=0,varyaxisangle=0, fontsizeratio=1,symbolsize=4,strPalette="Dark2",
                       blnShowVarXLegend=F,blnShowClass1Legend=F,varClass1LegendLabels=NA,blnShowClass2Legend=F,varClass2LegendLabels=NA,
```

```
                    blnSavePlot=F,fn=NA,figwidth=4000,figheight=4000,figres=400,blnReturnPlot=T,varFacetgrid=NA,
                    blnShowMean=T,blnLinkMean=T,LinkMeanLineType="dotdash",MeanColor="red",
                    ShapeValues=NA,LegendWidth=NA,LegendHeight=NA,LegendLineSize=NA,
                    annLabel=NA,annX=0,annY=0,annHJust=0,annSize=7,annColor="black",
                    blnShowBoxPlotValues=T,bxplotDigits=3,bxplotWidth=5,bxplotVjust=-0.3,bxplotHjust=-0.3,bxplot-
Size=5,bxplotColor="black")
    require(gridExtra)
    tiff(CH4_Boxplot, width = 4000, height = 8000, bg = "white", res = 400, compress = "lzw")
    grid.arrange(g1,g2,ncol=1)
    dev.off()
    if (file.exists(CH4_Boxplot))
    {
      newpage(T)
      cat(paste("#RetrieveGraph#{", CH4_Boxplot, "}", sep = ""))
    }
  }



  # +++++++++++++++
  # Robust Analyses
  # +++++++++++++++
  # MAD = Median Absolute Deviation
  newpage(T)
  library(MASS)
  median.CI <- function(x, alpha = 0.05)
  {
    # http://www.dst.unive.it/rsr/BelVenTutorial.pdf
    x <- x[is.na(x) == F]
    se.med <- sqrt((pi/2) * (mad(x)^2/length(x)))
    lower <- median(x) - qnorm(1 - alpha/2) * se.med
    upper <- median(x) + qnorm(1 - alpha/2) * se.med
    return(c(lower, upper))
  }

  get.rlm <- function(x, alpha = 0.05, k2 = 1.5)
  {
    fit <- try(rlm(x ~ 1, k2 = 1.5, scale.est = "proposal 2", method = "MM"), silent = True)
    mu <- summary(fit)$coefficients[1]
    se <- summary(fit)$coefficients[2]
    lower <- fit$coef[1] - qnorm(1 - alpha/2) * se
    upper <- fit$coef[1] + qnorm(1 - alpha/2) * se
    return(c(mu, se, lower, upper))
  }

  header <- paste("Robust Data Analyses", sep = "")
  headersize <- nchar(header)
  cat(paste("#Title#", header, "\n", string("=", headersize), sep = ""), "\n\n")

  cat(paste("Source                    Statistics              L/d       g/d     Mcal/d      MJ/d      % GEI    g/kg DM\n",
string("=", 102), "\n", sep = ""))
```

```
    if (anim.species == "Cattle" & anim.type == "Milk")
    {
      cat(paste("Dairy*                                ", sep = ""))
    } else
    {
      cat(paste("Dairy                                 ", sep = ""))
    }

    cat(paste("10% Trimmed Avg.", g_(mean(dairy_L_d, trim = 0.1, na.rm = T)), " ", g_(mean(dairy_g_d, trim = 0.1, na.rm = T)), " ", g_(mean(dairy_Mcal_d, trim = 0.1, na.rm = T)), " ", g_(mean(dairy_MJ_d, trim = 0.1, na.rm = T)), " ", g_(mean(dairy_pGEI, trim = 0.1, na.rm = T)), " ", g_(mean(dairy_g_kg, trim = 0.1, na.rm = T)), "\n", sep = ""))
    cat(paste("                    20% Trimmed Avg.", g_(mean(dairy_L_d, trim = 0.2, na.rm = T)), " ", g_(mean(dairy_g_d, trim = 0.2, na.rm = T)), " ", g_(mean(dairy_Mcal_d, trim = 0.2, na.rm = T)), " ", g_(mean(dairy_MJ_d, trim = 0.2, na.rm = T)), " ", g_(mean(dairy_pGEI, trim = 0.2, na.rm = T)), " ", g_(mean(dairy_g_kg, trim = 0.2, na.rm = T)), "\n", sep = ""))
    cat(paste("                    Median Abs. Dev.", g_(mad(dairy_L_d, na.rm = T)), " ", g_(mad(dairy_g_d, na.rm = T)), " ", g_(mad(dairy_Mcal_d, na.rm = T)), " ", g_(mad(dairy_MJ_d, na.rm = T)), " ", g_(mad(dairy_pGEI, na.rm = T)), " ", g_(mad(dairy_g_kg, na.rm = T)), "\n", sep = ""))
    cat(paste("                    Lower median CI ", g_(median.CI(dairy_L_d)[1]), " ", g_(median.CI(dairy_g_d)[1]), " ", g_(median.CI(dairy_Mcal_d)[1]), " ", g_(median.CI(dairy_MJ_d)[1]), " ", g_(median.CI(dairy_pGEI)[1]), " ", g_(median.CI(dairy_g_kg)[1]), "\n", sep = ""))
    cat(paste("                    Upper median CI ", g_(median.CI(dairy_L_d)[2]), " ", g_(median.CI(dairy_g_d)[2]), " ", g_(median.CI(dairy_Mcal_d)[2]), " ", g_(median.CI(dairy_MJ_d)[2]), " ", g_(median.CI(dairy_pGEI)[2]), " ", g_(median.CI(dairy_g_kg)[2]), "\n", sep = ""))
    cat(paste("                    Huber's mu      ", g_(huber(dairy_L_d)$mu), " ", g_(huber(dairy_g_d)$mu), " ", g_(huber(dairy_Mcal_d)$mu), " ", g_(huber(dairy_MJ_d)$mu), " ", g_(huber(dairy_pGEI)$mu), " ", g_(huber(dairy_g_kg)$mu), "\n", sep = ""))
    cat(paste("                    Huber's s       ", g_(huber(dairy_L_d)$s), " ", g_(huber(dairy_g_d)$s), " ", g_(huber(dairy_Mcal_d)$s), " ", g_(huber(dairy_MJ_d)$s), " ", g_(huber(dairy_pGEI)$s), " ", g_(huber(dairy_g_kg)$s), "\n", sep = ""))
    cat(paste(string("-", 102), "\n", sep = ""))
    rlm_dairy_L_d <- get.rlm(dairy_L_d)
    rlm_dairy_g_d <- get.rlm(dairy_g_d)
    rlm_dairy_Mcal_d <- get.rlm(dairy_Mcal_d)
    rlm_dairy_MJ_d <- get.rlm(dairy_MJ_d)
    rlm_dairy_pGEI <- get.rlm(dairy_pGEI)
    rlm_dairy_g_kg <- get.rlm(dairy_g_kg)
    cat(paste("       Robust Linear Model:Mean          ", g_(rlm_dairy_L_d[1]), " ", g_(rlm_dairy_g_d[1]), " ", g_(rlm_dairy_Mcal_d[1]), " ", g_(rlm_dairy_MJ_d[1]), " ", g_(rlm_dairy_pGEI[1]), " ", g_(rlm_dairy_g_kg[1]), "\n", sep = ""))
    cat(paste("       Robust Linear Model:Std. Error    ", g_(rlm_dairy_L_d[2]), " ", g_(rlm_dairy_g_d[2]), " ", g_(rlm_dairy_Mcal_d[2]), " ", g_(rlm_dairy_MJ_d[2]), " ", g_(rlm_dairy_pGEI[2]), " ", g_(rlm_dairy_g_kg[2]), "\n", sep = ""))
    cat(paste("       Robust Linear Model:Lower 95% CI  ", g_(rlm_dairy_L_d[3]), " ", g_(rlm_dairy_g_d[3]), " ", g_(rlm_dairy_Mcal_d[3]), " ", g_(rlm_dairy_MJ_d[3]), " ", g_(rlm_dairy_pGEI[3]), " ", g_(rlm_dairy_g_kg[3]), "\n", sep = ""))
    cat(paste("       Robust Linear Model:Upper 95% CI  ", g_(rlm_dairy_L_d[4]), " ", g_(rlm_dairy_g_d[4]), " ", g_(rlm_dairy_Mcal_d[4]), " ", g_(rlm_dairy_MJ_d[4]), " ", g_(rlm_dairy_pGEI[4]), " ", g_(rlm_dairy_g_kg[4]), "\n", sep = ""))
    cat(paste(string("=", 102), "\n", sep = ""))

    if (anim.species == "Cattle" & anim.type != "Milk")
    {
      cat(paste("Beef*                                 ", sep = ""))
    } else
    {
```

```
    cat(paste("Beef                          ", sep = ""))
  }
  cat(paste("10% Trimmed Avg.", g_(mean(beef_L_d, trim = 0.1, na.rm = T)), " ", g_(mean(beef_g_d, trim = 0.1, na.rm = T)), " ", g_(mean(beef_Mcal_d, trim = 0.1, na.rm = T)), " ", g_(mean(beef_MJ_d, trim = 0.1, na.rm = T)), " ", g_(mean(beef_pGEI, trim = 0.1, na.rm = T)), " ", g_(mean(beef_g_kg, trim = 0.1, na.rm = T)), "\n", sep = ""))
  cat(paste("                    20% Trimmed Avg.", g_(mean(beef_L_d, trim = 0.2, na.rm = T)), " ", g_(mean(beef_g_d, trim = 0.2, na.rm = T)), " ", g_(mean(beef_Mcal_d, trim = 0.2, na.rm = T)), " ", g_(mean(beef_MJ_d, trim = 0.2, na.rm = T)), " ", g_(mean(beef_pGEI, trim = 0.2, na.rm = T)), " ", g_(mean(beef_g_kg, trim = 0.2, na.rm = T)), "\n", sep = ""))
  cat(paste("                    Median Abs. Dev.", g_(mad(beef_L_d, na.rm = T)), " ", g_(mad(beef_g_d, na.rm = T)), " ", g_(mad(beef_Mcal_d, na.rm = T)), " ", g_(mad(beef_MJ_d, na.rm = T)), " ", g_(mad(beef_pGEI, na.rm = T)), " ", g_(mad(beef_g_kg, na.rm = T)), "\n", sep = ""))
  cat(paste("                    Lower median CI ", g_(median.CI(beef_L_d)[1]), " ", g_(median.CI(beef_g_d)[1]), " ", g_(median.CI(beef_Mcal_d)[1]), " ", g_(median.CI(beef_MJ_d)[1]), " ", g_(median.CI(beef_pGEI)[1]), " ", g_(median.CI(beef_g_kg)[1]), "\n", sep = ""))
  cat(paste("                    Upper median CI ", g_(median.CI(beef_L_d)[2]), " ", g_(median.CI(beef_g_d)[2]), " ", g_(median.CI(beef_Mcal_d)[2]), " ", g_(median.CI(beef_MJ_d)[2]), " ", g_(median.CI(beef_pGEI)[2]), " ", g_(median.CI(beef_g_kg)[2]), "\n", sep = ""))
  cat(paste("                    Huber's mu      ", g_(huber(beef_L_d)$mu), " ", g_(huber(beef_g_d)$mu), " ", g_(huber(beef_Mcal_d)$mu), " ", g_(huber(beef_MJ_d)$mu), " ", g_(huber(beef_pGEI)$mu), " ", g_(huber(beef_g_kg)$mu), "\n", sep = ""))
  cat(paste("                    Huber's s       ", g_(huber(beef_L_d)$s), " ", g_(huber(beef_g_d)$s), " ", g_(huber(beef_Mcal_d)$s), " ", g_(huber(beef_MJ_d)$s), " ", g_(huber(beef_pGEI)$s), " ", g_(huber(beef_g_kg)$s), "\n", sep = ""))
  cat(paste(string("-", 102), "\n", sep = ""))
  rlm_beef_L_d <- get.rlm(beef_L_d)
  rlm_beef_g_d <- get.rlm(beef_g_d)
  rlm_beef_Mcal_d <- get.rlm(beef_Mcal_d)
  rlm_beef_MJ_d <- get.rlm(beef_MJ_d)
  rlm_beef_pGEI <- get.rlm(beef_pGEI)
  rlm_beef_g_kg <- get.rlm(beef_g_kg)
  cat(paste("       Robust Linear Model:Mean          ", g_(rlm_beef_L_d[1]), " ", g_(rlm_beef_g_d[1]), " ", g_(rlm_beef_Mcal_d[1]), " ", g_(rlm_beef_MJ_d[1]), " ", g_(rlm_beef_pGEI[1]), " ", g_(rlm_beef_g_kg[1]), "\n", sep = ""))
  cat(paste("       Robust Linear Model:Std. Error    ", g_(rlm_beef_L_d[2]), " ", g_(rlm_beef_g_d[2]), " ", g_(rlm_beef_Mcal_d[2]), " ", g_(rlm_beef_MJ_d[2]), " ", g_(rlm_beef_pGEI[2]), " ", g_(rlm_beef_g_kg[2]), "\n", sep = ""))
  cat(paste("       Robust Linear Model:Lower 95% CI  ", g_(rlm_beef_L_d[3]), " ", g_(rlm_beef_g_d[3]), " ", g_(rlm_beef_Mcal_d[3]), " ", g_(rlm_beef_MJ_d[3]), " ", g_(rlm_beef_pGEI[3]), " ", g_(rlm_beef_g_kg[3]), "\n", sep = ""))
  cat(paste("       Robust Linear Model:Upper 95% CI  ", g_(rlm_beef_L_d[4]), " ", g_(rlm_beef_g_d[4]), " ", g_(rlm_beef_Mcal_d[4]), " ", g_(rlm_beef_MJ_d[4]), " ", g_(rlm_beef_pGEI[4]), " ", g_(rlm_beef_g_kg[4]), "\n", sep = ""))
  cat(paste(string("=", 102), "\n", sep = ""))

  if (anim.species == "Cattle")
  {
    cat(paste("Dairy or Beef*                ", sep = ""))
  } else
  {
    cat(paste("Dairy or Beef                 ", sep = ""))
  }
  cat(paste("10% Trimmed Avg.", g_(mean(dairy_beef_L_d, trim = 0.1, na.rm = T)), " ", g_(mean(dairy_beef_g_d, trim = 0.1, na.rm = T)), " ", g_(mean(dairy_beef_Mcal_d, trim = 0.1, na.rm = T)), " ", g_(mean(dairy_beef_MJ_d, trim = 0.1, na.rm = T)), " ", g_(mean(dairy_beef_pGEI, trim = 0.1, na.rm = T)), " ", g_(mean(dairy_beef_g_kg, trim = 0.1, na.rm = T)), "\n", sep = ""))
  cat(paste("                    20% Trimmed Avg.", g_(mean(dairy_beef_L_d, trim = 0.2, na.rm = T)), " ", g_(mean(dairy_beef_g_d, trim = 0.2, na.rm = T)), " ", g_(mean(dairy_beef_Mcal_d, trim = 0.2, na.rm = T)), " ",
```

```
g_(mean(dairy_beef_MJ_d, trim = 0.2, na.rm = T)), " ", g_(mean(dairy_beef_pGEI, trim = 0.2, na.rm = T)), " ",
g_(mean(dairy_beef_g_kg, trim = 0.2, na.rm = T)), "\n", sep = ""))
  cat(paste("                    Median Abs. Dev.", g_(mad(dairy_beef_L_d, na.rm = T)), " ", g_(mad(dairy_beef_g_d, na.rm = T)), " ", g_(mad(dairy_beef_Mcal_d, na.rm = T)), " ", g_(mad(dairy_beef_MJ_d, na.rm = T)), " ", g_(mad(dairy_beef_pGEI, na.rm = T)), " ", g_(mad(dairy_beef_g_kg, na.rm = T)), "\n", sep = ""))
  cat(paste("                    Lower median CI ", g_(median.CI(dairy_beef_L_d)[1]), " ", g_(median.CI(dairy_beef_g_d)[1]), " ", g_(median.CI(dairy_beef_Mcal_d)[1]), " ", g_(median.CI(dairy_beef_MJ_d)[1]), " ", g_(median.CI(dairy_beef_pGEI)[1]), " ", g_(median.CI(dairy_beef_g_kg)[1]), "\n", sep = ""))
  cat(paste("                    Upper median CI ", g_(median.CI(dairy_beef_L_d)[2]), " ", g_(median.CI(dairy_beef_g_d)[2]), " ", g_(median.CI(dairy_beef_Mcal_d)[2]), " ", g_(median.CI(dairy_beef_MJ_d)[2]), " ", g_(median.CI(dairy_beef_pGEI)[2]), " ", g_(median.CI(dairy_beef_g_kg)[2]), "\n", sep = ""))
  cat(paste("                    Huber's mu      ", g_(huber(dairy_beef_L_d)$mu), " ", g_(huber(dairy_beef_g_d)$mu), " ", g_(huber(dairy_beef_Mcal_d)$mu), " ", g_(huber(dairy_beef_MJ_d)$mu), " ", g_(huber(dairy_beef_pGEI)$mu), " ", g_(huber(dairy_beef_g_kg)$mu), "\n", sep = ""))
  cat(paste("                    Huber's s       ", g_(huber(dairy_beef_L_d)$s), " ", g_(huber(dairy_beef_g_d)$s), " ", g_(huber(dairy_beef_Mcal_d)$s), " ", g_(huber(dairy_beef_MJ_d)$s), " ", g_(huber(dairy_beef_pGEI)$s), " ", g_(huber(dairy_beef_g_kg)$s), "\n", sep = ""))
  cat(paste(string("-", 102), "\n", sep = ""))
  rlm_dairy_beef_L_d <- get.rlm(dairy_beef_L_d)
  rlm_dairy_beef_g_d <- get.rlm(dairy_beef_g_d)
  rlm_dairy_beef_Mcal_d <- get.rlm(dairy_beef_Mcal_d)
  rlm_dairy_beef_MJ_d <- get.rlm(dairy_beef_MJ_d)
  rlm_dairy_beef_pGEI <- get.rlm(dairy_beef_pGEI)
  rlm_dairy_beef_g_kg <- get.rlm(dairy_beef_g_kg)
  cat(paste("        Robust Linear Model:Mean              ", g_(rlm_dairy_beef_L_d[1]), " ", g_(rlm_dairy_beef_g_d[1]), " ", g_(rlm_dairy_beef_Mcal_d[1]), " ", g_(rlm_dairy_beef_MJ_d[1]), " ", g_(rlm_dairy_beef_pGEI[1]), " ", g_(rlm_dairy_beef_g_kg[1]), "\n", sep = ""))
  cat(paste("        Robust Linear Model:Std. Error        ", g_(rlm_dairy_beef_L_d[2]), " ", g_(rlm_dairy_beef_g_d[2]), " ", g_(rlm_dairy_beef_Mcal_d[2]), " ", g_(rlm_dairy_beef_MJ_d[2]), " ", g_(rlm_dairy_beef_pGEI[2]), " ", g_(rlm_dairy_beef_g_kg[2]), "\n", sep = ""))
  cat(paste("        Robust Linear Model:Lower 95% CI      ", g_(rlm_dairy_beef_L_d[3]), " ", g_(rlm_dairy_beef_g_d[3]), " ", g_(rlm_dairy_beef_Mcal_d[3]), " ", g_(rlm_dairy_beef_MJ_d[3]), " ", g_(rlm_dairy_beef_pGEI[3]), " ", g_(rlm_dairy_beef_g_kg[3]), "\n", sep = ""))
  cat(paste("        Robust Linear Model:Upper 95% CI      ", g_(rlm_dairy_beef_L_d[4]), " ", g_(rlm_dairy_beef_g_d[4]), " ", g_(rlm_dairy_beef_Mcal_d[4]), " ", g_(rlm_dairy_beef_MJ_d[4]), " ", g_(rlm_dairy_beef_pGEI[4]), " ", g_(rlm_dairy_beef_g_kg[4]), "\n", sep = ""))
  cat(paste(string("=", 102), "\n", sep = ""))
  cat("Robust Linear Model used method='MM', scale.est='proposal 2', and k2=1.5\n")



  # ++++++++++++++++
  # Cluster Analysis
  # ++++++++++++++++
  # http://www.statmethods.net/advstats/cluster.html
  # http://cran.cnr.berkeley.edu/web/views/Cluster.html
  # http://wiki.math.yorku.ca/index.php/R:_Cluster_analysis

  values <- c(CH4_Axelsson1949_DMI, CH4_Axelsson1949_DCHO, CH4_MoeTyrrell1979, CH4_Millsetal2003_linear1, CH4_Millsetal2003_linear2, CH4_Millsetal2003_linear3, CH4_Millsetal2003_linear4, CH4_Millsetal2003_nonlinear1, CH4_Millsetal2003_non-
```

```
linear2, CH4_Millsetal2003_nonlinear3, CH4_Ellisetal2007_Eq1d, CH4_Ellisetal2007_Eq2d, CH4_Ellisetal2007_Eq3d, CH4_Ellise-
tal2007_Eq4d, CH4_Ellisetal2007_Eq5d, CH4_Ellisetal2007_Eq6d, CH4_Ellisetal2007_Eq7d, CH4_Ellisetal2007_Eq8d,
CH4_RaminHuhtanen2013_Linear, CH4_RaminHuhtanen2013_Quad,
                CH4_Moraesetal2014_GE, CH4_Moraesetal2014_diet, CH4_Moraesetal2014_animal, CH4_Mutianetal2018_Eq1, CH4_Mu-
tianetal2018_Eq2, CH4_Mutianetal2018_Eq3, CH4_Mutianetal2018_Eq4, CH4_Mutianetal2018_Eq5, CH4_Mutianetal2018_Eq6, CH4_Mu-
tianetal2018_Eq7, CH4_Mutianetal2018_Eq8, CH4_Mutianetal2018_Eq9, CH4_Mutianetal2018_Eq10, CH4_Mutianetal2018_Eq11,
                CH4_BlaxterClapperton1965, CH4_Ellisetal2007_Eq1b, CH4_Ellisetal2007_Eq2b, CH4_Ellisetal2007_Eq3b, CH4_Ellise-
tal2007_Eq4b, CH4_Ellisetal2007_Eq5b, CH4_Ellisetal2007_Eq6b, CH4_Ellisetal2007_Eq7b, CH4_Ellisetal2007_Eq8b, CH4_Ellise-
tal2007_Eq9b, CH4_Ellisetal2007_Eq10b, CH4_Ellisetal2007_Eq11b, CH4_Ellisetal2007_Eq12b, CH4_Ellisetal2007_Eq13b, CH4_Ellise-
tal2007_Eq14b, CH4_Ellisetal2009_EqA, CH4_Ellisetal2009_EqB, CH4_Ellisetal2009_EqC,
                CH4_Ellisetal2009_EqD, CH4_Ellisetal2009_EqE, CH4_Ellisetal2009_EqF, CH4_Ellisetal2009_EqG, CH4_Ellise-
tal2009_EqH, CH4_Ellisetal2009_EqI, CH4_Ellisetal2009_EqJ, CH4_Ellisetal2009_EqK, CH4_Ellisetal2009_EqL, CH4_Ellise-
tal2009_EqM, CH4_Ellisetal2009_EqN, CH4_Ellisetal2009_EqO, CH4_Ellisetal2009_EqP, CH4_Ellisetal2009_EqQ, CH4_Ellise-
tal2009_EqR, CH4_Ellisetal2009_EqS, CH4_Ellisetal2009_EqT, CH4_Ellisetal2009_EqU, CH4_Ellisetal2009_EqV, CH4_Ellise-
tal2009_EqW, CH4_Ellisetal2009_EqX, CH4_Ellisetal2009_EqW1,
                CH4_Ellisetal2009_EqW2, CH4_Ellisetal2009_EqW3, CH4_Yanetal2009_Eq1a, CH4_Yanetal2009_Eq1b, CH4_Ya-
netal2009_Eq1c, CH4_Yanetal2009_Eq2a, CH4_Yanetal2009_Eq2b, CH4_Yanetal2009_Eq3a, CH4_Yanetal2009_Eq3b, CH4_Yanetal2009_Eq3c,
CH4_Moraesetal2014_GE, CH4_Moraesetal2014_diet, CH4_Moraesetal2014_animal, CH4_Kriss1930, CH4_BratzlerForbes1940,
CH4_IPCC_Tier2, CH4_Ellisetal2007_Eq1c, CH4_Ellisetal2007_Eq2c, CH4_Ellisetal2007_Eq3c, CH4_Ellisetal2007_Eq4c, CH4_Ellise-
tal2007_Eq5c, CH4_Ellisetal2007_Eq6c,
                CH4_Ellisetal2007_Eq7c, CH4_Ellisetal2007_Eq8c, CH4_Ellisetal2007_Eq9c, CH4_Ellisetal2007_Eq10c, CH4_Ric-
cietal2013_GEI, CH4_Riccietal2013_DMI, CH4_Riccietal2013_DEI, CH4_Riccietal2013_MEI)
  labels <- c("Axelsson1949_DMI", "Axelsson1949_DCHO", "MoeTyrrell1979", "Millsetal2003_linear1", "Millsetal2003_linear2",
"Millsetal2003_linear3", "Millsetal2003_linear4", "Millsetal2003_nonlinear1", "Millsetal2003_nonlinear2", "Millsetal2003_non-
linear3", "Ellisetal2007_Eq1d", "Ellisetal2007_Eq2d", "Ellisetal2007_Eq3d", "Ellisetal2007_Eq4d", "Ellisetal2007_Eq5d", "El-
lisetal2007_Eq6d", "Ellisetal2007_Eq7d", "Ellisetal2007_Eq8d", "RaminHuhtanen2013_Linear", "RaminHuhtanen2013_Quad", "Moraese-
tal2014_GE_D",
                "Moraesetal2014_diet_D", "Moraesetal2014_animal_D", "CH4_Mutianetal2018_Eq1", "CH4_Mutianetal2018_Eq2", "CH4_Mu-
tianetal2018_Eq3", "CH4_Mutianetal2018_Eq4", "CH4_Mutianetal2018_Eq5", "CH4_Mutianetal2018_Eq6", "CH4_Mutianetal2018_Eq7",
"CH4_Mutianetal2018_Eq8", "CH4_Mutianetal2018_Eq9", "CH4_Mutianetal2018_Eq10", "CH4_Mutianetal2018_Eq11",
                "BlaxterClapperton1965", "Ellisetal2007_Eq1b", "Ellisetal2007_Eq2b", "Ellisetal2007_Eq3b", "Ellisetal2007_Eq4b",
"Ellisetal2007_Eq5b", "Ellisetal2007_Eq6b", "Ellisetal2007_Eq7b", "Ellisetal2007_Eq8b", "Ellisetal2007_Eq9b", "Ellise-
tal2007_Eq10b", "Ellisetal2007_Eq11b", "Ellisetal2007_Eq12b", "Ellisetal2007_Eq13b", "Ellisetal2007_Eq14b", "Ellise-
tal2009_EqA", "Ellisetal2009_EqB", "Ellisetal2009_EqC", "Ellisetal2009_EqD", "Ellisetal2009_EqE", "Ellisetal2009_EqF",
                "Ellisetal2009_EqG", "Ellisetal2009_EqH", "Ellisetal2009_EqI", "Ellisetal2009_EqJ", "Ellisetal2009_EqK", "El-
lisetal2009_EqL", "Ellisetal2009_EqM", "Ellisetal2009_EqN", "Ellisetal2009_EqO", "Ellisetal2009_EqP", "Ellisetal2009_EqQ",
"Ellisetal2009_EqR", "Ellisetal2009_EqS", "Ellisetal2009_EqT", "Ellisetal2009_EqU", "Ellisetal2009_EqV", "Ellisetal2009_EqW",
"Ellisetal2009_EqX", "Ellisetal2009_EqW1", "Ellisetal2009_EqW2", "Ellisetal2009_EqW3", "Yanetal2009_Eq1a", "Yanetal2009_Eq1b",
"Yanetal2009_Eq1c",
                "Yanetal2009_Eq2a", "Yanetal2009_Eq2b", "Yanetal2009_Eq3a", "Yanetal2009_Eq3b", "Yanetal2009_Eq3c", "Moraese-
tal2014_GE_B", "Moraesetal2014_diet_B", "Moraesetal2014_animal_B", "Kriss1930", "BratzlerForbes1940", "IPCC_Tier2", "Ellise-
tal2007_Eq1c", "Ellisetal2007_Eq2c", "Ellisetal2007_Eq3c", "Ellisetal2007_Eq4c", "Ellisetal2007_Eq5c", "Ellisetal2007_Eq6c",
"Ellisetal2007_Eq7c", "Ellisetal2007_Eq8c", "Ellisetal2007_Eq9c", "Ellisetal2007_Eq10c", "Riccietal2013_GEI", "Ric-
cietal2013_DMI", "Riccietal2013_DEI",
                "Riccietal2013_MEI")
  CH4df <- data.frame(values, row.names = labels)
  is.na(CH4df) <- sapply(CH4df, is.infinite)  # Remove infinite
  CH4df <- na.omit(CH4df)
  CH4df <- scale(CH4df)

  ok <- check.necessary.packages(c("fpc"), FALSE, FALSE)
```

```
  if (ok == TRUE)
  {
    library(fpc)
    nc <- pamk(CH4df)$nc
  } else nc <- 7
  if (nc < 3) nc <- 3

  CH4_plot <<- createfilename(outputpath, "/Plot_Methane", "TIF")

  # Ward Hierarchical Clustering
  CH4_d <- dist(CH4df, method = "euclidean")
  tiff(CH4_plot, width = 8400, height = 5600, bg = "white", res = 560, compress = "lzw")
  if (as.numeric(R.version$major) <= 3 & as.numeric(R.version$minor) <= 0.3)
  {
    # Ward (1963)
    CH4_fit <- hclust(CH4_d, method = "ward")
    plot(CH4_fit, main = "Cluster Dendrogram for Methane Predictions", xlab = "Ward's Distance (Ward, 1963)", sub = paste("(with ", nc, " K-Means Clusters)", sep = ""))
  } else
  {
    # Murtagh, F., and P. Legendre. 2014. Ward's hierarchical agglomerative clustering method: Which algorithms implement ward's criterion? Journal of Classification. 31 (3):274-295.
    CH4_fit <- hclust(CH4_d, method = "ward.D2")
    plot(CH4_fit, main = "Cluster Dendrogram for Methane Predictions", xlab = "Ward's Distance (Murtagh and Legendre, 2014; J. Classification 31:274)", sub = paste("(with ", nc, " K-Means Clusters)", sep = ""))
  }

  # http://www.statmethods.net/advstats/cluster.html
  #wss<-(nrow(CH4df)-1)*sum(apply(CH4df,2,var))
  #for (i in 2:15) wss[i]<-sum(kmeans(CH4df, centers=i)$withinss)
  #plot(1:15, wss, type="b", xlab="Number of Clusters",ylab="Within groups sum of squares")

  groups <- cutree(CH4_fit, k = nc)
  rect.hclust(CH4_fit, k = nc, border = "red")
  dev.off()

  if (file.exists(CH4_plot))
  {
    newpage(T)
    cat(paste("#RetrieveGraph#{", CH4_plot, "}", sep = ""))
  }



  # ++++++++++
  # References
  # ++++++++++
  newpage(T)
  cat(paste("REFERENCES:\n\n", sep = ""))
  cat(paste("Axelsson, J. 1949. The amount of produced methane energy in the European metabolic\n", "   experiments with adult cattle. Ann. R. Agric. Coll. Sweden. 16:404-419.\n", "Bellio, R., and L. Ventura. 2005. An Introduction to Robust Estimation
```

```
with R Functions.\n", "   Available at: http://www.dst.unive.it/rsr/BelVenTutorial.pdf\n", "Blaxter, K. L. and J. L. Clapper-
ton. 1965. Prediction of the amount of methane produced\n", "   by ruminants. Br. J. Nutr. 19:511-522.\n", "Bratzler, J. W.,
and E. B. Forbes. 1940. The estimation of methane production by cattle.\n",
            "   J. Nutr. 19:611-613.\n", "Ellis, J. L., E. Kebreab, N. E. Odongo, B. W. McBride, E. K. Okine and J. France.
2007.\n", "   Prediction of methane production from dairy and beef cattle. J. Dairy Sci. 90:3456-\n", "   3467.\n", "Ellis, J.
L., E. Kebreab, N. E. Odongo, K. Beauchemin, S. McGinn, J. D. Nkrumah, S. S.\n", "   Moore, R. Christopherson, G. K. Murdoch,
B. W. McBride, E. K. Okine, and J. France.\n", "   2009. Modeling methane production from beef cattle using linear and nonlin-
ear\n",
            "   approaches. J. Anim. Sci. 87:1334-1345.\n", "Intergovernmental Panel on Climate Change. 2006. 2006 IPCC Guide-
lines for National\n", "   Greenhouse Gas Inventories: Agriculture, Forestry and Other Land Use. H. S. Eggleston,\n", "   L.
Buendia, K. Miwa, T. Ngara and K. Tanabe, eds. vol. 4. Institute for Global\n", "   Environmental Strategies (IGES), Hayama,
Hanagawa, Japan. 678 p.\n", "   Available at: http://www.ipcc-nggip.iges.or.jp/public/2006gl/vol4.html.\n", "Kriss, M. 1930.
Quantitative relations of the dry matter of the food consumed, the heat\n",
            "   production, the gaseous outgo, and the insensible loss in body weight of cattle. J.\n", "   Agric. Res.
40:283\u0096295\n", "Mills, J. A. N., E. Kebreab, C. M. Yates, L. A. Crompton, S. B. Cammell, M. S. Dhanoa,\n", "   R. E. Ag-
new, and J. France. 2003. Alternative approaches to predicting methane\n", "   emissions from dairy cows. J. Anim. Sci.
81:3141-3150.\n", "Moe, P. W. and H. F. Tyrrell. 1979. Methane production in dairy cows. J. Dairy Sci. 62:\n", "   1583-
1586.\n", "Moraes, L. E., A. B. Strathe, J. G. Fadel, D. P. Casper, and E. Kebreab. 2014. Prediction\n",
            "   of enteric methane emissions from cattle. Global Change Biology. 20:2140-2148.\n", "Mutian, N., E. Kebreab, A.
N. Hristov, J. Oh, C. Arndt, A. Bannink, A. R. Bayat,\n","   A. F. Brito, T. Boland, D. Casper, L. A. Crompton, J. Dijkstra,
M. A. Eugène,\n","   P. C. Garnsworthy, M. N. Haque, A. L. F. Hellwing, P. Huhtanen, M. Kreuzer,\n","   B. Kuhla, P. Lund, J.
Madsen, C. Martin, S. C. McClelland, M. McGee, P. J. Moate,\n","   S. Muetzel, C. Muñoz, P. O'Kiely, N. Peiren, C. K. Reyn-
olds, A. Schwarm, \n",
            "   K. J. Shingfield, T. M. Storlien, M. R. Weisbjerg, D. R. Yáñez-Ruiz, and\n","   Z. Yu. 2018. Prediction of
enteric methane production, yield, and intensity in dairy\n","   cattle using an intercontinental database. Global Change
Biol. 24 (8):3368-3389.\n", "Ramin, M., and P. Huhtanen. 2013. Development of equations for predicting methane\n", "   emis-
sions from ruminants. J. Dairy Sci. 96:2476-2493.\n", "Ricci, P., J. A. Rooke, I. Nevison, and A. Waterhouse. 2013. Methane
emissions from beef\n",
            "   and dairy cattle: Quantifying the effect of physiological stage and diet characteristics.\n", "   J. Anim.
Sci. 91:5379-5389.\n", "Wilkerson, V. A., D. P. Casper, and D. R. Mertens. 1995. The prediction of methane\n",
            "   production of Holstein cows by several equations. J. Dairy Sci. 78:2402-2414.\n", "Yan, T., M. G. Porter, and
C. S. Mayne. 2009. Prediction of methane emission from beef\n", "   cattle using data measured in indirect open-circuit respi-
ration calorimeters. Animal.\n", "   3:1455-1462.\n",sep = ""))


  # End user-script
  #newpage(T)
}
```

Appendix 2. R Script for Calculating Nitrogen Balance

```
main<-function()
{
  # Assuming DMI of 22.4 kg/d, milk yield of 35.8 kg/d, milk protein of 3.03%, and diet CP of 17.5
  #out1<-JonkerKohnErdman1998(22.4,17.6,(35.8*(3.03/100)/6.25)*1000,0,T)
  #out2<-JonkerKohnErdman1998(0,17.6,(35.8*(3.03/100)/6.25)*1000,20.17,T)

  # Assuming
  #out3<-WilkersonMertensCasper1997(1,607,33,163,22.8,16.1,33.8,16.2,T) #Lactating cow
  #out4<-WilkersonMertensCasper1997(2,680,62,0,0,15.9,35.7,6.8,T) #Dry cow
  #out4<-WilkersonMertensCasper1997(3,298,0,0,0,18.2,53.9,5.4,T) #Replacement heifer


  # COmparison... Jonker versus Wilkerson, assuming DMI=22.4, MY=35.8, DIM=132,
  #               CP=17.5, NDF=33.8, BW=598, and DP=33, using Jonker's data
  #out1<-JonkerKohnErdman1998(22.4,17.5,(35.8*(3.03/100)/6.25)*1000,0,T)
  #out3<-WilkersonMertensCasper1997(1,598,33,132,35.8,17.5,33.8,22.4,T)

  isz<-function(a,b)
  {
    if (length(a)==length(b)) c<-b else c<-rep(b,length(a))
    value<-ifelse(c!=0,a/c,0)
    return(value)
  }

  Waldripetal2013<-function(type=1,anim.diet.DMI.rate,anim.diet.CP.conc,RN=0,FN=0,showreports=T)
  {
    #Waldrip, H. M., R. W. Todd, and N. A. Cole. 2013. Prediction of nitrogen excretion by beef cattle: A meta-analysis. J.
Anim. Sci. 91:4290-4302.
    # NI = N intake, g/d
    # FN = Fecal N, g/d
    # UN = Urinary N, g/d
    # NB = N balance, g/d
    # RN = Retained N, g/d

    # NB = RN = NI - FN - UN
    # AN = NI - FN
    NI<-((anim.diet.DMI.rate*anim.diet.CP.conc/100)/6.25)*1000
    if (FN==0 & RN==0)
    {
      FN<-24.28+0.154*NI
      UN<-0.56*NI-21.18
      RN<-NB<-NI-FN-UN
      footnote<-"Note: fecal N and urinay N computed from N intake."
    } else
    {
      if (FN==0 & RN!=0)
      {
        NB<-RN
        if (type==1)
```

```
          {
            UN<-(0.0017*NI+0.29)*(NI-NB)
            footnote<-"Note: urinary N computed from N intake and retained N,\n        using Waldrip et al. (2013)."
          } else
          {
            UN<-(0.2331*log(NI)-0.6244)*(NI-NB)
            footnote<-"Note: urinary N computed from N intake and retained N,\n        using Waldrip et al. (unpublished)."
          }
          FN<-NI-RN-UN
        } else
        {
          if (FN!=0 & RN==0)
          {
            UN<-0.56*NI-21.18
            NB<-RN<-NI-FN-UN
            footnote<-"Note: urinary N computed from N intake."
          } else
          {
            NB<-RN
            UN<-NI-NB-FN
            footnote<-"Note: urinary N computed from NI, RN, and FN."
          }
        }
      }
      AN<-NI-FN


      text<-paste("Nitrogen Balance (Waldrip et al., 2013)\n",
                  "========================================================\n\n",
                  "                                  g/d      % NI      % AN\n",
                  "--------------------------------------------------------\n",
                  "Nitrogen intake (NI)        : ",formatC(NI,format="f",digits=2,width=6),"\n",
                  "Absorbed nitrogen (AN)      : ",formatC(AN,format="f",digits=2,width=6),"   ",formatC(isz(AN*100,NI),format="f",digits=2,width=6),"\n",
                  "Retained N (RN, N Balance)  : ",formatC(RN,format="f",digits=2,width=6),"   ",formatC(isz(RN*100,NI),format="f",digits=2,width=6),"   ",formatC(isz(RN*100,AN),format="f",digits=2,width=6),"\n",
                  "Fecal nitrogen (FN)         : ",formatC(FN,format="f",digits=2,width=6),"   ",formatC(isz(FN*100,NI),format="f",digits=2,width=6),"\n",
                  "Urinary nitrogen (UN)       : ",formatC(UN,format="f",digits=2,width=6),"   ",formatC(isz(UN*100,NI),format="f",digits=2,width=6),"   ",formatC(isz(UN*100,AN),format="f",digits=2,width=6),"\n",
                  "--------------------------------------------------------\n",footnote,"\n\n",sep="")

      if (showreports==T) cat(text)
      return(c(UN,FN,NB,AN))
    }

    Dongetal2014<-function(anim.diet.DMI.rate,anim.diet.CP.conc,RN=0,FN=0,showreports=T)
    {
      # Dong, R. L., G. Y. Zhao, L. L. Chai, and K. A. Beauchemin. 2014. Prediction of urinary and fecal nitrogen excretion by beef cattle. J. Anim. Sci. 92 (10):4669-4681.
      # NI = N intake, g/d
```

```
      # FN = Fecal N, g/d
      # UN = Urinary N, g/d
      # NB = N balance, g/d
      # RN = Retained N, g/d

      # NB = RN = NI - FN - UN
      # AN = NI - FN
      NI<-((anim.diet.DMI.rate*anim.diet.CP.conc/100)/6.25)*1000
      if (FN==0 & RN==0)
      {
        FN<-16.23+0.19*NI
        UN<-0.55*NI-17.55
        RN<-NB<-NI-FN-UN
        footnote<-"Note: fecal N and urinay N computed from N intake."
      } else
      {
        if (FN==0 & RN!=0)
        {
          NB<-RN
          UN<-(0.001*NI+0.417)*(NI-NB)
          footnote<-"Note: urinary N computed from N intake and retained N."
          FN<-NI-RN-UN
        } else
        {
          if (FN!=0 & RN==0)
          {
            UN<-0.55*NI-17.55
            NB<-RN<-NI-FN-UN
            footnote<-"Note: urinary N computed from N intake."
          } else
          {
            NB<-RN
            UN<-NI-NB-FN
            footnote<-"Note: urinary N computed from NI, RN, and FN."
          }
        }
      }
      AN<-NI-FN


      text<-paste("Nitrogen Balance (Dong et al., 2014)\n",
                   "=====================================================\n\n",
                   "                                    g/d      % NI      % AN\n",
                   "-----------------------------------------------------\n",
                   "Nitrogen intake (NI)          : ",formatC(NI,format="f",digits=2,width=6),"\n",
                   "Absorbed nitrogen (AN)        : ",formatC(AN,format="f",digits=2,width=6),"   ",formatC(isz(AN*100,NI),for-
mat="f",digits=2,width=6),"\n",
                   "Retained N (RN, N Balance)    : ",formatC(RN,format="f",digits=2,width=6),"   ",formatC(isz(RN*100,NI),for-
mat="f",digits=2,width=6),"   ",formatC(isz(RN*100,AN),format="f",digits=2,width=6),"\n",
                   "Fecal nitrogen (FN)           : ",formatC(FN,format="f",digits=2,width=6),"   ",formatC(isz(FN*100,NI),for-
mat="f",digits=2,width=6),"\n",
```

```
                    "Urinary nitrogen (UN)        : ",formatC(UN,format="f",digits=2,width=6),"   ",formatC(isz(UN*100,NI),format="f",digits=2,width=6),"   ",formatC(isz(UN*100,AN),format="f",digits=2,width=6),"\n",
                    "-------------------------------------------------------\n",footnote,"\n\n",sep="")

      if (showreports==T) cat(text)
      return(c(UN,FN,NB,AN))
    }


  JonkerKohnErdman1998<-function(anim.diet.DMI.rate=0,anim.diet.CP.conc,
                                 anim.milk.N.rate,anim.milk.UN.conc=0,showreports=T)
    {
      # Based on Jonker et al. (1998; J. Dairy Sci. 81:2681-2692)
      if (anim.diet.DMI.rate>0)
      {
        # Assume DMI is known and estimate urinary N (UN), fecal (FN), milk urea N (MUN)
        anim.diet.N.rate<-((anim.diet.DMI.rate*anim.diet.CP.conc/100)/6.25)*1000
        anim.urine.N.rate<-anim.diet.N.rate*0.83-(anim.milk.N.rate+97)
        anim.milk.UN.conc<-anim.urine.N.rate/12.54
        fc.diet.N.rate<-anim.diet.N.rate-anim.urine.N.rate-anim.milk.N.rate
        footnote<-"Note: DMI was used to back calculate MUN."
      } else
      {
        # Assume MUN is known and estimate UN, FN, MN
        anim.urine.N.rate<-12.54*anim.milk.UN.conc
        anim.diet.N.rate<-(anim.urine.N.rate+anim.milk.N.rate+97)/0.83
        fc.diet.N.rate<-anim.diet.N.rate-anim.urine.N.rate-anim.milk.N.rate
        anim.diet.DMI.rate<-((anim.diet.N.rate*6.25)/(anim.diet.CP.conc/100))/1000
        footnote<-"Note: DMI was predicted from NI."
      }

      anim.absorbed.N.rate<-anim.diet.N.rate-fc.diet.N.rate

      text<-paste("Nitrogen Balance (Jonker et al., 1998)\n",
                  "=====================================================\n\n",
                  "                               g/d     % NI     % AN\n",
                  "-----------------------------------------------------\n",
                  "Nitrogen intake (NI)         : ",formatC(anim.diet.N.rate,format="f",digits=2,width=6),"\n",
                  "Absorbed nitrogen (AN)       : ",formatC(anim.absorbed.N.rate,format="f",digits=2,width=6),"
 ",formatC(isz(anim.absorbed.N.rate*100,anim.diet.N.rate),format="f",digits=2,width=6),"\n",
                  "Fecal nitrogen (FN)          : ",formatC(fc.diet.N.rate,format="f",digits=2,width=6),"
 ",formatC(isz(fc.diet.N.rate*100,anim.diet.N.rate),format="f",digits=2,width=6),"\n",
                  "Urinary nitrogen (UN)        : ",formatC(anim.urine.N.rate,format="f",digits=2,width=6),"
 ",formatC(isz(anim.urine.N.rate*100,anim.diet.N.rate),format="f",digits=2,width=6),"
 ",formatC(isz(anim.urine.N.rate*100,anim.absorbed.N.rate),format="f",digits=2,width=6),"\n",
                  "Milk nitrogen (MN)           : ",formatC(anim.milk.N.rate,format="f",digits=2,width=6),"
 ",formatC(isz(anim.milk.N.rate*100,anim.diet.N.rate),format="f",digits=2,width=6),"
 ",formatC(isz(anim.milk.N.rate*100,anim.absorbed.N.rate),format="f",digits=2,width=6),"\n",
                  "-----------------------------------------------------\n",
                  "Manure nitrogen (FN + UN)   : ",formatC(anim.urine.N.rate+fc.diet.N.rate,format="f",digits=2,width=6),"
 ",formatC(isz((anim.urine.N.rate+fc.diet.N.rate)*100,anim.diet.N.rate),format="f",digits=2,width=6),"\n\n",
```

```
                  "Milk urea nitrogen (MUN), mg/dl : ",formatC(anim.milk.UN.conc,format="f",digits=2,width=6),"\n",
                  "Dry matter intake (DMI), kg/d   : ",formatC(anim.diet.DMI.rate,format="f",digits=2,width=6),"\n",
                  "--------------------------------------------------\n",footnote,"\n\n",sep="")

    if (showreports==T) cat(text)
    return(c(anim.diet.DMI.rate,anim.diet.N.rate,anim.urine.N.rate,anim.milk.N.rate,anim.milk.UN.conc,fc.diet.N.rate))
  }

  WilkersonMertensCasper1997<-function(type=1,anim.SBW,anim.pregnancy.days,anim.lactation.days,
                                       anim.lactation.milk.rate,anim.diet.CP.conc,
                                       anim.diet.NDF.conc,anim.diet.DMI.rate,
                                       showreports=T)
  {
    # Based on Wilkerson et al. (1997; J. Dairy Sci. 80:3193-3204)

    MatrixFromList<-function(listX) t(sapply(listX, function(x, n) c(x, rep(NA, n))[1:n], n = max(sapply(listX, length))))

    # Coefficients from Table 6
    Coef<-MatrixFromList(
      list(
        c(-1.103,-1.283,-0.000922,0.0013,1.497,0.0862,0.00249,0.00215,-2.351,-0.549,-0.00442,0.00336),
        c(0,0,0,0,-0.0372,0.0028,-0.00007,-0.0000405,0.0825,0.00738,0.0000766,-0.000118),
        c(0.745,0.687,-0.000101,-0.000151,-0.124,-0.179,0.0000366,-0.00106,0.791,0.298,0.0019,-0.000779),
        c(-0.00282,-0.00504,0.000000234,-0.00000299,0,0,0,0,-0.00747,-0.00233,-0.0000193,0.0000105),
        c(-0.0743,-0.0571,-0.0000379,0.000154,-0.0179,-0.0155,-0.0000337,-0.0000553,0.174,0.0101,0.000136,-0.0000681),
        c(0,0,0,0,0.00586,0.00206,-0.0000581,0.00000397,0,0,0,0),
        c(-0.0165,-0.0378,0.000118,-0.000175,0,0,0,0,0,0,0,0),
        c(0.0000379,0.0000789,-0.000000173,0.000000379,0,0,0,0,0,0,0,0),
        c(0.0391,-0.0864,-0.00289,-0.0016,0,0,0,0,0,0,0,0),
        c(-0.00724,-0.000407,0.0000501,0.0000373,0,0,0,0,0,0,0,0),
        c(0.00406,0.0032,0.00000393,-0.0000113,0,0,0,0,-0.00784,-0.000979,0.000000488,-0.00000114),
        c(0,0,0,0,0.000384,0.000495,0.00000069,0.00000189,0,0,0,0),
        c(4.047,4.03,-0.00211,0.00181,2.603,2.476,-0.0012,0.00804,-4.995,-0.00195,-0.00943,0.00116),
        c(-0.0373,-0.0798,0.00131,0.000549,-0.0132,-0.0366,0.00145,0.0000249,0.327,0.107,0.00154,0.000672)
      )
    )

    vars<-c(anim.diet.CP.conc,anim.diet.CP.conc^2,anim.diet.NDF.conc,
            anim.diet.NDF.conc^2,anim.SBW,anim.pregnancy.days,anim.lactation.days,anim.lactation.days^2,
            anim.lactation.milk.rate,anim.lactation.milk.rate*anim.diet.NDF.conc,
            anim.SBW*anim.diet.CP.conc,anim.SBW*anim.diet.NDF.conc,
            anim.diet.DMI.rate,anim.diet.DMI.rate*anim.diet.CP.conc)

    # Four columns for total manure, total feces, Total manure N, total feces N)
    # for lactating cows, dry cows, and growing/replacement heifers
    results<-vars%*%Coef

    text1<-paste("Manure Production and Composition (Wilkerson et al., 1997)\n",
                 "============================================================\n\n",
                 "Daily                         Lactating cows      Dry cows          Heifers     \n",
                 "                              --------------    --------------    --------------\n",
```

```
                    "                      DM, kg    N, g    DM, kg    N, g    DM, kg    N, g\n",
                    "----------------------------------------------------------------------\n",
                    "Manure  (feces + urine)  : ",
                    formatC(results[1],format="f",digits=2,width=6),"  ",formatC(results[3]*1000,format="f",digits=2,width=6),"  ",
                    formatC(results[5],format="f",digits=2,width=6),"  ",formatC(results[7]*1000,format="f",digits=2,width=6),"  ",
                    formatC(results[9],format="f",digits=2,width=6),"  ",formatC(results[11]*1000,format="f",digits=2,width=6),"\n",

                    "Feces                    : ",
                    formatC(results[2],format="f",digits=2,width=6),"  ",formatC(results[4]*1000,format="f",digits=2,width=6),"  ",
                    formatC(results[6],format="f",digits=2,width=6),"  ", formatC(results[8]*1000,format="f",digits=2,width=6),"  ",
                    formatC(results[10],format="f",digits=2,width=6),"  ",formatC(results[12]*1000,format="f",digits=2,width=6),"\n",

                    "Urine  (by difference)   : ",
                    formatC(results[1]-results[2],format="f",digits=2,width=6),"  ",formatC((results[3]-results[4])*1000,format="f",digits=2,width=6),"    ",
                    formatC(results[5]-results[6],format="f",digits=2,width=6),"  ",formatC((results[7]-results[8])*1000,format="f",digits=2,width=6),"    ",
                    formatC(results[9]-results[10],format="f",digits=2,width=6),"  ",formatC((results[11]-results[12])*1000,format="f",digits=2,width=6),"\n",
                    "----------------------------------------------------------------------\n\n",sep="")

    text2<-paste("Daily per 1000 kg SBW  Lactating cows      Dry cows           Heifers   \n",
                    "                      ---------------    ---------------    --------------\n",
                    "                      DM, kg    N, g    DM, kg    N, g    DM, kg    N, g\n",
                    "----------------------------------------------------------------------\n",
                    "Manure  (feces + urine)  : ",
                    formatC(results[1]*(1000/anim.SBW),format="f",digits=2,width=6),"  ",formatC(results[3]*1000*(1000/anim.SBW),format="f",digits=2,width=6),"    ",
                    formatC(results[5]*(1000/anim.SBW),format="f",digits=2,width=6),"  ",formatC(results[7]*1000*(1000/anim.SBW),format="f",digits=2,width=6),"    ",
                    formatC(results[9]*(1000/anim.SBW),format="f",digits=2,width=6),"  ",formatC(results[11]*1000*(1000/anim.SBW),format="f",digits=2,width=6),"\n",

                    "Feces                    : ",
                    formatC(results[2]*(1000/anim.SBW),format="f",digits=2,width=6),"  ",formatC(results[4]*1000*(1000/anim.SBW),format="f",digits=2,width=6),"    ",
                    formatC(results[6]*(1000/anim.SBW),format="f",digits=2,width=6),"  ", formatC(results[8]*1000*(1000/anim.SBW),format="f",digits=2,width=6),"    ",
                    formatC(results[10]*(1000/anim.SBW),format="f",digits=2,width=6),"  ",formatC(results[12]*1000*(1000/anim.SBW),format="f",digits=2,width=6),"\n",

                    "Urine  (by difference)   : ",
                    formatC((results[1]-results[2])*(1000/anim.SBW),format="f",digits=2,width=6),"  ",formatC((results[3]-results[4])*1000*(1000/anim.SBW),format="f",digits=2,width=6),"    ",
```

```
                    formatC((results[5]-results[6])*(1000/anim.SBW),format="f",digits=2,width=6),"    ",formatC((results[7]-results[8])*1000*(1000/anim.SBW),format="f",digits=2,width=6),"    ",
                    formatC((results[9]-results[10])*(1000/anim.SBW),format="f",digits=2,width=6),"    ",formatC((results[11]-results[12])*1000*(1000/anim.SBW),format="f",digits=2,width=6),"\n",
                    "-----------------------------------------------------------\n\n",sep="")

    footnote<-"Manure is wet feces plus urine without bedding material."
    if (type==1)  #Lactating cows
    {
      text<-paste("Manure Production and Composition (Wilkerson et al., 1997)\n",
                    "=========================================================\n\n",
                    "Lactating cows              Daily              per 1000 kg BW\n",
                    "                            --------------     --------------\n",
                    "                            kg          N, g   kg          N, g\n",
                    "-----------------------------------------------------------\n",
                    "Dry matter intake       : ",
                    formatC(anim.diet.DMI.rate,format="f",digits=2,width=6),"    ",formatC((anim.diet.DMI.rate*(anim.diet.CP.conc/100)*1000)/6.25,format="f",digits=2,width=6),"    ",
                    formatC(anim.diet.DMI.rate*(1000/anim.SBW),format="f",digits=2,width=6),"    ",formatC((anim.diet.DMI.rate*(anim.diet.CP.conc/100)*1000)/6.25*(1000/anim.SBW),format="f",digits=2,width=7),"\n",
                    "Manure (feces + urine) : ",
                    formatC(results[1],format="f",digits=2,width=6),"    ",formatC(results[3]*1000,format="f",digits=2,width=6),"    ",
                    formatC(results[1]*(1000/anim.SBW),format="f",digits=2,width=6),"    ",formatC(results[3]*1000*(1000/anim.SBW),format="f",digits=2,width=6),"\n",
                    "Feces                  : ",
                    formatC(results[2],format="f",digits=2,width=6),"    ",formatC(results[4]*1000,format="f",digits=2,width=6),"    ",
                    formatC(results[2]*(1000/anim.SBW),format="f",digits=2,width=6),"    ",formatC(results[4]*1000*(1000/anim.SBW),format="f",digits=2,width=6),"\n",
                    "Urine (by difference)  : ",
                    formatC(results[1]-results[2],format="f",digits=2,width=6),"    ",formatC((results[3]-results[4])*1000,format="f",digits=2,width=6),"    ",
                    formatC((results[1]-results[2])*(1000/anim.SBW),format="f",digits=2,width=6),"    ",formatC((results[3]-results[4])*1000*(1000/anim.SBW),format="f",digits=2,width=6),"\n",
                    "-----------------------------------------------------------\n",footnote,"\n\n",sep="")
    }

    if (type==2)  # Dry cows
    {
      text<-paste("Manure Production and Composition (Wilkerson et al., 1997)\n",
                    "=========================================================\n\n",
                    "Dry cows                    Daily              per 1000 kg BW\n",
                    "                            --------------     --------------\n",
                    "                            kg          N, g   kg          N, g\n",
                    "-----------------------------------------------------------\n",
                    "Dry matter intake       : ",
                    formatC(anim.diet.DMI.rate,format="f",digits=2,width=6),"    ",formatC((anim.diet.DMI.rate*(anim.diet.CP.conc/100)*1000)/6.25,format="f",digits=2,width=6),"    ",
                    formatC(anim.diet.DMI.rate*(1000/anim.SBW),format="f",digits=2,width=6),"    ",formatC((anim.diet.DMI.rate*(anim.diet.CP.conc/100)*1000)/6.25*(1000/anim.SBW),format="f",digits=2,width=7),"\n",
```

```
                      "Manure  (feces + urine)  : ",
                      formatC(results[5],format="f",digits=2,width=6),"   ",formatC(results[7]*1000,format="f",digits=2,width=6),"
",
                      formatC(results[5]*(1000/anim.SBW),format="f",digits=2,width=6),"   ",formatC(re-
sults[7]*1000*(1000/anim.SBW),format="f",digits=2,width=6),"\n",
                      "Feces                    : ",
                      formatC(results[6],format="f",digits=2,width=6),"   ", formatC(results[8]*1000,format="f",digits=2,width=6),"
",
                      formatC(results[6]*(1000/anim.SBW),format="f",digits=2,width=6),"   ", formatC(re-
sults[8]*1000*(1000/anim.SBW),format="f",digits=2,width=6),"\n",
                      "Urine  (by difference)   : ",
                      formatC(results[5]-results[6],format="f",digits=2,width=6),"   ",formatC((results[7]-results[8])*1000,for-
mat="f",digits=2,width=6),"      ",
                      formatC((results[5]-results[6])*(1000/anim.SBW),format="f",digits=2,width=6),"   ",formatC((results[7]-re-
sults[8])*1000*(1000/anim.SBW),format="f",digits=2,width=6),"\n",
                      "-------------------------------------------------------------\n",footnote,"\n\n",sep="")
     }

     if (type==3)  # Growing and replacement heifers
     {
       text<-paste("Manure Production and Composition (Wilkerson et al., 1997)\n",
                      "=============================================================\n\n",
                      "Replacement heifers      Daily              per 1000 kg BW\n",
                      "                         --------------     --------------\n",
                      "                         kg         N, g    kg         N, g\n",
                      "-------------------------------------------------------------\n",
                      "Dry matter intake        : ",
                      formatC(anim.diet.DMI.rate,format="f",digits=2,width=6),"
",formatC((anim.diet.DMI.rate*(anim.diet.CP.conc/100)*1000)/6.25,format="f",digits=2,width=6),"      ",
                      formatC(anim.diet.DMI.rate*(1000/anim.SBW),format="f",digits=2,width=6),"
",formatC((anim.diet.DMI.rate*(anim.diet.CP.conc/100)*1000)/6.25*(1000/anim.SBW),format="f",digits=2,width=7),"\n",
                      "Manure  (feces + urine)  : ",
                      formatC(results[9],format="f",digits=2,width=6),"   ",formatC(results[11]*1000,format="f",digits=2,width=6),"
",
                      formatC(results[9]*(1000/anim.SBW),format="f",digits=2,width=6),"   ",formatC(re-
sults[11]*1000*(1000/anim.SBW),format="f",digits=2,width=6),"\n",
                      "Feces                    : ",
                      formatC(results[10],format="f",digits=2,width=6),"   ",formatC(results[12]*1000,format="f",dig-
its=2,width=6),"      ",
                      formatC(results[10]*(1000/anim.SBW),format="f",digits=2,width=6),"   ",formatC(re-
sults[12]*1000*(1000/anim.SBW),format="f",digits=2,width=6),"\n",
                      "Urine  (by difference)   : ",
                      formatC(results[9]-results[10],format="f",digits=2,width=6),"   ",formatC((results[11]-results[12])*1000,for-
mat="f",digits=2,width=6),"      ",
                      formatC((results[9]-results[10])*(1000/anim.SBW),format="f",digits=2,width=6),"   ",formatC((results[11]-
results[12])*1000*(1000/anim.SBW),format="f",digits=2,width=6),"\n",
                      "-------------------------------------------------------------\n",footnote,"\n\n",sep="")
     }


     if (showreports==T) cat(text)
```

```
      return(results)
    }

    newpage(T)
    header<-paste("Nitrogen Balance for Cattle using Empirical Equations (EXPERIMENTAL)",sep="")
    headersize<-nchar(header)
    cat(paste(header,"\n",string("=",headersize),sep=""),"\n\n")
    anim.milk.N.rate<-((anim.lactation.milk.rate*anim.lactation.milk.protein.conc/100)/6.25)*1000
    anim.diet.NDF.conc<-anim.diet.NDF.rate*100/anim.diet.DMI.rate
    if (exists("anim.diet.CP.conc")==FALSE) anim.diet.CP.conc<-isz(anim.diet.CP.rate*100,anim.diet.DMI.rate)

    if (anim.species=="Cattle")
    {
      if (anim.type=="Milk")
      {
        if (anim.stage_type=="Lactating")
        {
          out1<-JonkerKohnErdman1998(anim.diet.DMI.rate,anim.diet.CP.conc,anim.milk.N.rate,0,T)
          cat("\n\n")
          out2<-WilkersonMertensCasper1997(1,anim.SBW,anim.pregnancy.days,anim.lactation.days,anim.lactation.milk.rate,
                                          anim.diet.CP.conc,anim.diet.NDF.conc,anim.diet.DMI.rate,T) #Lactating cow
        }
        if (anim.stage_type=="Dry")
        {
          out1<-WilkersonMertensCasper1997(2,anim.SBW,anim.pregnancy.days,0,0,anim.diet.CP.conc,
                                          anim.diet.NDF.conc,anim.diet.DMI.rate,T) #Dry cow
        }
        if (anim.stage_type=="Replacement")
        {
          out1<-WilkersonMertensCasper1997(3,anim.SBW,anim.pregnancy.days,0,0,anim.diet.CP.conc,
                                          anim.diet.NDF.conc,anim.diet.DMI.rate,T) #Replacement heifer
        }
      } else
      {
        FN<-0
        RN<-0
        out1<-Waldripetal2013(1,anim.diet.DMI.rate,anim.diet.CP.conc,FN=0,RN=0,showreports=T)
        cat("\n\n")
        if (FN==0 & RN!=0)
        {
          out2<-Waldripetal2013(2,anim.diet.DMI.rate,anim.diet.CP.conc,FN=0,RN=0,showreports=T)
          cat("\n\n")
        }
        out3<-Dongetal2014(anim.diet.DMI.rate,anim.diet.CP.conc,FN=0,RN=0,showreports=T)
      }
    } else
    {
      cat ("N balance not implemented for small ruminants.")
    }

    #References:
```

```
    #newpage(T)
    cat(paste("REFERENCES:\n\n",sep=""))
    cat(paste("Dong, R. L., G. Y. Zhao, L. L. Chai, and K. A. Beauchemin. 2014. Prediction of urinary and\n",
              "    fecal nitrogen excretion by beef cattle. J. Anim. Sci. 92 (10):4669-4681.\n",
              "Jonker, J. S., R. A. Kohn, and R. A. Erdman. 1998. Using milk urea nitrogen to predict nitrogen\n",
              "    excretion and utilization efficiency in lactating dairy cows. J. Dairy Sci. 81:2681-2692.\n",
              "Wilkerson, V. A., D. R. Mertens, and D. P. Casper. 1997. Prediction of excretion of manure and\n",
              "    nitrogen by Holstein dairy cattle. J. Dairy Sci. 80:3193-3204.\n",
              "Waldrip, H. M., R. W. Todd, and N. A. Cole. 2013. Prediction of nitrogen excretion by beef\n",
              "    cattle: A meta-analysis. J. Anim. Sci. 91 (9):4290-4302.\n",
              sep=""))
  }
```

Appendix 3. R Script for Calculating Relative Feed Value Indices

```r
main<-function()
{
  #isz<-function(a,b)
  #{
  #  if (length(a)==length(b)) c<-b else c<-rep(b,length(a))
  #  value<-ifelse(c!=0,a/c,0)
  #  return(value)
  #}

  newpage(T)
  #cat(paste("Relative Feed Value Indices\n",string("=",27),"\n\n",sep=""))

  # Moore, J. E. 1994. Forage quality indices: Development and application. Pages 967-998 in Forage Quality,
  #     Evaluation, and Utilization. G. C. Fahey Jr., M. Collins, D. R. Mertens and L. E. Moser, eds. American
  #     Society of Agronomy, Madison, WI.

  # Nutritive Value Indices-1960 (RVI))
  # ++++++++++++++++++++++++++++++++++
  if (anim.species=="Cattle") NVI.SDMI<-140 else NVI.SDMI<-80
  # Feed level
  ifelse(anim.SBW>0,anim.fd.DMI.rate*1000/(anim.SBW^0.75))
  fd.NVI.RI<-isz(anim.fd.DMI.rate*1000,(anim.SBW^0.75))*100/NVI.SDMI
  if (exists("anim.fd.DEm.rate")==TRUE) fd.NVI<-fd.NVI.RI*isz(anim.fd.GE.rate,anim.fd.DEm.rate) else fd.NVI<-
fd.NVI.RI*isz(anim.fd.GE.rate,anim.fd.DE.rate)
  # Diet level
  diet.NVI.RI<-isz(anim.diet.DMI.rate*1000,(anim.SBW^0.75))*100/NVI.SDMI
  if (exists("anim.diet.DEm.rate")==TRUE) diet.NVI<-diet.NVI.RI*isz(anim.diet.GE.rate,anim.diet.DEm.rate) else diet.NVI<-
diet.NVI.RI*isz(anim.diet.GE.rate,anim.diet.DE.rate)

  # Fill Unit (FiU) and Feed Unit (FdU)-1978
  # ++++++++++++++++++++++++++++++++++++++++++
  if (anim.species=="Cattle")
  {
    if (anim.type=="Milk" & anim.stage_type=="Lactating") FiU.STD<-140  else FiU.STD<-95 #g/kg metabolic BW
  } else FiU.STD<-75 #g/kg metabolic BW
  if (anim.stage_type=="Lactating") FdU.STD<-1700 else FdU.STD<-1820
  # Feed level
  fd.FiU<-isz(FiU.STD,isz(anim.fd.DMI.rate*1000,(anim.SBW^0.75)))
  if (anim.stage_type=="Lactating")
  {
    fd.FdU<-anim.fd.NEl.frac*1000/FdU.STD
  } else
  {
    fd.FdU<-anim.fd.NEg.frac*1000/FdU.STD
  }
  # Diet level
  diet.FiU<-isz(FiU.STD,isz(anim.diet.DMI.rate*1000,(anim.SBW^0.75)))
  if (anim.stage_type=="Lactating")
  {
```

```
    diet.FdU<-anim.diet.NEl.frac*1000/FdU.STD
  } else
  {
    diet.FdU<-anim.diet.NEg.frac*1000/FdU.STD
  }


  # Moore, J. E., and D. J. Undersander. 2002. Relative forage quality: An alternative to relative
  #     feed value and quality index. Pages 16-29 in Proceedings of the 13th Annual Florida Ruminant
  #     Nutrition Symposium, Gainesville, FL. University of Florida. Available at:
http://dairy.ifas.ufl.edu/rns/2002/moore.pdf.

  # Relative Feed Value-1976 (RFV)
  # +++++++++++++++++++++++++++++++
  # RFV compute base digestible DM intake as 40 or 69 g/kg metabolic BW for sheep or cattle, respectively
  # RFV compute base digestible DM intake as 1.29% of BW
  # RFV.DMI has to be computed either as g/metabolic BW or % of BW
  # Feed level: % BW
  fd.RFV.DMI<-isz(120,anim.fd.NDF.conc)
  fd.RFV.DDM<-88.9-0.779*anim.fd.ADF.conc
  fd.RFV1<-fd.RFV.DMI*fd.RFV.DDM/1.29 # Uses 120% of NDF
  fd.RFV2<-isz(anim.fd.DMI.rate*100,anim.SBW)*fd.RFV.DDM/1.29 # Uses user-inputted DMI as % of BW
  # Feed level - g/kg metabolic BW
  if (anim.species=="Cattle") RFV.DDMI<-69 else RFV.DDMI<-40
  fd.RFV3<-isz(anim.fd.DMI.rate*1000,(anim.SBW^0.75))*fd.RFV.DDM/RFV.DDMI # Uses user-inputted DMI as % of BW
  # Diet level: % BW
  diet.RFV.DMI<-isz(120,isz(anim.diet.NDF.rate*100,anim.diet.DMI.rate))
  diet.RFV.DDM<-88.9-0.779*isz(anim.diet.ADF.rate*100,anim.diet.DMI.rate)
  diet.RFV1<-diet.RFV.DMI*diet.RFV.DDM/1.29 # Uses 120% of NDF
  diet.RFV2<-isz(anim.diet.DMI.rate*100,anim.SBW)*diet.RFV.DDM/1.29 # Uses user-inputted DMI as % of BW
  # Diet level - g/kg metabolic BW
  if (anim.species=="Cattle") RFV.DDMI<-69 else RFV.DDMI<-40
  diet.RFV3<-isz(anim.diet.DMI.rate*1000,(anim.SBW^0.75))*diet.RFV.DDM/RFV.DDMI # Uses user-inputted DMI as % of BW

  # Quality Index-1984 (QI)
  # +++++++++++++++++++++++
  if (anim.species=="Cattle") QI.TDNm<-36 else QI.TDNm<-29
  # Feed level
  fd.QI<-isz(anim.fd.aTDN.rate,(anim.SBW^0.75))*1000/QI.TDNm
  # Diet level
  diet.QI<-isz(anim.diet.aTDN.rate,(anim.SBW^0.75))*1000/QI.TDNm

  # Relative Forage Quality (RFQ)
  # ++++++++++++++++++++++++++++++
  # Feed level
  fd.RFQ.DMI<-120/(anim.fd.NDF.conc)
  fd.RFQ1<-fd.RFQ.DMI*anim.fd.aTDN.conc/1.23
  fd.RFQ2<-(anim.diet.DMI.rate*100/anim.SBW)*anim.fd.aTDN.conc/1.23
  # Diet level
  diet.RFQ.DMI<-120/(anim.diet.NDF.rate*100/anim.diet.DMI.rate)
  diet.RFQ1<-diet.RFQ.DMI*anim.diet.aTDN.conc/1.23
```

```
    diet.RFQ2<-(anim.diet.DMI.rate*100/anim.SBW)*anim.diet.aTDN.conc/1.23

    # Report
    # ++++++
    fds<-feeds3
    RVQI<-fds["FeedName.x"]
    names(RVQI)<-"FeedName"
    RVQI["NVI"]<-fd.NVI
    RVQI["RFV1"]<-fd.RFV1
    RVQI["RFV2"]<-fd.RFV2
    RVQI["RFV3"]<-fd.RFV3
    RVQI["FiU"]<-fd.FiU
    RVQI["FdU"]<-fd.FdU
    RVQI["QI"]<-fd.QI
    RVQI["RFQ1"]<-fd.RFQ1
    RVQI["RFQ2"]<-fd.RFQ2

    RVQI_Diet<-data.frame("FeedName"="Ration")
    RVQI_Diet["NVI"]<-diet.NVI
    RVQI_Diet["RFV1"]<-diet.RFV1
    RVQI_Diet["RFV2"]<-diet.RFV2
    RVQI_Diet["RFV3"]<-diet.RFV3
    RVQI_Diet["FiU"]<-diet.FiU
    RVQI_Diet["FdU"]<-diet.FdU
    RVQI_Diet["QI"]<-diet.QI
    RVQI_Diet["RFQ1"]<-diet.RFQ1
    RVQI_Diet["RFQ2"]<-diet.RFQ2

    RVQI<-rbind(RVQI,RVQI_Diet)
    description<-paste("NIV = Nutritive Value Index (Crampton et al., 1960)\n",
                       "   . NVI > 70: better nutritive 'forage' value than early-cut, dehydrated legume hay\n",
                       "RFV = Relative Forage Value (Rohweder et al., 1978)\n",
                       "   . RFV > 100: better quality than full bloom alfalfa\n",
                       "   . RFV1 uses predicted DMI from NDF as % of BW\n",
                       "   . RFV2 uses user-inputted DMI as % of BW\n",
                       "   . RFV3 uses user-inputted DMI as g/kg of metabolic BW\n",
                       "FiU = Fill Unit (INRA, 1989)\n",
                       "   . Average pasture grass cut at the grazing stage of the first growth which,\n",
                       "     by definition, contains 1 Fill Unit per kg of DM\n",
                       "   . FiU > 1: animals consuming less than expected\n",
                       "   . FiU < 1: animals consuming more than expected\n",
                       "FdU = Feed Unit (INRA, 1989)\n",
                       "   . The Feed Unit is the ratio of the NE concentration of a feed to the NE\n",
                       "     concentration of standard barley grain for a particular type of production:\n",
                       "     1,700 or 1,820 kcal/kg for lactating or growing animals, respectively\n",
                       "   . FdU > 1: feed or diet has more net energy value than barley grain\n",
                       "   . FdU < 1: feed or diet has less net energy value than barley grain\n",
                       "QI = Quality Index (Moore et al., 1984)\n",
                       "   . QI < 1: weight loss, QI = 1: same weight, QI > 1: weight gain)\n",
                       "RFQ = Relative Forage Quality (Moore and Undersander, 2002)\n",
                       "   . RFQ1 uses predicted DMI from NDF\n",
```

```
                    "    . RFQ2 uses observed DMI\n",
                    "\n",sep="")
    footnote<-paste("NVI Standard Dry Matter Intake: ",formatC(NVI.SDMI,format="f",digits=2)," g/kg metabolic BW\n",
                    "RFV Base Digestible DM Intake : ",formatC(RFV.DDMI,format="f",digits=2)," g/kg metabolic BW\n",
                    "QI Maintenance TDN requirement: ",formatC(QI.TDNm,format="f",digits=2)," g/kg metabolic BW\n",
                    "FiU Standard Fill Unit        : ",formatC(FiU.STD,format="f",digits=2)," g/kg metabolic BW\n",
                    "FdU Standard Feed Unit        : ",formatC(FdU.STD,format="f",digits=2)," kcal/kg DM",sep="")
    report(RVQI,"Relative Feed Value Indices",description,footnote,3,2,1,9,FALSE,FALSE,FALSE,FALSE,TRUE,FALSE,FALSE)


    #References:
    #newpage(T)
    cat("\n")
    cat(paste("REFERENCES:\n\n",sep=""))
    cat(paste("Crampton, E. W., E. Donefer, and L. E. Lloyd. 1960. A nutritive value index for forages.\n",
              "   J. Anim. Sci. 19:538-544.\n",
              "Rohweder, D. A., R. F. Barnes, and N. Jorgensen. 1978. Proposed hay grading standards\n",
              "   based on laboratory analyses for evaluating quality. J. Anim. Sci. 47:747-759.\n",
              "Institut National de la Recherche Agronomique. 1989. Ruminant nutrition. Recommended\n",
              "   allowances and feed tables. Institut National de la Recherche Agronomique, John Libbey\n",
              "   Eurotext, Montrouge, France.\n",
              "Moore, J. E. 1994. Forage quality indices: Development and application.\n",
              "   Pages 967-998 in Forage Quality, Evaluation, and Utilization. G. C. Fahey\n",
              "   Jr., M. Collins, D. R. Mertens and L. E. Moser, eds. American Society of\n",
              "   Agronomy, Madison, WI.\n",
              "Moore, J. E., and D. J. Undersander. 2002. Relative forage quality: An alternative\n",
              "   to relative feed value and quality index. Pages 16-29 in Proceedings of the 13th\n",
              "   Annual Florida Ruminant Nutrition Symposium, Gainesville, FL. University of Florida.\n",
              "   Available at: http://dairy.ifas.ufl.edu/rns/2002/moore.pdf.\n",
              sep=""))


    # End user-script
    #newpage(T)
}
```

Appendix 4. R Script for Calculating Empirical Dry Matter Intake of Goats

```
main <- function()
{
  if (anim.species != "Goats") return(invisible(FALSE))

  newpage(T)

  header <- paste("Prediction of Dry Matter Intake of Goats using Empirical Equations", sep = "")
  headersize <- nchar(header)
  cat(paste("#Title#", header, "\n", string("=", headersize), sep = ""), "\n\n")

  if (exists("anim.FBW"))
    BW <- anim.FBW  # kg
  if (exists("anim.MSBW"))
    MW <- anim.MSBW  # kg
  if (exists("anim.age"))
    age <- anim.age * 30.4/7  # weeks
  if (exists("anim.diet.DE.frac"))
    DE <- anim.diet.DE.frac
  if (exists("anim.diet.ME.frac"))
    ME <- anim.diet.ME.frac
  if (exists("anim.diet.GE.frac"))
    GE <- anim.diet.GE.frac
  if (exists("anim.diet.ADF.rate"))
    ADF <- isz(anim.diet.ADF.rate, anim.diet.DMI.rate)  # g/g
  if (exists("anim.diet.CP.rate"))
    CP <- isz(anim.diet.CP.rate, anim.diet.DMI.rate)  # g/g
  if (exists("anim.diet.aDMD.conc"))
    DMD <- anim.diet.aDMD.conc/100  # g/g
  if (exists("anim.lactation.milk.rate"))
    MY <- anim.lactation.milk.rate  # kg/d
  if (exists("anim.diet.Forage.frac"))
    FOR <- anim.diet.Forage.frac  #g/g
  qm <- isz(ME, GE)
  if (anim.stage_type == "Lactating")
  {
    if (exists("anim.EB.SWG.rate"))
      ADG <- ifelse(anim.EB.SWG.rate < 0, 0, anim.EB.SWG.rate)
    if (exists("anim.lactation.FCM.rate"))
      FCM <- anim.lactation.FCM.rate
  } else
  {
    if (exists("anim.SWG"))
      ADG <- anim.SWG * 1000  # g/d
  }

  # Lu, C. D., and M. J. Potchoiba. 1990. Feed intake and weight gain of growing goats fed diets of various energy and protein
levels. J. Anim. Sci. 68 (6):1751-1759.
  DMI_LuPotchoiba1990.vect <- rep(NA, 5)
  if (age >= 17 & age <= 20)
```

```
    DMI_LuPotchoiba1990.vect[1] <- 1042.2 - 297.3 * DE + 25.4 * BW + 1.7 * ADG  # g/d, goats from 17 to 20 weeks
  if (age >= 21 & age <= 26)
    DMI_LuPotchoiba1990.vect[2] <- 1611 - 466.9 * DE + 28.3 * BW + 1.2 * ADG  # g/d, goats from 21 to 26 weeks
  if (age >= 25 & age <= 28)
    DMI_LuPotchoiba1990.vect[3] <- 1966.7 - 590.7 * DE + 29.1 * BW + 1.4 * ADG  # g/d, goats from 25 to 28 weeks
  if (age >= 29 & age <= 32)
    DMI_LuPotchoiba1990.vect[4] <- -901.6 + 5482.5 * ADF + 23.4 * BW + 1.1 * ADG  # g/d, goats from 29 to 32 weeks
  if (age >= 17 & age <= 32)
    DMI_LuPotchoiba1990.vect[5] <- 1748.7 - 495.7 * DE + 18.4 * BW + 3 * ADG  # g/d, goats from 17 to 32 weeks
  DMI_LuPotchoiba1990_min <- ifelse(all(is.na(DMI_LuPotchoiba1990.vect))==TRUE,"NA",min(DMI_LuPotchoiba1990.vect, na.rm = T))
  DMI_LuPotchoiba1990_avg <- ifelse(all(is.na(DMI_LuPotchoiba1990.vect))==TRUE,"NA",mean(DMI_LuPotchoiba1990.vect, na.rm = T))
  DMI_LuPotchoiba1990_max <- ifelse(all(is.na(DMI_LuPotchoiba1990.vect))==TRUE,"NA",max(DMI_LuPotchoiba1990.vect, na.rm = T))

  # Luo, J., A. L. Goetsch, I. V. Nsahlai, J. E. Moore, M. L. Galyean, Z. B. Johnson, T. Sahlu, C. L. Ferrell, and F. N. Owens. 2004. Voluntary feed intake by lactating, Angora, growing and mature goats. Small Ruminant Res. 53 (3):357-378.
  DMI_Luoetal.vect <- rep(NA, 5)
  if (anim.stage_type == "Growing/Finishing" | anim.stage_type == "Replacement")
  {
    DMI_Luoetal.vect[1] <- 0.4585 + 0.0229 * BW + 1.9349 * ADG - 0.0417 * (ME * 4.184)
    DMI_Luoetal.vect[2] <- 0.4605 + 0.0203 * BW + 1.9815 * ADG - 0.0387 * (ME * 4.184)
    DMI_Luoetal.vect[3] <- 0.5029 + 0.0168 * BW + 2.8545 * ADG - 20.5651 * ADG/BW - 0.035 * (ME * 4.184)
    DMI_Luoetal.vect[4] <- 0.4413 + 0.0214 * BW + 2.078 * ADG - 0.0394 * (ME * 4.184)
  } else
  {
    if (anim.stage_type == "Lactating")
    {
      DMI_Luoetal.vect[1] <- (1.1853 + 0.0117 * BW + 0.4343 * FCM - 0.072 * (ME * 4.184) + 1.3565 * (ADG/1000)) * 1000  # g/d
      DMI_Luoetal.vect[2] <- (2.0801 + 0.0115 * BW + 0.4621 * FCM - 0.159 * (ME * 4.184) + 1.5823 * (ADG/1000)) * 1000  # g/d
      DMI_Luoetal.vect[3] <- (2.0423 + 0.0119 * BW + 0.4641 * FCM - 0.1583 * (ME * 4.184) + 1.6866 * (ADG/1000)) * 1000  # g/d
      DMI_Luoetal.vect[4] <- (2.3971 + 0.0092 * BW + 0.4912 * FCM - 0.1819 * (ME * 4.184) + 1.4896 * (ADG/1000)) * 1000  # g/d
      DMI_Luoetal.vect[5] <- (1.7317 + 0.0095 * BW + 0.4445 * FCM - 0.1142 * (ME * 4.184) + 1.3075 * (ADG/1000)) * 1000  # g/d
    } else
    {
      DMI_Luoetal.vect[1] <- (0.3544 + 0.0217 * BW + 2.0562 * (ADG/1000) - 0.0324 * (ME * 4.184)) * 1000  # g/d
      DMI_Luoetal.vect[2] <- (0.3494 + 0.0165 * BW + 4.826 * (ADG/1000) - 101.8 * (ADG/1000)/BW - 0.0387 * (ME * 4.184) + 0.0194 * (CP * 100)) * 1000  # g/d
    }
  }
  DMI_Luoetal_min <- ifelse(all(is.na(DMI_Luoetal.vect))==TRUE,"NA",min(DMI_Luoetal.vect, na.rm = T))
  DMI_Luoetal_avg <- ifelse(all(is.na(DMI_Luoetal.vect))==TRUE,"NA",mean(DMI_Luoetal.vect, na.rm = T))
  DMI_Luoetal_max <- ifelse(all(is.na(DMI_Luoetal.vect))==TRUE,"NA",max(DMI_Luoetal.vect, na.rm = T))

  # AFRC
  if (anim.stage_type == "Growing/Finishing")
  {
    # Agricultural and Food Research Council. 1998. The Nutrition of Goats. CABI Publishing, Wallingford, UK.
    DMI_AFRC <- (76.7 * BW^0.75) * (-0.666 + 1.333 * ME - 0.266 * ME^2)  # g/d for growing/finishin goats
  } else
  {
    # Agricultural and Food Research Council. 1993. Energy and Protein Requirements of Ruminants. Agricultural and Food Research Council. CABI Publishing, Wallingford, UK.
```

```
    DMI_AFRC <- (130.9 * qm + 0.384 * BW - 18.75) * BW^0.75  # g/d for dry mature goats
  }

  # Institut National de la Recherche Agronomique. 2007. Alimentation des bovins, ovins et caprins. Besoins des animaux. Valeurs des aliments. Editions Quae, Versailles, France.
  DMI_INRA <- (-0.308 + 0.0435 * BW + 0.0037 * ADG) * 1000

  # National Research Council. 2007. Nutrient Requirements of Small Ruminants: Sheep, Goats, Cervids, and New World Camelids. (6th ed.). Nutrient requirements of small ruminants. National Academy Press, Washington, DC.
  DMI_NRC.vect <- rep(NA, 2)
  DMI_NRC.DMD_factor <- (1 - 1.7 * (0.8 - DMD))
  if (anim.stage_type == "Lactating")
  {
    # RNS does not have DIM for sheep/goats; thus, days in this stage will be used as a proxy for DIM
    # DIM <- seq(0,100,1)
    # plot(DIM,1 + 0.025 * DIM ^ (1.4 * exp(-0.05 * DIM)))
    T <- anim.stage.days
    DMI_NRC.MY_factor_single <- 1 + 0.025 * 1 * T^(1.4 * exp(-0.05 * T))  # Single kid
    DMI_NRC.MY_factor_twin <- 1 + 0.025 * 1.35 * T^(1.4 * exp(-0.05 * T))  # Twin kids
    DMI_NRC.vect[1] <- 1000 * (0.04 * MW * (BW/MW)) * (1.7 - BW/MW) * DMI_NRC.DMD_factor * DMI_NRC.MY_factor_single
    DMI_NRC.vect[2] <- 1000 * (0.04 * MW * (BW/MW)) * (1.7 - BW/MW) * DMI_NRC.DMD_factor * DMI_NRC.MY_factor_twin
  } else DMI_NRC.vect[1] <- 1000 * (0.04 * MW * (BW/MW)) * (1.7 - BW/MW) * DMI_NRC.DMD_factor
  DMI_NRC_min <- ifelse(all(is.na(DMI_NRC.vect)) == TRUE, "NA", min(DMI_NRC.vect, na.rm = T))
  DMI_NRC_avg <- ifelse(all(is.na(DMI_NRC.vect)) == TRUE, "NA", mean(DMI_NRC.vect, na.rm = T))
  DMI_NRC_max <- ifelse(all(is.na(DMI_NRC.vect)) == TRUE, "NA", max(DMI_NRC.vect, na.rm = T))

  # Pulina, G., T. Bettati, F. A. Serra, and A. Cannas. 1996. Razio-O: Costruzione e validazione di un software per l'alimentazione degli ovini da latte. Pages 11-14 in Atti Congresso Nazionale della Società Italiana di Patologia e di Allevamento degli Ovini e dei Caprini, 12. Varese, Italy.
  if (anim.stage_type == "Lactating")
  {
    DMI_Pulina1996 <- 1000 * (0.42 * MY + 0.024 * BW^0.75 + 0.4 * ADG + 0.7 * FOR)
  } else
  {
    if (anim.stage_type == "Dry")
    {
      DMI_Pulina1996 <<- (130.9 * qm + 0.384 * BW - 18.75) * BW^0.75
    } else
    {
      if (anim.sex == "Male" | (anim.sex == "Castrated male" & anim.age > 12))
      {
        DMI_Pulina1996 <<- 1000 * (0.522 + 0.0135 * BW)
      } else
      {
        DMI_Pulina1996 <<- (104.7 * qm + 0.307 * BW - 15) * BW^0.75
      }
    }
  }

  cat(paste("Source                          Min, g/d    Max, g/d    Avg, g/d\n", string("=", 63), "\n", sep = ""))
```

```
  cat(paste("Lu and Potchoiba (1990)                ", formatC(DMI_LuPotchoiba1990_min, format = "f", width = 8, digits = 2), "    ", formatC(DMI_LuPotchoiba1990_max, format = "f", width = 8, digits = 2), "    ", formatC(DMI_LuPotchoiba1990_avg, format = "f", width = 8, digits = 2), "\n", sep = ""))
  cat(paste("Luo et al. (2004)                      ", formatC(DMI_Luoetal_min, format = "f", width = 8, digits = 2), "    ", formatC(DMI_Luoetal_max, format = "f", width = 8, digits = 2), "    ", formatC(DMI_Luoetal_avg, format = "f", width = 8, digits = 2), "\n", sep = ""))
  cat(paste("NRC (2007)                             ", formatC(DMI_NRC_min, format = "f", width = 8, digits = 2), "    ", formatC(DMI_NRC_max, format = "f", width = 8, digits = 2), "    ", formatC(DMI_NRC_avg, format = "f", width = 8, digits = 2), "\n", sep = ""))
  if (anim.stage_type == "Lactating")
  {
    cat(paste("AFRC (1993)                            ", string(" ", 11 * 2), formatC(DMI_AFRC, format = "f", width = 8, digits = 2), "\n", sep = ""))
  } else
  {
    cat(paste("AFRC (1998)                            ", string(" ", 11 * 2), formatC(DMI_AFRC, format = "f", width = 8, digits = 2), "\n", sep = ""))
  }
  cat(paste("Pulina et al. (1996)                   ", string(" ", 11 * 2), formatC(DMI_Pulina1996, format = "f", width = 8, digits = 2), "\n", sep = ""))
  cat(paste("INRA (2007)                            ", string(" ", 11 * 2), formatC(DMI_INRA, format = "f", width = 8, digits = 2), "\n", sep = ""))
  cat(paste(string("=", 63), "\n\n\n", sep = ""))

  cat(paste("REFERENCES:\n\n", sep = ""))
  cat(paste("Agricultural and Food Research Council. 1993. Energy and Protein Requirements of Ruminants.\n     Agricultural and Food Research Council. CABI Publishing, Wallingford, UK.\n",
   "Agricultural and Food Research Council. 1998. The Nutrition of Goats. CABI Publishing,\n     Wallingford, UK.\n",
   "Institut National de la Recherche Agronomique. 2007. Alimentation des bovins, ovins et caprins.\n     Besoins des animaux. Valeurs des aliments. Editions Quae, Versailles, France.\n",
   "Lu, C. D., and M. J. Potchoiba. 1990. Feed intake and weight gain of growing goats fed diets\n     of various energy and protein levels. J. Anim. Sci. 68 (6):1751-1759.\n",
   "Luo, J., A. L. Goetsch, I. V. Nsahlai, J. E. Moore, M. L. Galyean, Z. B. Johnson, T. Sahlu, \n     C. L. Ferrell, and F. N. Owens. 2004. Voluntary feed intake by lactating, Angora, growing\n     and mature goats. Small Ruminant Res. 53 (3):357-378.\n",
   "National Research Council. 2007. Nutrient Requirements of Small Ruminants: Sheep, Goats, Cervids,\n     and New World Camelids. (6th ed.). Nutrient requirements of small ruminants. National Academy\n     Press, Washington, DC.\n",
   "Pulina, G., T. Bettati, F. A. Serra, and A. Cannas. 1996. Razio-O: Costruzione e validazione di\n     un software per l'alimentazione degli ovini da latte. Pages 11-14 in Atti Congresso Nazionale\n     della Società Italiana di Patologia e di Allevamento degli Ovini e dei Caprini, 12. Varese,\n     Italy.\n", sep=""))
  return(invisible(TRUE))
}
```

Appendix 5. R Script for Calculating Area Under the Curve

```
# Version 6.3
getauc<-function(x,y,ybase,splnmeth="fmm",nval=NA,lbl=NA,ylbl=NA,xlbl=NA,plot=T,fnprefix="",
                   replacefile=F,wd=1200,ht=6000,res=600,interpolmethod="spline",draw.polygon=F,
                   psymbol=1,psize=1)
{
  library(rootSolve)
  library(MESS)
  subarea<-function(x,y2,r1,r2)
  {
    r11<-r1
    r12<-r21<-r11+(r2-r1)/2
    r22<-r2
    cat(paste("      Splitting: ",r11," to ",r12," to ",r22,"\n",sep=""))
    area1<-try(auc(x,y2,type=interpolmethod,from=r11,to=r12),silent=TRUE)
    area2<-try(auc(x,y2,type=interpolmethod,from=r21,to=r22),silent=TRUE)
    if (is.numeric(area1) & is.numeric(area2))
    {
      cat(paste("      1st Area + 2nd Area = ",area1+area2,"\n",sep=""))
      return(area1+area2)
    } else
    {
      # Break once more
      if (is.numeric(area1)==FALSE)
      {
        area1<-subarea(x,y2,r11,r12)
      } else
      {
        cat(paste("      1st Area = ",area1,"\n",sep=""))
      }
      if (is.numeric(area2)==FALSE)
      {
        area2<-subarea(x,y2,r21,r22)
      } else
      {
        cat(paste("      2nd Area = ",area2,"\n",sep=""))
      }
      if (is.na(area1) | is.na(area2)) return(NA) else return(area1+area2)
    }
  }
  if (anyNA(y)==F)
  {
    if (length(x)<5)
    {
      cat(paste("Calculating ",lbl," (< 5 points)\n",sep=""))
      return(list("ybase"=ybase,"ymin"=NA,"ymax"=NA,"xmin"=NA,"xmax"=NA,
                  "roots"=NA,"auc"=NA,"tuc"=NA,"aac"=NA,"tab"=NA,"freq"=NA))
    }
    cat(paste("Calculating ",lbl,sep=""))
    y.min<-min(y)
```

```
    y.max<-max(y)
    x.min<-min(x)
    x.max<-max(x)
    y2<-y-ybase
    if (replacefile==T & plot==T) fn<-paste(getwd(),"/",fnprefix,"plot 1.tiff",sep="")
    if (replacefile==F & plot==T) fn<-funcSerialFilename(paste(getwd(),"/",fnprefix,"plot.tiff",sep=""))
    if (is.na(nval)) nval<-10*length(x)
    splfunc<-splinefun(x,y2,method=splnmeth,ties=mean)
    roots<-uniroot.all(splfunc,c(min(x),max(x)),n=nval)
    roots<-roots[order(roots)]
    # Add first and last X points as roots
    roots<-c(x[1],roots)
    roots<-c(roots,x[length(x)])
    if(length(roots)<2)
    {
      cat(" (< 2 roots)\n")
      if (plot==T)
      {
        tiff(fn,width=wd,height=ht,res=res,bg="white",compress="lzw")
        par(mfrow=c(2,1),bty="l")
        if (is.na(lbl)==T) lbl<-""
        if (is.na(ylbl)==T) ylbl1<-"Y values" else ylbl1<-ylbl
        if (is.na(xlbl)==T) xlbl1<-"X values" else xlbl1<-xlbl
        ylbl1<-paste(ylbl1," (base = ", ybase, ")", sep="")
        plot(x,y,main=lbl,xlab=xlbl1,ylab=ylbl1,
             sub=paste("Y: [min, max] = [",formatC(min(y),digits=3,width=7,format="f"),", ",formatC(max(y),digits=3,width=7,format="f"), "], ",
                       "X: [min, max] = [",formatC(min(x),digits=3,width=7,format="f"),", ",formatC(max(x),digits=3,width=7,format="f"), "]", sep=""))
        abline(h=ybase)
        s<-spline(x,y,n=nval,ties=mean)
        lines(s)
        # replot the points
        points(x,y,col="dodgerblue4",pch=psymbol,cex=psize)

        # Difference plot
        if (is.na(ylbl)==T) ylbl2<-paste("Y values - ",ybase,sep="") else ylbl2<-paste(ylbl," - ",ybase,sep="")
        if (is.na(xlbl)==T) xlbl2<-"X values" else xlbl2<-xlbl
        plot(x,y2,xlab=xlbl2,ylab=ylbl2)
        abline(h=0)
        abline(v=roots,lty=3)
        lines(spline(x,y2,n=nval))
        # replot the points
        points(x,y2,col="firebrick",pch=psymbol,cex=psize)
        dev.off()
      }
      return(list("ybase"=ybase,"ymin"=y.min,"ymax"=y.max,
                  "xmin"=x.min,"xmax"=x.max,"roots"=NA,
                  "auc"=NA,"tuc"=NA,"aac"=NA,"tac"=NA,"freq"=NA))
    }
    # tb = time between
```

```
  below.areasum<-0
  below.tbsum<-0
  below.freqsum<-0
  below.df<-data.frame(t=numeric(),area=numeric(),tb=numeric())
  below.df[nrow(below.df)+1,]<-c(0,0,0)
  above.areasum<-0
  above.tbsum<-0
  above.freqsum<-0
  above.df<-data.frame(t=numeric(),area=numeric(),tb=numeric())
  above.df[nrow(above.df)+1,]<-c(0,0,0)
  areaOK<-TRUE
  # progress bar
  # https://ryouready.wordpress.com/2009/03/16/r-monitor-function-progress-with-a-progress-bar/
  pb.total<-length(roots)-1
  pb.title<-ifelse(is.na(lbl)==T,"Processing",paste("Processing ",lbl,sep=""))
  pb<-tkProgressBar(title=pb.title,min=0,max=pb.total,width=300)
  for (i in 1:(length(roots)-1))
  {
    setTkProgressBar(pb,i,label=paste("Calculating area (",round(i/pb.total*100, 0),"% done)",sep=""))
    r1<-roots[i]
    r2<-roots[i+1]
    if (r1<r2)
      {
      areacalc<-try(auc(x,y2,type=interpolmethod,from=r1,to=r2),silent=TRUE)
      if (!is.numeric(areacalc))
      {
        # Break the interval in half the try to solve it
        cat("\n")
        cat(paste("    * sub-splitting roots (",i," and ",i+1,") ", r1," and ", r2, "\n",sep=""))
        areal<-subarea(x,y2,r1,r2)
        if (is.na(areal))
        {
          areacalc<-0
          areaOK<-FALSE
        } else
        {
          cat(paste("       Total Area = ",areal,"\n",sep=""))
          areacalc<-areal
        }
      }
      if (areacalc>0)
      {
        above.areasum<-above.areasum+areacalc
        above.freqsum<-above.freqsum+1
        above.tbsum<-above.tbsum+(r2-r1)
        above.df[nrow(above.df)+1,]<-c(r2,above.areasum,above.tbsum)
      } else
      {
        below.areasum<-below.areasum-areacalc   #areacalc is negative for below
        below.freqsum<-below.freqsum+1
        below.tbsum<-below.tbsum+(r2-r1)
```

```
          below.df[nrow(below.df)+1,]<-c(r2,below.areasum,below.tbsum)
        }
      }
    }
    if (areaOK==FALSE)
    {
      below.areasum<--1
      below.tbsum<--1
      below.freqsum<--1
      above.areasum<--1
      above.tbsum<--1
      above.freqsum<--1
      cat(" (FAILED)\n")
    } else cat(" (OK)\n")
    if (plot==T)
    {
      setTkProgressBar(pb,0,label=paste("Creating graphics (",round(0, 0),"% done)",sep=""))
      tiff(fn,width=wd,height=ht,res=res,bg="white",compress="lzw")
      layout(matrix(c(1,1,2,3), 2, 2, byrow = TRUE))
      if (is.na(lbl)==T) lbl<-""
      if (is.na(ylbl)==T) ylbl1<-"Y values" else ylbl1<-ylbl
      if (is.na(xlbl)==T) xlbl1<-"X values" else xlbl1<-xlbl
      ylbl1<-paste(ylbl1," (base = ", ybase, ")", sep="")
      plot(x,y,main=lbl,xlab=xlbl1,ylab=ylbl1,type="n",
        sub=paste("Y: [min, max] = [",formatC(min(y),digits=3,width=7,format="f"),", ",formatC(max(y),digits=3,width=7,format="f"), "], ",
                  "X: [min, max] = [",formatC(min(x),digits=3,width=7,format="f"),", ",formatC(max(x),digits=3,width=7,format="f"), "]", sep=""))
      # replot the points
      points(x,y,col="dodgerblue4",pch=psymbol,cex=psize)
      # reference line
      abline(h=ybase)
      # draw spline lines
      s<-spline(x,y,n=nval,ties=mean)
      lines(s,col="dodgerblue4")
      setTkProgressBar(pb,33,label=paste("Creating graphics (",round(33, 0),"% done)",sep=""))
      # draw polygon
      if (draw.polygon==T)
      {
        for (i in 1:(length(roots)-1))
        {
          setTkProgressBar(pb,i,label=paste("Drawing polygons (",round(i/pb.total*100, 0),"% done)",sep=""))
          nval2<-max(3,3*length(which(x>roots[i] & x<roots[i+1])))
          s2<-spline(x,y,n=nval2,xmin=roots[i],xmax=roots[i+1],ties=mean)
          if (sum(s2$y-ybase)<0)
          {
            polygon(c(roots[i],s2$x,roots[i+1]),c(ybase,s2$y,ybase),col=rgb(1,0,0,0.1),border=NA)
          } else
          {
            polygon(c(roots[i],s2$x,roots[i+1]),c(ybase,s2$y,ybase),col=rgb(0,0,1,0.1),border=NA)
          }
```

```
            }
        }
        # Cumulative area and tb for above and below the base
        if (is.na(ylbl)==T) ylbl2<-"Cummulative area" else ylbl2<-paste("Cumulative area of ",ylbl,sep="")
        if (is.na(xlbl)==T) xlbl2<-"X values" else xlbl2<-xlbl
        subl<-paste("Roots = ",length(roots), ", ",
                    "AAC = ",formatC(above.areasum,digits=3,width=7,format="f"), ", ",
                    "AUC = ",formatC(below.areasum,digits=3,width=7,format="f"), sep="")
        plot(c(above.df$t,below.df$t),c(above.df$area,-below.df$area),type="n",xlab=xlbl2,ylab=ylbl2,sub=subl)
        abline(h=0)
        lines(above.df$t,above.df$area,col=rgb(0, 0, 1, 0.7),lwd=2)
        lines(below.df$t,-below.df$area,col=rgb(1, 0, 0, 0.7),lwd=2)
        polygon(c(0,above.df$t,max(above.df$t)),c(0,above.df$area,0),col=rgb(0, 0, 1, 0.2),border=NA)
        polygon(c(0,below.df$t,max(below.df$t)),c(0,-below.df$area,0),col=rgb(1, 0, 0, 0.2),border=NA)

        setTkProgressBar(pb,66,label=paste("Creating graphics (",round(66, 0),"% done)",sep=""))
        if (is.na(ylbl)==T) ylbl2<-"Cummulative time" else ylbl2<-paste("Cumulative time of ",ylbl,sep="")
        if (is.na(xlbl)==T) xlbl2<-"X values" else xlbl2<-xlbl
        subl<-paste("TAC = ",formatC(above.tbsum,digits=3,width=7,format="f"), ", ",
                    "TUC = ",formatC(below.tbsum,digits=3,width=7,format="f"), ", ",
                    "Frequency = ",formatC(above.freqsum,digits=0,width=2,format="f"), sep="")
        plot(c(above.df$t,below.df$t),c(above.df$tb,-below.df$tb),type="n",xlab=xlbl2,ylab=ylbl2,sub=subl)
        abline(h=0)
        lines(above.df$t,above.df$tb,col=rgb(0, 0, 1, 0.7),lwd=2)
        lines(below.df$t,-below.df$tb,col=rgb(1, 0, 0, 0.7),lwd=2)
        polygon(c(0,above.df$t,max(above.df$t)),c(0,above.df$tb,0),col=rgb(0, 0, 1, 0.2),border=NA)
        polygon(c(0,below.df$t,max(below.df$t)),c(0,-below.df$tb,0),col=rgb(1, 0, 0, 0.2),border=NA)
        setTkProgressBar(pb,100,label=paste("Creating graphics (",round(100, 0),"% done)",sep=""))
        dev.off()
      }
      close(pb)
      output<-list("ybase"=ybase,"ymin"=y.min,"ymax"=y.max,
                   "xmin"=x.min,"xmax"=x.max,"roots"=length(roots),
                   "auc"=below.areasum,"tuc"=below.tbsum,
                   "aac"=above.areasum,"tac"=above.tbsum,
                   "freq"=above.freqsum)
      return(output)
    } else
    {
      cat(paste("Calculating ",lbl," (No points?)",sep=""))
      return(list("ybase"=ybase,"ymin"=y.min,"ymax"=y.max,
                  "xmin"=x.min,"xmax"=x.max,"roots"=NA,
                  "auc"=NA,"tuc"=NA,"aac"=NA,"tac"=NA,"freq"=NA))
    }
  }
```

Appendix 6. R Script for Calculating Distribution Overlap

```r
getDistOverlap<-function(dista,distb,plotfn=NA,extendcol=NA)
{
  require(sfsmisc)
  require(scales)
  require(overlap)
  # http://stats.stackexchange.com/questions/97596/how-to-calculate-overlap-between-empirical-probability-densities
  a <- dista
  b <- distb

  # Approach 1
  # define limits of a common grid, adding a buffer so that tails aren't cut off
  lower <- min(c(a, b)) - 1
  upper <- max(c(a, b)) + 1

  # generate kernel densities
  da <- density(a, from=lower, to=upper)
  db <- density(b, from=lower, to=upper)
  d <- data.frame(x=da$x, a=da$y, b=db$y)

  # calculate intersection densities
  d$w <- pmin(d$a, d$b)

  # integrate areas under curves
  library(sfsmisc)
  total <- integrate.xy(d$x, d$a) + integrate.xy(d$x, d$b)
  intersection <- integrate.xy(d$x, d$w)

  # compute overlap coefficient
  overlap1 <- 2 * intersection / total

  # Approach 2
  # To use overplapTrue(){overlap} the scale must be in radian (i.e. 0 to 2pi)
  # To keep the *relative* value of a and b the same, combine a and b in the
  # same dataframe before rescaling. You'll need to load the 'scales' library.
  # But first add a "Source" column to be able to distinguish between a and b
  # after they are combined.
  a = data.frame( value = a, Source = "a" )
  b = data.frame( value = b, Source = "b" )
  d = rbind(a, b)
  library(scales)
  d$value <- rescale( d$value, to = c(0,2*pi) )

  # Now you can created the rescaled a and b vectors
  a <- d[d$Source == "a", 1]
  b <- d[d$Source == "b", 1]

  # You can then calculate the area of overlap as you did previously.
  # It should give almost exactly the same answers.
  # Or you can use either the overlapTrue() and overlapEst() function
```

```
  # provided with the overlap packages.
  # Note that with these function the KDE are fitted using von Mises kernel.
  library(overlap)
  # Using overlapTrue():
  # define limits of a common grid, adding a buffer so that tails aren't cut off
  lower <- min(d$value)-1
  upper <- max(d$value)+1
  # generate kernel densities
  da <- density(a, from=lower, to=upper, adjust = 1)
  db <- density(b, from=lower, to=upper, adjust = 1)
  # Compute overlap coefficient
  overlap2<-overlapTrue(da$y,db$y)


  # Using overlapEst():
  temp<-overlapEst(a, b, kmax = 3, adjust=c(0.8, 1, 4), n.grid = 500)
  overlap3<-as.numeric(temp[1])
  overlap4<-as.numeric(temp[2])
  overlap5<-as.numeric(temp[3])

  # You can also plot the two KDEs and the region of overlap using overlapPlot()
  # but sadly I haven't found a way of changing the x scale so that the scale
  # range correspond to the initial x value and not the rescaled value.
  # You can only change the maximum value of the scale using the xscale argument
  # (i.e. it always range from 0 to n, where n is set with xscale = n).
  # So if some of your data take negative value, you're probably better off with
  # a different plotting method. You can change the x label with the xlab
  # argument.
  if (is.na(plotfn)==FALSE)
  {
    tiff(plotfn,width=8000,height=8000,bg="white",res=800,compress="lzw")
    if (is.na(extendcol)==FALSE)
    {
      overlapPlot(a,b,xscale=10,linetype=c(1,1),linecol=c("red","blue"),linewidth=c(2,2),rug=TRUE,olapcol="grey70",extend=extendcol,xlab="Scaled Values",main="")
    } else
    {
      overlapPlot(a,b,xscale=10,linetype=c(1,1),linecol=c("red","blue"),linewidth=c(2,2),rug=TRUE,olapcol="grey70",xlab="Scaled Values",main="")
    }
    dev.off()
  }
  out<-c(overlap1,overlap2,overlap3,overlap4,overlap5)
  out<-out[!is.na(out)]
  return(invisible(out))
}

```

References

Agricultural and Food Research Council. 1993. Energy and Protein Requirements of Ruminants. Agricultural and Food Research Council. CABI Publishing, Wallingford, UK.

Allen, M. S., and B. J. Bradford. 2006. Metabolic regulation of feed intake in cattle: A conceptual model. Page 10 in The 3rd Workshop on Adapting the Cornell Net Carbohydrate and Protein System to Tropic Conditions. P. B. Arcuri, ed. Juiz de Fora, MG, Brazil. EMBRAPA.

Argyle, J. L., and R. L. Baldwin. 1988. Modeling of rumen water kinetics and effects of rumen pH changes. J. Dairy Sci. 71 (5):1178-1188. doi: 10.3168/jds.S0022-0302(88)79672-1

Bach, A., S. Calsamiglia, and M. D. Stern. 2005. Nitrogen metabolism in the rumen. J. Dairy Sci. 88 (E. Suppl.):E9-E21. doi: 10.3168/jds.S0022-0302(05)73133-7

Beauchemin, K. A., and W. Z. Yang. 2005. Effects of physically effective fiber on intake, chewing activity, and ruminal acidosis for dairy cows fed diets based on corn silage. J. Dairy Sci. 88 (6):2117-2129. doi: 10.3168/jds.S0022-0302(05)72888-5

Bodine, T. N., and H. T. Purvis II. 2003. Effects of supplemental energy and/or degradable intake protein on performance, grazing behavior, intake digestibility, and fecal and blood indices by beef steers grazed on dormant native tallgrass prairie. J. Anim. Sci. 81:304-317.

Boston, R. C., D. G. Fox, C. J. Sniffen, R. Janczewski, R. Munson, and W. Chalupa. 2000. The conversion of a scientific model describing dairy cow nutrition and production to an industry tool: The CPM Dairy project. Pages 361-377 in Modelling Nutrient Utilization in Farm Animals. J. P. McNamara, J. France and D. Beever, eds. CABI Publishing, Oxford

Bowen, M. K., D. P. Poppi, and S. R. McLennan. 2017. Efficiency of rumen microbial protein synthesis in cattle grazing tropical pastures as estimated by a novel technique. Anim. Prod. Sci. 57 (8):1702-1712. doi: 10.1071/AN15535

Bowen, M. K., D. P. Poppi, and S. R. McLennan. 2018. Effect of quantity and source of rumen nitrogen on the efficiency of microbial protein synthesis in steers consuming tropical forage. Anim. Prod. Sci. 58 (5):811-817. doi: 10.1071/AN15739

Cannas, A., L. O. Tedeschi, D. G. Fox, A. N. Pell, and P. J. Van Soest. 2004. A mechanistic model for predicting the nutrient requirements and feed biological values for sheep. J. Anim. Sci. 82 (1):149-169. doi: 10.2527/2004.821149x

Cannas, A., and P. J. Van Soest. 2000. Simple allometric models to predict rumen feed passage rate in domestic ruminants. Pages 49-62 in Modelling Nutrient Utilization in Farm Animals. J. P. McNamara, J. France and D. E. Beever, eds. CABI Publishing, Wallingford, Oxon, UK

Castillo, A. R., E. Kebreab, D. E. Beever, and J. France. 2000. A review of efficiency of nitrogen utilisation in lactating dairy cows and its relationship with environmental pollution. J. Anim. Feed Sci. 9:1-32.

Commonwealth Scientific and Industrial Research Organization. 2007. Nutrient Requirements of Domesticated Ruminants. Commonwealth Scientific and Industrial Research Organization, Collingwood, VIC.

Corbett , J. L. 1987. Energy and protein utilization by grazing animals. Pages 341-355 in Temperate Pastures: Their Production, Use and Management. J. L. Wheeler, C. J. Pearson and G. E. Robards, eds. Australian Wool Corporation and CSIRO Publishing, Melbourne, Australia

Corbett, J. L., E. P. Furnival, M. W. Inskip, and F. S. Pickering. 1982. Protein digestion in grazing sheep. Pages 141-143 in Forage Protein in Ruminant Animal Production. D. J. Thomson, D. E. Beever and R. G. Gunn, eds. British Society of Animal Production and the British Grassland Society, Thames Ditton, UK

Cotanch, K. W., and R. J. Grant. 2006. Measuring physically effective fiber on-farm to predict cow response. Pages 151-160 in Proc. of the Cornell Nutrition Conference for Feed Manufacturers. Syracuse, NY. New York State College of Agriculture & Life Sciences, Cornell University.

Crampton, E. W. 1957. Interrelations between digestible nutrient and energy content, voluntary dry matter intake, and the overall feeding value of forages. J. Anim. Sci. 16 (3):546-552. doi: 10.2527/1957.163546x

Crampton, E. W., E. Donefer, and L. E. Lloyd. 1960. A nutritive value index for forages. J. Anim. Sci. 19 (2):538-544. doi: 10.2527/jas1960.192538x

Crawley, M. J. 2007. The R Book. John Wiley & Sons Ltd., West Sussex, England.

DelCurto, T., R. C. Cochran, D. L. Harmon, A. A. Beharka, K. A. Jacques, G. Towne, and E. S. Vanzant. 1990. Supplementation of dormant tallgrass-prairie forage: I. Influence of varying supplemental protein and(or) energy levels on forage utilization characteristics of beef steers in confinement. J. Anim. Sci. 68 (2):515-531. doi: 10.2527/1990.682515x

Dong, R. L., G. Y. Zhao, L. L. Chai, and K. A. Beauchemin. 2014. Prediction of urinary and fecal nitrogen excretion by beef cattle. J. Anim. Sci. 92 (10):4669-4681. doi: 10.2527/jas.2014-8000

Eisemann, J. H., and L. O. Tedeschi. 2016. Predicting the amount of urea nitrogen recycled and used for anabolism in growing cattle. J. Agric. Sci. 154 (06):1118-1129. doi: 10.1017/S0021859616000228

Everitt, B. S., and T. Hothorn. 2010. A Handbook of Statistical Analyses using R. (2nd ed.). CRC Press, Boca Raton, FL.

Faria, J. C., P. Grosjean, E. G. Jelihovschi, R. Pietrobon, and P. S. Farias 2015. Tinn-R Editor -- GUI for R Language and Environment. Editus Editora da UESC, Ilhéus, BA, Brazil.

Fox, D. G., C. J. Sniffen, and J. D. O'Connor. 1988. Adjusting nutrient requirements of beef cattle for animal and environmental variations. J. Anim. Sci. 66 (6):1475-1495. doi: 10.2527/jas1988.6661475x

Fox, D. G., and L. O. Tedeschi. 2002. Application of physically effective fiber in diets for feedlot cattle. Pages 67-81 in Proc. of the Plains Nutrition Council Conference. San Antonio, TX. Available at: http://amarillo.tamu.edu/facultystaff/tmc/pnc/. Accessed on: May 25, 2016

Fox, D. G., L. O. Tedeschi, T. P. Tylutki, J. B. Russell, M. E. Van Amburgh, L. E. Chase, A. N. Pell, and T. R. Overton. 2004. The Cornell Net Carbohydrate and Protein System model for evaluating herd nutrition and nutrient excretion. Anim. Feed Sci. Technol. 112 (1):29-78. doi: 10.1016/j.anifeedsci.2003.10.006

Fox, D. G., M. E. Van Amburgh, and T. P. Tylutki. 1999. Predicting requirements for growth, maturity, and body reserves in dairy cattle. J. Dairy Sci. 82 (9):1968-1977. doi: 10.3168/jds.S0022-0302(99)75433-0

Gallo, S. B., and L. O. Tedeschi. 2021. Developing a continuous adjustment factor for dry matter intake of gestating and lactating ewes. Sci. Agric. 78 (2):e20190082. doi: 10.1590/1678-992X-2019-0082

Galyean, M. L., and L. O. Tedeschi. 2014. Predicting microbial protein synthesis in beef cattle: Relationship to intakes of total digestible nutrients and crude protein. J. Anim. Sci. 92 (11):5099-5111. doi: 10.2527/jas.2014-8098

Grant, R. J., and K. W. Cotanch. 2005. Physically effective fiber for dairy cows: Current perspectives. Pages 61-70 in Proc. of the Cornell Nutrition Conference for Feed Manufacturers. Syracuse, NY. New York State College of Agriculture & Life Sciences, Cornell University.

Guo, K., A. Mimosi, R. Fortina, and I. Zoccarato. 2004. A computer model to predict the nitrogen excretion in growing-finishing cattle. Livest. Prod. Sci. 88:273-284.

Guo, K., and I. Zoccarato. 2005. A dynamic model to predict the nitrogen excretion in growing-finishing cattle. Ecol. Modell. 187 (2–3):219-231. doi: 10.1016/j.ecolmodel.2004.10.017

Horton, N. J., and K. Kleinman. 2011. Using R for Data Management, Statistical Analysis, and Graphics. CRC Press, Boca Raton, FL.

Huhtanen, P., J. I. Nousiainen, M. Rinne, K. Kytola, and H. Khalili. 2008. Utilization and partition of dietary nitrogen in dairy cows fed grass silage-based diets. J. Dairy Sci. 91 (9):3589-3599. doi: 10.3168/jds.2008-1181

Institut National de la Recherche Agronomique. 1989. Ruminant Nutrition; Recommended allowances and feed tables. INRA, John Libbey Eurotext, Montrouge, France.

Jonker, J. S., R. A. Kohn, and R. A. Erdman. 1998. Using milk urea nitrogen to predict nitrogen excretion and utilization efficiency in lactating dairy cows. J. Dairy Sci. 81:2681-2692.

Kauffman, A. J., and N. R. St-Pierre. 2001. The relationship of milk urea nitrogen to urine nitrogen excretion in Holstein and Jersey cows. J. Dairy Sci. 84 (10):2284-2294. doi: 10.3168/jds.S0022-0302(01)74675-9

Kebreab, E., J. France, R. E. Agnew, T. Yan, M. S. Dhanoa, J. Dijkstra, D. E. Beever, and C. K. Reynolds. 2003. Alternatives to linear analysis of energy balance data from lactating dairy cows. J. Dairy Sci. 86 (9):2904-2913. doi: 10.3168/jds.S0022-0302(03)73887-9

Kebreab, E., A. B. Strathe, J. Dijkstra, J. A. N. Mills, C. K. Reynolds, L. A. Crompton, T. Yan, and J. France. 2010. Energy and protein interactions and their effect on nitrogen excretion in dairy cows. Pages 417-425 in Proceedings of the 3rd International Symposium on Energy and Protein Metabolism and Nutrition. EAAP Publication No. 127. G. M. Crovetto, ed. Parma, Italy. Wageningen Academic Publishers.

Kohn, R. A., K. F. Kalscheur, and E. Russek-Cohen. 2002. Evaluation of models to estimate urinary nitrogen and expected milk urea nitrogen. J. Dairy Sci. 85 (1):227-233. doi: 10.3168/jds.S0022-0302(02)74071-X

Kononoff, P. J., and A. J. Heinrichs. 2003. The effect of reducing alfalfa haylage particle size on cows in early lactation. J. Dairy Sci. 86 (4):1445-1457. doi: 10.3168/jds.S0022-0302(03)73728-X

Lammers, B. P., D. R. Buckmaster, and A. J. Heinrichs. 1996. A simple method for the analysis of particle sizes of forage and total mixed rations. J. Dairy Sci. 79 (5):922-928. doi: 10.3168/jds.S0022-0302(96)76442-1

Lapierre, H., and G. E. Lobley. 2001. Nitrogen recycling in the ruminant: A review. J. Dairy Sci. 84:E223-E236. doi: 10.3168/jds.S0022-0302(01)70222-6

Lee, S. J., I. K. Nuberg, and W. S. Pitchford. 2017. Maternal body composition in seedstock herds. 1. Grazing management strategy influences perspectives on optimal balance of production traits and maternal productivity. Anim. Prod. Sci. 58 (1):117-124.

Leng, R. A., and J. V. Nolan. 1984. Nitrogen metabolism in the rumen. J. Dairy Sci. 67 (5):1072-1089.

Mertens, D. R. 1985a. Effect of fiber on feed quality of dairy cows. Pages 209-224 in Proc. of the 46th Minnesota Nutrition Conference. St. Paul, MN. University of Minnesota.

Mertens, D. R. 1985b. Factors influencing feed intake in lactating cows: From theory to application using neutral detergent fiber. Pages 1-18 in Proc. of the Georgia Nutrition Conference for the Feed Industry. Atlanta, GA.

Mertens, D. R. 1987. Predicting intake and digestibility using mathematical models of ruminal function. J. Anim. Sci. 64 (5):1548-1558. doi: 10.2527/jas1987.6451548x

Mertens, D. R. 1997. Creating a system for meeting the fiber requirements of dairy cows. J. Dairy Sci. 80 (7):1463-1481. doi: 10.3168/jds.S0022-0302(97)76075-2

Moore, J. E. 1994. Forage quality indices: Development and application. Pages 967-998 in Forage Quality, Evaluation, and Utilization. G. C. Fahey Jr., M. Collins, D. R. Mertens and L. E. Moser, eds. American Society of Agronomy, Madison, WI. doi: 10.2134/1994.foragequality.c24

Moore, J. E., M. H. Brant, W. E. Kunkle, and D. I. Hopkins. 1999. Effects of supplementation on voluntary forage intake, diet digestibility, and animal performance. J. Anim. Sci. 77 (Suppl. 2):122-135. doi: 10.2527/1999.77suppl_2122x

Moore, J. E., W. E. Kunkle, and W. F. Brown. 1991. Forage quality and the need for protein and energy supplementation. Pages 1-12 in Proceedings of the 40th Annual Florida Beef Cattle Short Course. Gainesville, FL. University of Florida. Available at: http://animal.ifas.ufl.edu/beef_extension/bcsc/1991/pdf/moore.pdf. Accessed on: April 17, 2017

Moore, J. E., and D. J. Undersander. 2002. Relative forage quality: An alternative to relative feed value and quality index. Pages 16-29 in Proceedings of the 13th Annual Florida Ruminant Nutrition Symposium. Gainesville, FL. University of Florida. Available at: http://dairy.ifas.ufl.edu/rns/2002/moore.pdf

Mouriño, F., R. Akkarawongsa, and P. J. Weimer. 2001. Initial pH as determinant of cellulose digestion rate by mixed ruminal microorganisms in vitro. J. Dairy Sci. 84 (4):848-859. doi: 10.3168/jds.S0022-0302(01)74543-2

National Academies of Sciences, Engineering, and Medicine. 2016. Nutrient Requirements of Beef Cattle. (8th ed.). Animal Nutrition Series. National Academy Press, Washington, DC. doi: 10.17226/19014

National Research Council. 1985. Ruminant Nitrogen Usage. National Academy Press, Washington, DC. doi: 10.17226/615

National Research Council. 1996. Nutrient Requirements of Beef Cattle. (7th ed.). Nutrient Requirements of Domestic Animals. National Academy Press, Washington, DC.

National Research Council. 2000. Nutrient Requirements of Beef Cattle. (updated 7th ed.). Nutrient Requirements of Domestic Animals. National Academy Press, Washington, DC. doi: 10.17226/9791

Nennich, T. D., J. H. Harrison, L. M. VanWieringen, D. Meyer, A. J. Heinrichs, W. P. Weiss, N. R. St-Pierre, R. L. Kincaid, D. L. Davidson, and E. Block. 2005. Prediction of manure and nutrient excretion from dairy cattle. J. Dairy Sci. 88 (10):3721-3733.

Nennich, T. D., J. H. Harrison, L. M. VanWieringen, N. R. St-Pierre, R. L. Kincaid, M. A. Wattiaux, D. L. Davidson, and E. Block. 2006. Prediction and evaluation of urine and urinary nitrogen and mineral excretion from dairy cattle. J. Dairy Sci. 89 (1):353-364.

Nolan, J. V., and R. C. Dobos. 2005. Nitrogen transactions in ruminants. Pages 177-206 in Quantitative Aspects of Ruminant Digestion and Metabolism. J. Dijkstra, J. M. Forbes and J. France, eds. (2nd ed.). CABI Publishing, Wallingford, UK

Nousiainen, J., K. J. Shingfield, and P. Huhtanen. 2004. Evaluation of milk urea nitrogen as a diagnostic of protein feeding. J. Dairy Sci. 87 (2):386-398. doi: 10.3168/jds.S0022-0302(04)73178-1

Oba, M., and M. S. Allen. 2003. Effects of diet fermentability on efficiency of microbial nitrogen production in lactating dairy cows. J. Dairy Sci. 86 (1):195-207. doi: 10.3168/jds.S0022-0302(03)73600-5

Pitt, R. E., J. S. Van Kessel, D. G. Fox, A. N. Pell, M. C. Barry, and P. J. Van Soest. 1996. Prediction of ruminal volatile fatty acids and pH within the net carbohydrate and protein system. J. Anim. Sci. 74 (1):226-244. doi: 10.2527/1996.741226x

Reed, K. F., L. E. Moraes, D. P. Casper, and E. Kebreab. 2015. Predicting nitrogen excretion from cattle. J. Dairy Sci. 98 (5):3025-3035. doi: 10.3168/jds.2014-8397

Rohweder, D. A., R. F. Barnes, and N. Jorgensen. 1978. Proposed hay grading standards based on laboratory analyses for evaluating quality. J. Anim. Sci. 47 (3):747-759. doi: 10.2527/jas1978.473747x

Santos, F. A. P., J. E. P. Santos, C. B. Theurer, and J. T. Huber. 1998. Effects of rumen-undegradable protein on dairy cow performance: A 12-year literature review. J. Dairy Sci. 81:3182-3213.

Satter, L. D., and L. L. Slyter. 1974. Effect of ammonia concentration on ruminal microbial protein production in vitro. Br. J. Nutr. 32 (2):199-208. doi: 10.1079/BJN19740073

Schuba, J., K. H. Südekum, E. Pfeffer, and A. Jayanegara. 2017. Excretion of faecal, urinary urea and urinary non-urea nitrogen by four ruminant species as influenced by dietary nitrogen intake: A meta-analysis. Livest. Sci. 198:82-88. doi: 10.1016/j.livsci.2017.01.017

Schwab, C. G., P. Huhtanen, C. W. Hunt, and T. Hvelplund. 2005. Nitrogen requirements of cattle. Pages 13-70 in Nitrogen and Phosphorus Nutrition of Cattle: Reducing the Environmental Impact of Cattle Operations. E. Pfeffer and A. N. Hristov, eds. CABI Publishing, Wallingford, UK. doi: 10.1079/9780851990132.0013

Seo, S., L. O. Tedeschi, C. G. Schwab, and D. G. Fox. 2006. Development and evaluation of empirical equations to predict feed passage rate in cattle. Anim. Feed Sci. Technol. 128 (1-2):67-83. doi: 10.1016/j.anifeedsci.2005.09.014

Sinclair, L. A., P. C. Garnsworth, J. R. Newbold, and P. J. Buttery. 1993. Effect of synchronizing the rate of dietary energy and nitrogen release on rumen fermentation and microbial protein synthesis in sheep. J. Agric. Sci. 120:251-263.

Smith, R. H. 1969. Nitrogen metabolism and the rumen. J. Dairy Res. 36 (2):313-331. doi: 10.1017/S0022029900012802

Spek, J. W., J. Dijkstra, G. van Duinkerken, W. H. Hendriks, and A. Bannink. 2013. Prediction of urinary nitrogen and urinary urea nitrogen excretion by lactating dairy cattle in northwestern Europe and North America: A meta-analysis. J. Dairy Sci. 96 (7):4310-4322.

Stern, M. D., and W. H. Hoover. 1979. Methods for determining and factors affecting rumen microbial protein synthesis: A review. J. Anim. Sci. 49 (6):1590-1603. doi: 10.2527/jas1979.4961590x

Strasia, C. A., and D. R. Gill. 1990. Formulating feedlot diets. Fact Sheet. No. 1600. Great Plains Beef Cattle Handbook. Oklahoma State University, Stillwater, OK. 6p.

Tamminga, S. 1991. Matching carbohydrate and protein degradation for maximal microbial protein production. Page 7 in Proceedings of Ralston Purina International Scientific Advisory Board. Paris, France.

Tedeschi, L. O., A. Cannas, and D. G. Fox. 2010. A nutrition mathematical model to account for dietary supply and requirements of energy and nutrients for domesticated small ruminants: The development and evaluation of the Small Ruminant Nutrition System. Small Ruminant Res. 89 (2-3):174-184. doi: 10.1016/j.smallrumres.2009.12.041

Tedeschi, L. O., A. Cannas, S. G. Solaiman, R. A. M. Vieira, and N. K. Gurung. 2012. Development and evaluation of empirical equations to predict ruminal fractional passage rate of forages in goats. J. Agric. Sci. 150 (1):95-107. doi: 10.1017/S0021859611000591

Tedeschi, L. O., and D. G. Fox. 2020. The Ruminant Nutrition System: Volume I - An Applied Model for Predicting Nutrient Requirements and Feed Utilization in Ruminants. (3rd ed.). XanEdu, Ann Arbor, MI.

Teetor, P. 2011. R Cookbook: Proven Recipes for Data Analysis, Statistics, and Graphics. O'Reilly, Sebastopol, CA.

Verzani, J. 2011. Getting Started with RStudio. O'Reilly, Cambridge, UK.

Waldo, D. R. 1968. Nitrogen metabolism in the ruminant. J. Dairy Sci. 51 (2):265-275.

Waldrip, H. M., R. W. Todd, and N. A. Cole. 2013. Prediction of nitrogen excretion by beef cattle: A meta-analysis. J. Anim. Sci. 91 (9):4290-4302. doi: 10.2527/jas.2012-5818

Walker, N. D., C. J. Newbold, and R. J. Wallace. 2005. Nitrogen metabolism in the rumen. Pages 71-115 in Nitrogen and Phosphorus Nutrition of Cattle: Reducing the Environmental Impact of Cattle Operations. E. Pfeffer and A. N. Hristov, eds. CABI Publishing, Wallingford, UK

Wickham, H. 2009. ggplot2 Elegant Graphics for Data Analysis. Use R! Springer, New York, NY.

Wilkerson, V. A., D. R. Mertens, and D. P. Casper. 1997. Prediction of excretion of manure and nitrogen by Holstein dairy cattle. J. Dairy Sci. 80:3193-3204.

Williams, C. B. 1988. Development of a Simulation Model to Provide Decision Support in Dairy Herd Nutritional Management. Dissertation, Cornell University, Ithaca, NY. Available at: http://search.proquest.com/pqdtglobal/docview/303695798/15B15A838B3744C8PQ/1?accountid=7082. Accessed on: December 11, 2019

Yan, T., J. P. Frost, T. W. J. Keady, R. E. Agnew, and C. S. Mayne. 2007. Prediction of nitrogen excretion in feces and urine of beef cattle offered diets containing grass silage. J. Anim. Sci. 85 (8):1982-1989. doi: 10.2527/jas.2006-408

Yang, W. Z., and K. A. Beauchemin. 2005. Effects of physically effective fiber on digestion and milk production by dairy cows fed diets based on corn silage. J. Dairy Sci. 88 (3):1090-1098. doi: 10.3168/jds.S0022-0302(05)72776-4

Yang, W. Z., and K. A. Beauchemin. 2006. Effects of physically effective fiber on chewing activity and ruminal pH of dairy cows fed diets based on barley silage. J. Dairy Sci. 89 (1):217-228. doi: 10.3168/jds.S0022-0302(06)72086-0

Zhai, S., J. Liu, Y. Wu, and J. Ye. 2007. Predicting urinary nitrogen excretion by milk urea nitrogen in lactating Chinese Holstein cows. Anim. Sci. J. 78 (4):395-399. doi: 10.1111/j.1740-0929.2007.00452.x